Cardiovascular Complications of COVID-19

Umair Mallick

Cardiovascular Complications of COVID-19

Risk, Pathogenesis and Outcomes

Springer

Umair Mallick
Kingston Hospital NHS Foundation Trust
London
London, UK

ISBN 978-3-030-90064-9 ISBN 978-3-030-90065-6 (eBook)
https://doi.org/10.1007/978-3-030-90065-6

This Springer imprint is published by the registered company Springer Nature Switzerland AG
The registered company address is: Gewerbestrasse 11, 6330 Cham, Switzerland

Contents

Chapter 1
The Epidemiology of CoViD19 and Cardiovascular Diseases

Key Questions

- What are the important epidemiological links between the CoViD19 and cardiovascular diseases?
- Cardiovascular disease or CoViD19, which comes first?
- What is the burden of cardiovascular risk factors in the CoViD19?
- What is the role of pre-existing cardiovascular diseases in the CoViD19?
- What is the connection between the critical CoViD19 complications and pre-existing cardiovascular diseases?
- What is the role of cardiovascular complications in CoViD19 mortality?

1.1 Introduction

The Coronavirus Disease (CoViD19) has emerged as a severe and unanticipated pandemic raising alarm bells at a global scale. The pandemic appeared in the later part of 2019 in association with a range of highly prevalent and complex comorbidities and serious complications including fatalities. The pathogen that causes CoViD19 is a novel Coronavirus referred to as "Severe Acute Respiratory Syndrome Coronavirus 2 (SARS Cov 2)", which appears to have originated in the Wuhan city in Hubei province in China. The initial outbreak of the CoViD19 in the Wuhan city evolved into an epidemic in China, rapidly acquiring the shape of a global pandemic, with serious health and economic implications across the world.

The spectrum of severity of the CoViD19 accompanies a variety of risk factors, ranging from demographic factors such as gender, the age, to several high-risk conditions including heart failure, hypertension, diabetes mellitus, chronic lung conditions, and malignancies. The data are currently emerging from well-designed

U. Mallick, *Cardiovascular Complications of COVID-19*,
https://doi.org/10.1007/978-3-030-90065-6_1

clinical studies from the healthcare centers across the globe, treating patients with CoViD19. The evidence suggests that the widescale prevalence of cardiometabolic diseases and the aging population, serve as a fertile ground for the serious complications associated with the growing pandemic of CoViD19. However, this argument accompanies an uncertainty due to the paucity of the literature systematically addressing the novel coronavirus disease in relation to the cardiometabolic diseases and risk factors, at this stage of the pandemic. This warrants a greater understanding of the CoViD19, associated comorbidities, and the risk factors. A multifaceted approach is strongly needed to accurately identify, assess and analyze these risk factors, and determine their clinical and pathogenetic significance, in the context of CoViD19, to help reach concrete conclusions. Such data are fundamental to the development of robust strategies and evidence-based mitigation plans to help lower the risk of complications in patients with cardiovascular illnesses exposed to CoViD19. This evidence can be further used for the development of the expert clinical guidelines to support the clinicians to improve management of patients with CoViD19 in clinical practice, which will eventually result in reducing the growing threat of the fatal outcomes emerging from the combined impact of the CoViD19 and cardiovascular diseases (Tables 1.1 and 1.2).

We provide an overview of the CoViD19 and the causal mechanisms, in association with the common and potentially fatal cardiovascular diseases (CVD) frequently met in patients with complicated CoViD19, and demonstrate the pathogenetic mechanisms involved in defining critical components of this relationship, a dilemma currently being debated by the scientists and clinicians worldwide. We take this further by focusing on the the core of this relationship and the CoViD19 outcomes based upon the currently available data (Fig. 1.1).

Table 1.1 Risk factors for cardiovascular complications in CoViD19

Background risk factors	Factors related to the acuity of COVID19
Age and male gender	Severity of viral disease
Hypertension	Hyperimmune inflammatory response
Pre-existing CVD	RAS dysregulation
Diabetes mellitus	Hemostatic dysregulation
Raised BMI/obesity	Metabolic dysregulation
	Cellular stress mechanisms

CVD, cardiovascular disease; BMI, body mass index

Table 1.2 Cardiovascular complications in CoViD19

Complication	Subtypes
Cardiac injury	Myo/pericarditis, Myocardial injury Stress cardiomyopathy
Acute coronary syndromes	ST elevation ACS Non-ST Elevation ACS
Hypertension	
Heart failure	Left ventricular failure Right heart failure, Congestive heart failure
Cardiac arrhythmias	Atrial/ventricular, Sudden cardiac death
Thromboembolic complications	Arterial and venous thromboembolism Microvascular disease Intestinal thrombosis, Stroke
Cardiogenic shock	

ACS, acute coronary syndromes

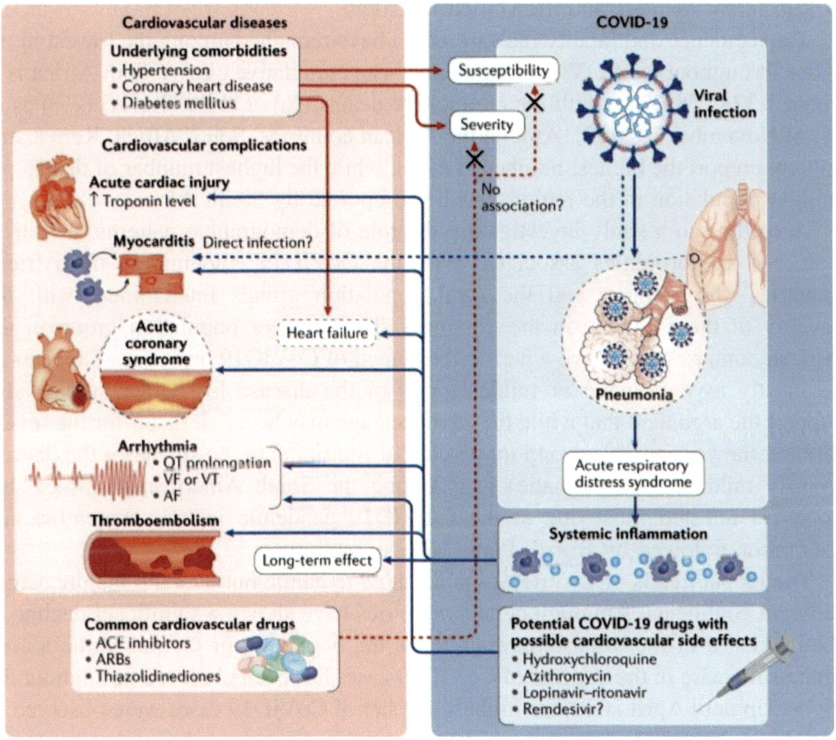

Fig. 1.1 Bidirectional interaction between cardiovascular diseases and COVID-19. AF, atrial fibrillation; VF, ventricular fibrillation; VT, ventricular tachycardia. *Source* Figure 2. Nishiga, M., Wang, D.W., Han, Y., Lewis, D.B. and Wu, J.C., 2020. COVID-19 and cardiovascular disease: from basic mechanisms to clinical perspectives. Nature Reviews Cardiology, 17(9), pp. 543–558. https://www.nature.com/articles/s41569-020-0413-9. By Springer Nature Group

1.2 Epidemiology

According to the estimates from the World Health Organization statistics, as of 1st of November 2020, the new coronavirus disease COVID19 has infected about 46 million individuals and caused 1.2 million related deaths globally (WHO weekly update epidemiology 1st of November). Most of the COVID19 cases have been observed in Europe, with the cumulative cases (%) at 11,088,612 (24%), followed by the Americas 20,477,535 (45%), South-East Asia 9,251,788 (20%), and Eastern Mediterranean 3,092,037 (7%), and the cumulative deaths (%) at 285,402 (24%), 639,353 (54%), 144,194 (12%), and 78,599 (7%), respectively.

The countries with more than 1 million confirmed COVID19 cases as of 1st of November 2020, are the United States, India, Brazil, Russian Federation, France, Spain, Argentina, Colombia, and the United Kingdom. In the United Kingdom alone, the number of individuals infected with CoViD19 is about 1,213,367 and there are approximately 49,238 related deaths [1]. The countries with cumulative deaths of more than 40,000 as of 1st of November 2020 include the United States, Brazil, India, Mexico, and the United Kingdom.

The incidence and fatality rates in Africa have remained among the lowest in the globe throughout the COVID19 pandemic. The cumulative cases (%) in Africa is at about 1,324,258 (3%), with the cumulative deaths (%) at about 29,785 (2%) as of 1st of November 2020 [2]. Among the African countries, South Africa, Kenya, and Ethiopia report the highest number of cases, while the highest number of deaths per million population in the region, has been reported by South Africa.

According to a study investigating the role of demographic patterns, urbanization, and comorbidities associated with the CoViD19 epidemic in the African countries, the younger and the rural population groups interconnect with the severity of the epidemic in the continent. The younger population group in the African countries may have a part in the spread of CoViD19 however, it appears to be mostly asymptomatic or milder forms of the disease [3]. Other studies also support the argument that while the advanced age may be a risk factor for the severe disease, the younger age group may strongly contribute to the spread of the disease (mostly mild or asymptomatic) [4]. Among the South American countries, the countries affected most due to the COVID19 pandemic include Argentina and Columbia, followed by Brazil, Peru, Mexico, and others [2].

The global trends of CoViD19 spread show dynamic but a mixed picture across different continents. Although certain countries have shown a significant decline in the incidence of the disease, overall, since the beginning of the pandemic a continuous increase in the number of CoViD19 cases has been observed throughout the globe. Up until April 2020, the highest number of CoViD19 cases were observed in the USA, about 307,318 infected cases and 8,358 related deaths, and remains the highest at 9,868,389 cases and 236,042 deaths (as of 1st of November 2020). Although the number of cases in India stood at relatively lower levels up until April 2020, these showed a continuous rise in the early part of the second semester. As of 1st of November 2020, India appears to have the second-highest number of

CoViD19 cases 8,591,730 and 127,059 deaths and is further followed by Brazil 5,664,115 cases and 162,397 fatalities. During the earlier months of the pandemic (April 2020), the USA was followed by Spain, with 130,759 cases and 12,418 confirmed deaths, and further by Italy with approximately 128,948 cases and 15,889 fatalities [5]. Since April 2020, the incidence of CoViD19 significantly declined in these countries and remained at the low levels for approximately five to six months, however, reflected a new rising trend that continues.

In China, the incidence of CoViD19 reached peak levels in the first week of February 2020, thereafter showing a rapid decline by the end of the month. The daily cumulative index (DCI) of COVID-19 (cumulative cases/no. of days between the first reported case and 29 February 2020) was (1320.85) [6]. As of April 2020, about 83,005 CoViD19 cases and 3,340 related deaths, had been reported in China. Although by the 1st of November 2020, the total number of cases reached 92,271 and 4,748 fatalities, the rise in number has been relatively smaller as compared to other countries. Overall, the CoViD19 related morbidity and mortality trends in the Chinese population indicate a decline, and the number of new cases has remained consistently relatively smaller since February 2020 [5, 7].

The mortality rates due to CoViD19 vary in different population groups, ranging between 10.5% in Italy [8] and as low as 2.5% in China [9]. The most critical complications of CoViD19 such as ARDS (Acute Respiratory Distress Syndromes), cardiac injury, multi-organ failure, appear to be directly associated with mortality. Several demographic factors and conventional cardiometabolic risk factors including diabetes mellitus, as well as lung disease, and cancer appear to precondition these critical complications in patients with CoViD19.

Cardiovascular diseases (CVD) remain the number one cause of death and disability worldwide. It is estimated that about 17.9 million people die each year from cardiovascular diseases alone, representing about 31% of all caused deaths globally [10]. Several classical cardiovascular risk factors such as older age, hypertension, diabetes mellitus, smoking and others, appear to be highly prevalent among patients who develop CoViD19 complications.

1.2.1 Cardiovascular Disease or CoViD19, Which Comes First?

There is a growing body of evidence suggesting that patients with CoViD19 have a significantly high burden of cardiovascular diseases and risk factors such as hypertension, coronary heart disease diabetes mellitus, and others [11–13]. It is, however, not clear whether the cardiovascular diseases increase the susceptibility towards CoViD19 or associated complications, or the stress related to CoViD19 unfolds masked cardiovascular diseases, exacerbates the preexisting cardiovascular diseases, or directly results in neo cardiovascular complications.

1.2.2 The Burden of Cardiovascular Risk Factors in CoViD19

The demographic data from several CoViD19 studies reflect a relatively higher prevalence of cardiovascular diseases in patients hospitalized with complicated CoViD19. A retrospective single-center cohort of 99 patients admitted with CoViD19 pneumonia in China revealed that 40% of patients had a background of cardiovascular or cerebrovascular disease [14]. Another retrospective cohort of 138 consecutive patients admitted with CoViD19 revealed a high prevalence of hypertension 31.2% (43), cardiovascular disease 14.2% (20), and diabetes mellitus 10.1% (14) [15]. This was further confirmed in another retrospective observational study of 191 patients hospitalized with CoViD19 indicating that hypertension 30% (58) and diabetes mellitus 19% (36), as the most common background risk factors in patients with severe CoViD19 [13].

The important risk factors for cardiovascular diseases, among several others, also include older age and male gender. In the older age group, an increased prevalence of the CoViD19 complications is reported, with considerably higher rates of morbidity and mortality. The existing evidence suggests that among patients in the older age group, admitted with the CoViD19, the rates of cardiovascular, and other critical complications, including Acute Respiratory Distress Syndromes (ARDS), multi-organ failure (MOF), and death, are much elevated [16].

A report of a large-scale study of 72,314 cases with the CoViD19 in China, revealed that 3% (1408) of the subjects were older adults age $\geq$ 80 years. The rates of associated morbidity and mortality significantly increased with age, rising to 8.0% (312 of 3918) among patients 70–79 years, and 14.8% (208 of 1408) in patients over the age of 80 years. The mortality was higher in patients with pre-existing cardiovascular diseases, diabetes, chronic respiratory disease, hypertension, and cancer, in mostly older subjects [17].

Similarly, trends in the gender disparity seen in CoViD19 and the related cardiovascular complications appear to indicate higher CoViD19 complications in the male subjects as compared to the females [18]. An analysis of the CoViD19 studies reveals a gender dichotomy with a higher prevalence of CoViD19 in the male subjects, although deviations exist. Regardless, the gender disparity is reflected in the mortality trends and appears consistent across all age groups. The overall data seem to indicate that there might be a sex predisposition to COVID-19, with men more susceptible to the disease and its complications. The relationship between the gender disparity observed in the CoViD19 complications appears complex, and several factors such as biological, socioeconomic, and others may account for this difference.

Overall, multiple studies have shown comparable data, and confirm the presence of a higher burden of the cardiometabolic risk factors in patients with CoViD19, among which hypertension and diabetes mellitus are most common [13, 19]. The male gender and older age appear to be consistently related to the CoViD19 complications, and in close parity with the associated cardiovascular risk.

1.2.3 *Role of the Pre-existing Cardiovascular Diseases in CoViD19*

Several clinical studies investigating CoViD19 indicate that acute myocardial injury, myocarditis, acute coronary syndromes, heart failure, hypertension, and arrhythmias are important common cardiovascular complications observed in CoViD19 patients. Evidence shows that patients with a previous history of cardiovascular diseases or those with a higher burden of cardiovascular and metabolic risk factors are prone to developing such cardiovascular complications in CoViD19.

In a single-center retrospective case series study of 187 patients hospitalized with CoViD19, about 27.8% (52 of 187) had a myocardial injury, their mean age was 71 years, 63.5% (33 of 52) of these were hypertensives, 32.7% (17 of 52) had coronary heart disease and 30.8% (16 of 52) were diabetics [12]. According to another retrospective cohort study of 416 hospitalized patients with CoViD19, about 19.7% (82 of 416) had evidence of a myocardial injury [20]. These patients were much older (mean age 74 years), and had a higher prevalence of hypertension 59.8% (49), coronary artery disease 29.3% (24), heart failure 14.6% (12), and diabetes 24.4% (20) than those without the myocardial injury [12, 20].

1.2.4 *Critical CoViD19 Complications and Pre-existing Cardiovascular Disease*

The data show that patients with pre-existing cardiovascular diseases, also appear to be highly susceptible to the critical complications of the CoViD19 as well as higher fatalities. There appears to be a higher burden of cardiovascular and metabolic risk factors such as raised body mass index (BMI) and pre-existing cardiovascular diseases in the critically ill and deceased CoViD19 patients [21]. In a retrospective study of 799 patients admitted with CoViD19 in China, data analysis of 274 patients (113 deceased, 161 recovered patients), revealed a higher rate of acute cardiac injury (72/94; 77%) and heart failure (41/83; 49%) among patients with CoViD19 with previously established cardiovascular comorbidities [11]. Similarly, in another study of a retrospective cohort of 138 patients hospitalized with CoViD19 who received critical care therapy, patients had a higher burden of cardiovascular diseases and risk factors such as hypertension 58.3%, cardiovascular disease 25%, and diabetes mellitus 22% [15].

The above data suggest that pre-existing cardiovascular and metabolic disease in CoViD19 may be a hallmark of severe cardiovascular complications including acute cardiac injury that appears to be a common critical cardiovascular complication in severe CoViD19. Therefore, the presence of these risk factors or the pre-existing cardiovascular diseases may be recognized as a precaution or an early warning sign, indicating the development of severe CoViD19 or possibly associated critical cardiovascular complications, ringing the alarm bells to the treating clinicians. The authors of a meta-analysis of eight retrospective studies of patients hospitalized with CoViD19 in China suggest that an underlying cardiovascular disease and hypertension could be considered markers of risk of severity of the illness, in patients infected with SARS CoV-2 [22].

1.2.5 *Role of Cardiovascular Complications in CoViD19 Mortality*

The burden of cardiovascular diseases is higher among fatal cases of the CoViD19 as compared to the survivors, further suggesting an interlink between preexisting cardiovascular diseases and the associated risk factors as co determinants of the increased CoViD19 mortality [11–13]. Several studies suggest that pre-existing cardiovascular diseases in patients with CoViD19 may predict fatality. According to a report of the clinical outcomes in 72,314 confirmed cases of COVID-19, the overall case fatality rate (CFR) was 2.3% in the entire cohort but significantly higher in those with pre-existing cardiovascular comorbidities, i.e., for cardiovascular disease 10.5%, diabetes mellitus 7.3%, and for hypertension 6.0% [23].

In a retrospective study of 799 patients admitted with CoViD19 in China, data analysis of 274 patients (113 deceased, 161 recovered patients) showed that hypertension, cardiovascular diseases, and the cerebrovascular diseases were much more frequent among the deceased patients 54 (48%), 16 (14%), and 4 (4%)) than among the recovered patients (39 (24%), 7 (4%), and 0 (0%) respectively [11]. The evidence further suggests that patients with CoViD19 previously naïve to cardiovascular illness, also have a significantly higher fatality rate due to the cardiac complications developing during the infection. The highest mortality rates were observed in the patients with raised markers of the myocardial injury who had underlying cardiovascular disease 69.4% (25 of 36). However, the mortality rates were also elevated in patients with elevated troponin (TnT) levels without a prior cardiovascular disease 37.5% (6 of 16) [12]. These data possibly suggest that the CoViD19 may directly increase the risk of cardiovascular complications thus the higher mortality.

1.3 Discussion

The evidence from the epidemiological surveys conducted to date strongly indicates that patients with severe CoViD19 exhibit a significant burden of cardiovascular and metabolic risk factors as well as pre-existing cardiovascular diseases. Hypertension, diabetes mellitus, and coronary heart disease appear to be important risk factors among promoters of these complications. A range of significant critical cardiovascular complications may also develop during the CoViD19, and present in a variety of forms and varying severity. The background cardiovascular risk factors and the pre-existing cardiovascular diseases, contribute to the development and the severity of these complications. The data further indicate that patients with severe CoViD19 previously naïve to cardiovascular diseases may develop neo cardiovascular complications. There is a higher likelihood of the occurrence of neo cardiovascular complications, in the presence of predisposing cardiovascular or metabolic risk factors. These complications may be critical or may prove fatal, especially when there is a higher burden of the predisposing risk factors. The pre-existing cardiovascular diseases or cardiometabolic risk factors such as hypertension and diabetes mellitus appear to have a much distinct role in the development of cardiovascular complications in CoViD19 patients. Furthermore, there appears to be a higher fatality rate among severe CoViD19 patients with a history of pre-existing cardiovascular diseases.

The overall interlink between cardiovascular diseases and the critical complications of the CoViD19 including death appears important and complex. Both, neo cardiovascular injury and pre-existing cardiovascular diseases, appear to have a distinct implication in the CoViD19. However, the exact impact of neo cardiovascular injury and pre-existing cardiovascular insults remains unclear.

Different risk factors tend to contribute differently to the severity of cardiovascular complications, and the fatality in patients with severe CoViD19. These may be attributed to the variations in the background demographic, clinical, and pathogenetic features and mechanisms related to each risk factor. The recent CoViD19 studies successfully identify these risk factors and the associated specific individual cardiovascular complications. However, to help understand how these complications may develop, the particular pathogenetic and specific viral mechanisms accompanying CoViD19 require a careful investigation and examination. Further well-designed studies are needed, using appropriately defined key cardiovascular indicators and outcomes. The impact of the neo cardiovascular injury and pre-existing cardiovascular insult should be explored in relationship with the CoViD19 outcomes [22].

1.4 Conclusion

The emergence of CoViD19 with a global spread, with Europe and the US as the epicenters of the disease, has shown remarkable dynamics and trends worldwide. The sharp rise in the number of cases in early 2020, followed by a decline, with shifting behavior between the populations across the continents and reemergence in certain countries, has resulted in an explosion of cases at a massive scale not seen previously. The epicenter of the pandemic has shown a shift in South America, mostly affecting Brazil, Peru, Chile, and Mexico, as of November 2020. The variabilities in the association of the demographic factors, comorbidities, and population traits, with the severity of the disease across the globe, reveal peculiar aspects of the CoViD19 pandemic, which have also resulted in variations in the fatality rates. The trends reflecting the association of CoViD19 with cardiovascular disease show a significant impact on the severity of the disease and the fatality and warrant the attention of scientists and researchers worldwide.

The cardiovascular disease or the CoViD19, whichever may come first, both the clinicians and the patients need to use a cautious approach. This is even more important for patients with a higher burden of cardiovascular and metabolic risk factors so that they may take early precautionary measures. It remains the duty of the clinicians not only to warn and educate the patients with cardiovascular diseases and risk factors about prevention of the CoViD19 but also to offer close monitoring and early use of aggressive management strategies when facing an existing combined threat of the CoViD19 and the heart disease.

Summary Box

- Cardiovascular diseases hold a significant share in the CoViD19 complications and the associated mortality.
- CoViD19 patients who develop complications are frequently known to have cardiovascular and metabolic risk factors.
- The most important risk factors for complications of CoViD19 include hypertension, diabetes mellitus, and a history of cardiovascular diseases.
- These cardiovascular complications of CoViD19 include acute cardiac injury, myocarditis, acute coronary syndromes, heart failure, and arrhythmias.
- Risk of developing cardiovascular complications in CoViD19 patients increases in the presence of background risk factors.
- Cardiovascular complications may also develop in patients previously naïve to cardiovascular diseases.
- Patients with a background of cardiovascular diseases, or a high-risk factor burden, should be educated regarding the preventive measures for CoViD19.
- Evidence-based, aggressive risk management practices need to be adapted, for managing CoViD19 patients with a history of cardiovascular diseases or a high-risk factor profile.

References

1. Coronavirus disease 2019 (COVID19) Situation report–77 (Data as reported by national authorities by 10:00 CET 6 April 2020). https://www.who.int/emergencies/diseases/novel-coronavirus-2019.
2. COVID-19 weekly epidemiological update data as received by WHO from national authorities, as of 1 November 2020, 10 a.m. CEST.

3. Diop BZ, Ngom M, Pougué Biyong C, et al. The relatively young and rural population may limit the spread and severity of COVID-19 in Africa: a modeling study. BMJ Glob Health. 2020;5:e002699. https://doi.org/10.1136/bmjgh-2020-002699.
4. Guan WJ, Ni ZY, Hu Y, Liang WH, Ou CQ, He JX, et al. Clinical characteristics of coronavirus disease 2019 in China N. Engl J Med. 2020.
5. https://who.sprinklr.com/region/wpro/country/cn. Accessed on April 2020.
6. Lai C-C, et al. Global epidemiology of coronavirus disease 2019: disease incidence, daily cumulative index, mortality, and their association with country healthcare resources and economic status. Int J Antimicrob Agents. 2020:105946.
7. WHO statistics dashboard: https://covid19.who.int/region/wpro/country/cn (Data last updated: 2020/11/10, 5:22 p.m. CET).
8. Report sulle caratteristiche dei pazienti positivi a COVID19 in Italia. Italian Report, March 26, 2020. https://www.epicentro.iss.it/coronavirus/bollettino/Bollettino-sorveglianza-integrata-COVID-19_26-marzo%202020.pdf.
9. Deng S-Q, Peng H-J. Characteristics of and public health responses to the coronavirus disease 2019 outbreak in China. J Clin Med. 2020;9(2):575.
10. Li B, Yang J, Zhao F, Zhi L, Wang X, Liu L, Zha Y. Prevalence and impact of cardiovascular metabolic diseases on COVD 19 in China. Clin Res Cardiol. 2020. PMID 32161990.
11. Chen T, et al. Clinical characteristics of 113 deceased patients with coronavirus disease 2019: retrospective study. BMJ. 2020;368. https://doi.org/10.1136/bmj.m1091 (Published 26 March 2020).
12. Guo T, Fan Y, Chen M, et al. Cardiovascular implications of fatal out comes of patients with coronavirus disease 2019 (COVID-19). JAMA Cardiol. Published online March 27, 2020. https://doi.org/10.1001/jamacardio.2020.1017.
13. Zhou F, Yu T, Du R, Fan G, Liu Y, Liu Z, Xiang J, Wang Y, Song B, Gu X, Guan L, Wei Y, Li H, Wu X, Xu J, Tu S, Zhang Y, Chen H, Cao B. Clinical course and risk factors for mortality of adult inpatients with COVID-19 in Wuhan, China: a retrospective cohort study. Lancet. 2020;395(10229):1054–1062. https://doi.org/10.1016/S0140-6736(20)30566-3. [Epub 2020 Mar 11. Erratum in: Lancet. 2020;395(10229):1038. Lancet. 2020;395(10229): 1038. PubMed PMID: 32171076.]
14. Chen N, Zhou M, Dong X, et al. Epidemiological and clinical characteristics of 99 cases of 2019 novel coronavirus pneumonia in Wuhan, China: a descriptive study. Lancet. 2020;395 (10223):507513. https://doi.org/10.1016/S0140-6736(20)30211-73.
15. Wang D, Hu B, Hu C, et al. Clinical characteristics of 138 hospitalized patients with 2019 novel coronavirus–infected pneumonia in Wuhan, China. JAMA. 2020;323(11):1061–1069. https://doi.org/10.1001/jama.2020.15854.
16. Yang X, Yu Y, Xu J, Shu H, Xia J, Liu H, et al. Clinical course and outcomes of critically ill patients with SARS-CoV-2 pneumonia in Wuhan, China: a single-centered, retrospective, observational study. Lancet Respira Med. 2020:S2213-600(20)30079-5. PubMed PMID: 32105632. eng.
17. Wu Z, McGoogan JM. Characteristics of and important lessons from the coronavirus disease 2019 (COVID-19) outbreak in China: summary of a report of 72 314 cases from the Chinese Center for disease control and prevention. JAMA Published Online First: 24 February 2020. https://doi.org/10.1001/jama.2020.2648.
18. Scully EP, Haverfield J, Ursin RL, Tannenbaum C, Klein SL. Considering how biological sex impacts immune responses and COVID-19 outcomes. Nat Rev Immunol. 2020;20(7): 442–447.
19. Huang C, Wang Y, Li X, et al. Clinical features of patients infected with 2019 novel coronavirus in Wuhan, China. Lancet. 2020;395(10223):497–506. https://doi.org/10.1016/S0140-6736(20)30183-52.
20. Shi S, Qin M, Shen B, et al. Association of cardiac injury with mortality in hospitalized patients with COVID-19 in Wuhan, China. JAMA Cardiol. Published online March 25, 2020. https://doi.org/10.1001/jamacardio.2020.095011

21. Peng YD, Meng K, Guan HQ, Leng L, Zhu RR, Wang BY, He MA, Cheng LX, Huang K, Zeng QT. Clinical characteristics and outcomes of 112 cardiovascular disease patients infected by 2019-nCoV. Zhonghua Xin Xue Guan Bing Za Zhi. 2020;48(0):E004. https://doi.org/10.3760/cma.j.cn112148-20200220-00105. [Epub ahead of print] Chinese. PubMed PMID: 32120458.
22. Yang J, et al. Prevalence of comorbidities in the novel Wuhan coronavirus (COVID-19) infection: a systematic review and meta-analysis. Int J Infect Dis. 2020.
23. Wu Z, Mc Googan JM. Characteristics of and important lessons from the coronavirus disease 2019(COVID-19) outbreak in China: summary of a report of 72314 cases from the Chinese Center for disease control and prevention. JAMA: Published; 2020.

Chapter 2
Virology of CoViD19

Key Questions

- Where does the SARS CoV2 come from?
- Which hosts are used by the virus?
- What are the main structural features of SARS CoV2?
- What are the main determinants of viral affinity and infectivity?
- Whar are the main featrures of variations in SARS CoV2?
- How does the SARS CoV2 enter the cell?

2.1 Viral Characteristics

2.1.1 Origins of SARS CoV2

The most recent common ancestor of the coronaviruses dates back about 10,000 years [1]. The Severe Acute Respiratory Syndrome Coronavirus 2 (SARS CoV2) discovered in late 2019 is a novel single-stranded enveloped RNA virus believed to have originated in bats which are already known to be the reservoirs of 4 out of 9 beta coronavirus species. The beta coronaviruses are associated with respiratory illnesses in humans and vary in infectivity, pathogeneity, and severity. These beta coronaviruses are divided into four lineages (A, B, C, and D), and pose a greater threat to human beings as they have high plasticity for receptor usage and a capability for adaptive mutations and recombination. The SARS CoV2 belongs to lineage B.

Similar to the SARS CoV2, two other coronaviruses such as SARS-CoV (2002) [2] and MERS CoV (2012) [3] resulted in severe epidemics, known as the Severe

U. Mallick, *Cardiovascular Complications of COVID-19*,
https://doi.org/10.1007/978-3-030-90065-6_2

Table 2.1 Comparison of SARS CoV and SARS CoV2

Pathogen	SARS CoV	SARS COV2
Immediate host	Paguma larvata	Pangolin, Mink (Possible)
Definitive host	Rhinolophus sinicus	Rhinolophus affinis (Possible)
Virus type	RNA virus	RNA virus
Species pathogen	β-coronavirus	β-coronavirus
Total genome length	29,751 nucleotides	29, 903 nucleotides
Latency	1–4 days on average	3–7 days on average
Receptor used	ACE2	ACE2
Receptor priming agent	TMPRSS2	TMPRSS2

Acute Respiratory Syndrome (SARS) and Middle East Respiratory Syndrome (MERS) respectively, with only SARS resulting in about 8096 cases and about 774 deaths [4]. A study involving evolutionary analysis of the SAS CoV 2 suggested that the ancestral origin of SARS CoV2 is likely to be from a divergent host species rather than SARS CoV [5].

2.1.2 *Hosts*

Subsequent to the discovery of the novel coronaviruses in 2005, in the horseshoe bats (genus Rhinolopus), many coronaviruses phylogenetically related to the SARS CoV (SARSr- CoVs) were discovered in the bats from different provinces in China and also from the European, African and Southeast Asian countries [6]. During the SARS outbreak, SARS CoV was found to have an intermediary host in civets, whereas, during the MERS outbreak, camels were identified as the intermediary hosts. The SARS CoV2 possibly uses the Malayan Pangolin as an intermediary host, before transferring to the humans [7]. The evolution of the bat strains may determine variability in the binding affinity with the human ACE2 receptors ie less binding affinity may produce less severe symptoms of the disease or may allow them to cross the barriers between the primary host and the intermediary host, and pose a greater threat to the humans [8].

2.1.3 *SARS CoV2 Structure*

The single-stranded RNA genome of SARS CoV2 contains 29,891 nucleotides, encoding for 9860 amino acids. It is enveloped round, elliptic or pleomorphic shape and has a diameter of 60–140 nm. The viral genome is wrapped in a nucleocapsid. It has an outer structural nucleocapsid protein (N) and glycoprotein spikes S of 9–12 nm. The coronaviruses have classical structural (spike S, membrane M,

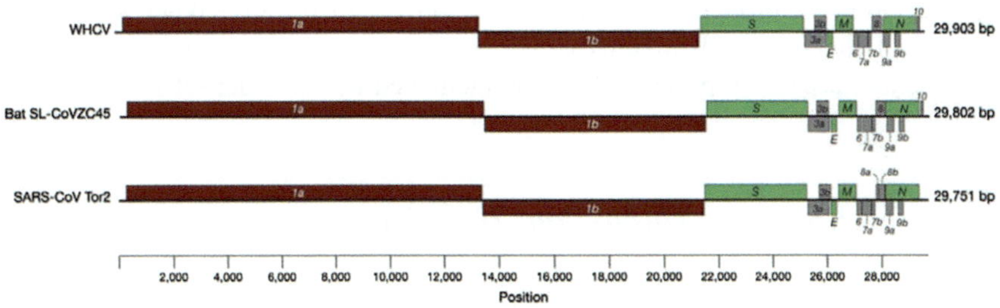

Fig. 2.1 Genome organization of SARS and SARS-like CoVs. The organization of genes for WHCV, bat SL-CoVZC45 and SARS-CoV Tor2. *Source* Figure 1. Wu, F., Zhao, S., Yu, B., Chen, Y.M., Wang, W., Song, Z.G., Hu, Y., Tao, Z.W., Tian, J.H., Pei, Y.Y. and Yuan, M.L., 2020. A new coronavirus associated with human respiratory disease in China. Nature, 579(7798), pp. 265–269. https://www.nature.com/articles/s41586-020-2008-3. By Springer Nature Group

envelope E, and nucleocapsid N proteins and accessory proteic chains) and non-structural proteins (NSP) that are connected with the pathophysiology and the virulence (Figs. 2.1 and 2.2). Evidence suggests that the NSP may block the innate host immune response [9].

In SARS COV the outer N protein is involved in the virion assembly and the virus transcription, whereas the S protein binds to the host cell receptors and replicates in the cytoplasm after gaining entry [10, 11]. The S protein is composed of two subunits (S1 and S2). The spike stalk S2 in SARSCoV2 contains a fusion peptide, a transmembrane domain, and a cytoplasmic domain. It is highly conserved approximately 99% identical to those of the tw bat SARS-like CoVs [12]. On the contrary, the spike receptor-binding domain (RBD) presents only a 40% amino acid identity with the other SARS CoVs. The nucleocapsid (N) protein is most abundant and is highly conserved, across the coronaviruses [13]. In SARS CoV2, the N protein has approximately 90% amino acid similarity as the SARS CoV [14].

The genomic structure of the SARS CoV2 is organized in a + ssRNA of approximately 30 kb in length. The total length of the DNA sequence of the SARS CoV2 is 29,903. The SARS CoV2 has a great structural similarity with these viruses, with 79.0% nucleotide identity to SARS-CoV and 51.8% identity to the MERS-CoV [15, 16]. The pathogenicity is linked with the genomic and structural features of the virus. In coronaviruses, the genomic structure has ++sRNA of approx. 30 kb length with +5 prime cap and −3 prime poly-A tail. It serves as the messenger RNA (mRNA), allowing the translation of the replicase/transcriptase and the viral structural proteins. The 2/3rd of the 5 prime end sequence, account for non-structural protein and 1/3rd for the structural proteins. The viral RNA serves the host to synthesize the polyprotein 1a/1ab (pp1a/pp1ab). The synthesis of the subgenomic RNAs (sgRNAs) sequences is facilitated by the replication-transcription complex (RCT) (in double-membrane vesicles). The open reading frames (ORFs) work as the templates for the production of the subgenomic mRNAs. The transcription regulatory sequences are located between the ORFs. The production of 16 non-structural proteins in the coronaviruses is guided by the ORF

1a and ORF 1b through the polypeptides "pp1a and pp1ab". Whereas the production of the structural proteins (spike, membrane, envelope, and nucleocapsid proteins and accessory proteic chains) is facilitated by the other ORFs (Fig. 2.2).

2.1.4 SARS CoV2 Affinity and Infectivity

Several arguments lead to the presence of variations in SARS CoV2. These include variations in the Ro (the universal basic reproductive number for virus spread) noted in relationship with the geographical spread of the virus. The mutations, recombination, and deletion play an important role in host switching and adaptation. The mutations in the viral proteins are linked with the infectivity and pathogenicity of these viruses. These determine the binding capacity of the virus with the host cell receptors.

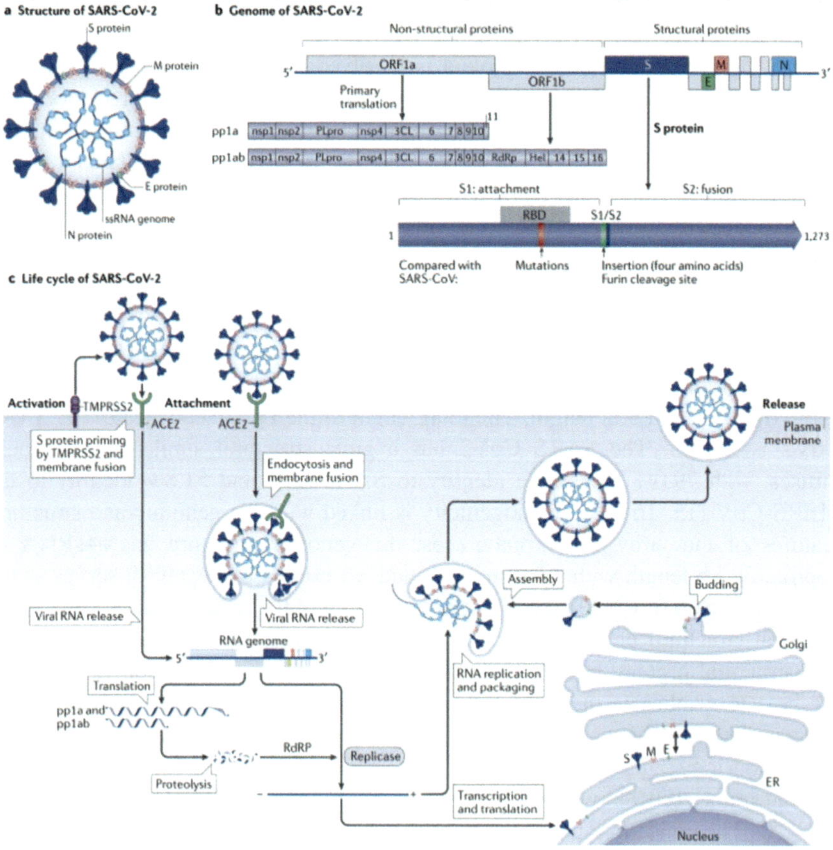

◂**Fig. 2.2** Structure, genome and life cycle of SARS-CoV-2. **a** Coronaviruses form an enveloped spherical particle that consists of four structural proteins (spike (S), envelope (E), membrane (M) and nucleocapsid (N)) and a positive-sense, single-stranded RNA (ssRNA) genome that is 30 kb in length. **b** The 5′-terminal two-thirds of the severe acute respiratory syndrome coronavirus 2 (SARS-CoV-2) genome encodes polyproteins pp1a and pp1ab, which are cleaved into 16 different non-structural proteins. Structural proteins are encoded in the 3′-terminal one-third of the genome. The S protein consists of two subunits; the S1 subunit contains a receptor-binding domain (RBD) that binds to angiotensin-converting enzyme 2 (ACE2) on the surface of host cells, whereas the S2 subunit mediates fusion between the membranes of the virus and the host cell. Compared with the S protein of SARS-CoV, the S protein of SARS-CoV-2 has two notable features. First, within the RBD of the S1 subunit, five of the six residues that are crucial for binding to human ACE2 are mutated. Second, an insertion of four amino acid residues at the boundary between the S1 and S2 subunits is present in SARS-CoV-2 but not in SARS-CoV, which introduces a novel furin cleavage site. **c** SARS-CoV-2 infection is triggered by the binding of the S protein to ACE2 on the surface of host cells, and the viral complex is incorporated into the cytoplasm either by direct fusion with the cell membrane or via endocytosis with later release into the cytoplasm from the endocytic vesicle. The S protein is cleaved at the S1/S2 boundary and the S2 subunit facilitates membrane fusion. The viral genome RNA is released into the cytoplasm, and the first open reading frame (ORF) is translated into polyproteins pp1a and pp1ab, which are then cleaved by viral proteases into small, non-structural proteins such as RNA-dependent RNA polymerase (RdRP). The viral genomic RNA is replicated by RdRP. Viral nucleocapsids are assembled from genomic RNA and N proteins in the cytoplasm, whereas budding of new particles occurs at the membrane of the endoplasmic reticulum (ER) Golgi intermediate compartment. Finally, the genomic RNA and structural proteins are assembled into new viral particles, leading to their release via exocytosis. 3CL, 3-chymotrypsin-like protease. *Source* Figure 1. Nishiga, M., Wang, D.W., Han, Y., Lewis, D.B. and Wu, J.C., 2020. COVID-19 and cardiovascular disease: from basic mechanisms to clinical perspectives. Nature Reviews Cardiology, 17(9), pp. 543–558. https://www.nature.com/articles/s41586-020-2008-3. By Springer Nature Group

The affinity of the SARS COV to bind with ACE2 is associated with viral infectivity. The adaptive mutations in the S protein of SARS-CoV have been linked with variations in binding with ACE2 receptors in the previous outbreaks. The mutations can have an impact on the binding affinity of the virus spike protein RBD and the ACE2, and therefore the infectivity. Different strains of the SARS CoV, have varying affinity and infectivity in the human ACE2 and the cells. For instance, the SARS COV epidemic strain "hTor02" with high affinity for the human ACE2 and high infectivity in human cells, promoted efficient transmission between the humans [17]. This paper describes the genetic evolution of human SARS- CoV during SARS outbreaks.

It has been demonstrated that SARS-CoV2 uses the ACE2 receptors more efficiently than the human SARS CoV (the year 2003), but less efficiently than human SARS-CoV (the year 2002) [18]. The affinity between the ACE2 and the RBD of the SARS-CoV2 is 10–20 times higher than that of the previous SARS-CoVs [19, 20]. The higher affinity may be associated with the increased infectivity and transmissibility of the SARS CoV2. The SARS CoV2 may also be susceptible to the novel mutations. Data show that a single N501T mutation may significantly enhance the binding affinity [18].

Furthermore, viral strain adaptations may occur in different phases of an epidemic. These genetic variabilities or adaptations may play a role in the modulation of the mechanisms involved in inhibiting the host defense.

2.1.5 SARS CoV2 Variability and Strains

The variabilities in the SARS CoV were found in two genes ie the S gene and the Orf8 gene. The components of the S gene (S1 and S2) and the amino-terminal domain S1-NTD and S1-CTD (carboxyl-terminal domain) that also acts as the RBD (Receptor Binding Domain), binds to the ACE2 and enters cells conferring the infectivity. Similarly, the Orf8 gene variations (Orf8a and Orf8b) owing to the deletion of a certain number of nucleotides, were associated with the viral strain adaptations involved in the early, middle, and late phase of the epidemic might even play a role in modulating the endoplasmic reticulum stress, including apoptosis and inhibiting the interferon responses in the host cells.

Several mechanisms are related to the adaptation of SARS CoV2 to the human host. The viral evolution is a result of the Nucleotide substitution [21]. The changing viral antigenicity is linked with the mutations in the spike surface glycoprotein. The identification and localization of the amino acids, that determine the conformational changes of the SARS CoV2 spike surface glycoprotein structure, remains poorly known. Following the rapid spread of the CoViD19 worldwide, the emergence of the genomic diversity of the SARS CoV2 over time, and possible mutations, have been explored in several studies. An analysis of the Eighty-six complete or near-complete genomes of the SARS-CoV2 revealed several mutations and deletions on the coding and non-coding regions of the SARS CoV2 [22].

The findings from another study examining the phylogenic relationships of 31 isolates, indicated that the SARS CoV2 were infected from different regions in the Wuhan (city of origin of SARS CoV2), and constantly evolved and disseminated in various geographical regions [23]. The possibility of an ongoing adaptation and the convergent evolution of the SARS CoV2 was revealed in an analysis of a dataset of 7666 public genome assemblies. Out of the 198 filtered recurrent mutations in the SARS-CoV2 genome, about 80% produced non-synonymous changes at the protein level and a large number of the recurrent mutations (>15 events) in three sites in Orf1ab in the regions encoding the Nsp6, Nsp11, Nsp13, and one in the Spike protein [24]

2.2 Mechanism of Viral Entry in Cells

2.2.1 SARS CoV2 Viral Spike-ACE2 Signaling Mechanisms

The viral cell entry mechanism for the SARS CoV2 has been well elucidated. Once, the virus is transmitted to the human host and gains contact with the internal environment, the viral host cell interaction initiates the signaling mechanisms. A variety of immunoinflammatory mechanisms and mediators are involved in the host response. The ACE2 is the primary host cell receptor known to be involved in the viral cell entry mechanism. The viral spike stalk binds with the ACE2 receptor helped by the coreceptors.

Evidence suggests that following the viral contact with the epithelial cells, multiple signaling pathways are activated that promote viral spike and ACE2 receptor interaction and inflammatory mechanisms involving the cytokines and receptors [25–28]. In addition to the S gene, chemokines are also involved in the process of viral entry into the host cell. For instance, the viral protein spike- ACE2 signaling pathway involves a cytokine called the Chemokine (C–C motif) ligand 2 (CCL2), which has the CCR1 and the CCR2 receptors. These receptors are associated with the inflammatory reaction and finally the pulmonary fibrosis [29]. The infected lung epithelial cells activate the casein kinase II (CKII), which helps the virus binding to the ACE2. It is also known to be involved in the activation of the ERK1/2 and the API. This further upregulates the expression of the CCL2. Furthermore, the expression of the CCL2 is also upregulated by the ACE2 through intracellular signaling pathways and activation of the ERK1/2 through interaction with the Ras and the protein kinase C, and therefore promoting lung fibrosis.

2.2.2 SARS COV, Cell Entry, and Receptors

Several specific receptors and co-receptors are utilized by the coronaviruses to gain entry into the host cells. Among the receptors notable ones have been identified as the ACE2, CD209 (Dendritic Cell-Specific ICAM 3 Grabbing Non-Integrin 1), CELEC (C-type lectin domain family 4 members G and M). The SARS CoV primarily infects the ciliated bronchial epithelial cells and type II pneumocytes. The angiotensin-converting enzyme 2 (ACE2) is used by the SARS coronavirus (SARS-CoV) as the main receptor [30]. Whereas the MERS- CoV uses the dipeptidyl peptidase 4 (DPP4; also known as CD26) and infects the unciliated bronchial epithelial cells and type II pneumocytes [8]. Previous studies demonstrated a crucial role of the angiotensin-converting enzyme 2 (ACE2) in SARS coronavirus-induced lung injury [31].

The range of receptors and coreceptors involved in the SARS COV and the ACE2 binding, is a critical determinant for the host range for the SARS CoV [32, 33].

In addition to the ACE2 other receptors include CD209 (Dendritic Cell-Specific ICAM 3 Grabbing Non-Integrin 1), CELEC (C-type lectin domain family 4 members G and M), and co-receptors include peptidases such as ANPEP, DPP4, and possibly ENPEP [34] however, only ACE2 appears to have a definite role.

The co-receptors are used to prime the S proteins of the viral spike and promote the entry into the cell. Evidence suggests that SARS CoV uses the endosomal cysteine proteases cathepsin B and L (CatB/L) [35] and the serine protease TMPRSS2 as co-receptors [36–38].

2.2.3 SARS CoV2 Similarities with SARS COV and MERS

The SARS CoV2 is known to have a great structural similarity with other coronaviruses, known to have resulted in previous outbreaks, with 79.0% nucleotide identity to SARS-CoV and 51.8% identity to MERS-CoV [15, 16]. The nucleocapsid (N) protein (most abundant in coronaviruses is highly conserved across CoVs [13]. The N protein in SARS-CoV-2 shares ~90% amino acid identity with that in SARS-CoV [14]. In addition, there are several other aspects these viruses can be compared, for example, use of receptors, co-receptors, route of transmission, transmissibility, case fatality, and others, however, these aspects are beyond the scope of this book. Despite sharing similarities in the identity, the SARS CoV2 and SARS COV, it remains unclear whether sequence similarities between them, translate into similar biological properties, including the pandemic potential [41] (Table 2.1).

2.2.4 SARS CoV2, Cell Entry and Receptors

As observed in the SARS COV infection, the SARS CoV2 also appears to use ACE2 for cell entry, however, the role of other receptors such as DPP4 or aminopeptidase N (APN) in viral cell entry could not be confirmed [39]. Furthermore, the presence of a variety of co-factors has also been shown to facilitate viral cell entry. Early evidence shows that the auxiliary proteins or co-receptors such as TMPRSS2 (a serine protease), help the SARS CoV2 binding to the ACE2 receptor to gain entry into the cells [18]. This was further confirmed in later studies showing that SARS CoV2 may use auxiliary proteins or co-receptors to gain entry into the cells such as TMPRSS2 a priming agent that helps binding viral spike S proteins with the receptors on the surface of the host cell [40]. In addition to the TMPRSS2, the presence of other factors has also been suggested that may assist SARS CoV2 viral cell entry process. Research has shown that the use of a protease inhibitor to block the SARS CoV2 binding mechanism with the ACE2, is able to limit but not fully terminate this process, suggesting that in addition to the mechanism of priming of the SARS CoV2 viral spike S protein via TMPRSS2, some other factors may also be involved [40]. These may include other cellular attachment-promoting factors such as CatB/L through which SARS CoV2 may exploit cell entry. In addition to this, other factors also appear to influence the viral capability to interact with ACE2 to gain cell entry and capacity for transmissibility of the virus, such as Gln493 and Asn501 (viral RBM residues) or pathways such as binding to the glycan in the respiratory tract [39, 40].

2.3 Summary

In summary, the SARS CoV2 is a novel coronavirus that is closely related to the coronaviruses involved in the previous coronavirus outbreaks. However, several variations in the structure and genomics appear to be associated with the diversity in the structural proteins, non-structural proteins, and the spike stalk protein. Such variations may also be closely related to the differences in the pathogenetic mechanisms and may have important clinical implications.

The mechanisms of the viral cell entry used by the coronaviruses largely coincide. The viral structural and host cell receptors and the auxiliary factors remain the major players in this process. The evidence suggests that the SARS CoV2 mainly uses ACE2 as a human cell receptor to gain entry into the cells. The cofactors, among which the TMPRSS2 appears to have more convincing supporting evidence, facilitate this process. The viral binding affinity of the SARS CoV2, with the ACE2 receptors, has shown to be superior to the SARS CoV.

The SARS CoV2 is subject to adaptive mutations. The adaptations to the human host and SARS CoV2 genome mutations may give rise to a variety of viral strains. The phenotypic implications as a result of the SARS CoV2 genetic variations may also have significant virological, biochemical, immunological consequences. The infectivity, pathogenicity, and disease severity may vary due to these differences. Furthermore, the variations associated with the modulation of the host defense mechanisms, and those observed in complex viral host cell signaling mechanisms that also involve immune mediators, and inflammatory pathways, may play an important role in the complicated CoViD19.

Overall, the precise mechanisms responsible for the specific changes that determine variations in SARS CoV2 related affinity, transmissibility, and fatality need to be better understood. These mechanisms may have important implications for the prevention and treatment of COVID19 and its complications. The viral cell entry mechanism for SARS CoV2 involving ACE2 and the associated factors, has been subject to therapeutic experimental explorations and is being further explored.

Although the scientific community has widely recognized that the interaction between human and the viral host species such as bats is closely related to the emergence of the novel coronavirus disease, recognition of the precise origins, and identification of the specific mechanisms behind the rapid global spread of the CoViD19 remains a vital challenge to the scientific community. The COVID19 pandemic may partly be explained by several viral and host evolutionary complexities, as well as the intermediary links. The environmental degradation, an ever-expanding human interaction with the remote environments, and the resulting consequences appear to be of greater significance. A concerted global collaborative effort is vital, to effectively explore and answer these important questions.

Summary Box

- The SARS CoV2 is a positive single-stranded RNA beta coronavirus that derives from the lineage B of the beta coronaviruses.
- The bats serve as the hosts and pangolins as possible intermediary hosts for the SARS CoV2.
- The SARS CoV2 viral structure is made of structural proteins (spike S, membrane M, envelope E, nucleocapsid N proteins, and accessory proteic chains) and non-structural proteins (NSP).
- The SARS CoV2 has 79.0% nucleotide identity similar to the SARS-CoV and 51.8% to the MERS-CoV.
- The mutations and variabilities of the SARS CoV2 are correlated with the spread, virulence, and fatality.
- The main viral host interaction is promoted by the viral s-stalk protein of the SARS CoV2.
- The mechanism of the viral cell entry is facilitated by the host cell receptors and the coreceptors, among which the ACE2 and TMPRSS2 play a major role.
- The SARS CoV2 uses the ACE2 receptors more efficiently than the human SARS CoV.
- Numerous factors including, environmental degradation, close human and viral host interactions, appear to be related to the emergence and spread of the novel coronavirus disease.
- The precise mechanisms concerning SARS CoV2 characteristics, infectivity, and virulence, as well as viral host interactions, need to be further defined.

References

1. Wertheim JO, Chu DKW, Peiris JSM, Kosakovsky Pond SL, Poon LLM. A case for the ancient origin of coronaviruses. J Virol. 2013;87 (12):7039–7045. https://doi.org/10.1128/JVI.03273-12..
2. Ksiazek TG, et al. A novel coronavirus associated with severe acute respiratory syndrome. N Engl J Med. 2003;348:1953–66.
3. Badawi A, Ryoo SG. Prevalence of comorbidities in the Middle East respiratory syndrome coronavirus (MERS-CoV): a systematic review and meta-analysis. Int J Infect Dis. 2016;49:129–33.

4. WHO. Summary of probable SARS cases with onset of illness from 1 November 2002 to 31 July 2003. 2004. https://www.who.int/csr/sars/country/table2004_04_21/en/.
5. Ji W, Wang W, Zhao X, Zai J, Li X. Homologous recombination within the spike glycoprotein of the newly identified coronavirus may boost cross-species transmission from snake to human. J Med Virol. 2020;92:433–40.
6. Cui J, Li F, Shi ZL. Origin and evolution of pathogenic coronaviruses. Nature Reviews Microbiology. 2019 Mar;17(3):181–92.
7. Lam TTY, Shum MHH, Zhu HC, Tong YG, Ni XB, Liao YS. Identifying SARS-CoV-2 related coronaviruses in Malayan pangolins. Nature. 2020 Feb 26 [Epub ahead of print].
8. Lei J, Kusov Y, Hilgenfeld R. Nsp3 of coronaviruses: Structures and functions of a large multi-domain protein. Antiviral Res. 2018;149:58–74.
9. Perlman S, Netland J. Coronaviruses post SARS: Update on replication and pathogenesis. Nat Rev Microbiol. 2009;7:439–50.
10. Ding Y, Wang H, Shen H, Li Z, Geng J, Han H, Cai J, Li X, Kang W, Weng D, et al. The clinical pathology of severe acute respiratory syndrome (SARS): a report from China. J Pathol. 2003;200:282–9.
11. Chan JFW, Kok KH, Zhu Z, Chu H, To KKW, Yuan S, Yuen KY. Genomic characterization of the 2019 novel human-pathogenic coronavirus isolated from a patient with atypical pneumonia after visiting Wuhan. Emerg Microbes Infect. 2020;9:221–36.
12. Menachery VD, Graham RL, Baric RS. Jumping species—a mechanism for coronavirus persistence and survival. Curr Opin Virol. 2017;23:1–7.
13. Gralinski LE, Menachery VD. Return of the coronavirus: 2019-nCoV. Viruses 2020;12:135.
14. Ren LL, Wang YM, Wu ZQ, Xiang ZC, Guo L, Xu T. Identification of a novel coronavirus causing severe pneumonia in human: a descriptive study. Chin Med J (Engl). 2020 [Epub ahead of print].
15. Chan JFW, Kok KH, Zhu Z, Chu H, To KKW, Yuan S, Yuen KY. Genomic characterization of the 2019 novel human-pathogenic coronavirus isolated from a patient with atypical pneumonia after visiting Wuhan. Emerg Microbes Infect. 2020;9:221–236.
16. Chinese SMEC. Molecular evolution of the SARS coronavirus during the course of the SARS epidemic in China. Science. 2004;303:1666–9.
17. Wan Y, Shang J, Graham R, Baric RS, Li F. Receptor recognition by novel coronavirus from Wuhan: an analysis based on decade-long structural studies of SARS. J Virol. 2020.
18. Wrapp D, Wang N, Corbett KS, Goldsmith JA, Hsieh CL, Abiona O, Graham BS, McLellan JS. Cryo-EM structure of the 2019-nCoV spike in the prefusion conformation. Science 2020;367:1260–63.
19. Yan R, Zhang Y, Li Y, Xia L, Zhou Q. Structure of dimeric full-length human ACE2 in complex with B0AT1. BioRxiv 2020.
20. Lauring AS, Andino R. Quasispecies theory and the behavior of RNA viruses. PLoS Pathog 2010;6, Article e1001005, https://doi.org/10.1371/journal.ppat.1001005.
21. Phan T. Genetic diversity and evolution of SARS-CoV-2 Infection. Genetics Evol. 2020; 81:104260. ISSN 1567-1348, https://doi.org/10.1016/j.meegid.2020.104260, http://www.sciencedirect.com/science/article/pii/S1567134820300915.
22. Zhang J, Ma K, Li H, Liao M, Qi W.The continuous evolution and dissemination of 2019 novel human coronavirus. J Infect. 2020;80(6):671–693. ISSN 0163-4453, https://doi.org/10.1016/j.jinf.2020.02.001. http://www.sciencedirect.com/science/article/pii/S0163445320300839.
23. van Dorp L, Acman M, Richard D et al. Emergence of genomic diversity and recurrent mutations in SARS-CoV-2 [published online ahead of print, 2020 May 5]. Infect Genet Evol. 2020;104351. https://doi.org/10.1016/j.meegid.2020.104351.
24. Cheung CY, Poon LL, Ng IH, Luk W, Sia SF, Wu MH. Cytokine responses in severe acute respiratory syndrome coronavirus-infected macrophages in vitro: possible relevance to pathogenesis. J Virol. 2005;79:7819–26.
25. Heurich A, Hofmann-Winkler H, Gierer S, Liepold T, Jahn O, Pohlmann S. TMPRSS2 and ADAM17 cleave ACE2 differentially and only proteolysis by TMPRSS2 augments entry

driven by the severe acute respiratory syndrome coronavirus spike protein. J Virol. 2014;88:1293–307.
26. Chen IY, Chang SC, Wu HY, Yu TC, Wei WC, Lin S. Upregulation of the chemokine (C-C motif) ligand 2 via a severe acute respiratory syndrome coronavirus spike–ACE2 signaling pathway. J Virol. 2010;84:7703–12.
27. Gharaee-Kermani M, Denholm EM, Phan SH. Costimulation of fibroblast collagen and transforming growth factor β1 gene expression by monocyte chemoattractant protein-1 via specific receptors. J Biol Chem. 1996;271:17779–84.
28. Li W, Moore MJ, Vasilieva N, Sui J, Wong SK, Berne MA, Somasundaran M, Sullivan JL, Luzuriaga K, Greenough TC, Choe H, Farzan M. Angiotensin-converting enzyme 2 is a functional receptor for the SARS coronavirus. Nature 2003;426:450–454.
29. Kuba K, Imai Y, Rao S, Gao H, Guo F, Guan B, et al. A crucial role of angiotensin converting enzyme 2 (ACE2) in SARS coronavirus-induced lung injury. Nat Med. 2005;11(8):875–9. https://doi.org/10.1038/nm1267.PMID16007097.
30. Li F. Receptor recognition and cross- species infections of SARS coronavirus. Antiviral Res. 2013;100:246–54.
31. Li WH et al. Animal origins of the severe acute respiratory syndrome coronavirus: insight from ACE2-S- protein interactions. J Virol. 2006;80:4211–19.
32. Qi F, Qian S, Zhang S, Zhang Z. Single cell RNA sequencing of 13 human tissues identify cell types and receptors of human coronaviruses. Biochem Biophys Res Commun. 2020: S0006–291X(20)30523–4. https://doi.org/10.1016/j.bbrc.2020.03.044. [Epub ahead of print] PubMed PMID: 32199615).
33. Simmons G, Gosalia DN, Rennekamp AJ, Reeves JD, Diamond SL, Bates P. Inhibitors of cathepsin L prevent severe acute respiratory syndrome coronavirus entry. Proc Natl Acad Sci U S A. 2005;102(33):11876–81. Epub 2005 Aug 4. PubMed PMID: 16081529; PubMed Central PMCID: PMC1188015.
34. Shulla A, Heald-Sargent T, Subramanya G, Zhao J, Perlman S, Gallagher T. A transmembrane serine protease is linked to the severe acute respiratory syndrome coronavirus receptor and activates virus entry. J Virol. 2011;85:873–82.
35. Glowacka I, Bertram S, Müller MA, Allen P, Soilleux E, Pfefferle S, Steffen I, Tsegaye TS, He Y, Gnirss K et al. Evidence that TMPRSS2 activates the severe acute respiratory syndrome coronavirus spike protein for membrane fusion and reduces viral control by the humoral immune response. J Virol. 2011;85:4122–34.
36. Matsuyama S, Nagata N, Shirato K, Kawase M, Takeda M, Taguchi F. Efficient activation of the severe acute respiratory syndrome coronavirus spike protein by the transmembrane protease TMPRSS2. J Virol. 2010;84:12658–64.
37. Zhou P, Yang XL, Wang XG, Hu B, Zhang L, Zhang W, Si HR, Zhu Y, Li B, Huang CL, Chen HD, Chen J, Luo Y, Guo H, Jiang RD, Liu MQ, Chen Y, Shen XR, Wang X, Zheng XS, Zhao K, Chen QJ, Deng F, Liu LL, Yan B, Zhan FX, Wang YY, Xiao GF, Shi ZL. A pneumonia outbreak associated with a new coronavirus of probable bat origin. Nature. 2020 Mar;579(7798):270–273. doi: https://doi.org/10.1038/s41586-020-2012-7. Epub 2020 Feb 3. PubMed PMID: 32015507; PubMed Central PMCID: PMC7095418.
38. Hoffmann M, Kleine-Weber H, Schroeder S, Krüger N, Herrler T, Erichsen S, Schiergens TS, Herrler G, Wu NH, Nitsche A, Müller MA, Drosten C, Pöhlmann S.SARS-CoV-2 Cell entry depends on ACE2 and TMPRSS2 and is blocked by a clinically proven protease inhibitor. Cell. 2020 Mar 4. pii: S0092–8674(20)30229–4. doi:https://doi.org/10.1016/j.cell.2020.02.052. [Epub ahead of print] PubMed PMID: 32142651; PubMed Central PMCID: PMC7102627.
39. Li W, Hulswit RJG, Widjaja I, Raj VS, McBride R, Peng W, Widagdo W, Tortorici MA, van Dieren B, Lang Y, et al. Identification of sialic acid-binding function for the Middle East respiratory syndrome coronavirus spike glycoprotein. Proc Natl Acad Sci USA. 2017;114: E8508–17.

40. Park YJ, Walls AC, Wang Z, Sauer MM, Li W, Tortorici MA, Bosch BJ, DiMaio F, Veesler D. Structures of MERS-CoV spike glycoprotein in complex with sialoside attachment receptors. Nat Struct Mol Biol. 2019;26:1151–7.
41. Letko M, Marzi A, Munster V. Functional assessment of cell entry and receptor usage for SARS-CoV-2 and other lineage B betacoronaviruses. Nat Microbiol. 2020;5:562–569. https://doi.org/10.1038/s41564-020-0688-y.

Chapter 3
An Introduction to the Clinical and Diagnostic Features, and CoViD19 Complications

Key Questions

- What are the main clinical characteristics of the CoViD19?
- What are the frequently associated complications of CoViD19?
- How do we diagnose the CoViD19?
- What are the important hematological and biochemical characteristics of CoViD19?
- What are the common radiological features of CoViD19?

3.1 Introduction

The CoViD19 is associated with a wide variety of clinical features. The clinical presentation of patients with CoViD19 ranges from being asymptomatic to the appearance of severe symptoms related to the infection and the affected body systems, indicating a significant heterogeneity [1]. According to the severity of symptoms the disease is classified as mild, moderate, server and critical (Table 3.1). According to a report highlighting the epidemiological characteristics of the first 425 confirmed CoViD19 cases in Wuhan, the median age of the patients was 59 years (range, 15–89) and the mean incubation period was 5.2 days (95% confidence interval [CI], 4.1–7.0), with the 95th percentile of the distribution at 12.5 days [2]. In a study, the median time from disease onset to death amongst the deceased patients was 16 (interquartile range 12.0–20.0) days [26]. In another study, the median time to death was 18·5 days [7]. According to a summary report of 72,314 cases, 46,672 with the confirmed disease, the percentage of patients with the symptomatic, severe, and mild disease was around 81% (36,160), 14% (6,168), and critical 5% (2,087) cases, respectively. The case fatality rate was 2.3% (1,023 44,672 confirmed cases) [3].

U. Mallick, *Cardiovascular Complications of COVID-19*,
https://doi.org/10.1007/978-3-030-90065-6_3

Table 3.1 CoViD19 severity and features (CDC)

Mild	Severe	Critical
Non-pneumonia and mild pneumonia cases	Dyspnea, respiratory frequency ≥ 30/min, blood O_2 sat $\leq 93\%$, PaO_2/FiO_2 ratio <300, lung infiltrates >50% within 24–48 h	Respiratory failure, septic shock, and/or multiple organ dysfunction or failure, death
80.9%	13.8%	4.7%

Centers for Disease Control and Prevention. COVID-19 Overview and Infection Prevention and Control Priorities in non-US Healthcare Settings. Updated Feb. 26, 2021. COVID-19 Overview and Infection Prevention and Control Priorities in non-US Healthcare Settings | CDC. Accessed on 06–26–2021

Table 3.2 Clinical symptomatology CoViD19

Symptoms
Fever or chills
Cough
Shortness of breath or difficulty breathing
Fatigue
Headache
Nasal congestion or runny nose
Muscle or body aches
Sore throat
New loss of smell or taste
Nausea or vomiting
Diarrhea

Centers for Disease Control and Prevention. COVID-19 Overview and Infection Prevention and Control Priorities in non-US Healthcare Settings. Last updated on Feb. 26, 2021. COVID-19 Overview and Infection Prevention and Control Priorities in non-US Healthcare Settings | CDC. Accessed on 06–26–2021. *Content Source* National Center for Immunization and Respiratory Diseases (NCIRD), Division of Viral Diseases. Copyright info: https://www.cdc.gov/other/agencymaterials.html

The asymptomatic CoViD19 is more common in the younger population group and may be associated with a higher risk of spread by the younger adults. The presence of asymptomatic CoViD19 and the risk of pre-symptomatic transmission have been investigated in several studies. A meta-analysis of 504 patients from 34 studies of asymptomatic CoViD19 found that more than half of the patients (62.2%) had abnormalities in the CT imaging of the lungs. The radiological findings were more frequently observed in the age group (39.14 ± 26.70 years), as compared to the younger age group (19.59 ± 7.17 years) [4]. Another study investigating infectiousness profile in 94 cases with laboratory-confirmed CoViD19, showed that 44% (95% confidence interval, 30–57%) of secondary cases were infected during the index cases' presymptomatic stage [5]. The CoViD19, although, is a highly contagious novel coronavirus disease, however most cases (about 81%) exhibit a mild form of the disease. The mortality rates for CoViD19 are much lower as compared to the MERS (9.6%) or SARS (34.5%), with the majority of the patients showing good recovery [6]. The asymptomatic form of the CoViD19 appears to be complex and contagious and may accompany overt hematological/ radiological presence.

In this chapter, we provide the readers, key information related to the clinical forms of the CoViD19, the symptomatology, and an overview of the diagnostic features of the disease (Fig. 3.1). We also provide an evidence-based summary of the COViD19 complications, together with associated hematological and radiological abnormalities. We further present a focus on pathological characteristics of the cardiovascular complications of the CoViD19, highlighting the macro and microscopic cardiac and vascular involvement of the disease, as well as the associated thrombotic process, as evidenced in the emerging literature.

3.2 Clinical Symptomatology

Most commonly, CoViD19 presents with respiratory symptoms such as dry cough, along with signs of infection such a fever, myalgia, or gastrointestinal symptoms. In a retrospective cohort of 799 patients admitted with CoViD19, an analysis of 274 patients, fever was detected in 91% (241/274) patients, cough 68% (185/274), myalgia 22% (62/274), and gastrointestinal symptoms 6–28% (16–77/274) patients. Similarly, another multi-center retrospective cohort study of 119 hospitalized CoViD19 patients showed that about 94% (180) patients had fever, 79% (151) patients had a cough, 15% (29) had myalgia, and about 5% (9) had gastrointestinal symptoms [7] (Tables 3.1 and 3.3).

In general, the CoViD19 patients with milder forms of the disease present with a low fever, mild fatigue, and without signs or symptoms of respiratory infection. As the disease progresses to a severe form, dyspnea and or hypoxia may develop, further evolving with features of the sepsis and septic shock (ARDS, shock, metabolic acidosis, coagulation dysfunction, and multiple organ functional failure), indicating the critical stage of the disease. Deviations in the symptomatology may exist in the critical subjects presenting with mild symptoms such as low-grade fever or absence of fever. The alterations in the taste and smell may exist in some patients [8].

3.3 Sepsis and Complications of CoViD19

A systemic extension of the local viral injury in CoViD19 may result in a variety of complications of varying severity (Fig. 3.2). The common and critical complications include pneumonia, ARDS (Acute Respiratory Distress Syndrome), SIRS (Systemic Inflammatory Response Syndrome), renal impairment, liver failure, disseminated intravascular coagulopathy, multi-organ failure, shock, and death. Similarly, several cardiovascular complications have been reported and may include

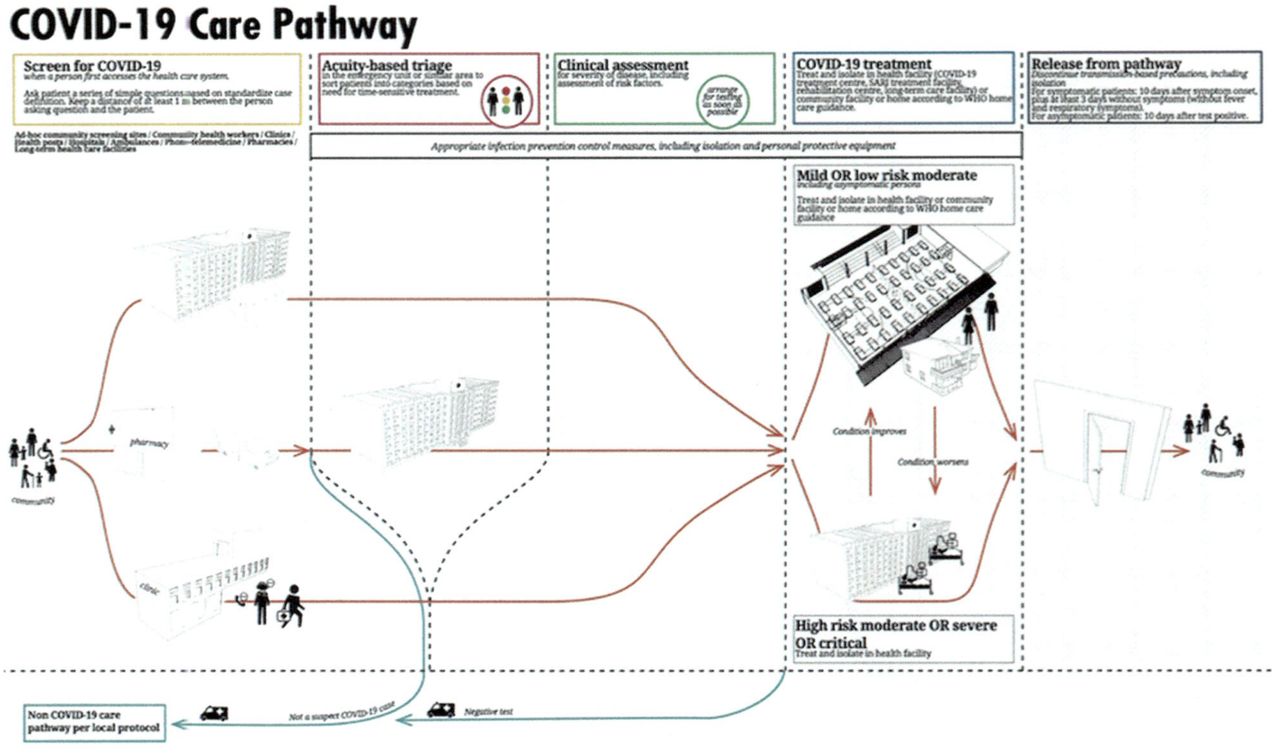

Fig. 3.1 CoViD19 Care pathway. *Source* World Health Organization. WHO REFERENCE NUMBER: WHO/2019-nCoV/clinical/2021.1. Annex 1 CoViD19 Care pathway. Clinical management of COVID-19 patients: living guidance, 25 January 2021 COVID-19: Clinical care. Vol.16 Published on 3/16/21. Clinical management of COVID-19 patients: living guidance, 25 January 2021||Annex 1: COVID-19 care pathway (magicapp.org). Accessed on 06.26.2021. COPYRIGHT: CC BY-NC-SA 3.0 IGO

Table 3.3 CoViD19 severity (WHO)

Critical CoViD19	Severe CoViD19	Non-severe CoViD19
Defined by the criteria for acute respiratory distress syndrome (ARDS), sepsis, septic shock, or other conditions that would normally require the provision of life-sustaining therapies such as mechanical ventilation (invasive or non-invasive) or vasopressor therapy	Defined by any of: • Oxygen saturation <90% on room air • Respiratory rate >30 breaths/min in adults and children >5 years old; ≥ 60 breaths/min in children <2 months old; ≥ 50 in children 2–11 months old; and ≥ 40 in children 1–5 years old • Signs of severe respiratory distress (accessory muscle use, inability to complete full sentences, and, in children, very severe chest wall indrawing, grunting, central cyanosis, or presence of any other general danger signs)	Defined as absence of any criteria for severe or critical COVID-19

According to the panel suggesting the recommendations in this table, the oxygen saturation threshold of 90% to define severe COVID-19 is arbitrary and should be interpreted cautiously. For example, clinicians must use their judgment to determine whether a low oxygen saturation is a sign of severity or is normal for a given patient with chronic lung disease. Similarly, a saturation >90–94% on room air is abnormal (in patient with normal lungs) and can be an early sign of severe disease, if patient is on a downward trend. Generally, if there is any doubt, the panel suggested erring on the side of considering the illness as severe

World Health Organization. WHO REFERENCE NUMBER: WHO/2019-nCoV/clinical/2021.1. Clinical management of COVID-19 patients: living guidance, 25 January 2021 COVID-19: Clinical care. COVID-19 Clinical management: living guidance (who.int). Accessed on 06.26. 2021. Copyright info: Creative Commons—Attribution-NonCommercial-ShareAlike 3.0 IGO—CC BY-NC-SA 3.0 IGO

myocardial injury, acute, fulminant myocarditis, heart failure, arrhythmias, and others.

The evidence suggests a frequent association of sepsis with complicated CoViD19. Sepsis and septic shock are defined as life-threatening organ dysfunction as a result of the dysregulated host response to suspected or proven infection, involving organ dysfunction [28]. According to the definition, sepsis accompanies persistent hypotension, hyper- or hypothermia, leukocytosis or leukopenia, and thrombocytopenia [9]. The CoViD19 patients presenting with sepsis may exhibit signs and symptoms of systemic involvement and multi-organ dysfunction often indicating a poor survival. These include dry skin, severe dyspnea, hypoxemia, tachycardia, hypotension, altered mental function, decreased urine output, and others. A multicenter retrospective study of 191 patients hospitalized with CoViD19 showed, about 59% (112/191) of the overall cohort, and 100% (54/54) of the non-survivors, had sepsis. Among the survivors, about 42% (58/137) had sepsis, indicating a high prevalence in this study. Septic shock was seen in 20% (38/191)

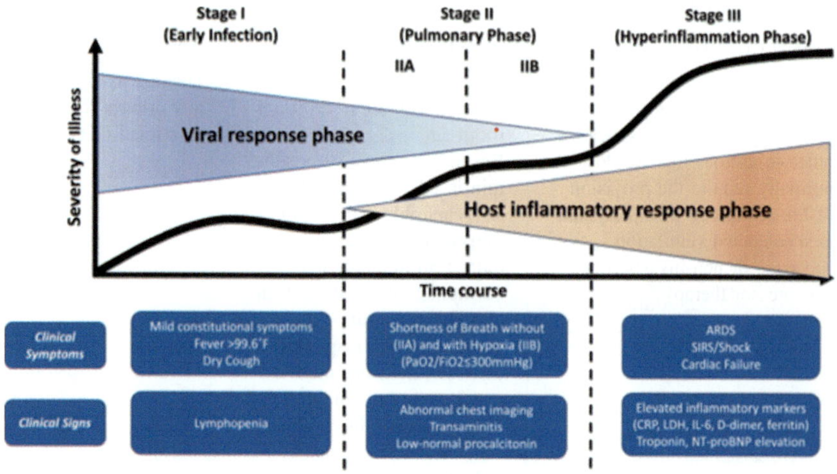

Fig. 3.2 Proposed classification of CoViD19 disease stages. Classification of COVID-19 disease states. The figure illustrates 3 escalating phases of COVID-19 disease progression, with associated signs, symptoms. ARDS, acute respiratory distress syndrome; CRP, C-reactive protein; JAK, janus kinase; LDH, lactate dehydrogenase; NT-proBNP, N-terminal pro B-type natriuretic peptide; SIRS, systemic inflammatory response syndrome; GM-CSF, Granulocyte Macrophage Colony Stimulating Factor. *Modified from source* Siddiqi, H.K. and Mehra, M.R., 2020. COVID-19 illness in native and immunosuppressed states: a clinical–therapeutic staging proposal. *The Journal of Heart and Lung Transplantation*, *39*(5), p. 405. Accessible on: https://www.ncbi.nlm.nih.gov/pmc/articles/PMC7118652/. Accessed on June 28, 2021. Copyright © Published by Elsevier Inc. on behalf of International Society for Heart and Lung Transplantation

and 70% (38/54) of the overall cohort and non-survivors, respectively, whereas none of the survivors had septic shock. Similarly, higher frequency of systemic complications was observed, such as ARDS 31% (59/191), heart failure 23% (44/191), acute cardiac injury17% (33/191), acute kidney injury 15% (28/191) and coagulopathy 19% (37/191) in the overall cohort. The non-survivors had much higher rates of complications such as sepsis 100% (54/54), ARDS 93% (50/54), heart failure 52% (28/54), the acute cardiac injury 59% (32/54), acute kidney injury and coagulopathy both 50% (27/54) among others. In this study, the median time from the onset of illness (ie, before admission) to the discharge, was 22·0 days, whereas the median time to death was 18·5 days and half of the non-survivors experienced a secondary infection [7].

Multiple other studies report a high prevalence of the CoViD19 complications in associaton with mortality. According to a retrospective study of 799 patients admitted with CoViD19 in China, the data analysis of 274 patients (113 deceased, 161 recovered patients) showed that acute respiratory distress syndrome was detected in 72% (196/274) patients and was more commonly found among the deceased than the recovered patients 100% (113/113) versus 52% (83/161), respectively. In this study other systemic complications commonly found in the deceased patients as compared to the survivors indicating an association with the clinical outcome included, sepsis 100% (113), acute kidney injury 25% (28/113), DIC 17% (19/113), shock 41% (46/113), and acute liver injury 9% (10/113). Other clinical complications reported included acute cardiac injury 77% (72/94); heart failure 49% (41/83), alkalosis 40% (14/35), hyperkalemia 37% (42), and hypoxic encephalopathy 20% (23) [10].

In another retrospective cohort analysis of 138 consecutive patients admitted with CoViD19, about 36 patients received ICU care, and the most common complications included ARDS 61.1% (22), arrhythmia 44.4% (16), shock 33.6% (11), acute cardiac injury 22.2% (8) and acute kidney injury 8.3% (3) [11].

In summary, data from numerous studies reflect features, associations, and outcomes of the complications of CoViD19, indicating that worsening of the disease often associated with sepsis, may adverse involve multiple body systems, including the pulmonary and cardiovascular systems. The severe respiratory compromise appears to be a serious and frequent association of the complicated CoViD19 that may result in death. The deceased patients more frequently manifest features of sepsis, ARDS, and cardiac complications of varying severity and forms.

3.4 Important Diagnostic Features

3.4.1 Viral Sampling

The SARS CoV2 can be found in a variety of clinical samples. In patients with CoViD19, viral specimens may include oral, nasopharyngeal, the lower respiratory tract, and blood samples [12, 13]. Besides, the use of gastrointestinal sites, such as fecal and anal sampling, has also been reported [14]. However, less viral loads have been reported in the fecal samples as compared to the respiratory samples [13]. In addition, in the gastrointestinal tract, the virus had been detected in the gastric, duodenal, and rectal epithelia [15].

In a study involving viral sampling from multiple sites of 205 patients with COVID-19, the lower respiratory tract samples most often tested positive for the SARS-CoV-2. The live virus was also detected in the feces, thereby, implying that SARS CoV2 may be transmitted by the fecal route. A small percentage of the blood samples had positive PCR (Polymerase Chain Reaction) test results, suggesting systemic involvement of the virus [16].

The reverse transcription assay (RT PCR) is commonly used for the diagnosis and monitoring of the infection with SARS CoV2. A systematic review and meta-analysis using real-time reverse transcription-polymerase chain reaction (qRT-PCR), involving 8136 poled samples, reported wide use (69.6%) of nasopharyngeal swabs with a positive rate (PR) of 45.5% (95% CI: 31.2–59.7%). The lower respiratory tract (LRT) samples had a positive rate of 71.3% (95% confidence interval [CI]: 60.3–82.3%) [17].

Although the RT PCR is the gold standard diagnostic test for CoViD19, droplet digital PCR (ddPCR) may be better for the detection of low-viral-load samples with a higher value for assessment of disease progression and prognosis. According to a report, quantitative monitoring of the viral load in lower respiratory tract samples helps to monitor the disease progression, especially in patients with low viral load. The lapse of time since the onset of clinical symptomatology and the clinical presentation help guiding the viral sampling [18]. The sampling of the respiratory specimens, at the least, is recommended by the WHO guidelines [19].

Other tests that may assist in the diagnosis of SARS CoV2 infection include Antigen Testing for SARS-CoV2 Infection for nucleoprotein (N protein) or spike protein (S protein), and serologic or antibody testing. The antigen testing is less sensitive to RT PCR and has almost similar specificity but a limited diagnostic value in CoViD19 patients, although may be useful in the early symptomatic disease (NIH CoViD19 treatment guidelines Ref.).

The serological tests, based on the detection of antibodies such as IgM, IgG, IgA, and/or total antibodies, or a combination of IgM and IgG antibodies, may assist in diagnosing the SARS CoV2 inflection in conjunction with other tests such as NAAT and the antigen testing. Several expert professional societies provide guidance for the use of these tests in real practice in CoViD19 [20–25].

3.4.2 Biochemical and Hematological Features

Several hematological and biochemical abnormalities are associated with different stages of the CoViD19 severity (Fig. 3.3). The early form of CoViD19 is associated with normal or low white cell count, with lymphocytopenia reflecting a negative evolution of the disease. The pathological features of sepsis reflect multi-organ involvement, metabolic, and coagulation disorders. These may include increased urea, creatinine, electrolyte imbalance, deranged liver enzymes, hyperbilirubinemia, thrombocytopenia, coagulopathy, metabolic dysregulation such as acidosis, raised serum lactate levels, and others. According to the laboratory data of CoViD19 patients from a retrospective study of 799 hospitalized patients, data of 113 deceased and 161 survivors were analyzed, leukocytosis, lymphopenia, and thrombocytopenia were more common in the deceased versus recovered patients 56 (50%) versus 6 (4%), 103 (91%) versus 76 (47%) respectively, as well as the markers of liver, kidney and cardiac injury. Similarly, concentrations of the interleukin 2 receptor, interleukin 6, interleukin 8, interleukin 10, and tumor necrosis factor α were significantly higher in the deceased patients than in the recovered patients. Furthermore, the study also reported higher concentrations of the procalcitonin, high sensitivity C-reactive protein, ferritin, D dimers, and elevated erythrocyte sedimentation rate in the deceased as compared to the recovered patients [26]. In another retrospective cohort study of 138 consecutive patients admitted with CoViD19, lymphopenia 70.3% (97), prolonged prothrombin time 58% (80), and elevated lactate dehydrogenase 39.9% (55), were commonly reported [11].

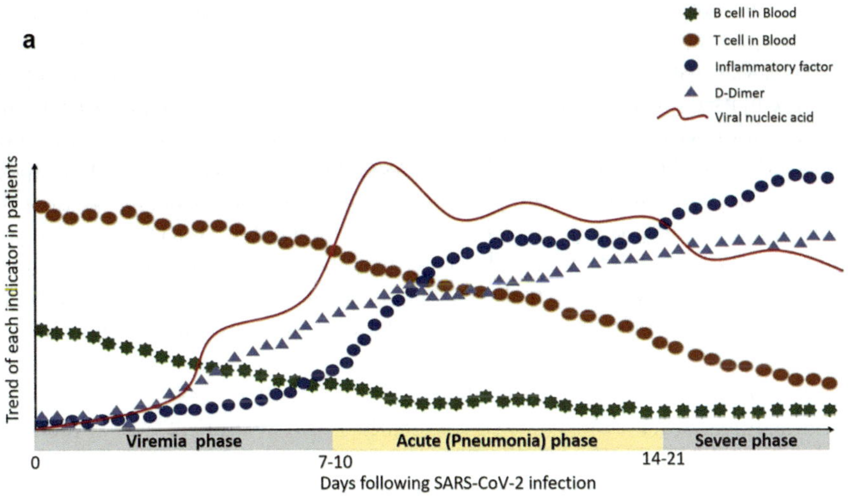

Fig. 3.3 Hypothetical pathogenesis of COVID-19. The X-axis refers to days after SARS-CoV-2 infection. The disease course is divided into three phases. The Y-axis shows the trend of T cells, B cells, inflammatory factors, D-dimer and viral load in patients. A The trend of each indicator in severe COVID-19 patients. *Source* Figure 1. Cao, W. and Li, T., 2020. COVID-19: towards understanding of pathogenesis. Cell research, 30(5), pp. 367–369. https://www.nature.com/articles/s41422-020-0327-4. By Springer Published Group

Furthermore, the hyperinflammatory picture manifested by the cytokine storm, hyper feritinemia, raised D dimer levels, and coagulopathy, is commonly associated with the multi-organ failure and critical complications of CoViD19, including the fatality. The elevated levels of several acute cytokines including IL-1B, IL6, IL8, IFN-γ, IP-10, and monocyte chemoattractant protein 1 (MCP-1), may mark poor prognosis [32–34]. The cytokine storm in severe CoViD19 cases is manifested by consumption of CD4+ and CD8+ T cells, and the decrease in regulatory T cells, and elevated pro-inflammatory cytokinesCytokines (TNF-α, IL-1β, IL-6), chemokines (IL-8) [35, 36]. Several studies have reported an increase in cytokine levels including IL-2, IL-7, IL-10, granulocyte-colony stimulating factor (G-CSF), granulocyte macrophage-colony stimulating factor (GM-CSF), interferon-inducible protein-10 (IP10), monocyte chemotactic protein 1 (MCP1), macrophage inflammation, Inflammation protein-1α, IFN-γ [26, 37, 38] (Table 3.4).

Several CoViD19 studies and case records report the presence of coagulation abnormalities in complicated CoViD19 patients. A single-center study of 183 consecutive patients, admitted with CoViD19 pneumonia, reported elevated levels of abnormal coagulation markers such as D dimers and FDP (Fibrinogen Degradation Products), which were common among the non-survivors. In this study, about 71.4% (15/21) of the non-survivors had DIC (Disseminated Intravascular Coagulopathy), as compared to the survivors 0.6% (1/162). A mortality rate of 11.5% (21) was observed in this study [27].

Various short and long-term outcome predicting models have been validated in the clinical practice, to help clinicians make decisions, and also used in clinical research. For instance, the Sequential Organ Failure Assessment (SOFA) score, is commonly used for risk stratification and determination of prognosis, in critically ill patients with sepsis, in the intensive care settings. Based on the laboratory and clinical data, the Sequential Organ Failure Assessment (SOFA) score has been used in multiple studies, investigating the mortality risk in patients with CoViD19 with multi-organ damage, as a prognostic tool, to predict the ICU (Intensive Care Unit) mortality [29]. According to a multi-center retrospective cohort study of 191 hospitalized CoViD19 patients, high sequential Organ Failure Assessment (SOFA) score and raised d-dimer greater than 1 μg/mL, were associated with a poor prognosis [7].

Overall, the biochemical, immunological, and hematological abnormalities associated with complicated CoViD19 reflect differences in the stages of the disease and may hold a prognostic significance. The presence of lymphopenia is a marker of the negative evolution of the disease and reflects infection of the T cells [30]. The IL6 and IL10 are important immune markers of the critical stage of the disease in patients with CoViD19 [31]. The Procalcitonin and CRP may be used to monitor disease evolution, however, the presence of superadded bacterial infections may result in deviations in the measurements (Table 3.4).

Table 3.4 Laboratory features of CoViD19

Common lab features	Association with worse outcomes
Lymphopenia	+
Thrombocytopenia	+
Elevated D dimers	+
Elevated aminotransaminase levels	+
Elevated lactate dehydrogenase levels	+
Elevated inflammatory markers (e.g., ferritin, C-reactive protein, erythrocyte sedimentation rate)	+
Elevated coagulation markers increased (PT)	+
Elevated cardiac and other markers (Troponin, CPK)	+
Elevated immune markers (interleukin 6 [IL-6] and tumor necrosis factor [TNF]-alpha)	+
Elevated markers of acute kidney injury	+

Sources COVID-19: Management in hospitalized adults. Authors: Arthur Y Kim, Rajesh T Gandhi. Editor: Martin S Hirsch, Deputy Editor: Allyson Bloom. Topic 128323 Version 35.0. Accessible on: https://www.uptodate.com/contents/covid-19-clinical-features?topicRef=126981&source=related_link#H2249070035. Accessed on 28 June, 2021. Last updated on June 02, 2021. © 2021 UpToDate, Inc. and/or its affiliates. All Rights Reserved

3.4.3 Radiological Features

The radiological presence of CoViD19 is usually a sign of the advanced disease, however, abnormalities may be found in the asymptomatic form of the disease [4, 39] (Fig. 3.4). The radiological features of pneumonia in CoViD19 may include ground glass shadowing or consolidation type lesions that present as unilateral or bilateral shadowing, or the reticular nodular type shadowing, involving a subsegmental, segmental, lobar, or an entire portion of a lung.

The later stages of the disease are usually marked by septal thickening, bronchiectasis, pleural thickening, and subpleural involvement, although less commonly observed. The occurrence of pleural/pericardial effusions, enlarged lymph nodes, development of cavitation, the CT halo sign, or pneumothorax is rare, mark the progression of the disease. The ground glass opacification appears to be a more common radiological feature in CoViD19 pneumonia, with the critical patients more often exhibiting these signs. In a retrospective multi-center retrospective cohort study of 191 CoViD19 patients admitted in the hospital, a majority 75% (143) patients had bilateral pulmonary infiltration. According to the type of

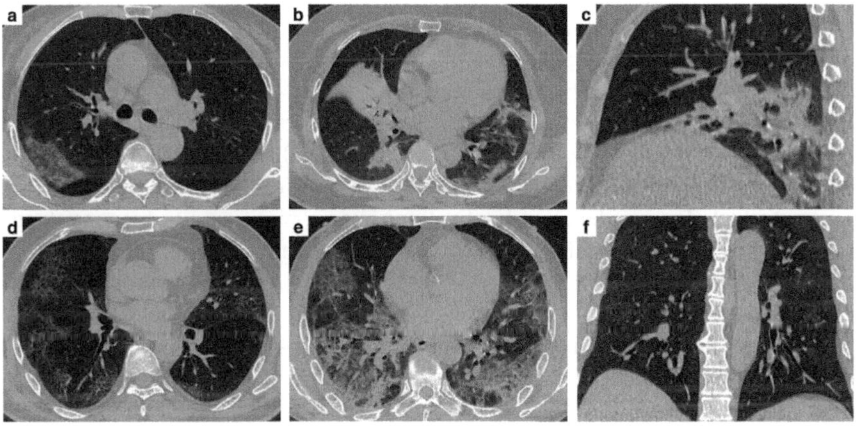

Fig. 3.4 Representative chest CT images of patients with COVID-19 pneumonia. **a** Subpleural patchy areas of GGO with crazy-paving sign in the right middle lobe. **b** Multiple patchy areas of consolidation in the right middle lobe, left upper lobe, and bilateral lower lobes and air bronchogram in the right middle lobe. **c** Multiple patchy areas of organizing pneumonia in the right middle and lower lobes on the sagittal image with CT severity score of 9 for the right lung. **d** Bilateral and peripheral multiple patchy areas of GGO with reticular and intralobular septal thickening. **e** Multiple mixed distributed pure GGO, GGO with consolidation, and interlobular septal thickening in bilateral lungs. **f** Bilateral multiple patchy and thin areas of GGO in the posterior parts of the lungs. *Source* Figure 2. Feng, Z., Yu, Q., Yao, S., Luo, L., Zhou, W., Mao, X., Li, J., Duan, J., Yan, Z., Yang, M. and Tan, H., 2020. Early prediction of disease progression in COVID-19 pneumonia patients with chest CT and clinical characteristics. Nature communications, 11(1), pp. 1–9. https://www.nature.com/articles/s41467-020-18786-x. By Springer Nature Group

radiological lesions, the ground-glass opacification 71% (136) appeared more common than the lesions appearing as consolidation 59% (112). Furthermore, the occurrence of these lesions was more common in the survivors versus the non-survivors [7]. In another retrospective study of CoViD19 patients hospitalized with pneumonia, all 138 patients had bilateral pulmonary infiltrates as patchy shadows or ground-glass opacity [11]. Several CoViD19 studies report a relationship between the appearance of the radiological findings and patients' age. In patients, less than 50 years of age, ground-glass opacification (GGO) was present in 77% of the patients, versus 55% of patients above age 50 years. The consolidative opacities were present in 23% of patients age less than 50 years versus 45% above, $p < 0.001$ [40].

In patients with CoViD19, a bilateral spread of the radiological disease appears to be a common feature among severely ill patients and the non-survivors. In a single-center retrospective cohort of 99 patients admitted with CoViD19, 75% (74) patients showed bilateral pneumonia, 14 (14%) patients showed multiple mottling and ground-glass opacity, and one (1%) patient had a pneumothorax [38]. Furthermore, in another retrospective study of 799 patients admitted with CoViD19, data of 113 deceased and 161 were analyzed. The study showed bilateral involvement on the chest radiographs in 100% (113) of the deceased patients versus 94% of (152) of the survivors. In this study bilateral ground-glass opacity and subsegmental areas of consolidation were found on the chest computed tomography of the deceased patients on admission that rapidly extended as bilateral high-density mass shadows [26]. Another retrospective study of 417 patients admitted with CoViD19 showed a higher incidence of bilateral versus unilateral pneumonia, 70.7% (295/417) versus 17.3% (72/417), in the overall cohort. The patients were divided into two groups according to the severity of the disease, mild-moderate, and severe-critical. The incidence of bilateral pneumonia was found to be consistently higher in the severe-critical group when compared with unilateral pneumonia i.e. mild-moderate bilateral pneumonia 64.9% (211/417) versus mild-moderate unilateral pneumonia 20.6% (67/417) and sever-critical cases bilateral pneumonia 91.3% (84/417) versus severe-critical unilateral pneumonia 5.43% (5). These values were statistically significant ≤ 0.001 [41]. Moreover, a systemic review of 919 patients from 30 studies of CoViD19 patients, reported that bilateral and multifocal involvement with a peripheral or posterior distribution (or both), were most commonly found among the CoViD19 patients. The bilateral and multi-lobar involvement and subsegmental consolidative opacities were the signs of the severity of the disease [42].

In summary, the CoViD19 may present with a variety of radiological appearances at different stages of the disease. Although the absence of a respiratory infection is a feature of the milder cases, the possibility of the subtle presence of the radiological abnormalities warrants early imaging in patients with CoViD19.The radiological findings of the ARDS appear to be a marker of the critical stage of the disease in most of the studies and show a similar pattern of the radiological features in CoViD19. Although the markers of the advanced disease, such as ground-glass opacification and consolidation, are the most common radiological findings, a bilateral extension of the disease appears to be a hallmark of the critical stage of CoViD19. The evolution of the disease severity may be recognized, by a progressive increase in the number and size of the lesions in multifocal consolidation, fibrotic transformation with septal thickening, and the development of a crazy-paving pattern. Attempts have been made to develop predictive models and scoring systems, based on the clinical and CT imaging features of the CoViD19 patients [43, 44], however require a cautious approach [45].

Most studies in patients with complicated CoViD19 appear to show that the radiological findings associated with the ARDS reflect a critical stage of the CoViD19, and exhibit a similar pattern of radiological features. The most common radiological findings that mark advanced disease, are ground-glass opacification and consolidation. The bilateral extension of the disease appears to be another hallmark of the critical stage of the disease in patients with CoViD19. Similarly, several dynamics of the radiological features may indicate the evolution of CoViD19 severity. These include a progressive increase in size and the number of the lesions in multifocal consolidation, fibrotic conversion reflected by septal thickening, and the appearance of a crazy-paving pattern. The presence of a radiological disease in asymptomatic patients with CoViD19 may present a risk to the patient and a challenge to the treating healthcare professionals. The asymptomatic form of the disease may have significant implications in the management of the disease at a larger scale, especially in the spread of the disease in the community (Tables 3.5 and 3.6).

3.5 Summary

In the early phase of the pandemic, rapid and effective recognition of the clinical and diagnostic characteristics of CoViD19 emerged as the main challenge to clinicians and scientists worldwide. Multiple well-conducted studies around the globe that investigated the novel coronavirus disease have helped to describe the clinical and biochemical characteristics of the disease. The evidence base has further grown, and the national and international expert societies and the leading public health organizations have recognized and endorsed several findings from the literature. Several coordinated efforts of the expert groups have facilitated the development of a consensus and publication of practical recommendations in protocols and guidelines to help the healthcare professionals effectively diagnose, manage, and treat patients with CoViD19.

The CoViD19 may present in an asymptomatic form or may manifest in the mild, moderate, severe, or critical forms with several clinical complications such as sepsis, shock, multi-organ failure, and death. In CoViD19, the lungs appear to be the core of the disease, and the cardiovascular system is commonly affected. The radiological form of lung disease is usually a hallmark of the critical stage in CoViD19 patients. The blood markers reflecting inflammatory, immunological, and prothrombotic complications of the CoViD19 may help in recognizing the disease's

Table 3.5 Radiological chest CT features of CoViD19

Common features[a]	Less common features[a]	Typical features[b]	Intermediate features[b]	Atypical features[b]
GGO with or without consolidative abnormalities, consistent with viral pneumonia Chest CT abnormalities in COVID-19 are often bilateral, have a peripheral distribution, and involve the lower lobes	Crazy paving pattern (GGO with superimposed septal thickening), bronchiectasis, pleural effusion, pericardial effusion, and lymphadenopathy	Peripheral, bilateral GGO or Multifocal GGO of round morphology (with or without consolidation, or visible intralobular lines or "crazy- paving pattern")[b] Reverse halo sign or other findings of organizing pneumonia (observed later in the disease)	Absence of typical features, AND Presence of: Multifocal, diffuse, perihilar or unilateral GGO with or without consolidation lacking a specific distribution, and are non-rounded or non-peripheral Few and very small GGO with non-rounded or non-peripheral distribution	Absence of typical or intermediate features AND Presence of: Isolated lobar or segmental consolidation without GGO Discrete small nodules (centrilobular, "tree-in-bud") Lung cavitation Smooth interlobular septal thickening with pleural effusion

COVID-19: coronavirus disease 2019; CT: computed tomography; GGO: ground-glass opacity; RT-PCR: reverse transcription polymerase chain reaction

Associated CT findings for each category are based upon available literature at the time of writing in March 2020, noting the retrospective nature of many reports, including biases related to patient selection in cohort studies, examination timing, and other potential confounders

CT is not a substitute for RT-PCR, consider testing according to local recommendations and procedures for and availability of RT-PCR

[a] COVID-19: Clinical features Author: Kenneth McIntosh, Section Editor: Martin S Hirsch, Deputy Editor: Allyson Bloom. Available at: https://www.uptodate.com/contents/covid-19-clinical-features?topicRef=126981&source=related_link#H2249070035. Accessed on June 28–2021. Last updated on Jun 10, 2021. ©2021 UpToDate, Inc. All rights reserved. UpToDate Terms of Use: https://www.uptodate.com/legal/terms-of-use

[b] *Source* Simpson, S., Kay, F.U., Abbara, S., Bhalla, S., Chung, J.H., Chung, M., Henry, T.S., Kanne, J.P., Kligerman, S., Ko, J.P. and Litt, H., 2020. Radiological society of north America expert consensus document on reporting chest CT findings related to COVID-19: endorsed by the society of thoracic Radiology, the American college of Radiology, and RSNA. Radiology: Cardiothoracic Imaging, 2(2), p. e200152. © 2021 Radiological Society of North America. Radiological Society of North America, Inc. https://www.rsna.org/about/rsna-terms-of-use?_ga=2.262979020.1392014871.1624878128-864326882.1617991897. (RSNA), 820 Jorie Boulevard Suite 200, Oak Brook, IL 60523-2251. Available at: https://pubs.rsna.org/doi/10.1148/ryct.2020200152 (Accessed on June 28, 2021). Reproduced under the terms of the Creative Commons Attribution License

Table 3.6 Radiological features and CoViD19 severity

Early stage	Late stage	Indicators of severity of disease	Indicators of poor prognosis
Bilateral ground glass opacities, with a predominantly peripheral, subpleural location	Crazy paving and organizing pneumonia pattern	Intralobular reticulations can be seen superimposed on the ground glass opacities, resulting in a crazy-paving pattern	Extensive consolidation

Source Revel, M.P., Parkar, A.P., Prosch, H., Silva, M., Sverzellati, N., Gleeson, F. and Brady, A., 2020. COVID-19 patients and the Radiology department–advice from the European Society of Radiology (ESR) and the European Society of Thoracic Imaging (ESTI). European radiology, 30 (9), pp. 4903–4909. © 2021 Springer Nature Switzerland AG. Part of Springer Nature. https://link.springer.com/article/10.1007/s00330-020-06865-y. Accessed on June 28, 2021

evolution and severity. In addition to the biochemical indicators of the systemic SARS CoV2 infection, such as elevated serum markers of inflammation including CRP (C reactive protein), ESR (erythrocyte sedimentation rate), LDH (lactate dehydrogenase), or ferritin levels, the decline in the immune cells marked by lymphopenia or development of thrombocytopenia may predict a poor outcome. The raised immune markers of CoViD19 such as cytokines, and the indicators of the abnormal coagulation, such as raised D Dimer levels or a prolonged prothrombin time, showcase the inflammatory and thrombotic burden of CoViD19, respectively. An increase in the BUN (blood urea nitrogen), creatinine or the liver enzymes, or elevated serum troponin levels, or serum natriuretic peptides in patients with severe CoViD19, reflects the involvement of the kidneys, liver, or the heart, respectively. The radiological markers of the severe CoViD19 include the presence of bilateral pulmonary shadowing, ground-glass opacification, and consolidation on lung imaging such as computed tomography. Tthe SARS CoV2 viral detection methods, such as the RT PCR, should be used to detect the virus in the symptomatic patients or the asymptomatic individuals who have been in contact with a confirmed or suspected CoViD19 patient, and nasopharyngeal, nasal (anterior or mid turbinate), or perhaps the oropharyngeal specimens should be used. For futher reading readers are advised to refer to the guidelines [19–21] for the specific set of recommendations related to diagnosing CoViD19.

The diagnostic techniques in CoViD19 are further evolving to help provide rapid and efficient testing methods. The reverse transcriptase-polymerase chain reaction (RT PCR, a Nucleic Acid Amplification Test (NAAT)) is a gold-standard method for diagnosing CoViD19 and detects the viral RNA. The antigen testing for the SARS COV2 has also received the EUA (Emergency Use Authorization) from the Food and Drug Administration [46]. The role of the antibodies in diagnosing acute CoViD19, however, remains limited. The specific SARS CoV2 antibodies testing has low sensitivity but may help to detect a recent viral disease. Furthermore, the usefulness of the serum antibody levels as a marker for future CoViD19 disease protection requires a more comprehensive understanding.

The CoViD19 patients may have an inappropriate immune response and increased production of the cytokines. Measuring markers of immunity and the cytokine response may help guide the treatment of CoViD19 patients in clinical practice. Detecting the disease early in asymptomatic individuals through prompt recognition of the chief blood and radiological markers of the disease may be life-saving, particularly in the high-risk population groups such as diabetics, cardiac or immunocompromised patients. Efficient diagnostic strategies may help reduce the burden of severe CoViD19 and associated complications. However, further understanding of the immune mechanisms in CoViD19, rapid diagnostic methods, identification of markers of severity of the disease is needed to help identify early the patients at risk. Such measures can also help the development of effective short and long-term risk stratification methods and tools in the management of CoViD19 patients. Further efforts are underway to overcome these challenges faced by healthcare professionals in managing CoViD19 globally.

Summary Box

- About 80% of patients contracting SARS CoV2 remain asymptomatic, about 15% develop the viral disease, and 3 to 5% of patients develop complications.
- The incubation period of the SARS CoV2 is 12 to 16 days.
- Important common clinical symptoms include headaches, olfactive and gustatory dysfunction, fever, dry cough, muscle pains, and fatigue.
- Features of the critical CoViD19 include sepsis, shock with multi-organ failure involving kidneys, liver, heart, and brain in addition to lungs.
- The Nuclear Acid Amplification Testing method, the RT PCR is the gold standard for the detection of SARS CoV2.
- Prominent blood features of the CoViD19 include leukocytosis, lymphopenia, thrombocytopenia, and increased CRP, ferritin, LDH, and markers of abnormal coagulation
- Viral immune and pro-inflammatory responses lead to lymphopenia and cytokine storm.
- The cytokine storm in the severe case is manifested by elevated IL-1β, IL-2, IL-6, IL-7, IL-8, IL-10, granulocyte-colony stimulating factor (G-CSF), granulocyte macrophage-colony stimulating factor (GM-CSF), interferon-inducible protein-10 (IP10), monocyte chemotactic protein 1 (MCP1), macrophage inflammation protein-1α, IFN-γ, and TNF-α.
- The radiological features of the critical disease include ground glass shadowing, consolidation, and bilateral shadowing.

References

1. Guan WJ, Ni ZY, Hu Y, et al. Clinical characteristics of coronavirus disease 2019 in China N Engl J Med. 2020. Published online Feb 28. https://doi.org/10.1056/NEJMoa2002032.
2. Li Q, et al. Early transmission dynamics in Wuhan, China, of novel coronavirus–infected pneumonia. New Engl J Med. 2020.
3. Wu Z, Mc Googan JM. Characteristics of and important lessons from the coronavirus disease 2019 (COVID-19) outbreak in China: summary of a report of 72314 cases from the Chinese Center for Disease Control and Prevention. JAMA: Published; 2020.
4. Kronbichler A, et al. Asymptomatic patients as a source of COVID-19 infections: a systematic review and meta-analysis. Int J Infect Dis. 2020;98:180–6.
5. He X, et al. Temporal dynamics in viral shedding and transmissibility of COVID-19. Nat Med. 2020;26(5):672–5.
6. Zumla A, Chan JF, Azhar EI, Hui DS, Yuen KY. Coronaviruses—drug discovery and therapeutic options. Nat Rev Drug Discov. 2016;15(5):327–47.
7. Zhou F, Yu T, Du R. Clinical course and risk factors for mortality of adult inpatients with COVID-19 in Wuhan, China: a retrospective cohort study. Lancet. 2020.
8. Spinato G, Fabbris C, Polesel J, Cazzador D, Borsetto D, Hopkins C. Alterations in smell or taste in mildly symptomatic outpatients with SARS-CoV-2 infection. JAMA. 2020;323(20):2089–90.
9. Levy MM, et al. 2001 SCCM/ESICM/ACCP/ATS/SIS international sepsis definitions conference. Crit Care Med. 2003;31:1250–6.
10. Clinical characteristics of 113 deceased patients with coronavirus disease,. retrospective study. BMJ. 2019;2020:368. https://doi.org/10.1136/bmj.m1091 (Published 26 March 2020).
11. Wang D, Hu B, Hu C, Zhu F, Liu X, Zhang J, Wang B, Xiang H, Cheng Z, Xiong Y, Zhao Y, Li Y, Wang X, Peng Z. Clinical characteristics of 138 hospitalized patients with 2019 novel coronavirus-infected pneumonia in Wuhan, China. JAMA. 2020. https://doi.org/10.1001/jama.2020.1585. [Epub ahead of print] PubMed PMID: 32031570; PubMed Central PMCID: PMC7042881.
12. Zhang W, Du RH, Li B, et al. Molecular and serological investigation of 2019-nCoV infected patients: implication of multiple shedding routes. Emerg Microbes Infect. 2020;9(1):386–9. https://doi.org/10.1080/22221751.2020.1729071. PubMed Google Scholar Crossref.
13. Pan Y, Zhang D, Yang P, Poon LLM, Wang Q. Viral load of SARS-CoV-2 in clinical samples. Lancet Infect Dis. 2020;20(4):411–2. Published online February 24, 2020. https://doi.org/10.1016/S1473-3099(20)30113-4. PubMed Google Scholar.
14. Gao QY, Chen YX, Fang JY. 2019 novel coronavirus infection and gastrointestinal tract. J Dig Dis. 2020;21:125–6. https://doi.org/10.1111/751-2980.12851.
15. Xiao F, Tang M, Zheng X, et al. Evidence for gastrointestinal infection of SARS-CoV-2. medRxiv 2020. https://doi.org/10.1053/j.gastro.2020.02.055.
16. Wang W, et al. Detection of SARS-CoV-2 in different types of clinical specimens. JAMA. 2020;323(18):1843–4.
17. Bwire GM, et al. Detection profile of SARS-CoV-2 using RT-PCR in different types of clinical specimens: a systematic review and meta-analysis. J Med Virol. 2020.
18. Yu F, et al. Quantitative detection and viral load analysis of SARS-CoV-2 in infected patients. Clin Infect Dis. 2020.
19. Diagnostic testing for SARS-CoV-2, Interim Guidance, 11 September 2020 World Health Organisation. https://www.who.int/publications/i/item/diagnostic-testing-for-sars-cov-2. Accessed on 17 November 2020.
20. NIH CoViD19 treatment guidelines. Testing for SARS-CoV-2 Infection. Last Updated: November 3, 2020. https://www.covid19treatmentguidelines.nih.gov/overview/sars-cov-2-testing/. Accessed on December 11, 2020.
21. Hanson KE, et al. Infectious diseases society of America guidelines on the diagnosis of COVID-19. Clin Infect Dis. 2020.

22. Infectious Diseases Society of America Guidelines on the Diagnosis of COVID-19 Published by IDSA, 5/6/2020. Accessed December 11, 2020.
23. https://www.idsociety.org/covid-19-real-time-learning-network/diagnostics/antibody-testing/. Accessed December 11, 2020.
24. https://www.cdc.gov/coronavirus/2019-ncov/lab/serology-testing.html.
25. https://www.fda.gov/medical-devices/letters-health-care-providers/important-information-use-serological-antibody-tests-covid-19-letter-health-care-providers.
26. Chen T, Wu D, Chen H, Yan W, Yang D, Chen G, Ma K, Xu D, Yu H, Wang H, Wang T, Guo W, Chen J, Ding C, Zhang X, Huang J, Han M, Li S, Luo X, Zhao J, Ning Q. Clinical characteristics of 113 deceased patients with coronavirus disease 2019: retrospective study. BMJ. 2020;26(368):m1091. https://doi.org/10.1136/bmj.m1091. Erratum. In: BMJ. 2020 Mar 31;368:m1295. PubMed PMID: 32217556.
27. Tang N, Li D, Wang X, Sun Z. Abnormal coagulation parameters are associated with poor prognosis in patients with novel coronavirus pneumonia. J Thromb Haemost. 2020;18 (4):844–7. https://doi.org/10.1111/jth.14768.
28. Singer M, Deutschman CS, Seymour CW, Shankar-Hari M, Annane D, Bauer M, Bellomo R, Bernard GR, Chiche JD, Coopersmith CM, Hotchkiss RS, Levy MM, Marshall JC, Martin GS, Opal SM, Rubenfeld GD, van der Poll T, Vincent JL, Angus DC. The third international consensus definitions for sepsis and septic shock (Sepsis-3). JAMA. 2016;315 (8):801–10.
29. Seymour CW, Kennedy JN, Wang S, Chang CH, Elliott CF, Xu Z, Berry S, Clermont G, Cooper G, Gomez H, Huang DT, Kellum JA, Mi Q, Opal SM, Talisa V, van der Poll T, Visweswaran S, Vodovotz Y, Weiss JC, Yealy DM, Yende S, Angus DC. Derivation, validation, and potential treatment implications of novel clinical phenotypes for sepsis. JAMA. 2019;321(20):2003–17. [PMC free article: PMC6537818] [PubMed: 31104070].
30. Wang X, Xu W, Hu G, Xia S, Sun Z, Liu Z. SARS-CoV-2 infects T lymphocytes through its spike protein-mediated membrane fusion. Cell Mol Immunol. 2020;17(8):894.
31. Moore BJB, June CH. Cytokine release syndrome in severe COVID-19. Science. 2020;368 (490):473–4. And 113 BMJ study.
32. Ozsurekci Y, Aykac K, Er AG, Halacli B, Arasli M, Oygar PD, Gürlevik S, Cura Yayla BC, Karakaya J, Alp A, Topeli A. Predictive value of cytokine/chemokine responses for the disease severity and management in children and adult cases with COVID-19. J Med Virol. 2021;93(5):2828–37.
33. Luo Y, Mao L, Yuan X, Xue Y, Lin Q, Tang G, Song H, Wang F, Sun Z. Prediction model based on the combination of cytokines and lymphocyte subsets for prognosis of SARS-CoV-2 infection. J Clin Immunol. 2020;40(7):960–9.
34. Cabaro S, D'Esposito V, Di Matola T, Sale S, Cennamo M, Terracciano D, Parisi V, Portella G, Beguinot F, Atripaldi L, Sansone M. Cytokine signature and COVID-19 prediction models in the two waves of pandemics. 2021.
35. Qin C, Zhou L, Hu Z, Zhang S, Yang S, Tao Y, Xie C, et al. Dysregulation of immune response in patients with COVID-19 in Wuhan, China. Clin Infect Dis. 2020.
36. Liu J, Li S, Liu J, Liang B, Wang X, Wang H, Li W, et al. Longitudinal characteristics of lymphocyte responses and cytokine profiles in the peripheral blood of SARS-CoV-2 infected patients. EBioMed. 2020:102763.
37. Huang C, Wang Y, Li X, Ren L, Zhao J, Hu Y, Zhang L, et al. Clinical features of patients infected with 2019 novel coronavirus in Wuhan, China. The Lancet. 2020;395(10223):497–506.
38. Chen N, Zhou M, Dong X, Qu J, Gong F, Han Y, Qiu Y, et al. Epidemiological and clinical characteristics of 99 cases of 2019 novel coronavirus pneumonia in Wuhan, China: a descriptive study. The Lancet. 2020;395(10223):507–13.
39. Shi H, Han X, Jiang N, et al. Radiological findings from 81 patients with COVID-19 pneumonia in Wuhan, China: a descriptive study. Lancet Infect Dis. 2020;S1473–3099 (20):30086–3008.

40. Song F, Shi N, Shan F, et al. Emerging coronavirus 2019-nCoV pneumonia. Radiology. 2020 Feb 6 [Epub ahead of print].
41. Chen C, Wang H, Liang Z, et al. Predicting illness severity and short-term outcomes of COVID-19: a retrospective cohort study in China. 2020;1(1):100007. https://doi.org/10.1016/j.xinn.2020.04.007.
42. Salehi S, Abedi A, Balakrishnan S, Gholamrezanezhad A. Coronavirus disease 2019 (COVID-19): a systematic review of imaging findings in 919 patients [published online ahead of print, 2020 Mar 14]. AJR Am J Roentgenol. 2020:1–7. https://doi.org/10.2214/AJR.20.23034.
43. Qin L, et al. A predictive model and scoring system combining clinical and CT characteristics for the diagnosis of COVID-19. Eur Radiol. 2020;30(12):6797–807.
44. Francone M, et al. Chest CT score in COVID-19 patients: correlation with disease severity and short-term prognosis. Eur Radiol. 2020;30(12):6808–17.
45. Wynants L, et al. Prediction models for diagnosis and prognosis of covid-19: systematic review and critical appraisal. BMJ. 2020;369.
46. https://www.fda.gov/medical-devices/coronavirus-disease-2019-covid-19-emergency-use-authorizations-medical-devices/in-vitro-diagnostics-euas-antigen-diagnostic-tests-sars-cov-2#Individual%20EUAs. Accessed on December 16, 2021.

Chapter 4
The Pathological Features of CoViD19 Cardiovascular Complications

Key Questions

- What are the salient pathological features of CoViD19 complications?
- What are the key cardiovascular pathological features of CoViD19 complications?
- What is the histopathological evidence incriminating viral damage to the cardiac and vascular structures in CoViD19?
- What variations in the histopathological features may be observed in the myocardial injury in CoViD19?

4.1 Introduction

Several pathology reports, published in literature from autopsy series, and biopsies, have described morpho-pathological and histopathological characteristics of CoViD 19, linking pathogenetic mechanisms with the disease outcomes. The key morpho-pathological features from the autopsy of the deceased patients with CoViD 19 include organ damage, tissue destruction, and thrombotic disease. The lungs appear to be the focus of the core pathological findings in the complicated CoViD 19. Other organs, such as the heart, vasculature, liver, and kidneys, may also be affected in the advanced phase of the disease. In addition, the involvement of other organs and systems, such as the spleen, liver, testicles, blood, and others, had also been described in studies investigating CoViD19 pathology (Fig. 4.4). Reports of the gastro-intestinal tract involvement, with the presence of viral nucleocapsid membrane, and lymphocytic infiltration and interstitial edema, in the esophagus (excluding viral nucleocapsid membrane), stomach, duodenum, and rectum have been published [1].

U. Mallick, *Cardiovascular Complications of COVID-19*,
https://doi.org/10.1007/978-3-030-90065-6_4

Similarly, several reports describing renal implications of CoViD19 have been published. In these reports, a variety of COVID19 related pathology indicating the involvement of renal tubular, vascular, and glomerular structures with histopathological changes including, the cellular organellar abnormalities involving mitochondria, and endoplasmic reticulum, have been described. Development of severe acute tubular necrosis with lymphocyte and macrophage infiltration, acute proximal tubular injury, peritubular erythrocyte aggregation, and glomerular fibrin thrombi with ischemic collapse, among others, have been reported [2, 3]. Several mechanisms, such as virus-mediated injury, cytokine storm, Ang II pathway activation, dysregulation of complement, hypercoagulation, and microangiopathy, have been implicated in this process. Studies have demonstrated the presence of SARS-CoV-2 nucleocapsid protein in renal tubular structures [2] and virus-like particles in podocytes and renal tubular epithelial cells [3].

Acute Respiratory Distress Syndrome (ARDS) is an important feature of the complicated CoViD19 in the critical phase. The typical pulmonary findings in the ARDS include diffuse alveolar damage (DAD), characterized by hyaline membrane formation in the alveoli, in the acute stage (intra-alveolar proteinosis), and interstitial widening by edema and fibroblast proliferation with fibrin deposition in the organizing stage (Fig. 4.3). These processes accompany viral cytopathic change and immune cell infiltration, including lymphocytes. In a pathology report of three CoViD 19 deceased patients, lungs exhibited the core pathology of the disease. The pathological features in the lungs included alveolar exudative inflammation and interstitial inflammation, alveolar epithelium proliferation, and hyaline membrane formation [4].

The pathological features of cardiovascular involvement of patients with complicated CoViD 19 confirm the presence of macro and microvascular disease, with an emphasis on the pulmonary and coronary vascular territories. Data also suggest the involvement of other cardiac structures including the myocardium, pericardium, electrical conduction system that may result in a cardiovascular compromise in critical CoViD19 patients. The immunohistochemical and virology data reveal patterns of the myocardial injury observed in CoViD 19, indicating a variety of mechanisms and features such as involvement of cardiomyocyte and the interstitial tissue with edema, and presence of cytopathic acute inflammatory cells in the interstitial and perivascular tissue.

In this chapter, we provide an overview of the pathophysiological features associated with critical CoViD19 related cardiovascular complications such as myocardial injury, vascular injury, and thromboembolism and illustrate the associated histopathological evidence. We describe CoViD19 related histopathological abnormalities, frequently observed in a range of cardiovascular structures such as myocardial tissue, microvasculature, endothelial cells, and the coagulation system that may precipitate in the development of these complications.

4.2 Key Features of Cardiovascular Pathology

4.2.1 The Myocardial Injury in CoViD19

The pathological changes associated with complications of CoViD19 involving myocardium have been highlighted in several studies. Various patterns of myocardial involvement associated with CoViD19 may translate into different clinical forms of cardiac complications such as heart failure, arrhythmias, thromboembolism, or death. However, defining myocardial injury in CoViD19 patients may be a challenge and inconsistencies may lead to suboptimal conclusions (Table 4.1).

The myocardial injury may be reflected by myocarditis due to immune or inflammatory mechanisms or viral injury and may involve various cardiac structures. A variety of forms of myocarditis have been reported in patients with complicated CoViD19. An autopsy series of 21 CoViD19 patients reported an increased interstitial macrophage infiltration in 18 (86%) of the cases and showed the presence of lymphocytic myocarditis in 3 (14%) of the cases, mild pericarditis in 4 cases, and acute myocardial injury in the right ventricle in 4 cases. The authors concluded that the majority of CoViD19 cases had increased interstitial macrophage infiltration, and a variety of forms of myocarditis were present including, multifocal lymphocytic myocarditis and other forms of myocardial injury [5].

According to the data from a pathology report of three CoViD 19 deceased patients, the cardiac pathological features included cardiomyocyte hypertrophy, partial cardiomyocyte degeneration, necrosis, mild interstitial congestion, edema, and a small amount of lymphocytic, monocytic, and neutrophil immersion. In the myocardial tissue, the inflammatory cells were mainly macrophages and a small number of CD4-positive T-cells. The CD8-positive T-cells, CD20-positive-B cells, or virus components could not be detected [4].

In a report on the cardiopulmonary findings in a series of autopsies of four patients with CoViD 19, the pulmonary findings included diffuse alveolar damage

Table 4.1 Factors impacting the diagnosis of myocarditis[a] in CoViD19

Issues
• Severity stage of CoViD19
• Heterogeneity of CoViD19 symptoms
• Variabilities in ECG
• Frequent elevation in troponin and markers of inflammation
• Difficulties in obtaining cardiac and coronary imaging
• Superimposed cardiac and other pathologies

[a] Diagnostic criteria for myocarditis [33] is based on clinical presentation with features of ECG/Holter/stress test modifications, elevated myocardiocytolysis markers (TnT/TnI), functional and structural abnormalities on cardiac imaging (echo/angio/CMR), and abnormal features on tissue characterization by CMR such as edema and/or LGE of classical myocarditic pattern as per ESC guidelines, and features of myocardial inflammation (coexistence of T1 and T2-related criteria) [34] and exclusion of obstructive coronary artery disease

(DAD), with a mild to moderate mononuclear response consisting of notable CD4+ aggregates around thrombosed small vessels, and significantly associated hemorrhage. The authors suggested the involvement of thrombotic microangiopathy as a pathogenetic mechanism. The cardiac findings included the presence of right ventricular dilatation in a patient showing scattered myocyte degeneration, possibly related to both maladaptive cytokine pathways and platelet response, or capillary endothelial cell/microvascular dysfunction possible cause of individual cell necrosis. A typical pattern of viral myocarditis was not diagnosed in the absence of significant brisk lymphocytic inflammatory infiltrate [6].

The autopsy report of 23 CoViD 19 patients from 5 centers in the United States of America revealed the presence of major pulmonary thrombo-emboli with pulmonary infarcts and or hemorrhage in 5 of the 23 patients. The multifocal acute injury of the cardiac myocytes was a commonly observed cardiac lesion. In this series, one case confirmed the presence of lymphocytic myocarditis. In addition to the major pulmonary pathology, three cases had lymphocytic pericarditis together with the features of multifocal acute injury of the cardiomyocytes, without the inflammatory cellular infiltrates. These patients had significantly raised body mass index (BMI) and evidence of a chronic cardiac enlargement (BMIs of 33.8, 51.65, and 35.2 kg/m^2) [7].

4.2.2 *Endomyocardial Biopsy and Myocarditis*

Several autopsy series or case reports of patients with CoViD19 provide data from the endomyocardial biopsies giving evidence of pathological indicators of myocardial involvement associated with various forms of myocarditis implicating various mechanisms [5, 8, 9] (Table 4.2).

Table 4.2 Variabilities in the features of cardiac histology in CoViD19 studies

- Cardiac lymphocytic infiltrates, interstitial edema and limited foci of necrosis [21]
- Lymphocytic myocarditis [7, 25] with SARS CoV2 RNA particles [35]
- Eosinophilic myocarditis [36]
- Diffuse vasculitis [31] or inflammatory process impacting vascular wall with small arterial obliteration and damage [37]
- Individual myocardial cell necrosis without lymphocytic myocarditis [6]
- Interstitial macrophage infiltration in the myocardium without myocyte injury [5]
- Low-grade interstitial and endocardial inflammation and
- Virus particles in cardiac macrophages without involving cardiomyocytes and endothelia, or signs of myocardial necrosis [22]
- Myocardial presence of SARS-CoV-2 in interstitial cells or macrophages invading the myocardial tissue [38]

Although several studies demonstrate the involvement of the myocardium in CoViD 19 patients [10–12], the use of endomyocardial biopsy with pathological data linking SARS CoV2 and myocardial disease in diagnosing CoViD19 myocardial disease is limited [13] or may have inconsistencies, raising doubts about the actual incidence of myocarditis in CoViD19 [14, 15]. Limited use of the endomyocardial biopsy, a gold standard, may be due to the associated risks related to the invasive nature of the investigation and infectiousness of CoViD19.

The CoViD19 may directly or indirectly affect the myocardium and other cardiac structures through inflammatory and immune-mediated mechanisms involving cytokines or direct viral involvement. The EMB may help to distinguish between the pathological patterns associated with CoViD19 related myocardial injuries. A case study reporting evidence of SARS CoV2 mediated systemic inflammation affecting the myocardium confirmed a diagnosis of acute lympho-plasmo-histiocytic myocarditis. The endomyocardial biopsy report indicated the presence of interstitial edema, small foci of necrosis, interstitial and perivascular infiltrates composed of CD138+ CD79a+ CD20− plasmocytes, CD3+ CD8+ T-lymphocytes (7 cells/mm^2), few neutrophils, and a dense and diffuse infiltration by CD163+ macrophages [8].

The endomyocardial biopsy reports from series of CoViD 19 cases provide evidence of the development of heart failure or sudden death as a result of the involvement of the vessel walls and the electrical conduction system. The findings from the case series of the cardiac autopsies of 9 patients with myopericarditis related to the CoViD19, showed cardiogenic shock and sudden death as the main causes of death [16]. In this series, pericardial effusion was found, in 6 out of 9 patients. The macroscopic cardiac findings showed an increase in weight and the absence of significant epicardial coronary artery disease. The cardiac histological examination demonstrated, presence of lympho-nuclear infiltrates (CD68, CD45, Ro positive), with areas of focal necrosis in the adjacent myocytes (in the myocardium and the pericardium) in all patients, and in the intramural vessels (with vessel wall necrosis) in 6 patients who had died of the heart failure.

The development of TakoTsumbo cardiomyopathy has been incriminated in the CoViD19 [17–20]. The endomyocardial biopsy (EMB) was performed on 43 years old female presenting with a reverse Tako-Tsubo syndrome, in a patient with SARS CoV2 respiratory infection, in Italy. On the CTA (Computed Tomographic Arteriography), dynamic 3D volume-rendering reconstruction demonstrated hypokinesia of the left ventricle mid and basal segments, with normal apical contraction, suggesting a reverse Tako-Tsubo syndrome (TTS) pattern. Subsequently, CMR (Cardiac Magnetic Resonance) (day 7) showed persistent mild hypokinesia at basal and mid-left ventricular segments and recovery of systolic function (from 52% by CTA to 64% by CMR). Diffuse myocardial edema, associated with wall pseudo-hypertrophy, was observed on the week myocardial sites. The findings on the EMB showed an acute inflammatory process with diffuse T-lymphocytic inflammatory infiltrates (CD3þ >7/mm^2), extensive interstitial edema, and limited foci of necrosis. The signs of replacement fibrosis, contraction band necrosis, or TTS-associated microvascular abnormalities were absent. The SARS-CoV-2 genome could not be detected within the myocardium. A final diagnosis of acute virus-negative lymphocytic myocarditis, associated with the SARS-CoV-2 respiratory infection, was confirmed [21].

4.2.3 Endomyocardial Biopsy and Myocarditis with Viral Localization

The virological techniques (viral genome analysis via quantitative PCR) and immuno-histological techniques may help determine the etiology of the myocardial injury using the EMB. Vaious patterns of myocardial invovement may be observed in CoViD19 exhibiting myocardial inflammation with or without SARS CoV2 viral localization, and myocardial inflammation may be observed with or without myocardial injury. A vareity of inflammatory cells including CD68+ macrophages (D–F), CD3+ lymphocytes (G–I) or others may be observed (Figs. 4.1 and 4.2).

The viral particles were observed in the interstitial cells, which demonstrated loss of the cytoplasmic membrane integrity. The myocytes and the endothelia had no viral particles. The cardiac myocytes showed non-specific features consisting of focal myofibrillar lysis or lipid droplets, without significant myocyte hypertrophy or nuclear changes. A minimal focal interstitial fibrosis was observed, mainly in the perivascular zones. Small intramural vessels were free from vasculitis and thrombosis [22].

In a series of post mortem examination of 12 fatal CoViD 19 patients, the SARS-CoV-2 RNA was detected in the cardiac tissue of a patient with lymphocytic myocarditis [23].

Several endomyocardial biopsy reports confirm the presence of SARS CoV2 mRNA in the heart. According to a report, endomyocardial biopsies revealed the presence of SARS CoV2 mRNA in the myocardium in patients with negative nasopharyngeal swabs for SARS CoV2 [24]. A positive genome SARS CoV2 was detected using the RT PCR assay. The authors suggested a subacute clinical course of the myocarditis related to the CoViD19. Another single-center autopsy study investigated deaths of the first 12 consecutive COVID19 positive patients and reported the detection of SARS CoV2 mRNA in the myocardium in 5 out of 12 COVID19 patients [25].

4.2.4 The Vascular Injury, Microvascular Cardiac Involvement, and Thromboembolic Features

The CoViD19 impacts microvasculature in multiple vascular territories including lungs, heart, kidneys, and others. Several mechanisms may be implicated in the development of CoViD19 related microvascular disease. Research has shown the presence of endothelial dysfunction involving a range of mechanisms such as

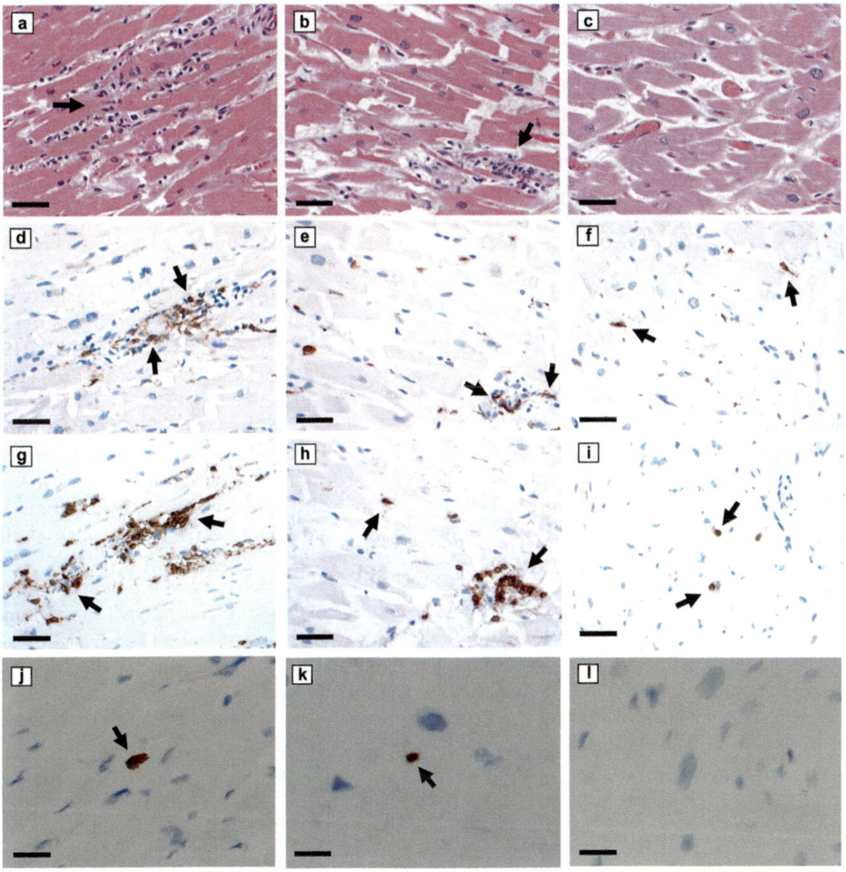

Fig. 4.1 Histology of the three pathologically defined patient groups. Depicted are histologic images of slides stained with H&E (**a–c**), immunohistochemistry for the macrophages marker CD68 (**d–f**), immunohistochemistry for the T-lymphocyte marker CD3 (**g–i**), and in situ hybridization for SARS-CoV-2 (**j–l**) for cases with myocarditis along with SARS-CoV-2+ cells in the myocardium (V+ M+, **a**, **d**, **g**, **j**), negative for myocarditis but with SARS-CoV-2+ cells in the myocardium (V+ M–, **b**, **e**, **h**, **k**), and negative for both myocarditis and myocardial SARS-CoV-2 + cells (V–M–, **c**, **f**, **i**, **l**). There is inflammation with myocardial injury (arrow) in the V+ M+ case (**a**) compared with inflammation (arrow) without injury in the V+ M– case (**b**). Arrows indicate CD68+ macrophages (**d–f**), CD3+ lymphocytes (**g–i**), and SARS-CoV-2+ cells (**j**, **k**). Scale bars represent 40 μm (**a–i**) and 80 μm (**j–l**). *Source* Figure 1. Bearse, M., Hung, Y.P., Krauson, A.J., Bonanno, L., Boyraz, B., Harris, C.K., Helland, T.L., Hilburn, C.F., Hutchison, B., Jobbagy, S. and Marshall, M.S., 2021. Factors associated with myocardial SARS-CoV-2 infection, myocarditis, and cardiac inflammation in patients with COVID-19. Modern Pathology, 34(7), pp. 1345–1357. Modern Pathology ISSN 1530-0285 (online). https://www.nature.com/articles/s41379-021-00790-1. By Springer Nature Group. Rightslink® by Copyright Clearance Center

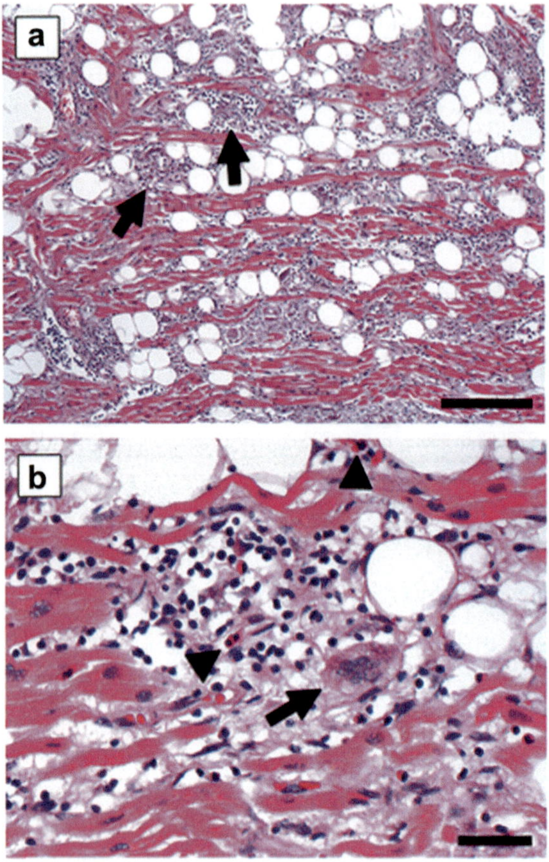

Fig. 4.2 Myocarditis with eosinophils and giant cells in a patient who died from COVID-19. *Source* Figure 3. Bearse, M., Hung, Y.P., Krauson, A.J., Bonanno, L., Boyraz, B., Harris, C.K., Helland, T.L., Hilburn, C.F., Hutchison, B., Jobbagy, S. and Marshall, M.S., 2021. Factors associated with myocardial SARS-CoV-2 infection, myocarditis, and cardiac inflammation in patients with COVID-19. Modern Pathology, 34(7), pp. 1345–1357. Modern Pathology ISSN 1530-0285 (online). https://www.nature.com/articles/s41379-021-00790-1. By Springer Nature Group. Rightslink® by Copyright Clearance Center

hyperinflammatory /immune response, oxidative stress, hypoxemic injury and others as well as vascular injury, coagulation abnormalities in patients with complicated CoViD19 [26–28]. The evidence of an underlying microvascular cardiac involvement in CoViD 19 patients with cardiovascular risk factors was shown in a case series of two patients. A 77 years old male subject with BMI 31.8 kg/m^2 and a history of hypertension had six days history of chills, fever, and shortness of breath and suffered a cardiac arrest. The post mortem examination showed microscopic evidence of acute cardiac ischemia and coronary atherosclerosis with a marked two-vessel disease. Coronary artery disease was identified as a contributory factor for death. The

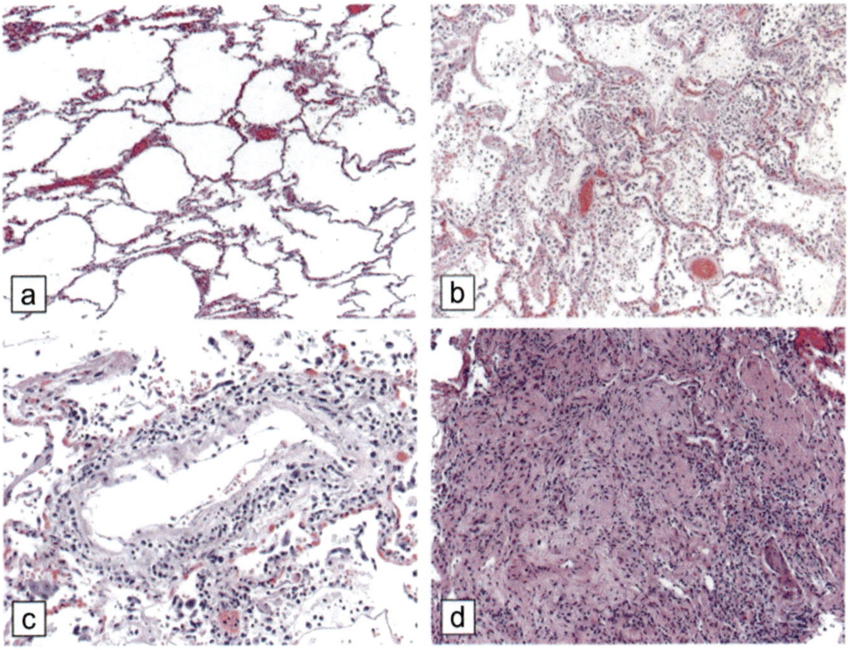

Fig. 4.3 Histopathologic findings of COVID-19 in the lung. **a** Normal lung with open alveoli and delicate alveolar septa containing thin capillaries lined by an attenuated alveolar epithelium (hematoxylin–eosin; original magnification × 200). **b** Acute diffuse alveolar damage (DAD) with hyaline membranes lining alveolar spaces, pneumocyte hyperplasia, desquamation of alveolar epithelial cells into the alveolar spaces, inflammatory infiltrates, and capillary congestion (hematoxylin–eosin; original magnification × 200). **c** Perivascular inflammation (hematoxylin–eosin; original magnification × 400). **d** Organizing pneumonia with granulation tissue plugs within the lumen of respiratory bronchioles (hematoxylin–eosin; original magnification × 200). *Source* Figure 1. Caramaschi, S., Kapp, M.E., Miller, S.E., Eisenberg, R., Johnson, J., Epperly, G., Maiorana, A., Silvestri, G. and Giannico, G.A., 2021. Histopathological findings and clinicopathologic correlation in COVID-19: a systematic review. Modern Pathology, pp. 1–20. https://www.nature.com/articles/s41379-021-00814-w. Rightslink® by Copyright Clearance Center

pulmonary pathology features included the classical characteristics of the DAD, with the presence of thrombi within a few small branches of the pulmonary artery [29].

The association of chronic coronary comorbidity with the fatality in CoViD 19 has been demonstrated in several autopsy studies. An autopsy report of 12 consecutive CoViD 19 deceased patients revealed a high incidence of thromboembolic events, suggesting an important role of coagulopathy in the CoViD19. Among these patients, coronary heart disease (50%) and asthma or chronic pulmonary obstructive disease (25%) were the most common chronic comorbidities. About 7 of 12 of the patients (58%) had a DVT (Deep Venous Thrombosis), whereas four patients had

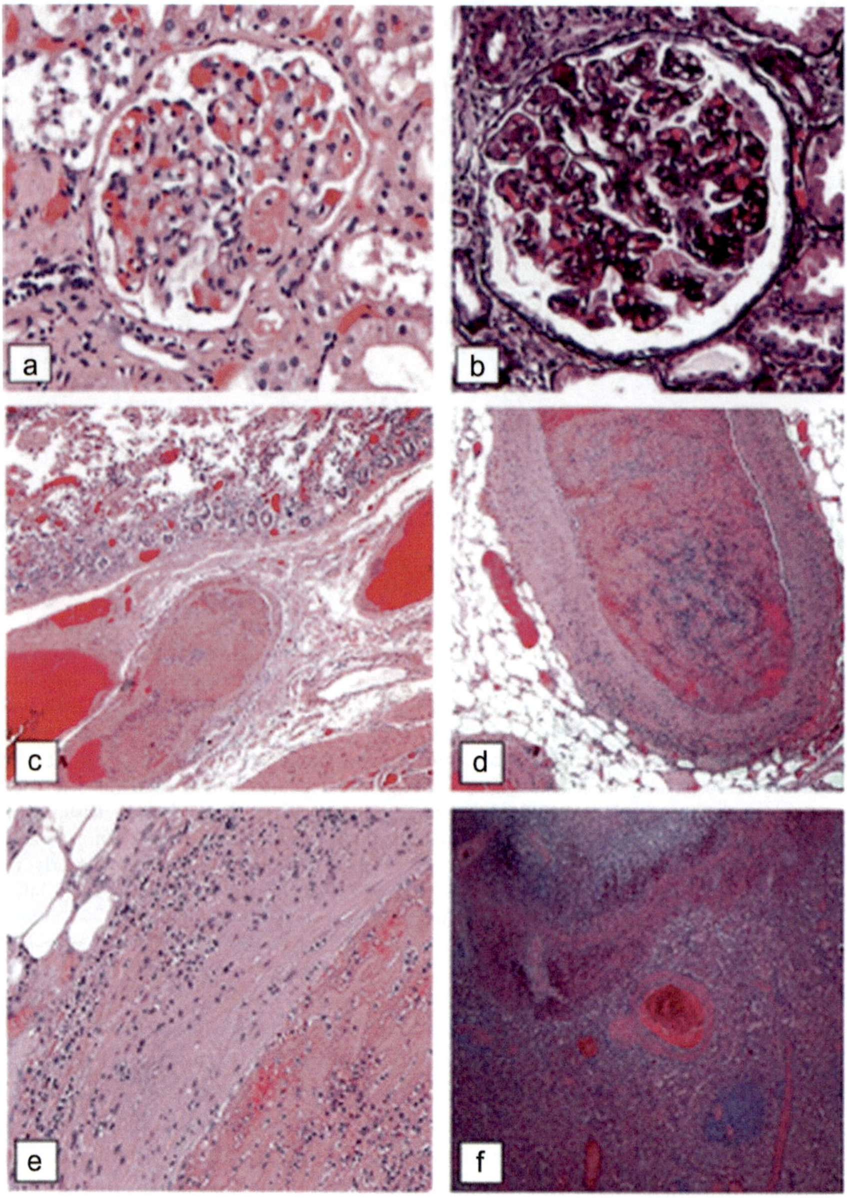
a
b
c
d
e
f

◂**Fig. 4.4** Histopathological features of multiple organs in CoViD19. Prinetd as Fig. 2: Histopathologic findings of COVID-19 in the kidney, small bowel and spleen. **a** Thrombotic microangiopathy with glomerular capillary loop and arteriole fibrin thrombi (hematoxylin–eosin; original magnification × 400). **b** Glomerulus with segmental capillary collapse and overlying podocyte hyperplasia (Jones methenamine silver; original magnification × 400). **c** Small bowel thrombus and mucosal ischemic changes (hematoxylin–eosin; original magnification × 100). **d** Spleen hilar thrombus (hematoxylin–eosin; original magnification × 200). **e** Detail of Fig. **d** with transmural vascular inflammation (hematoxylin–eosin; original magnification × 400). **f** Splenic thrombosis and infarct (hematoxylin–eosin; original magnification × 100). *Source* Figure 2. Caramaschi, S., Kapp, M.E., Miller, S.E., Eisenberg, R., Johnson, J., Epperly, G., Maiorana, A., Silvestri, G. and Giannico, G.A., 2021. Histopathological findings and clinico-pathologic correlation in COVID-19: a systematic review. Modern Pathology, pp. 1–20. https://www.nature.com/articles/s41379-021-00814-w. Rightslink® by Copyright Clearance Center

PE (Pulmonary Embolism), a direct cause of death. About eight 8 of 12 patients (67%) had histo-morphologically diffuse alveolar damage. In this study, about 6 of 10 patients had moderate viremia (<4 × 10/4 copies/mL), and all patients had high concentrations of SARS CoV2 RNA in the lungs. However, titers of the viral RNA in the liver, kidney, or heart, were higher in 5 of 12 patients, exceeding the viremia [25].

The autopsy report of 21 patients with CoViD19 showed the presence of vascular dysfunction. In this study, the presence of generalized thrombotic microangiopathy 3 of 21 (14%), pulmonary thrombotic microangiopathy 5 of 11 (45%), focal cardiomyocytes necrosis 3 of 21 (14%), myocardial hypertrophy 15 of 21 (71%), in addition to the senile amyloidosis 6 of 21 (29%), myocardial infarction 1 of 21 (5%), and the ulcerated plaques in the aorta (70%) of cases, were prominent histopathological findings. The pulmonary embolism, alveolar hemorrhage, and vasculitis were found, in 4 of 21 (19%), 3 of 21 (14%), and 1 of 21 (5%) patients, respectively. The study further showed the presence of cardiovascular risk factors, such as prior cardiovascular disease 15 of 21 (71%), hypertension 21 of 21 (100%), diabetes 7 of 21 (35%), and obesity, frequently among the patients in this study [30].

4.2.5 Endothelial Cell Infection and Apoptosis

The evidence of direct viral infection of the endothelial cell, and diffuse endothelial inflammation across vascular beds of different organs, was provided in a case series of two patients with CoViD19. The immunohistochemical and histological assessments revealed increased lymphocytes (CD3, LFA-1, and CD45R0), macrophages (Mac-1), and perforin-positive cytotoxic T cells, and absent cardiomyocyte necrosis. In a 71 years old male recipient of the renal transplant, known with hypertension and coronary artery disease, the endothelial cells showed the presence of viral inclusion structures. The examination further revealed an accumulation of the inflammatory cells as well as apoptotic bodies in the heart, small intestine, and lungs. The second case of a 58 years old diabetic, hypertensive, and obese patient with CoViD 19, developed significant cardiovascular complications such as right heart failure secondary to the ST-segment elevation myocardial infarction, leading to a fatal cardiac arrest. The post-mortem studies indicated lymphocytic endotheliitis in the lung, heart, kidney, and liver, as well as signs of liver cell necrosis. The histological examination showed an absence of lymphocytic myocarditis. The submucosal vessels in the small intestine showed evidence of endotheliitis [31]. Another series of post mortem examinations of 12 fatal CoViD 19 patients of older age and associated comorbidities confirmed the presence of viral particles in the kidneys in the tubular epithelium, endothelium, and podocytes without significant inflammation [23].

4.3 Summary

A large number of pathology reports, derived from biopsies or autopsy reports from individual cases or case series of patients with complications of CoViD19, have been published. The data demonstrate a systemic involvement of the disease that may affect various organs. However, the disease appears to have a major cardiovascular and pulmonary focus. The variations in the morphopathological forms, histology, and cytopathology may represent the evolutionary stages of the disease and the patterns of organ involvement.

The pathology reports of CoViD 19 patients with cardiovascular complications demonstrate the involvement of multiple cardiac structures in CoViD 19 patients, including myocardium, vascular structures, and the electrical conduction system. The studies help to identify and determine the extent, severity, and reversibility of the structural cellular damage, associated factors, and mechanisms that contribute to the development of cardiovascular complications in CoViD19 and may carry prognostic implications. The data promote a better understanding of myocardial injury, heart failure, sudden death, arrhythmias, thrombotic complications, and stress cardiomyopathies in the context of CoViD19. The data further strengthen the notion of the contribution of the burden of chronic cardiovascular disease and risk factors, including obesity, towards the development of complications in patients with CoViD 19.

The endomyocardial biopsy appears to be an important tool in investigating and defining the cardiac injury in CoViD 19, thus improving the diagnostic accuracy [32]. The reports confirm the presence of a variety of mechanisms such as direct myocardial viral damage, direct vascular viral injury, hyper inflammation, exaggerated immune response, microvascular disease, and prothrombotic mechanisms, which appear to be associated with the cardiovascular complications in CoViD 19. A multi-faceted approach involving novel histopathological diagnostic techniques, improved EMB techniques such as electro-anatomical voltage mapping to guide endomyocardial biopsy in combination with imaging, and genetic profiling methods, may be further explored. Similarly, a better characterization of EMB samples via phenomics (such as proteomics, viral diagnosis, and immune cell profiling),

MicroRNA (miRNA) profiling of the EMB, and other tools may help to reduce the diagnostic uncertainties associated with myocarditis associated with CoViD19.

The cardiovascular virulence of the SARS CoV 2 exhibits a spectrum of cardiovascular pathologies such as endotheliitis, myocarditis, a microvascular myocardial injury that appear to be particularly specific to this etiology. The presence of acute inflammatory, immunomodulatory cells, apoptosis, cellular necrosis in patients with CoViD 19 suggests a likely involvement of the signaling pathways, mediators, and mechanisms of cell death, associated with cardiovascular dysfunction and disease. A better understanding of these mechanisms may help clinicians devise improved strategies to diagnose, manage and treat patients with cardiovascular complications of CoViD19. Therefore, research is needed to establish these mechanisms, the frequencies, and associations to help to lower the mortality associated with the cardiovascular complications of CoViD19.

Summary Box

- In complicated CoViD19, the lungs are the central to the pathology, and appearance of ARDS is a step towards complication.
- The diffuse alveolar damage (DAD) is the main pathological feature of the ARDS, characterized by hyaline membrane formation in the alveoli, interstitial edema, fibroblast proliferation and fibrin deposition.
- Current evidence on CoViD19 cardiac pathology is limited, is based on research findings from the autopsies or endomyocardial biopsies, and histopathological observations.
- The CoViD19 cardiovascular pathology indicates presence of macro and microvascular disease, thrombo-embolic state, myocardial injury, with features of immuno-inflammation, with or without viral detection.
- The histopathological forms of CoViD19 related myocardial injury reveal viral myocarditis, reactive inflammatory myocarditis, and multifocal lymphocytic myocarditis among others.
- The cellular features CoViD19 myocardial injury include cardiomyocytes and interstitial tissue, with edema, cytopathic acute inflammatory cells in the interstitial and perivascular tissue, macrophages, features of multifocal lymphocytic myocarditis with CD4 or CD8 cells, lympho-nuclear infiltrates, focal necrosis in myocytes or intramural vasculature, and endothelial inflammation.
- The presence of elevated cytokines, direct viral damage, microvascular cardiac disease, vascular injury, endotheliitis, and thromboembolic phenomenon is associated with inflammatory and immune-mediated mechanisms in CoVid19.

References

1. Xiao F, et al. Evidence for gastrointestinal infection of SARS-CoV-2. Gastroenterology. 2020;158(6):1831–1833.
2. Diao B, Wang CH, Wang RS, Feng ZQ, Tan YJ, Wang HM, et al. Human kidney is a target for novel severe acute respiratory syndrome coronavirus 2 [SARS-CoV-2] infection [preprint posted online April 10, 2020]. medRxiv. https://doi.org/10.1101/2020.03.04.20031120.
3. Su H, et al. Renal histopathological analysis of 26 postmortem findings of patients with COVID-19 in China [published online ahead of print April 9, 2020]. Kidney Int. 2020;10.
4. Yao XH, Li TY, He ZC, et al. A pathological report of three COVID-19 cases by minimal invasive autopsies. Zhonghua Bing li xue za zhi Chin J Pathol. 2020;49(5):411–417. https://doi.org/10.3760/cma.j.cn112151-20200312-00193.
5. Basso C, et al. Pathological features of COVID-19-associated myocardial injury: a multicentre cardiovascular pathology study. Eur Heart J. 2020;41(39):3827–3835.
6. Fox SE, Akmatbekov A, Harbert JL, Li G, Brown JQ, Vander Heide RS. Pulmonary and cardiac pathology in Covid-19: the first autopsy series from New Orleans. Lancet Respir Med. 2020;8(7):681–6. https://doi.org/10.1101/2020.04.06.20050575.
7. Buja LM, Wolf DA, Zhao B, et al. The emerging spectrum of cardiopulmonary pathology of the coronavirus disease 2019 (COVID-19): report of 3 autopsies from Houston, Texas, and review of autopsy findings from other United States cities [published online ahead of print, 2020 May 7]. Cardiovasc Pathol. 2020;48:107233. https://doi.org/10.1016/j.carpath.2020.107233.
8. Nicol M, et al. Delayed acute myocarditis and COVID-19-related multisystem inflammatory syndrome. ESC Heart Fail. 2020.
9. Xu Z, Shi L, Wang Y, Zhang J, Huang L, Zhang C, et al. Pathological fndings of COVID-19 associated with acute respiratory distress syndrome. Lancet Respir Med. 2020. https://doi.org/10.1016/S2213-2600(20)30076-X.
10. Zeng J-H, et al. First case of COVID-19 complicated with fulminant myocarditis: a case report and insights. Infection. 2020;1.
11. Xu Z, Shi L, Wang Y, Zhang J, Huang L, Zhang C, et al. Pathological findings of COVID-19 associated with acute respiratory distress syndrome. Lancet Respir Med. 2020. https://doi.org/10.1016/S2213-2600(20)30076-X.
12. Deng Q, et al. Suspected myocardial injury in patients with COVID-19: evidence from front-line clinical observation in Wuhan, China. Int J Cardiol. 2020.
13. Ho JS, et al. Coronavirus-induced myocarditis: a meta-summary of cases. Heart Lung. 2020;49(6):681–5.
14. Ozieranski K, Tyminska A, Caforio ALP. Clinically suspected myocarditis in the course of coronavirus infection. Eur Heart J. 2020;41(22):2118–9.
15. Halushka MK, Vander Heide RS. Myocarditis is rare in COVID-19 autopsies: cardiovascular findings across 277 post-mortem examinations. Cardiovasc Pathol. 2020:107300.
16. Del Nonno F, et al. Virus-negative myopericarditis in human coronavirus infection: report from an autopsy series. Circ Heart Fail. 2020: CIRCHEARTFAILURE-120.
17. Meyer P, et al. Typical takotsubo syndrome triggered by SARS-CoV-2 infection. Eur Heart J. 2020;41(19):1860.
18. Giustino G, et al. Takotsubo cardiomyopathy in COVID-19. J Am Coll Cardiol. 2020;76(5):628–9.
19. Tsao CW, et al. COVID-19–associated stress (Takotsubo) cardiomyopathy. Circ Cardiovasc Imaging. 2020;13(7):e011222.
20. van Osch D, Asselbergs FW, Teske AJ. Takotsubo cardiomyopathy in COVID-19: a case report. Haemodynamic and therapeutic considerations. Eur Heart J Case Rep. 2020.

21. Sala S, Peretto G, Gramegna M, Palmisano A, Villatore A, Vignale D, De Cobelli F, Tresoldi M. Cappelletti AM, Basso C, Godino C, Esposito A. Acute myocarditis presenting as a reverse Tako-Tsubo syndrome in a patient with SARS-CoV-2 respiratory infection. Eur Heart J. 2020;41(19):1861–2. https://doi.org/10.1093/eurheartj/ehaa286.
22. Tavazzi G, Pellegrini C, Maurelli M, Belliato M, Sciutti F, Bottazzi A, Sepe PA, Resasco T, Camporotondo R, Bruno R, Baldanti F, Paolucci S, Pelenghi S, Iotti GA, Mojoli F, Arbustini E. Myocardial localization of coronavirus in COVID-19 cardiogenic shock. Eur J Heart Fail. 2020;22(5):911–915. https://doi.org/10.1002/ejhf.1828. epub ahead of print.
23. Bradley BT, Maioli H, Johnson R, Chaudhry I, Fink SL, Xu H, Najafian B, Marshall D, Lacy JM, Williams T, Yarid N. Histopathology and ultrastructural findings of fatal COVID-19 infections. MedRxiv. https://www.medrxiv.org/content/10.1101/2020.04.17.20058545v1.
24. Wenzel P, et al. Evidence of SARS-CoV-2 mRNA in endomyocardial biopsies of patients with clinically suspected myocarditis tested negative for COVID-19 in nasopharyngeal swab. Cardiovasc Res. 2020;116(10):1661–3.
25. Wichmann D, Sperhake JP, Lutgehetmann M, Steurer S, Edler C, Heinemann A, Heinrich F, Mushumba H, Kniep I, Schroder AS, Burdelski C, de Heer G, Nierhaus A, Frings D, Pfefferle S, Becker H, Bredereke-Wiedling H, de Weerth A, Paschen HR, Sheikhzadeh-Eggers S, Stang A, Schmiedel S, Bokemeyer C, Addo MM, Aepfelbacher M, Puschel K, Kluge S. Autopsy findings and venous thromboembolism in patients with covid-19: a prospective cohort study. Ann Intern Med. 2020. https://doi.org/10.7326/M20-2003.
26. Liu PP, et al. The science underlying COVID-19: implications for the cardiovascular system. Circulation. 2020;142(1):68–78. https://doi.org/10.1161/CIRCULATIONAHA.120.047549.
27. Rovas A, et al. Microvascular dysfunction in COVID-19: the MYSTIC study. Angiogenesis. 2020:1–13.
28. Roberts KA, et al. Vascular manifestations of COVID-19–thromboembolism and microvascular dysfunction. Front Cardiovasc Med. 2020;7.
29. Barton LM, Duval EJ, Stroberg E, Ghosh S, Mukhopadhyay S. COVID-19 autopsies, Oklahoma, USA. Am J Clin Pathol. 2020;153(6):725–3. https://doi.org/10.1093/ajcp/aqaa062.
30. Menter T, et al. Postmortem examination of COVID-19 patients reveals diffuse alveolar damage with severe capillary congestion and variegated findings in lungs and other organs suggesting vascular dysfunction. Histopathology. 2020;77(2):198–209.
31. Varga Z, Flammer AJ, Steiger P, et al. Endothelial cell infection and endotheliitis in COVID-19. The Lancet. 2020;395(10234):1417–8. https://doi.org/10.1016/S0140-6736(20)30937-5.
32. Kociol RD, et al. Recognition and initial management of fulminant myocarditis: a scientific statement from the American heart association. Circulation. 2020;141:e69–92.
33. Caforio AL, Pankuweit S, Arbustini E, Basso C, Gimeno-Blanes J, Felix SB, Fu M, Heliö T, Heymans S, Jahns R, Klingel K. Current state of knowledge on aetiology, diagnosis, management, and therapy of myocarditis: a position statement of the European society of cardiology working group on myocardial and pericardial diseases. Eur Heart J. 2013;34(33):2636–48.
34. Ferreira VM, Schulz-Menger J, Holmvang G, Kramer CM, Carbone I, Sechtem U, Kindermann I, Gutberlet M, Cooper LT, Liu P, Friedrich MG. Cardiovascular magnetic resonance in nonischemic myocardial inflammation: expert recommendations. J Am Coll Cardiol. 2018;72(24):3158–76.
35. Bradley BT, Maioli H, Johnston R, Chaudhry I, Fink SL, Xu H, Najafian B, Deutsch G, Lacy JM, Williams T, Yarid N. Histopathology and ultrastructural findings of fatal COVID-19 infections in Washington State: a case series. The Lancet. 2020;396(10247):320–32.
36. Craver R, Huber S, Sandomirsky M, McKenna D, Schieffelin J, Finger L. Fatal eosinophilic myocarditis in a healthy 17-year-old male with severe acute respiratory syndrome coronavirus 2 (SARS-CoV-2c). Fetal Pediatr Pathol. 2020;39(3):263–8.

37. Escher F, Pietsch H, Aleshcheva G, Bock T, Baumeier C, Elsaesser A, Wenzel P, Hamm C, Westenfeld R, Schultheiss M, Gross U. Detection of viral SARS-CoV-2 genomes and histopathological changes in endomyocardial biopsies. ESC Heart Fail. 2020;7(5):2440–7.
38. Lindner D, Fitzek A, Bräuninger H, Aleshcheva G, Edler C, Meissner K, Scherschel K, Kirchhof P, Escher F, Schultheiss HP, Blankenberg S. Association of cardiac infection with SARS-CoV-2 in confirmed COVID-19 autopsy cases. JAMA Cardiol. 2020;5(11):1281–5.

Chapter 5
Treatment Options in CoViD19

Key Questions

- What are the treatment options in the COViD19?
- What are the important therapeutic target mechanisms and agents for CoViD19?
- Which novel therapeutic options are under exploration for the treatment of CoViD19?
- What are the basics of the vaccine therapy in CoViD19?

5.1 Introduction

The critical complications of CoViD19 and the complex pathogenetic nature of the disease require a multifaceted approach to help effectively combat the disease.

A range of combating strategies have been introduced in clinical practice since the beginning of the CoViD19 pandemic (Table 5.1). These strategies refer to preventive interventions, drug treatments, or supportive therapies that may directly target the pathogen or modify the associated pathogenetic mechanisms or related stress. Although such measures have been of benefit in the fight for the prevention and treatment of the disease and the complications, definite treatment options are not available.

The CoViD19 is an RNA viral disease involving a series of dysregulated pathophysiological mechanisms that are triggered by the viral entry into the

U. Mallick, *Cardiovascular Complications of COVID-19*,
https://doi.org/10.1007/978-3-030-90065-6_5

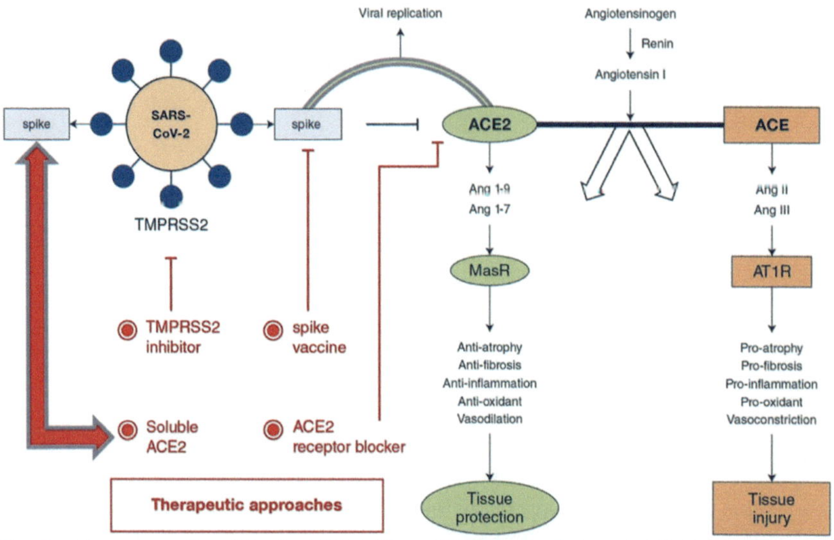

Fig. 1 Potential approaches to address ACE2-mediated COVID-19 following SARS-CoV-2 infection. The finding that SARS-CoV-2 and SARS-CoV use the ACE2 receptor for cell entry has important implications for understanding SARS-CoV-2 transmissibility and pathogenesis. SARS-CoV and likely SARS-CoV-2 lead to downregulation of the ACE2 receptor, but not ACE, through binding of the spike protein with ACE2. This leads to viral entry and replication, as well as severe lung injury. Potential therapeutic approaches include a SARS-CoV-2 spike protein-based vaccine; a transmembrane protease serine 2 (TMPRSS2) inhibitor to block the priming of the spike protein; blocking the surface ACE2 receptor by using anti-ACE2 antibody or peptides; and a soluble form of ACE2 which should slow viral entry into cells through competitively binding with SARS-CoV-2 and hence decrease viral spread as well as protecting the lung from injury through its unique enzymatic function. MasR—mitochondrial assembly receptor, AT1R—Ang II type 1 receptor

Fig. 5.1 SARS CoV2 receptors-based therapies. *Source* Figure 1. Zhang, H., Penninger, J.M., Li, Y., Zhong, N. and Slutsky, A.S., 2020. Angiotensin-converting enzyme 2 (ACE2) as a SARS-CoV-2 receptor: molecular mechanisms and potential therapeutic target. Intensive care medicine, 46(4), pp. 586–590. https://link.springer.com/article/10.1007/s00134-020-05985-9. Published by Springer Nature

organism, viral cell recognition process, induced cell injury, and others that lead to multi-organ dysfunction and death. These mechanisms accompany numerous mediators and pathways such as signaling pathways, immunoregulatory factors, inflammatory systems, prothrombotic processes, hemodynamic regulatory systems, intracellular mechanisms, and processes related to cell death.

The viral cell entry mechanism in CoViD19 has remained a particular focus of research throughout, especially due to the therapeutic potential. This important mechanism refers to the viral and cell receptor binding process, mainly involving the ACE2 receptor or other secondary receptors such as Cathepsin L, and the co-factors such as the TMPRSS2 that play an important role in the primary viral cell-binding process through the viral spike glycoproteins.

The data from recent research show that a variety of pathophysiological mechanisms are closely associated with the severity and complications of the CoViD19 may be subject to target for potential therapies. These include abnormal immunoregulatory processes, including the cytokine storm, hyperinflammatory reactions, prothrombotic processes, and others. The drugs mainly explored in

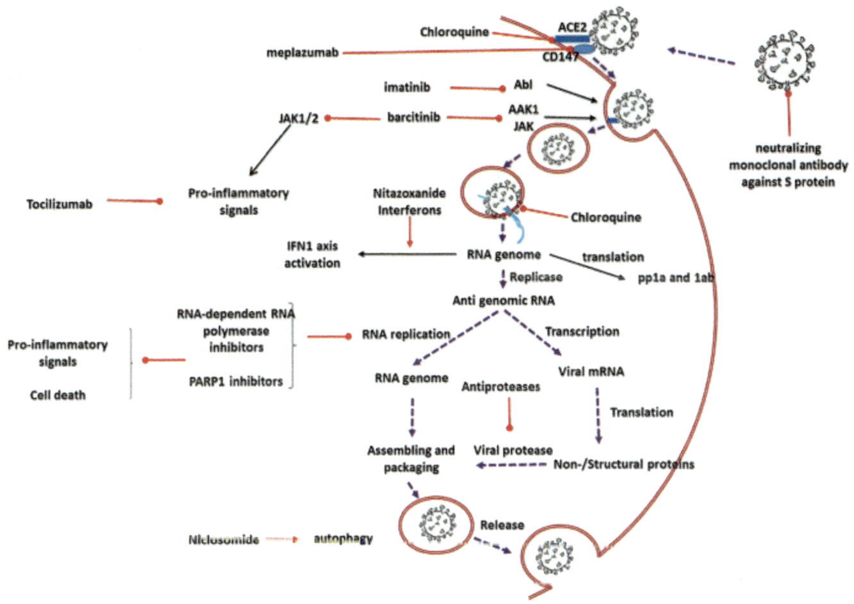

Fig. 5.2 Drugs against COVID19. Schematic represents the possible effects of proposed drugs on the severe acute respiratory syndrome coronavirus 2. AAK1, Ap2-associated protein kinase 1; Ab1, a non-receptor tyrosine kinase; ACE2, angiotensin-converting enzyme 2; IFN1, interferons type 1; JAK, Janus kinase; mRNA, messenger ribonucleic acid; PARP1, poly-ADP-ribose polymerase 1; RNA, ribonucleic acid; pp1a and 1ab, protein phosphatase 1a and 1ab. → activator effect; ● inhibitory effect; ⇢ viral cell cycle. *Source* Figure 2. Rameshrad, M., Ghafoori, M., Mohammadpour, A.H., Nayeri, M.J.D. and Hosseinzadeh, H., 2020. A comprehensive review on drug repositioning against coronavirus disease 2019 (COVID19). Naunyn-Schmiedeberg's archives of pharmacology, 393, pp. 1137–1152. https://link.springer.com/article/10.1007/s00210-020-01901-6. Published by Springer Nature

CoViD19 treatment impact virus-host interactions, inhibit the mechanism of viral assembly, influence innate host response, or the signaling pathways associated with the process of viral replication. Several therapeutic interventions based on these mechanisms are currently used in clinical practice to treat CoViD19 patients (Tables 5.2 and 5.3). The commonly used treatments include antiviral drugs, antiviral receptor binding agents, immunomodulators, and cytoprotective therapies. Other interventions, based on the novel exploratory mechanisms, are currently in the experimental stage. These mechanisms include NETs (Neutrophil Extracellular Traps, or related to NOD-like receptor protein 3 (NLRP3) inflammasome and others.

Furthermore, other therapies, such as those used for the treatment of cardiovascular diseases, cardioprotective drugs, and antithrombotics, have been shown to help minimize the severity and the associated risk due to CoViD19 complications. Several CoViD19 studies and expert groups have debated the role of ACE inhibitors /ARBs in the CoViD19 patients with cardiovascular diseases, which has been later validated by the expert guidelines. Similarly, the role of antithrombotic therapy

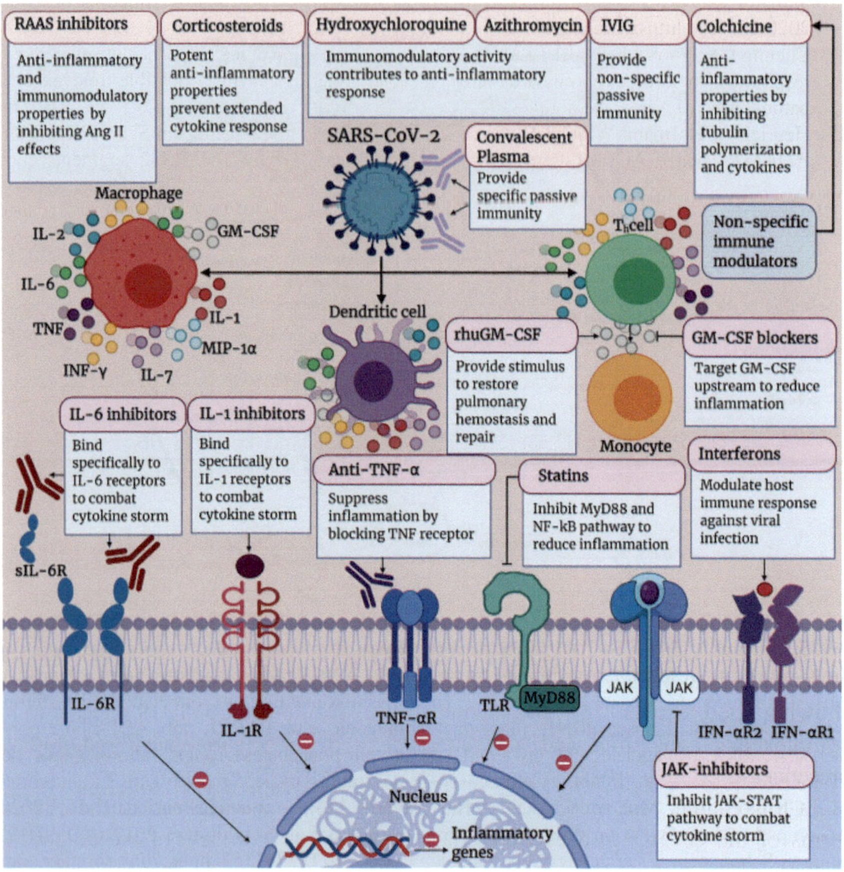

Fig. 5.3 Immunomodulation in COViD19. Schematic representation of the immunomodulators' site of action. Hydroxychloroquine, azithromycin, statins, RAASi and their combinations have not been reliably shown to be of benefit in hospitalized patients with COVID-19, and therefore are represented here to define a potential pathophysiological target for therapy. This should not be seen as endorsement for use of such agents. The use of hydroxychloroquine and azithromycin in COVID-19 patients may be associated with harm. Whether such agents are beneficial in other stages of infection remains a matter of study. Created with biorender.com. Ang II angiotensin II, GM-CSF granulocyte–macrophage colony-stimulating factor, IFN interferon, IL interleukin, IL-6R interleukin-6 receptor, IVIG intravenous immunoglobulin, JAK Janus kinase, JAK-STAT Janus kinase-signal transducer and activator of transcription, MIP-1α macrophage inflammatory protein 1-α, MyD88 myeloid differentiation primary response 88, NF-κB nuclear factor-κB, RAAS renin–angiotensin–aldosterone system, rhuGM-CSF recombinant human granulocyte–macrophage colony-stimulating factor, sIL-6R soluble IL-6 receptor, TLR toll-like receptor, TNF tumor necrosis factor reserve. *Source* Figure 1. Rizk, J.G., Kalantar-Zadeh, K., Mehra, M.R., Lavie, C.J., Rizk, Y. and Forthal, D.N., 2020. Pharmaco-immunomodulatory therapy in COVID-19. Drugs, pp. 1–26. https://link.springer.com/article/10.1007/s40265-020-01367-z. Published by Springer Nature

Table 5.1 Potential treatments in CoViD19

Potential therapeutic strategies in CoViD19
Antiviral drugs Immune based therapies (immunomodulators) Anti-inflammatory therapy Adjunctive therapy (anticoagulation, antibiotics and others)

Table 5.2 Potential therapeutic interventions impacting SARS CoV2 and disease progression

Drugs interfering with the fusion of the virus with host cells	Antivirals Serine protease inhibitors Interleukin inhibitors Antifibrinolytic homeostatics
Drugs targeting RAAS ACE2 AT1 receptor	Recombinant enzyme Cardioprotective angiotensin peptide (Ang 1-7) ACE inhibitors AT1 Receptor blockers
Drugs interfering with translocation of the virus within host cells	Anti-malarial or combination with antibiotic
Drugs interfering with the proteolysis mechanism of the virus within host cells	Antivirals Antiretrovirals Anticancer
Drugs interfering with replication, transcription, and translocation of virus genomic material	Antivirals Anticancer Anti-parasite Glucocorticoids
Drugs interfering with cytokine storm and compromised immune function	Anti-inflammatories Anticancer Immunosuppressants Antioxidants Antigout Antiangiogenics Acetylcholinesterase inhibitors
Drugs preventing the progression of CoViD19 in severe ARDS	Immunomodulators Anti inflammatories Antidepressants Vasoactive peptide analog

For further details please refer to Poduri, R., Joshi, G. and Jagadeesh, G., 2020. Drugs targeting various stages of the SARS-CoV-2 life cycle: exploring promising drugs for the treatment of Covid-19. Cellular signalling, 74, p.109721. https://doi.org/10.1016/j.cellsig.2020.109721.

to prevent and treat CoViD19 related complications is currently under exploration in several clinical trials [1].

A variety of conventional and non-conventional approaches are also under exploration for developing vaccines for the prevention of CoViD19. The vaccines

Table 5.3 Potential target mechanisms and drug types CoViD19

Potential target mechanisms	Drug types
Inhibitors of cell entry	Inhibitors of Angiotensin-Converting Enzyme 2 (ACE2) Antimalarial Drugs (Hydroxychloroquine) Inhibitors of Transmembrane Protease, Serine 2 (TMPRSS-2 (Nafamostat) Serine Subfamily Member 2 (TMPRSS-2) (Camostat Mesylate)
Inhibitors of replication, membrane fusion, and assembly of SARS CoV2	Lopinavir /Ritonavir Combination Umifenovir Favipiravir
Immunomodulators	Tocilizumab Interferon-β-1a Passive immune therapy (Convalescent Plasma)
Anti inflammatories	Corticosteroids JAK1/2 Inhibitors (Baricitinib) Specialized pro-resolving lipid autacoid mediators (SPMs) eg Resolvins, Protectins Maresins and Soluble epoxide hydrolase (sEH) inhibitors
Anticoagulant and antiplatelets	Low molecular weight heparin Heparin, Inhibitor of the TMPRSS-2 (Nafamostat)

Ref for further reading:
1. Panigrahy, D., Gilligan, M.M., Huang, S., Gartung, A., Cortés-Puch, I., Sime, P.J., Phipps, R.P., Serhan, C.N. and Hammock, B.D., 2020. Inflammation resolution: a dual-pronged approach to averting cytokine storms in COVID-19?. Cancer and Metastasis Reviews, 39(2), pp.337–340.
2. Manickam, M., Meenakshisundaram, S. and Pillaiyar, T., 2021. Activating endogenous resolution pathways by soluble epoxide hydrolase inhibitors for the management of COVID-19. Archiv der Pharmazie, p.e2100367.

are used for introducing a limited amount of disease-specific antigens into the human body to stimulate the immune system to produce the required amount of antibodies but without causing the disease. The process of development of vaccines includes multiple technology platforms such as nucleic acid (DNA and RNA), virus-like particles, peptides, viral vector (replicating and non-replicating), recombinant protein, live attenuated virus, and the inactivated virus. The DNA- and mRNA-based platforms offer promising potential and flexibility in terms of manipulation of the antigen, and potential for the speed, followed by the development of recombinant protein-subunit vaccines [2].

The prevention of the rapid spread of the CoViD19 pandemic remains a significant challenge to the medical and scientific community and other public health organizations worldwide. Various community and public health programs have been launched globally to help minimize the risk of viral contamination. The health experts and public health organizations recommend the use of rigorous preventive

Table 5.4 Drug interactions CoViD19 and cardiovascular drugs

CoViD19 drugs	Cardiovascular drugs
Ribavirin	Warfarin
Lopinavir/ritonavir	Anticoagulants (Apixaban, Rivaroxaban, Dabigatran, Edoxaban) Antiplatelets (Clopidogrel, Ticagrelor, Prasugrel) Statins (Atorvastatin, Rosuvastatin, Lovastatin, Simvastatin) Antiarrhythmics (QT-prolonging agents), Digoxin, Ivabradine Angiotensin Receptor-Neprilysin Inhibitor (Sacubitril) Angiotensin Receptor Blocker (Losartan, Valsartan) Diuretics (Indapamide)
Chloroquine/ hydroxychloroquine	Beta-blockers (Metoprolol, carvedilol, propranolol, labetalol) Antiarrhythmics (QT-prolonging agents) Digoxin
IL-6 inhibitors (Tocilizumab)	Warfarin, apixaban, rivaroxaban

The information presented here about the drug interactions in CoViD19 is not comprehensive and lacks specific details related to the actual impact. For specific details related to the drug interactions, and further recommendations please consult the relevant guidance.

1. Naksuk, N., Lazar, S. and Peeraphatdit, T., 2020. Cardiac safety of off-label COVID-19 drug therapy: a review and proposed monitoring protocol. European Heart Journal: Acute Cardiovascular Care, 9(3), pp. 215–221.
2. Talasaz, A.H., Kakavand, H., Van Tassell, B., Aghakouchakzadeh, M., Sadeghipour, P., Dunn, S. and Geraiely, B., 2020. Cardiovascular complications of COVID-19: pharmacotherapy perspective. Cardiovascular Drugs and Therapy, pp. 1–11.
3. Scavone, C., Mascolo, A., Rafaniello, C., Sportiello, L., Trama, U., Zoccoli, A., Bernardi, F.F., Racagni, G., Berrino, L., Castaldo, G. and Coscioni, E., 2021. Therapeutic strategies to fight COVID-19: Which is the status artis?. British Journal of Pharmacology

measures to stop the spread of the disease. These include physical preventive measures such as hand hygiene practices, the use of sanitizers and protective equipment (face masks, gloves, eye protection, bodysuits), physical distancing, and many others. Specially designed protocols and tools have been introduced in the healthcare centers and in public places to minimize the risk of disease contraction in the general population and those at high-risk subpopulation groups.

Several expert groups and societies have published expert guidances for the prevention and management of CoViD19 in the high-risk subpopulation groups such as the older age patients, diabetics, or individuals with a background of cardiovascular diseases, and several others, including with mental health issues. Overall, several strategies are in use and remain under exploration for the prevention and treatment of patients with CoViD19 globally. Some of the important therapeutic agents commonly used by health experts to treat patients with CoVD19 and the complications are provided below.

5.2 Antiviral Agents in CoViD19

The acute lung injury that is a core pathology in CoViD19 is a specific target of potential therapeutic interventions that may help reduce the severity and complications related to the pulmonary parenchymal and vascular injuries. The role of a variety of antiviral agents in the treatment of CoViD19 is currently under exploration.

A combination antiretroviral drug lopinavir/ritonavir, where lopinavir is a primary agent that inhibits the viral protease and ritonavir that increases the plasma concentration of lopinavir via inhibition of CYP3A4-mediated metabolism, has been investigated for the treatment of CoViD19. The randomized, controlled, open-label trial in 199 patients hospitalized with CoViD19, assigned 99 patients to the lopinavir-ritonavir group and 100 to the standard-care group, showed no improvement in time to clinical improvement (hazard ratio for clinical improvement, 1.31; 95% confidence interval [CI], 0.95 to 1.80), or difference in 28-day mortality (19.2% vs. 25.0%; difference, − 5.8 percentage points; 95% CI, − 17.3 to 5.7) between the two groups and similar percentages of patients with detectable viral RNA at various time points [3].

Similarly, a randomized, controlled, open-label, platform trial of lopinavir-ritonavir for the treatment of CoViD19 patients admitted in the hospital, received either usual standard of care (3424 patients) or the routine standard of care with lopinavir-ritonavir (1616 patients), showed no benefits in 28-day mortality (374 (23%) versus 767 (22%) rate ratio 1·03, 95% CI 0·91–1·17; $p = 0{\cdot}60$), duration of hospital stay (median 11 days [IQR 5 to > 28]), or risk of progressing to invasive mechanical ventilation or death (risk ratio 1·09, 95% CI 0·99–1·20; $p = 0{\cdot}092$) [4].

However, in an open-label, prospective randomized phase II trial involving 127 patients admitted with CoViD19, the use of a triple combination of interferon beta 1b, lopinavir/ritonavir, and ribavirin as early triple antiviral therapy was safe and superior to lopinavir-ritonavir alone in alleviating symptoms and shortening the duration of the viral shedding and hospital stay, in patients with mild to moderate CoViD19 [5].

Another antiviral agent, remdesivir (a broad spectrum nucleotide analog that inhibits RNA replication by inhibiting RNA-dependent RNA polymerase activity in several RNA viruses), is being explored for the treatment of CoViD19. Although improvement in time to recovery has been observed, remdesivir has not shown any promising results in the treatment of CoViD19 [6–8].

The efficacy of remdesivir was analyzed in a randomized, double-blind, placebo-controlled, multi-centre trial in 237 patients with severe CoViD19. Although a reduction in the time to clinical improvement was observed, remdesivir was not associated with statistically significant clinical benefits in patients admitted with CoViD19. Overall, use of remdesivir was not associated with a difference in time to clinical improvement (hazard ratio 1·23 [95% CI 0·87–1·75]), although numerically, this treatment group had a faster time to clinical improvement as compared to the placebo arm, with symptom duration of 10 days or less (hazard ratio 1·52 [0·95–2·43]) [7, 9].

A double-blind, randomized, placebo-controlled trial of intravenous remdesivir in 1062 patients hospitalized with CoViD19 with lower respiratory tract infection, showed that remdesivir was superior to placebo in shortening the time to recovery. In the remdesivir treatment group, the patients had a median recovery time of 10 days (95% confidence interval [CI], 9 to 11), as compared with 15 days (95% CI, 13 to 18) among those who received placebo (rate ratio for recovery, 1.29; 95% CI, 1.12 to 1.49; $P < 0.001$, by a log-rank test) [10].

Similarly, other antiviral agents such as a viral envelope membrane fusion inhibitor umifenovir (Arbidol), a purine nucleotide RNA polymerase inhibitor favipiravir (Avigan), or antiretroviral drugs such darunavir-based regimens have shown no promising results in the treatment of CoViD19 [11, 12]. Other investigational products explored for the CoViD19 treatment include antiviral agents such as Toll-Like Receptor 3 (TLR 3) agonists (rintatolimod), nucleoside reverse transcriptor inhibitor (azvudine), viral RNA polymerase inhibitor (favipiravir), and several others.

In summary, although certain antiviral drugs, such as Remdesivir, have shown an acceleration in the recovery process in patients with CoViD19, the data does not show a significant benefit in the treatment of CoViD19. The Food and Drug Administration of the USA (FDA) has issued the emergency use authorization (EUA) for Remdesivir for the treatment of CoViD19 [13]. Further research is needed from robust clinical trials to assess the efficacy and safety of other antivirals such as oseltamivir, favipiravir, umifenovir, and others in patients with CoViD19.

5.2.1 Viral Cell Entry Inhibition and Viral Assembly Blockage

Another class of drugs, serine protease inhibitors, may halt SARS CoV2 spike protein activation, preventing the viral cell entry by blocking the TMPRSS2 activity [14]. A serine protease inhibitor, camostat mesylate, has been shown to block the TMPRSS2 activity and inhibit the SARS CoV entry into the cells [15]. A synthetic serine protease inhibitor (TMPRSS2) nafamostat (Fusan) that may play a role in the cell entry Mechanism of SARS CoV2 is undergoing further research [16–19]. The other investigational products, such as the recombinant human ACE2 (rhACE2; APN01, GSK2586881), use potential therapeutic target Angiotensin-Converting Enzyme 2 (ACE2), a SARS CoV2 receptor, are suggested for the treatment of patients with CoViD19 [20–23].

Similarly, Cathepsin L-selective Inhibitors may have an important potential role in the treatment of COVID19 patients. The inhibition of the Cathepsin L (CatL), an endosomal cysteine protease that mediates S1 subunit cleavage on SARS CoV2 glycoprotein spike to facilitate viral cell entry, is currently being explored [24, 25].

The activity of the Cathepsin L may also be hampered, by several other pharmaceutical agents, including the antimicrobials rifampicin and teicoplanin.

Other agents include a humanized anti CD147 antibody Meplazumab that inhibits CD147 (Basigin or EMMPRIN), a host cell expressing surface receptor involved in the viral cell entry process through interaction with SARS CoV2 glycoprotein receptor spike protein [26, 172]. Similarly, the AP2-associated protein kinase 1 (AAK1) and cyclin G associated kinase known as regulators of endocytosis during the process of viral cell entry may have a role in the treatment of CoViD19. The Janus kinase inhibitor baricitinib, efficiently binds with AAK1 and with cyclin G-associated kinase, may inhibit viral entry and the inflammation in patients with CoViD19 [27]. Baricitinib also inhibits the viral assembly process. The viral assembly process involves the coordinated interaction of various proteins. Several drugs may disrupt the essential viral protein–protein interactions such as lopinavir, ritonavir, and darunavir. These drugs inhibit translation and cleavage of polyproteins by proteases like $3CL^{pro}$, PL^{pro}, or others [28]. Further research is needed to explore the efficacy and safety of these agents in CoViD19 patients.

5.3 Amino Quinolones in CoViD19

Hydroxychloroquine a “Disease-Modifying Antirheumatic Drug” (DMARD) may impede the binding of ACE2 and SARS CoV2 spike protein, inhibit the antigen-presentation, and activation of T-cells, inhibit the cytosolic Toll-like receptor (TLR)-signaling, and production of pro-inflammatory cytokines (IL1 and TNF alpha). The beneficial role of hydroxychloroquine in CoViD19 relies on the mechanisms involving averting cytokine storm [29]. The substances, such as the 4 aminoquinolones (chloroquine and hydroxychloroquine), are actively explored in the treatment of CoViD19. The research shows that chloroquine can effectively block the SARS CoV2 infection in cultured cells [30]. A variety of mechanisms, such as an increase in the endosomal pH in the host intracellular organelles, inhibition of the autophagosome-lysosome fusion, or nonspecific inactivation of the enzymes that viruses require for replication, such as lysosomal cathepsins, may be involved in this process [31–35].

In addition, several other mechanisms, such as a direct effect on the protease synthesis (through CDP/Cux transcription factor at neutral pH) [34], immunomodulatory effect (the hydroxychloroquine being superior to the chloroquine, in countering the cytokine storm) [36] or interference with the glycosylation of the ACE2 receptor used by SARS CoV2 to enter the cells [37] and others such as antithrombotic activity and inhibition of the Neutrophil Extra Cellular Trap (NET) formation [38], has been demonstrated.

Although chloroquine/hydroxychloroquine is currently approved for off-label use for the treatment of patients with CoViD19 by the Food and Drug

Administration (FDA) [39] and Chinese National Medicine Products Association (NMPA) [40], use of this drug in CoViD19 is restricted and is only administered under close medical supervision (Ref Chinese + FDA). The United States Food and Drug Administration (FDA) issued an emergency use authorization (EUA) permitting chloroquine phosphate (medical grade) and hydroxychloroquine sulfate to be added to the strategic national stockpile (SNS) [41].

5.3.1 *Analysis of Body of Evidence on Amino Quinolones in CoViD19*

The evidence of potential benefits of chloroquine in patients with CoViD19 was initially provided in a report from an in vitro study, which showed that remdesivir and chloroquine are highly effective in the control of CoViD19 in vitro [42]. Subsequently, the positive effect of the hydroxychloroquine was demonstrated in a retrospective study of 1061 CoViD19 patients, which concluded that the administration of the hydroxychloroquine and azithromycin (HCQ + AZ) in combination before CoViD19 complications occur, is safe and is associated with a very low fatality rate in patients [43]. Similarly, a non-comparative, observational study showed a decline in the viral load in a cohort of 80 relatively mildly infected in-patients treated with a combination of hydroxychloroquine and azithromycin [44], further strengthening the notion of beneficial effects of the therapy in CoViD19 patients.

On the other hand, data from several studies in patients with CoViD19 show a lack of therapeutic benefit of the 4 aminoquinolones, alone or in combination, but also provide evidence of the potential toxicity associated with the treatment. An observational study included 181 patients admitted with severe CoViD19 requiring oxygen concluded that hydroxychloroquine is of no benefit in this population group [45]. Similarly, in a retrospective cohort study of 1438 patients admitted with CoViD19, the combination of azithromycin and hydroxychloroquine did not show a significant reduction in in-hospital mortality [46]. Other studies have shown the lack of additional benefits of virus elimination from adding hydroxychloroquine to the current standard of care in patients with mainly persistent mild to moderate CoViD19 [47]. In the second semester of the CoViD19 pandemic in the later part of 2020, multiple trials have been conducted further confirming the lack of benefit of 4 aminoquinolones in CoViD19 patients. These include an open-label trial [48], randomized controlled trials, completed [49, 50] and others that were discontinued due to the lack of an obvious benefit [51, 52]. Furthermore, an early administration of hydroxychloroquine in patients with COVID19, before hospitalization to assess the impact on hospitalization was tested in research studies and showed no significant benefit [53, 54].

Furthermore, multiple reports provide evidence of the toxicity of the "4 aminoquinolones" alone or in the form of combination therapy. An observational study of 1446 consecutive patients with CoViD19 showed the lack of benefit of hydroxychloroquine [55] or even harm [56], most likely due to the narrow therapeutic window that may result in cardiovascular, gastrointestinal, and retinal toxicity. Although several other CoViD19 studies suggest the presence of cardiac toxicity with the combination therapy of "4 aminoquinolones and azithromycin", the evidence of an increased risk of cardiac toxicity (QT interval prolongation) that may result in cardiac death when hydroxychloroquine and azithromycin are co-administered comes from other studies no related to the CoViD19 research [46, 57–59].

The body of evidence related to the use of 4 aminoquinolones in CoViD19 appears to have several, design and methodological flaws, and a variety of biases. Several reports have been published revealing such inadequacies in the clinical research related to the use of 4 aminoquinolones in CoViD19 that may impact the interpretability of findings of the research. The studies showing beneficial effects of hydroxychloroquine [43, 44] are mostly small, observational, poorly designed, inappropriate endpoints, are confounded, contain selection bias, are poorly analyzed, have data attrition, or are inappropriately reported [60], or even lack comparator control groups (single-armed) [43].

Similarly, in addition to the inherited weakness in the study design, several studies showing no benefit or harm associated with the therapy in patients with CoViD19 also carry several methodological, design, and reporting flaws [61, 62]. The study showing lack of beneficial effects of hydroxychloroquine therapy in CoViD19 patients appears to have several biases related to the patient selection and data attrition, [47] also observed in the other studies, showing harm associated with the therapy [45].

A critical appraisal of the evidence related to the effectiveness of chloroquine and hydroxychloroquine (with azithromycin) in CoViD19 included three randomized control trials and three observational studies. The authors identify poor-quality research related to the use of chloroquine/ hydroxychloroquine in CoViD19 and potential treatments, with limitations in research methodology that could impact clinical decision-making. These limitations include the poor, sparse, or underreporting of important patient outcomes [64]. Another critical analysis of the trials investigating chloroquine and hydroxychloroquine in CoViD19 indicates poor methodology, inadequate reporting, and flaws in the research endpoints [65]. Similarly, the trials conducted in patients with CoViD19 in the later part of 2020, investigating the benefits of 4 aminoquinolones in various settings, had lower strength of evidence due to the limitations and high risk of bias and showed no clear benefits. The overall evidence fails to support the usefulness of treatment with 4 aminoquinolones in CoViD19 patients [48, 66, 68]. In order to draw plausible conclusions about efficacy and safety of the treatment with 4 aminoquinolones in patients with CoViD19, sound clinical research, in the hierarchy of evidence base, is strongly needed.

Several ongoing trials are investigating the hydroxychloroquine in CoViD19 alone and in combination with other drugs such as Camostat Mesylate (a protease inhibitor) in a variety of settings, including in primary care [69, 70]. A randomized, placebo-controlled, double-blind trial aims to recruit approximately 2000 outpatients with early CoViD19, is investigating hydroxychloroquine plus azithromycin versus placebo in the prevention of hospital admission and death due to the CoViD19 [71]. Another ongoing trial, in the primary care settings, is aimed to evaluate the use of HCQ as a monotherapy, compared to the routine care, in 3000 older susceptible patients with CoViD19, including those in the care homes, to assess the impact on progression to a more severe disease involving hospital admission or death [72].

5.4 Immune-Based Therapies in CoViD19

5.4.1 Immunomodulatory Agents

Several immunomodulators such as corticosteroids, inter interleukin inhibitors, interferons, and kinase inhibitors may be used in the treatment of patients with CoViD19. The drugs with immunomodulatory properties affect immune system function, such as the IL6 inhibitors (IL6 receptor antagonists such as tocilizumab and sarilumab or monoclonal antibodies targeting IL-6 such as siltuximab) may be useful in patients with hypercytokinetic inflammatory presentation of CoViD19 [73], are under exploration in clinical research [74–79]. Similarly, several other immunomodulatory therapeutic agents are under exploration in the treatment of CoViD19. These include the IL-1 inhibitors, Kinase inhibitors such as Bruton's Tyrosine Kinase Inhibitors (acalabrutinib, ibrutinib, zanubrutinib), or Janus Kinase Inhibitors (baricitinib, ruxolitinib, tofacitinib), glucocorticoids, or others such as Interferon Alfa 2b or Interferon Beta-1a interferon-alpha, pegylated interferon λ1.

The Anti-IL-6R mAb bind to both the membrane-bound and soluble forms of the IL-6R, and may rapidly deplete the circulating levels of IL-6 in blood. The effectiveness of tocilizumab in patients with severe COVID19, has been demonstrated in several studies [80–82].

An observational study of 764 patients with COVID19 requiring ICU support who received tocilizumab showed a reduction in mortality (HR 0·64, 95% CI 0·47–0·87; p = 0·0040) [83]. However, a randomized, double-blind, placebo-controlled phase III trial investigating tocilizumab in patients with COVID19 associated pneumonia failed to show an improvement in the clinical status or a reduction in mortality [84]. Several gaps have been identified, in the study quality, such as the use of broad patient selection criteria, the timing of drug administration, and assessment of patient outcomes [85].

The IL6 inhibitors appear to have a scope in the suppression of the hyperinflammatory state of the disease. The potential role of these immunomodulatory agents needs further exploration with robust data for assessment of the efficacy, safety, and drug administration strategies [86].

The interferons are a family of cytokines with antiviral properties, may have a potential role in the early phase of CoViD19. Studies have explored the potential role of interferon-beta 1a in combination with antiviral therapy in patients with CoViD19. A prospective, open-label, randomized, phase 2 trial of 127 patients hospitalized with CoViD19 assessed the efficacy and safety of combined interferon beta-1b, lopinavir-ritonavir, and ribavirin. The study reported that early triple antiviral therapy was safe and superior to lopinavir-ritonavir alone in alleviating symptoms and shortening the duration of viral shedding and hospital stay in patients with mild to moderate COVID19 [88]. The data supporting the use of interferons in CoViD19 is insufficient, although there may be benefits of the interferon in the early phase of the disease and require careful assessment of the toxicity risk.

Another class of drugs Inhibitors of the JAK signaling pathway, potent anti-inflammatory agents, counter elevated cytokine levels. A selective JAK inhibitor, baricitinib, showed a decline in viral replication and the inflammatory response, [91], is undergoing further trials alone [92] and in combination with other drugs such as remdesevir [93].

Furthermore, the evidence of mortality benefits with dexamethasone in patients admitted in hospital with CoViD19 comes from a large randomized controlled trial investigating dexamethasone (n = 2104) versus standard care (n = 4321) (RR 0.83, 95% CI 0.74–0.92, p = 0.0007) [56] and other trials [87, 89]. The guidelines recommend the use of dexamethasone in CoViD19 patients requiring oxygen support [90]. Several trials are underway investigating dexamethasone in range of doses and severity of the disease in CoViD19 patients and combination with other therapies [94, 95].

5.4.2 Convalescent Plasma, and Antibody-Based Therapies

Several other blood-derived therapies for the treatment of CoViD19 may have a role in the treatment of CoViD19. These include convalescent plasma therapy, immunoglobulins (specific or non-specific to SARS CoV2), and Mesenchymal Stem Cells. The investigational convalescent plasma, collected from the individuals who have recovered from CoViD19 (COVID19 convalescent plasma), may contain antibodies to SARS CoV2, is under exploration for COVID19 treatment [93].

The Food and Drug Administration (FDA) has issued guidance to provide recommendations to the health care providers and the investigators on the administration and further study of the investigational convalescent plasma in CoViD19 [49]. Furthermore, the FDA has also provided Emergency Use Authorization (EUA) for convalescent plasma therapy in patients with CoViD19, based on data from several randomized or non-randomized, observational, and case series [87]. The efficacy and safety of the convalescent plasma for the treatment of COVID19 needs to be further established.

Another potential prophylactic and therapeutic option for COVID19, the Neutralizing monoclonal antibodies, which target the receptor-binding domain of SARSCoV2 spike protein, may hold potential and have received an emergency use authorization EUA for "bamlanivimab" a neutralizing monoclonal antibody (IgG1) therapy, from the FDA [89, 90]. The recombinant neutralizing human IgG1 monoclonal antibodies that have EUA from the FDA are Casirivimab and imdevimab (combination use) in patients with CoViD19 [94]. The immunoglobulins such as IVIG and neutralizing antibodies may have a role in the treatment of complications that develop with CoViD19 [95, 96]. Several ongoing trials are investigating role of IVIG in CoViD19 [96–98]. Further data related to the efficacy and safety of these drugs is needed from robust clinical research. Similarly, data supporting the role of mesenchymal stem cells for the treatment of CoViD19 is insufficient. These agents are not currently approved by the Food and Drug Administration (FDA) for the treatment of COVID19. Other potential investigational products, such as complement inhibitors, have also been proposed but supporting data is insufficient [103]. Besides, supportive treatments such as vitamin C, D may also be considered for the CoViD19 treatment, but data are lacking. Several ongoing trials are investigating these supplements in CoViD19 [100, 101].

5.5 Potential Anti-inflammatory Mechanisms

5.5.1 NOD-Like Receptor Protein 3 (NLRP3)-Anti-inflammasomes

Several studies propose the use of the anti-inflammasomes for the treatment of CoViD19 [101, 102]. The activation of the NOD-like receptor protein 3 (NLRP3) inflammasome is linked with the cytokine storm [103], known in association with the severe forms of CoViD19 [104–106]. In addition to the NLRP3 inflammasome signaling pathway, the pro-apoptotic mitochondrial signaling pathway associated with "Unfolded Proteins Response /Autophagy pathways" are important for the viral cycle of SARS CoV2 and may serve as a novel target for developing drugs for the treatment of CoViD19 [107].

Several drugs that interfere with immune response and immune mechanisms, tranilast [108], or others such as IL-6R and IL-1 receptor blocking agents anikara [109], NLRP3 inhibitors arglabin and MCC950 [110, 111], may display potential anti-inflammasome impact in CoViD19 [112].

5.5.2 *Neutrophil Extracellular Traps (NETs)-Anti NETosis Therapy*

Another novel mechanism that may serve as the potential therapeutic target in CoViD19 involves the Neutrophil Extracellular Traps (NETs). The Neutrophil Extracellular Traps (NETs) consisting of circulating free DNA and histones are related to inflammation, coagulation, and thrombosis both locally and systemically in a variety of conditions [113]. The NETs are a matrix of DNA decorated with neutrophils granule proteins, such as MPO (myeloperoxidase), cathepsin G, and neutrophil elastase that may sequestrate, kill and trap pathogens including viruses [114, 115].

The viruses can stimulate neutrophils to produce Neutrophil Extracellular Traps (NETs), a network structure formed by freely circulating DNA expelled by neutrophils, and a variety of proteins. This process leads to cell death, characterized by the destruction of the nuclear membrane before the plasmatic membrane that is not related to necrosis or apoptosis. In dysregulated forms, this process generates an extreme systemic response with the production of the cytokines, interferon I, and immune complexes, and may result in local and systemic damage. The NETs trap erythrocytes and activate platelets [116] may promote thrombosis via multiple mechanisms, such as degradation of the anticoagulant protein, TFPI (tissue factor pathway inhibitor) (augmenting TF activity and thrombin generation), and may activate platelets via TLR-2 and TLR-4 and enhance fibrin formation [117].

The patients with CoViD19 have high levels of circulating free (cf-DNA) and DNA-myeloperoxidase complexes [118]. The elevated levels of these freely circulating complexes correlate with the acuity of illness, inflammatory response, and severe disease. The circulating free RNA from SARS CoV2 may trigger a coagulation cascade. The evidence shows that cf-RNA serves as a cofactor for auto-activation of factor VII-activating protease, thereby initiating coagulation [119].

Low Molecular Weight Heparin [120], steroids [121], IVIg [122] and several other agents [123] induce a reduction of NET formation. The potential role of NETosis, the association between NETs activity and the mortality from CoViD19, as well as the associations between markers of NETosis and serum markers of inflammation and thrombosis, is currently under exploration in clinical research in the context of CoViD19, may serve as a new therapeutic target for the treatment of CoViD19 [124]. Potential role of Siglec-9 agonism to curb neutrophilic hyper inflammation in COVID19 as a promising therapeutic strategy has been suggested [125].

5.6 Anticoagulants

The CoViD19 is a hypercoagulability state and has a high inflammatory burden. Anticoagulation therapy has been suggested to have a role in the treatment of CoViD19 with benefits of improvement in mortality [126]. The use of anticoagulation therapy rapidly gained recognition in CoViD19 patients with moderate and severe disease. Prophylactic anticoagulation is recommended in the hospitalized CoViD19 patients [127, 128].

The antithrombin-mediated inhibition of FXa or thrombin by heparins or LMWH is a commonly used treatment in VTE prophylaxis, also in COVID19 patients. It has been suggested that the heparins have anti-inflammatory properties [129], and may bind to the SARS CoV2 spike protein and or down-regulate interleukin-6 (IL-6), therefore may have enhanced benefit in CoViD19 patients [130, 131].

A retrospective cohort study of 449 patients with severe CoViD19 showed the beneficial impact of low molecular weight heparin with better prognosis in severe CoViD19 (sepsis-induced coagulopathy criteria) or with markedly elevated serum D dimer levels. In the heparin using group, the 28 day mortality was lower than in the nonusers in patients with SIC score $\geq$ 4 (40.0% vs 64.2%, P = 0.029), or D-dimer > sixfold of the upper limit of normal (32.8% vs 52.4%, P = 0.017) [132].

Another potential anticoagulation mechanism that may serve as a potential target mechanism in CoViD19, currently under investigation, is based on Factor XII inhibition [133]. The anti-thrombo-inflammatory effects associated with this mechanism may provide added benefit in CoViD19 associated with the thrombo-inflammatory burden [134]. The role of antiplatelets including aspirin in sepsis and various settings of hyper-thrombotic states associated with sepsis has been advocated, and shown to have mortality benefits [135–137]. Antiplatelet therapy such as dipyridamole [138], and fibrinolytics such as tissue-type plasminogen activator (tPA) [139], may have a role in the treatment of severe COVID19. An inhibitor of the TMPRSS 2, Nafamostat, is known to have anti-platelet effects and antifibrinolytic actions, may have a role as combination therapy with heparin, in patients with CoViD19 [140]. The nafamostat is currently under investigation for the treatment of CoViD19 [141].

The hematological markers of thrombosis associated with CoViD19 such as D Dimers, partial prothrombin, and prothrombin times, may guide the use of anti-coagulation. The timing of the use of anticoagulation therapy has presented a challenge to clinicians treating patients with CoViD19. This might be due to the gaps and the uncertainties in recognition and understanding of the development of the thrombotic complications in connection with the early or late phase of the condition and is further augmented by the risks associated with the use of anticoagulation therapy. Preadmission anticoagulation or use of antiplatelets has been explored but no favorable effects have been found in CoVid19 patients [142]. Further research is needed to determine the interplay of multiple pathogenetic pathways involved in the development of prothrombotic complications in

CoViD19. The efficacy and safety of various anticoagulants and antiplatelet agents remain unclear in the treatment of CoViD19 and need to be investigated using randomized controlled trials. The therapeutic doses of the anticoagulants in hospitalized CoViD19 patients need to be established.

5.7 CoViD19 Vaccines

A large number of vaccine candidates for the prevention of CoViD19 are under exploration globally. Several breakthroughs have been reported with the successful completion of vaccine trials. Numerous platforms, such as nucleic acids (DNA and RNA), virus-like particles, protein subunits or peptides, viral vectors (replicated and non-replicated), recombinant proteins, attenuated live viruses and inactivated virus methods are being utilized to develop COVID19 vaccines. Recent developments in bioinformatics, proteomics, genomics, and system biology have led to advancements in the domain of vaccinology. Several bioinformatics tools and analytics, such as fusion of computational technologies with the recombinant DNA technology, reverse vaccinology, chemical conjugation of proteins to polysaccharides, as well as advances in the use of novel adjuvants and others, have facilitated the process of development of vaccines. For instance, scientists are now able to design vaccines, without having to grow specific microorganisms, from the information encoded in the genome. The recombinant DNA technique enabled the development of SARS CoV2 antigen and embedding within a primate adenovirus vector, once the genome sequence became available. The replication-competent version of other viruses (the vector) is used to shuttle the antigen-producing genes from the target pathogen to human cells. The S protein is the major target for COVID19 vaccine development.

Currently, 261 vaccines are tested; most of the vaccines are in the preclinical phase of development, while 11 vaccines have entered phase III clinical trials [143]. About 4 replicating viral vector-based vaccines, 4 inactivated, 2 peptide subunit, and one RNA-based vaccine have reached phase III clinical trials stage. One RNA-based vaccine is already in the phase IV stage [144].

The BioNTech BNT162 (b1/b2) is a lipid nanoparticle encapsulated mRNA based SARS CoV2 vaccine that contains nucleoside modified messenger RNA that encodes the receptor-binding domain of the SARS CoV2 spike protein, has gained authorization for Emergency use in the UK [145]. The efficacy of the vaccine against COVID19 is reported to be 95% based on the primary efficacy analysis of 170 confirmed cases (18 Nov 2020). These included 10 cases of severe COVID19, 9 of which occurred in the placebo group. The vaccine was 95% effective 28 days after the first dose [146].

The Moderna mRNA-1273 is RNA vaccine contains lipid nanoparticle-encapsulated nucleoside-modified messenger RNA (mRNA)-based vaccine encoding pre-fusion spike (S) protein has shown efficacy against COVID19 reported to be 94.5% based on the interim analysis of phase III trial enrolling 30,000 subjects, 95

CoViD19 cases of which 90 cases were observed in the placebo group and five were reported in the vaccine group. There were 11 cases of severe COVID19 all occurred in the placebo group [147]. Further reports are awaited from phase 2 [148] and phase 3 trials [149].

The Oxford ChAdOx1-S vaccine uses a replication-defective simian adenovirus to deliver recombinant SARS CoV2 spike (S) protein genes to human cells. The initial evidence of safety and tolerance of the ChAdOx1 nCoV-19 comes from phase I/II clinical trial (NCT04324606) [150]. A report based on interim data from 131 cases showed efficacy against COVID19 to be 62–90% [151]. According to the report, the vaccine could be up to 90% effective when a half dose is given, followed by a full dose one month later.

The Gamaleya Gam-COVID-Vac/Sputnik V is a non-replicating adenovirus (rAd26-S + rAd5-S) type vaccine is based on two components, the recombinant Ad26 (prime) (recombinant adenovirus vector based on the human adenovirus type 26) and recombinant Ad5 (boost) (adenovirus vector based on the human adenovirus type 5) viruses expressing full-length spike (S) protein has shown efficacy against COVID19 reported to be 92% based on interim data from 20 cases, is approved for early use in Russia, conditional on phase III results (11 Nov 2020) [152].

Another non-replicating viral vector based on Ad5 vector containing full-length spike (S) protein COVID19 vaccine has efficacy data pending, is approved for military use in China [153], is further tested in phase 2b and 3 trials [154].

Overall, three vaccines that have shown efficacy above 90% are based on RNA and non-replicating viral vector platforms. The Oxford ChAdOx1-S vaccine has already been made available for administration in the UK. Multiple phase-II and phase-III trials are underway that will reveal further efficacy and safety data on the vaccine development programs globally. The efficacy of these vaccines will be reflected by robust and durable immunity and the generalizability of the results to the global population.

5.8 Summary

Among several therapeutic approaches used in the treatment of CoViD19, the use of antiviral drugs has gained vast recognition despite evidence of the limited efficacy and the indications of possible safety precautions from clinical research. The treatments that influence the specific CoViD19 immune profile and the viral signaling mechanisms appear promising in CoViD19. The most commonly used treatments of CoViD19 include antivirals, glucocorticoids, and immunoglobulin.

The other drugs that modulate the immunopathogenesis of CoViD19 include agents that enhance lymphocytes (through NK cell-based therapy), immunomodulators, or convalescent plasma therapy or drugs that inhibit the inflammation (treatments based on mesenchymal stem cells (MSC) or the regulatory T (Treg) cells, the IL-6 signaling blockade, and inhibitors of Janus kinase (JAK)). Data from sound evidence base suggest that the use of dexamethasone can reduce the mortality in patients with severe CoViD19 [49], favoring the use of corticosteroids in CoViD19. Further data suggest that remdesivir, hydroxychloroquine, lopinavir/ritonavir, and interferon regimens have little or no effect on overall mortality, initiation of the ventilation, and duration of hospital stay among CoViD19 hospitalized patients [48].

Various stages of the CoViD19 are characterized by variations in the intensity and duration of complex immunological and inflammatory processes, warranting judicious use of anti-inflammatory and immunomodulatory drugs. Several strategies to counter the cytokine storm for the treatment of patients with CoViD19 exist in the literature. The impact of anti-inflammatory therapy in patients may vary, especially in the presence of pre-existing inflammatory conditions that may compromise optimized early immune response. The use of anti-inflammatory drugs in such patients in the early stage of CoViD19 may further compromise the innate immune response and may therefore be inappropriate. Furthermore, the argument that a swift production of type I interferon (IFNα/β) is associated with an early viral clearance may justify an early use of the antiviral drugs and other therapies to augment the IFNα/β to counter the cytokine storm early [156]. The treatment of CoViD19 patients may involve a variety of drug combinations. The appropriate use of the combination of antivirals and immunomodulators in the disease stage may result in better outcomes [157].

Overall, the main challenges associated with these treatments include judicious use of the drug in different stages of the disease and the timing of the therapeutic intervention, carefully selected patient population, optimal treatment duration, which are determinants of an efficient treatment strategy. Such a treatment strategy warrants a meticulous assessment of the clinical and laboratory parameters in making effective clinical decisions. Moreover, the therapeutic interventions in CoViD19 may be subject to limitations due to the cardiovascular safety of certain drugs and the interactions with drugs used in cardiovascular diseases (Table 5.4).

In patients with CoViD19, viral-induced immune impairment, hyper inflammation, and viral clearance are reflected by the clinical and pathological markers such as the viral load, markers of immune vulnerability (lymphocyte count, CD4 + and CD8 + T cell levels, signs of lymphocyte exhaustion, development of specific antibodies), require careful evaluation when immunosuppressors are considered [5]. The expert groups, such as the American Infectious Diseases Society [158], the Centers for Disease Control (CDC) [159], the World Health Organization (WHO) [160], the National Institute of Health (NIH) [161], and several other national societies have developed several CoViD19 treatment protocols and guidelines to help clinicians provide evidence-based best treatment options to the patients with CoViD19. Early use of antiviral drugs and interferon or combination therapies, timely suppression of inflammation, and early suppression of pro-inflammatory cytokines, improving antibodies and lymphopenia, are promising therapeutic tactics in CoViD19 [162–171].

The interim reports of CoViD19 vaccine trials require a cautious interpretation at this stage. The conventional route for evaluation of a pharmaceutical agent to the drug approval involves well-designed (randomized, blinded, and controlled), phase I to IV clinical trials in addition to the preclinical studies. The advanced phase trials assess efficacy and safety in the larger population. For instance, the phase III trials usually involve larger sample sizes, and phase IV (the post-marketing) trials help to answer the rare efficacy or safety issues. Patients in the real-world scenario may behave differently than in the trial population, may have different demographic, clinical, and disease characteristics, and may be treated differently. Therefore, the efficacy of the experimental drug may dilute. The expedited development of the CoViD19 vaccine may be subject to such limitations. For instance, the interim analysis of the phase III vaccine trial of the mRNA-1273 vaccine involves a limited number of subjects (95 confirmed cases of 30,000 (0.32%) in the report [49]. Several other limitations may exist in the report. These include the unavailability of the data related to baseline and follow-up immune genesis and the outcome of the immune system response. Further data about disease incidence or efficacy of the vaccine against genetic variants of SARS CoV2 that may exist globally or the extent of viral testing in the study subjects are also important. These limitations and several others, such as selection and population bias in the trial and a pending peer-reviewed publication, warrant a cautious interpretation of the published report.

Furthermore, novel platforms for the development of vaccines remain largely untested. These include replication-defective simian adenovirus or replication-defective human adenovirus type 26 (used to deliver recombinant SARS CoV2 spike (S) protein genes to human cells (ChAdOx1-S)), or others that use complex lipid delivery system that prevents rapid degradation of the mRNA by the extra-cellular ribonucleases (mRNA-1273 and BNT162 (b1/b2)) [148]. Further data from several ongoing studies on a variety of vaccine candidates tested globally will shed light on the efficacy, tolerability, and safety of the CoViD19 vaccines across populations worldwide in the future.

Summary Box

- Recent research has revealed the implication of a myriad of pathogenetic mechanisms that could serve as a possible therapeutic target for the CoViD19 treatment.
- Promising mechanisms as potential therapeutic targets include viral cell entry, viral assembly, or those influencing immune dysfunction.
- Notable CoViD19 therapeutic agents include antivirals, immunomodulators with anti-cytokines, immunity enhancers (antibodies/immunoglobulins), and adjunctive medicines such as anticoagulants, corticosteroids.
- Among the antivirals, the inhibitors of replication, membrane fusion, and assembly of SARS CoV2 include lopinavir-ritonavir, remdesevir, umifenovir, and others

- The drugs targeting viral entry mechanisms involving inhibitors of Transmembrane Protease/Serine Subfamily Member 2 (TMPRSS2) include camostat, nafamostat, or rhACE2 (recombinant ACE2).
- Hydroxychloroquine and azithromycin have not shown any significant benefits in the treatment of CoViD19, are associated with cardiac risk.
- Among the immune-based therapies targeting specific CoViD19 immune profile, include anti cytokines, immunomodulators, immunosuppressors, immunity enhancers (passive and active).
- Anticoagulants lower the risk of thromboembolism in patients with CoViD19; dual therapy with nafamostat and heparin appears to inhibit viral entry and target hypercoagulation.
- Protocols and guidelines have been published recommending the use of evidence-based treatments for patients with CoViD19 include IADS, NIH, CDC.
- Several drug regulatory agencies (The FDA of the US, the EMEA of Europe, the National Medical Products Administration (NMPA) of China) have issued emergency use, expanded access, or authorization for compassionate use for several drugs for CoViD19.
- The drugs received EUA (Emergency Use Authorization) from the FDA include remdesevir, convalescent plasma, baricitinib with remdesevir, bamlanivimab, and casirivimab, and imdevimab (combination use).
- The development of the CoViD19 vaccine has resulted in a significant breakthrough with rapidly evolving data and administration of vaccines in the UK, China, and Russia.
- Further research is needed to establish the efficacy and safety of antivirals, immunomodulators, anti-inflammatory agents, and drugs targeting viral cell entry mechanisms with multiple trials underway.

References

1. ClinicalTrials.gov. Prevention of Arteriovenous Thrombotic Events in Critically-Ill COVID19 Patients Trial (COVID-PACT). Identifier: NCT04409834. Last updated June 1, 2020. https://clinicaltrials.gov/ct2/show/NCT04409834.
2. Lurie N, Saville M, Hatchett R, Halton J. Developing CoViD19 Vaccines at Pandemic Speed. N Engl J Med. 2020;382(21):1969–73. https://doi.org/10.1056/NEJMp2005630.
3. Cao Bin et al. A trial of lopinavir–ritonavir in adults hospitalized with severe CoViD19. New England Journal of Medicine. 2020.
4. Horby Peter W et al. Lopinavir–ritonavir in patients admitted to hospital with COVID19 (RECOVERY): a randomised, controlled, open-label, platform trial. The Lancet. 2020;396.10259 (2020):1345–52.
5. Hung IF, Lung KC, Tso EY, et al. Triple combination of interferon beta-1b, lopinavir-ritonavir, and ribavirin in the treatment of patients admitted to hospital with

COVID19: an open-label, randomised, phase 2 trial. Lancet. 2020;395(10238):1695–704. https://doi.org/10.1016/S0140-6736(20)31042-4.
6. Grein J, Ohmagari N, Shin D, et al. Compassionate Use of Remdesivir for Patients with Severe CoViD19 [published online ahead of print, 2020 Apr 10]. N Engl J Med. 2020; NEJMoa2007016. doi:https://doi.org/10.1056/NEJMoa2007016.
7. Wang Y, Zhang D, Du G, et al. Remdesivir in adults with severe COVID19: a randomised, double-blind, placebo-controlled, multicentre trial [published correction appears in Lancet. 2020 May 30;395(10238):1694. Lancet. 2020;395(10236):1569–78. doi:https://doi.org/10.1016/S0140-6736(20)31022-9.
8. National Institute of Health (NIH). NIH clinical trial shows remdesivir accelerates recovery from advanced COVID19. https://www.niaid.nih.gov/news-events/nih-clinical-trial-shows-remdesivir-accelerates-recovery-advanced-CoViD19. Accessed May 6, 2020.
9. Wang Y, Zhang D, Du G, et al. Remdesivir in adults with severe COVID19: a randomised, double-blind, placebo-controlled, multicentre trial [published correction appears in Lancet. 2020 May 30; 395(10238):1694]. Lancet. 2020; 395(10236):1569–1578. doi:10.1016/S0140-6736(20)31022-9.
10. Beigel John H et al. Remdesivir for the Treatment of CoViD19-Preliminary Report. New Engl J Med. 2020.
11. Lian N, Xie H, Lin S, Huang J, Zhao J, Lin Q. Umifenovir treatment is not associated with improved outcomes in patients with coronavirus disease 2019: a retrospective study. Clin Microbiol Infect 2020; Apr 25. doi:https://doi.org/10.1016/j.cmi.2020.04.026.
12. Chen C, Zhang Y, Huang J, et al. Favipiravir versus arbidol for COVID19: a randomized clinical trial. medRxiv 2020; April 15. doi:https://doi.org/10.1101/2020.03.17.20037432.
13. Johnson & Johnson Services, Inc. Lack of evidence to support use of darunavir-based treatments for SARS CoV2. https://www.jnj.com/lack-of-evidence-to-support-darunavir-based-hiv-treatments-for-coronavirus. Accessed June 4, 2020.
14. Coronavirus FDA. Update: FDA Issues Emergency Use Authorization for Potential COVID19 Treatment, 2020 (2020). Coronavirus (COVID19) Update: FDA Issues Emergency Use Authorization for Potential COVID19 Treatment | FDA. Accessed on Dec 03 2020.
15. Hoffmann M, Kleine-Weber H, Schroeder S, Krüger N, Herrler T, Erichsen S, Schiergens TS, Herrler G, Wu NH, Nitsche A, Müller MA, Drosten C, Pöhlmann S. SARS-CoV-2 Cell Entry Depends on ACE2 and TMPRSS2 and Is Blocked by a Clinically Proven Protease Inhibitor. Cell. 2020 Mar 4. pii: S0092-8674(20)30229–4. doi: https://doi.org/10.1016/j.cell.2020.02.052.
16. Kawase M, Shirato K, van der Hoek L, Taguchi F, Matsuyama S. Simultaneous treatment of human bronchial epithelial cells with serine and cysteine protease inhibitors prevents severe acute respiratory syndrome coronavirus entry. J Virol. 2012;86:6537–45.
17. Bittmann S, et al. TMPRSS2-Inhibitors Play a role in Cell Entry Mechanism of COVID19: An Insight into Camostat and Nefamostat. J Regen Biol Med. 2020;2(2):1–3.
18. https://www.clinicaltrials.gov/ct2/show/NCT04418128?term=nafamostat&cond=Corona+Virus+Infection&draw=2&rank=1 ClinicalTrials.gov Identifier: NCT04418128. Last updated June 09,2020. Accessed on December 10, 2020.
19. https://www.clinicaltrials.gov/ct2/show/NCT04352400?term=nafamostat&cond=Corona+Virus+Infection&draw=2&rank=2 ClinicalTrials.gov Identifier: NCT04352400. Last updated April 20,2020. Accessed on December 10, 2020.
20. Zhang H, Penninger JM, Li Y, Zhong N, Slutsky AS. Angiotensin-converting enzyme 2 (ACE2) as a SARS CoV2 receptor: molecular mechanisms and potential therapeutic target. Inten Care Med. 2020;46(4):586–90. https://doi.org/10.1007/s00134-020-05985-9.
21. Haschke M, Schuster M, Poglitsch M, Loibner H, Salzberg M, Bruggisser M, Penninger J, Krahenbuhl S. Pharmacokinetics and pharmacodynamics of recombinant human angiotensin-converting enzyme 2 in healthy human subjects. Clin Pharmacokinet. 2013;52:783–92. https://doi.org/10.1007/s40262-013-0072-7.

22. Khan A, Benthin C, Zeno B, Albertson TE, Boyd J, Christie JD, Hall R, Poirier G, Ronco JJ, Tidswell M, et al. A pilot clinical trial of recombinant human angiotensin-converting enzyme 2 in acute respiratory distress syndrome. Crit Care. 2017;21:234. https://doi.org/10.1186/s13054-017-1823-x.
23. Zhang H, Baker A. Recombinant human ACE2: acing out angiotensin II in ARDS therapy. Crit Care. 2017;21:305. https://doi.org/10.1186/s13054-017-1882-z.
24. Liu T, Luo S, Libby P, Shi GP. Cathepsin L-selective inhibitors: A potentially promising treatment for COVID19 patients [published online ahead of print, 2020 May 26]. Pharmacol Ther. 2020;107587. doi: https://doi.org/10.1016/j.pharmthera.2020.107587.
25. Zhao MM, Yang WL, Yang FY, Zhang L, Huang WJ, Hou W, Fan CF, Jin RH, Feng YM, Wang YC, Yang JK. Cathepsin L plays a key role in SARS-CoV-2 infection in humans and humanized mice and is a promising target for new drug development. Signal Transduction and Targeted Therapy. 2021;6(1):1–12.
26. Wang Ke et al. SARS CoV2 invades host cells via a novel route: CD147-spike protein. BioRxiv. 2020.
27. Richardson Peter et al. Baricitinib as potential treatment for 2019-nCoV acute respiratory disease. Lancet (London, England). 2020;395.10223:e30.
28. Ojha PK, Kar S, Krishna JG, Roy K, Leszczynski J. Therapeutics for COVID19: from computation to practices—where we are, where we are heading to. Molec Div. 2020;1–35.
29. Zhou D, Dai SM, Tong Q. COVID19: a recommendation to examine the effect of hydroxychloroquine in preventing infection and progression. J Antimicrob Chemother. 2020;75(7):1667–70.
30. Wang M, Cao R, Zhang L, Yang X, Liu J, Xu M, Shi Z, Hu Z, Zhong W, Xiao G. Remdesivir and chloroquine effectively inhibit the recently emerged novel coronavirus (2019-nCoV) in vitro Cell Res. 2020;1–3. https://doi.org/10.1038/s41422-020-0282-0.
31. Salata C, Calistri A, Parolin C, Baritussio A, Palù G. Antiviral activity of cationic amphiphilic drugs. Expert Rev Anti Infect Ther. 2017;15:483–92. https://doi.org/10.1080/14787210.2017.1305888pmid:28286997.
32. Tang TT, Lv LL, Pan MM, Wen Y, Wang B, Li ZL, Wu M, Wang FM, Crowley SD, Liu BC. Hydroxychloroquine attenuates renal ischemia/reperfusion injury by inhibiting cathepsin mediated NLRP3 inflammasome activation. Cell Death Dis. 2018;9:351.
33. Shivanna V, Kim Y, Chang KO. Endosomal acidification and cathepsin L activity is required for calicivirus replication. Virology. 2014;464–465:287–295; Wang et al., 2020a.
34. Goulet B, Baruch A, Moon NS, Poirier M, Sansregret LL, Erickson A, Bogyo M, Nepveu A. A cathepsin L isoform that is devoid of a signal peptide localizes to the nucleus in S phase and processes the CDP/Cux transcription factor. Mol Cell. 2004;14:207–19.
35. Mauthe M, Orhon I, Rocchi C, Zhou X, Luhr M, Hijlkema KJ, Coppes RP, Engedal N, Mari M, Reggiori F. Chloroquine inhibits autophagic flux by decreasing autophagosome-lysosome fusion. Autophagy. 2018;14(8):1435–1455.
36. Xueting Yao, Fei Ye, Miao Zhang, Cheng Cui, Baoying Huang, Peihua Niu, Xu Liu, Li Zhao, Erdan Dong, Chunli Song, Siyan Zhan, Roujian Lu, Haiyan Li, Wenjie Tan, Dongyang Liu. In Vitro antiviral activity and projection of optimized dosing design of hydroxychloroquine for the treatment of severe acute respiratory syndrome coronavirus 2 (SARS CoV2). Clin Infec Dis. ciaa237. https://doi.org/10.1093/cid/ciaa237.
37. Vincent MJ, Bergeron E, Benjannet S, et al. Chloroquine is a potent inhibitor of SARS coronavirus infection and spread. Virol J. 2005;2:69. Doi:https://doi.org/10.1186/1743-422X-2-69 pmid:16115318.
38. Boone BA, Murthy P, Miller-Ocuin J, Doerfer WR, Ellis JT, Liang X, Ross MA, Wallace CT, Sperry JL, Lotze MT, Neal MD, Zeh HJ 3rd. Chloroquine reduces hypercoagulability in pancreatic cancer through inhibition of neutrophil extracellular traps. BMC Cancer. 2018;18:678.
39. Letter to Dr Rick Bright re: request for Emergency Use Authorization for use of chloroquine phosphate or hydroxychloroquine sulfate supplied from the strategic national stockpile for

treatment of 2019 coronavirus disease. Published March 28, 2020. Accessed August 3, 2020. https://www.fda.gov/media/136534/download.
40. National Health Commission of the People's Republic of China. COVID-19 Treatment Guideline, the 8th Edition 2020.essed 2 Mar 2021.
41. https://www.fda.gov/emergency-preparedness-and-response/mcm-legal-regulatory-and-policy-framework/emergency-use-authorization.
42. Wang Manli et al. Remdesivir and chloroquine effectively inhibit the recently emerged novel coronavirus (2019-nCoV) in vitro. Cell Res. 2020;30(3):269–271. doi:https://doi.org/10.1038/s41422-020-0282-0.
43. Million M, Lagier JC, Gautret P, et al. Early treatment of COVID19 patients with hydroxychloroquine and azithromycin: a retrospective analysis of 1061 cases in Marseille, France [published online ahead of print, 2020 May 5 Travel Med Infect Dis. 2020;101738. doi:https://doi.org/10.1016/j.tmaid.2020.101738.
44. Gautret P, Lagier JC, Parola P, et al. Clinical and microbiological effect of a combination of hydroxychloroquine and azithromycin in 80 CoViD19 patients with at least a six-day follow up: a pilot observational study. Travel Med Infect Dis. 2020;34. https://doi.org/10.1016/j.tmaid.2020.101663pmid:32289548.
45. Mahévas M, Tran V-T, Roumier M, et al. Clinical efficacy of hydroxychloroquine in patients with CoViD19 pneumonia who require oxygen: observational comparative study using routine care data. BMJ. 2020;369:m1844. doi:https://doi.org/10.1136/bmj.m1844 pmid:32409486.
46. Rosenberg ES, Dufort EM, Udo T, et al. Association of Treatment With Hydroxychloroquine or Azithromycin With In-Hospital Mortality in Patients With COVID19 in New York State. JAMA. Published online May 11, 2020. doi:https://doi.org/10.1001/jama.2020.8630.
47. Tang Wei, Cao Zhujun, Han Mingfeng, Wang Zhengyan, Chen Junwen, Sun Wenjin et al. Hydroxychloroquine in patients with mainly mild to moderate coronavirus disease 2019: open label, randomised controlled trial. BMJ. 2020;369:m1849.
48. Cavalcanti Alexandre B et al. Hydroxychloroquine with or without Azithromycin in Mild-to-Moderate CoViD19. New England J Med. 2020;383(21):2041–2052.
49. Horby Peter et al. Dexamethasone in hospitalized patients with CoViD19-preliminary report. The New England Journal of Medicine. 2020.
50. Horby Peter et al. Effect of Hydroxychloroquine in Hospitalized Patients with COVID19: preliminary results from a multi-centre, randomized, controlled trial. MedRxiv. 2020.
51. National Institutes of Health (NIH) NIH halts clinical trial of hydroxychloroquine NIH (20 June 2020). https://www.nih.gov/news-events/news-releases/nih-halts-clinical-trial-hydroxychloroquine. Accessed 01 December 2020.
52. World Health Organization. WHO discontinues hydroxychloroquine and lopinavir/ritonavir treatment arms for COVID19. Geneva, Switzerland: WHO. Available at: https://www.who.int/news-room/detail/04-07-2020-who-discontinueshydroxychloroquine-and-lopinavir-ritonavir-treatment-arms-forCoViD19. Accessed July 6 (2020):2020
53. Mitjà Oriol et al. Hydroxychloroquine for early treatment of adults with mild CoViD19: a randomized-controlled trial. Clinical Infectious Diseases. 2020.
54. Skipper Caleb P et al. Hydroxychloroquine in nonhospitalized adults with early COVID19: a randomized trial. Ann Int Med. 2020;173.8:623–631.
55. Geleris J, Sun Y, Platt J, et al. Observational study of hydroxychloroquine in hospitalized patients with CoViD19. N Engl J Med. 2020. https://doi.org/10.1056/NEJMoa2012410 pmid:32379955.
56. Borba MGS, Val FFA, Sampaio VS, et al. Chloroquine diphosphate in two different dosages as adjunctive therapy of hospitalized patients with severe respiratory syndrome in the context of coronavirus (SARS CoV2) infection: Preliminary safety results of a randomized, double-blinded, phase IIb clinical trial (CloroCoViD19 Study). medRxiv [Preprint] 2020. doi:https://doi.org/10.1101/2020.04.07.20056424.

57. Chorin E, Dai M, Shulman E, et al. The QT interval in patients with COVID19 treated with hydroxychloroquine and azithromycin [published online ahead of print, 2020 Apr 24]. Nat Med. 2020;https://doi.org/10.1038/s41591-020-0888-2. doi:https://doi.org/10.1038/s41591-020-0888-2.
58. Ray WA, Murray KT, Hall K, Arbogast PG, Stein CM. Azithromycin and the risk of cardiovascular death. N Engl J Med. 2012;366(20):1881–90. https://doi.org/10.1056/NEJMoa1003833.
59. Mercuro Nicholas J et al. Risk of QT interval prolongation associated with use of hydroxychloroquine with or without concomitant azithromycin among hospitalized patients testing positive for coronavirus disease 2019 (COVID19). JAMA cardiology. 2020.
60. Eliesbik. Thoughts on the Gautret et al. paper about Hydroxychloroquine and Azithromycin treatment of COVID19 infections. Science Integrity Digest. 2020. https://scienceintegritydigest.com/2020/03/24/thoughts-on-the-gautret-et. Accessed 17 May 2020, https://pubpeer.com/publications/B4044A446F35DF81789F6F20F8E0EE.
61. Emani Venkata R et al. Randomized controlled trials for COVID19: evaluation of optimal randomization methodologies-need for the data validation of the completed trials, and to improve the ongoing and future randomized trial designs. Int J Antim Agents.2020;106222.
62. Hernandez, Adrian V., et al. "Update alert: hydroxychloroquine or chloroquine for the treatment or prophylaxis of COVID19." *Annals of internal medicine* 173.4 (2020): W78-W79.
63. Tang Wei, Cao Zhujun, Han Mingfeng, Wang Zhengyan, Chen Junwen, Sun Wenjin et al. Hydroxychloroquine in patients with mainly mild to moderate coronavirus disease 2019: open label, randomised controlled trial BMJ. 2020;369:m1849.
64. Alexander PE, Debono VB, Mammen MJ, et al. COVID19 coronavirus research has overall low methodological quality thus far: case in point for chloroquine/hydroxychloroquine [published online ahead of print, 2020 Apr 21]. J Clin Epidemiol. 2020;S0895–4356(20):30371–1. doi:https://doi.org/10.1016/j.jclinepi.2020.04.016.
65. Ferner Robin E, Aronson Jeffrey K. Chloroquine and hydroxychloroquine in CoViD19. BMJ. 2020;369:m1432.
66. Skipper Caleb P et al. Hydroxychloroquine in nonhospitalized adults with early COVID19: a randomized trial. Annals Int Med. 2020;173(8):623631.
67. Hernandez Adrian V et al. Update alert 2: hydroxychloroquine or chloroquine for the treatment or prophylaxis of COVID19. Annals Int Med. 2020;173(7):W128–9.
68. Schluger NW. The saga of hydroxychloroquine and COVID19: a cautionary tale. Ann Intern Med. 2020;173(8):662–3.
69. ClincalTrials.gov. Open Label Study to Compare Efficacy, Safety and Tolerability of Hydroxychloroquine Combined With Azithromycin Compared to Hydroxychloroquine Combined With Camostat Mesylate and to "no Treatment" in SARS CoV2 Virus (COSTA). Identifier NCT04355052. Last updated April 21, 2020. https://clinicaltrials.gov/ct2/show/NCT04355052.
70. ClincalTrials.gov. Combination Therapy With Camostat Mesilate + Hydroxychloroquine for COVID19 (CLOCC). Identifier NCT04338906. Last updated Apr 08. 2020. https://clinicaltrials.gov/ct2/show/NCT04338906.
71. Clinicaltrial.gov. Evaluating the efficacy of hydroxychloroquine and azithromycin to prevent hospitalization or death in persons with CoViD19. 2020. https://clinicaltrials.gov/ct2/show/NCT04358068.
72. http://www.isrctn.com/ISRCTN86534580 PRINCIPLE: a trial evaluating treatments for suspected COVID19 in people aged 50 years and above with pre-existing conditions and those aged 65 years and above. ISRCTN86534580, https://doi.org/10.1186/ISRCTN86534580. Last updated/05/2020.
73. Crisafulli Salvatore et al. Potential role of anti-interleukin (IL)-6 drugs in the treatment of COVID19: rationale, clinical evidence and risks. BioDrugs. 34(4):415–22.

74. ClinicalTrials.gov. Tocilizumab in COVID19 Pneumonia (TOCIVID-19) (TOCIVID19). Identifier: NCT04317092. Last updated April 7, 2020. https://www.clinicap-;/ltrials.gov/ct2/show/NCT04317092.
75. ClinicalTrials.gov.Tocilizumab vs CRRT in Management of Cytokine Release Syndrome (CRS) in COVID19 (TACOS). Identifier: NCT04306705. Last updated March 17, 2020. https://clinicaltrials.gov/ct2/show/NCT04306705.
76. Anti Interlukin-6 Receptor mAB. Accessed on December 4, 2020. http://www.tizianalifesciences.com/drug-pipeline/anti-il-6r/.
77. ClinicalTrials.gov. Tocilizumab for SARS-CoV2 Severe Pneumonitis. Identifier: NCT04315480. Last updated April 13, 2020. https://clinicaltrials.gov/ct2/show/NCT04315480.
78. ClinicalTrials.gov. Evaluation of the Efficacy and Safety of Sarilumab in Hospitalized Patients With COVID19. Identifier: NCT04315298. Last updated April 6, 2020. https://www.clinicaltrials.gov/ct2/show/NCT04315298.
79. ClinicalTrials.gov. Study on the Use of Sarilumab in Patients With COVID19 Infection. Identifier: NCT04386239. Last updates May 13, 2020. https://clinicaltrials.gov/ct2/show/NCT04386239. Anti Interlukin-6 Receptor mAB Tiziana Life Sciences Accessed on 4 December 2020).
80. Alattar Rand et al. Tocilizumab for the Treatment of Severe COVID-19. J Med Virol. 2020.
81. Sciascia S, et al. Pilot prospective open, single-arm multicentre study on off-label use of tocilizumab in severe patients with COVID19. Clin Exp Rheumatol. 2020;38(3):529–32.
82. Xu Xiaoling et al. Effective treatment of severe COVID19 patients with tocilizumab. Proc Nat Acad Sci. 2020;117(20):10970–5.
83. Biran Noa et al. Tocilizumab among patients with COVID19 in the intensive care unit: a multicentre observational study. Lancet Rheumatol. 2020;2(10):e603–12.
84. Roche. Roche provides an update on the phase III COVACTA trial of Actemra/RoActemra in hospitalised patients with severe COVID19 associated pneumonia. [cited 2020 Jul 29]. Available from: https://www.roche.com/investors/updates/inv-update-2020-07-29.htm.
85. Furlow Bryant. COVACTA trial raises questions about tocilizumab's benefit in COVID19. Lancet Rheum. 2020;2(10):e592.
86. Zhou Zeyun, Christina C Price. Overview on the use of IL-6 agents in the treatment of patients with cytokine release syndrome (CRS) and pneumonitis related to COVID19 disease. Expert opinion on investigational drugs. 2020.
87. Villar Jesús et al. Dexamethasone treatment for the acute respiratory distress syndrome: a multicentre, randomised controlled trial. Lancet Resp Med. 2020;8(3):267–76.
88. Hung Ivan Fan-Ngai et al. Triple combination of interferon beta-1b, lopinavir-ritonavir, and ribavirin in the treatment of patients admitted to hospital with COVID19: an open-label, randomised, phase 2 trial. Lancet (London, England). 2020;395(10238):1695–1704. doi: https://doi.org/10.1016/S0140-6736(20)31042-4.
89. Fernandez-Cruz Ana et al. Impact of glucocorticoid treatment in sars cov2 infection mortality: a retrospective controlled cohort study. medrxiv. 2020.
90. NIH COVID19 treatment guidelines. NIH. https://www.covid19treatmentguidelines.nih.gov/whats-new/ Updated on December 03 2020 Accessed on December 11, 2020.
91. Wu Dandan, Xuexian O Yang. TH17 responses in cytokine storm of COVID19: an emerging target of JAK2 inhibitor Fedratinib. J Microb Immunol Infect. 2020. ClinicalTrials.gov Identifier: NCT04640168 Last updated on November 23, 2020. Accessed on December 10, 2020.
92. https://www.clinicaltrials.gov/ct2/show/NCT04421027?term=baricitinib&cond=Corona+Virus+Infection&draw=2&rank=3 ClinicalTrials.gov Identifier: NCT04421027. Last updated on June 09, 2020. Accessed on December 10, 2020.
93. https://www.clinicaltrials.gov/ct2/show/NCT04640168?term=baricitinib&cond=Corona+Virus+Infection&draw=2&rank=5 ClinicalTrials.gov Identifier: NCT04640168 Last updated on Accessed on November 23, 2020. December 10, 2020.

94. https://www.clinicaltrials.gov/ct2/show/NCT04452565?term=dexamethasone&cond=COVID19&draw=5&rank=13 ClinicalTrials.gov Identifier: NCT04452565. Last updated on September 07, 2020. Accessed on December 11, 2020.
95. https://www.clinicaltrials.gov/ct2/show/NCT04509973?term=dexamethasone&cond=COVID19&draw=6&rank=4 ClinicalTrials.gov Identifier: NCT04509973. Last updated on September 01, 2020. Accessed on December 11, 2020.
96. Chen Long et al. Convalescent plasma as a potential therapy for COVID19. Lanc Infect Dis. 2020;20(4):398–400.
97. https://www.fda.gov/vaccines-blood-biologics/investigational-new-drug-ind-or-device-exemption-ide-process-cber/recommendations-investigational-CoViD19-convalescent-plasma.
98. Food and Drug Administration. EUA 26382: Emergency Use Authorization (EUA) decision memo. 2020. Available at: https://www.fda.gov/media/141480/download. Accessed December 07, 2020.
99. https://www.fda.gov/news-events/press-announcements/coronavirus-CoViD19-update-fda-authorizes-monoclonal-antibody-treatment-CoViD19 Immediate Release: November 09, 2020 Accessed on December 07 2020.
100. U.S. Food and Drug Administration. Letter of FDA Emergency Use Authorization to Eli Lilly and Company dated November 10, 2020. In: Phillips C, Eli Lilly and Company, 2020.
101. https://www.fda.gov/media/143891/download Issued on November 21, 2020 Accessed on December 09, 2020.
102. Galeotti Caroline, Srini V Kaveri, Jagadeesh Bayry. Intravenous immunoglobulin immunotherapy for coronavirus disease-19 (COVID-19). Clin Transl immunol. 2020;9(10):e1198.
103. https://www.clinicaltrials.gov/ct2/show/NCT04432324?term=IVIG&cond=Corona+Virus+Infection&draw=2&rank=1 ClinicalTrials.gov Identifier: NCT04432324. Last updated on October 12, 2020. Accessed on December 09, 2020.
104. https://www.clinicaltrials.gov/ct2/show/NCT04480424?term=IVIG&cond=Corona+Virus+Infection&draw=2&rank=3 ClinicalTrials.gov Identifier: NCT04480424. Last updated on November 24, 2020. Accessed on December 10, 2020.
105. https://www.clinicaltrials.gov/ct2/show/NCT04521309?term=IVIG&cond=Corona+Virus+Infection&draw=2&rank=4 ClinicalTrials.gov Identifier: NCT04521309. Last updated on November 27, 2020. Accessed on December 10, 2020 https://www.clinicaltrials.gov/ct2/show/NCT04546581?term=IVIG&cond=Corona+Virus+Infection&phase=2&draw=2&rank=1 ClinicalTrials.gov Identifier: NCT04546581. Last updated on December 09, 2020. Accessed on December 10, 2020.
106. Bergeron-Lafaurie A, Azoulay E, Peffault de Latour R, Assistance Publique - Hôpitaux de Paris. CORIMUNO19-ECU: Trial Evaluating Efficacy and Safety of Eculizumab (Soliris) in Patients With COVID19 Infection, Nested in the CORIMUNO-19 Cohort (CORIMUNO19-ECU). Available at: https://clinicaltrials.gov/ct2/show/NCT04346797 ClinicalTrials.gov Identifier: NCT04346797 Last updated on April 27, 2020 Accessed on December 07, 2020.
107. Administration of Intravenous Vitamin C in Novel Coronavirus Infection (COVID19) and Decreased Oxygenation - Full Text View - ClinicalTrials.gov ClinicalTrials.gov Identifier: NCT04357782. Last updated on September 18, 2020. Accessed on December 10, 2020.
108. Paniri Alireza, Haleh Akhavan-Niaki. Emerging role of IL-6 and NLRP3 inflammasome as potential therapeutic targets to combat COVID19: role of lncRNAs in cytokine storm modulation. Life Sci. 2020;118114.
109. Zhang Wen et al. The use of anti-inflammatory drugs in the treatment of people with severe coronavirus disease 2019 (COVID19): the experience of clinical immunologists from China. Clin Immunol. 2020;108393.
110. Lin L et al. An NLRP3 inflammasome-triggered cytokine storm contributes to streptococcal toxic shock-like syndrome (STSLS). PLoS Pathog. 2019;15.
111. Chen Guang et al. Clinical and immunological features of severe and moderate coronavirus disease 2019. J Clin Invest. 2020;130(5).

112. Pedersen Savannah F, Ya-Chi Ho. SARS CoV2: a storm is raging. J Clin Invest. 2020;130 (5).
113. Chen C et al. Thalidomide combined with low-dose glucocorticoid in the treatment of COVID19 Pneumonia. 1–6 (2020). Preprints.
114. Nabirotchkin S, Peluffo AE, Bouaziz J, Cohen D. Focusing on the Unfolded Protein Response and Autophagy Related Pathways to Reposition Common Approved Drugs against COVID19. Preprints 2020, 2020030302. doi: https://doi.org/10.20944/preprints202003.0302.v1.
115. Saeedi-Boroujeni A, Mahmoudian-Sani MR, Nashibi R, Houshmandfar S, Tahmaseby Gandomkari S, Khodadadi A. Tranilast: a potential anti-Inflammatory and NLRP3 inflammasome inhibitor drug for COVID19. Immunoph Immunotoxic. 2021;1–12.
116. Cavalli G, De Luca G, Campochiaro C, Della-Torre E, Ripa M, Canetti D, Oltolini C, Castiglioni B, Din CT, Boffini N, Tomelleri A. Interleukin-1 blockade with high-dose anakinra in patients with COVID19, acute respiratory distress syndrome, and hyperinflammation: a retrospective cohort study. Lancet Rheumat. 2020;2(6):e325–31.
117. Tan HY, Yong YK, Shankar EM, Paukovics G, Ellegård R, Larsson M, Kamarulzaman A, French MA, Crowe SM. Aberrant inflammasome activation characterizes tuberculosis-associated immune reconstitution inflammatory syndrome. J Immunol. 2016;196(10):4052–63.
118. Abderrazak A, Couchie D, Mahmood DFD, Elhage R, Vindis C, Laffargue M, Matéo V, Büchele B, Ayala MR, El Gaafary M, Syrovets T. Anti-inflammatory and antiatherogenic effects of the NLRP3 inflammasome inhibitor arglabin in ApoE2. Ki mice fed a high-fat diet. Circulation. 2015;131(12):1061–70.
119. Freeman TL, Swartz TH. Targeting the NLRP3 inflammasome in severe COVID19. Front Immun. 2020;11:1518.
120. Li B, Liu Y, Hu T, Zhang Y, Zhang C, Li T, Wang C, Dong Z, Novakovic VA, Hu T, Shi J. Neutrophil extracellular traps enhance procoagulant activity in patients with oral squamous cell carcinoma. J Cancer Res Clin Oncol. 2019;145:1695–707.
121. Brinkmann Volker et al. Neutrophil extracellular traps kill bacteria. Science. 2004;303 (5663):1532–5.
122. Narasaraju Teluguakula et al. Excessive neutrophils and neutrophil extracellular traps contribute to acute lung injury of influenza pneumonitis. Am J Pathol. 2011;179(1):199–210.
123. Fuchs Tobias A et al. Extracellular DNA traps promote thrombosis. Proc Nat Acad Sci. 2010;107(36):15880–5.
124. Massberg Steffen et al. Reciprocal coupling of coagulation and innate immunity via neutrophil serine proteases. Nat Med. 2010;16(8):887–96.
125. Zuo Y, Yalavarthi S, Shi H, Gockman K, Zuo M, Madison JA, Blair CN, Weber A, Barnes BJ, Egeblad M, Woods RJ, Kanthi Y, Knight JS. Neutrophil extracellular traps in COVID19. JCI Insight. 2020. https://doi.org/10.1172/jci.insig ht.138999.
126. Nakazawa F, Kannemeier C, Shibamiya A, Song Y, Tzima E, Schubert U, Koyama T, Niepmann M, Trusheim H, Engelmann B, Preissner KT. Extracellular RNA is a natural cofactor for the (auto-)activation of factor VII-activating protease (FSAP). Biochem J. 2005;385:831–8.
127. Manfredi AA, Rovere-Querini P, D'Angelo A, Maugeri N. Low molecular weight heparins prevent the induction of autophagy of activated neutrophils and the formation of neutrophil extracellular traps. Pharmacol Res. 2017;123:146–56.
128. Zhang G, Zhang X, Huang H, Ji Y, Li D, Jiang W. Saquinavir plus methylprednisolone ameliorates experimental acute lung injury. Brazil J Med Biol Res. 2018;51(10).
129. Uozumi R, Iguchi R, Masuda S, Nishibata Y, Nakazawa D, Tomaru U, Ishizu A. Pharmaceutical immunoglobulins reduce neutrophil extracellular trap formation and ameliorate the development of MPO-ANCA-associated vasculitis. Mod Rheumat. 2019.
130. Cicco S, Cicco G, Racanelli V, Vacca A. Neutrophil extracellular traps (NETs) and damage-associated molecular patterns (DAMPs): two potential targets for COVID19 treatment. Med Inflam. 2020.

131. ClinicalTrials.gov. CoViD19: Possible Role of Neutrophil Extracellular Traps (NETSINCOVID) Identifier: NCT04412382. Last updated June 02, 2020.
132. Delaveris CS, Wilk AJ, Riley NM, Stark JC, Yang SS, Rogers AJ, Ranganath T, Nadeau KC, Stanford COVID19 Biobank, Blish CA, Bertozzi CR. Synthetic Siglec-9 agonists inhibit neutrophil activation associated with COVID19. ACS Cent Sci. 2021;7(4):650–7.
133. Tang Ning et al. Anticoagulant treatment is associated with decreased mortality in severe coronavirus disease 2019 patients with coagulopathy. J Thromb Haemost. 2020;18(5):1094–9.
134. Connors JM, Levy JH. COVID19 and its implications for thrombosis and anticoagulation. Blood J Am Soc Hematol. 2020;135(23):2033–40.
135. Cuker A, Tseng EK, Nieuwlaat R, Angchaisuksiri P, Blair C, Dane K, Davila J, DeSancho MT, Diuguid D, Griffin DO, Kahn SR. American Society of Hematology 2021 guidelines on the use of anticoagulation for thromboprophylaxis in patients with COVID19. Blood Adv. 2021;5(3):872–88.
136. Poterucha TJ, Libby P, Goldhaber SZ. More than an anticoagulant: do heparins have direct anti-inflammatory effects? Thromb Haemost. 2017;117(03):437–44.
137. Mycroft-West CJ, Su D, Elli S, Li Y, Guimond SE, Miller GJ, Turnbull JE, Yates EA, Guerrini M, Fernig DG, de Lima MA. The 2019 coronavirus (SARS CoV2) surface protein (Spike) S1 Receptor Binding Domain undergoes conformational change upon heparin binding. BioRxiv. 2020.
138. Mummery RS, Rider CC. Characterization of the heparin-binding properties of IL-6. J Immunol. 2000;165(10):5671–9.
139. Tang N, Bai H, Chen X, Gong J, Li D, Sun Z. Anticoagulant treatment is associated with decreased mortality in severe coronavirus disease 2019 patients with coagulopathy. J Thromb Haemost. 2020;18:1094–9. https://doi.org/10.1111/jth.14817.
140. URL: https://www.clinicaltrials.gov. Unique identifier: NCT03712228.
141. Maas C, Renné T. Coagulation factor XII in thrombosis and inflammation. Blood. 2018;131(17):1903–9.
142. Ouyang Y, Wang Y, Liu B, Ma X, Ding R. Effects of antiplatelet therapy on the mortality rate of patients with sepsis: a meta-analysis. J Crit Care. 2019;50:162–8.
143. Wang Y, Ouyang Y, Liu B, Ma X, Ding R. Platelet activation and antiplatelet therapy in sepsis: a narrative review. Thromb Res. 2018;166:28–36.
144. Wang L, Li H, Gu X, Wang Z, Liu S, Chen L. Effect of antiplatelet therapy on acute respiratory distress syndrome and mortality in critically ill patients: a meta-analysis. PLoS One. 2016;11(5):e0154754.
145. Liu Xiaoyan et al. Potential therapeutic effects of dipyridamole in the severely ill patients with COVID19. Acta Pharmaceutica Sinica B. 2020.
146. Whyte Claire S et al. Fibrinolytic abnormalities in acute respiratory distress syndrome (ARDS) and versatility of thrombolytic drugs to treat COVID-19. J Thromb Haemost. 2020.
147. Asakura H, Ogawa H. Potential of heparin and nafamostat combination therapy for COVID-19. J Thromb Haemost. 2020;18(6):1521–2.
148. https://www.clinicaltrials.gov/ct2/show/NCT04352400?term=NCT04352400&draw=2&rank=1. NCT04352400. Last updated on Apr 20 2020, accessed on December 07, 2020.
149. Russo V, Di Maio M, Attena E, Silverio A, Scudiero F, Celentani D, Lodigiani C, Di Micco P. Clinical impact of pre-admission antithrombotic therapy in hospitalized patients with COVID19: a multicenter observational study. Pharmacol Res. 2020;159:104965.
150. Parker Edward PK, Madhumita Shrotri, Beate Kampmann. Keeping track of the SARS CoV2 vaccine pipeline. Nat Rev Immunol. 2020;20(11):650.
151. COVID19 vaccine tracker. London School of Hygiene and Tropical Medicine. https://vac-lshtm.shinyapps.io/ncov_vaccine_landscape/ Accessed on December 07, 2020
152. https://www.pfizer.com/news/press-release/press-release-detail/pfizer-and-biontech-achieve-first-authorization-world.

153. NEWS/ Pfizer and BioNTech Achieve First Authorization in the World for a Vaccine to Combat COVID19. PFIZER AND BIONTECH ACHIEVE FIRST AUTHORIZATION IN THE WORLD FOR A VACCINE TO COMBAT COVID19 Published on December 02, 2020. https://www.pfizer.com/news/press-release/press-release-detail/pfizer-and-biontech-achieve-first-authorization-world. Accessed on December 07, 2020.
154. Moderna's COVID19 Vaccine Candidate Meets its Primary Efficacy Endpoint in the First Interim Analysis of the Phase 3 COVE Study. Moderna. Published on November 16, 2020. https://investors.modernatx.com/news-releases/news-release-details/modernas-CoViD19-vaccine-candidate-meets-its-primary-efficacy. Accessed on December 07 2020.
155. Dose-Confirmation Study to Evaluate the Safety, Reactogenicity, and Immunogenicity of mRNA-1273 COVID19 Vaccine in Adults Aged 18 Years and Older. https://www.clinicaltrials.gov/ct2/results?cond=&term=NCT04405076&cntry=&state=&city=&dist= Last updated on July 10, 2020. ClinicalTrials.gov number, NCT04405076 Accessed on December 07, 2020.
156. Jackson Lisa A et al. An mRNA vaccine against SARS CoV2—preliminary report. New England J Med. 2020;383(20):1920–31.
157. Folegatti Pedro M et al. Safety and immunogenicity of the ChAdOx1 nCoV-19 vaccine against SARS CoV2: a preliminary report of a phase 1/2, single-blind, randomised controlled trial. The Lancet. 2020;396(10249):467–78.
158. AZD1222 vaccine met primary efficacy endpoint in preventing COVID19. Published on 23 November 2020. https://www.astrazeneca.com/media-centre/press-releases/2020/azd1222hlr.html Accessed on December 07 2020.
159. THE FIRST INTERIM DATA ANALYSIS OF THE SPUTNIK V VACCINE AGAINST COVID19 PHASE III CLINICAL TRIALS IN THE RUSSIAN FEDERATION DEMONSTRATED 92% EFFICACY. Moscow, 11.11.2020. https://sputnikvaccine.com/newsroom/pressreleases/the-first-interim-data-analysis-of-the-sputnik-v-vaccine-against-CoViD19-phase-iii-clinical-trials-/ Accessed on December 07 2020.
160. Health News. Reuters. Published on June 29 2020. https://uk.reuters.com/article/us-health-coronavirus-china-vaccine/cansinos-CoViD19-vaccine-candidate-approved-for-military-use-in-china-idUKKBN2400DZ Accessed on December 07, 2020.
161. Zhu Feng-Cai et al. Immunogenicity and safety of a recombinant adenovirus type-5-vectored COVID19 vaccine in healthy adults aged 18 years or older: a randomised, double-blind, placebo-controlled, phase 2 trial. The Lancet. 2020;396(10249):479–88.
162. World Health Organization. Therapeutics and COVID19: living guideline, 20 November 2020. No. WHO/2019-nCov/remdesivir/2020.1. World Health Organization, 2020.
163. Feuillet Vincent, Bruno Canard, Alain Trautmann. Combining antivirals and immunomodulators to fight COVID19. Trends in Immunology. 2020.
164. Hung IF, Lung KC, Tso EY et al. Triple combination of interferon beta-1b, lopinavir-ritonavir, and ribavirin in the treatment of patients admitted to hospital with COVID19: an open-label, randomised, phase 2 trial. Lancet. 2020;395(10238):1695–704. https://doi.org/10.1016/S0140-6736(20)31042-4.
165. De Stefano Ludovico et al. A "Window of Therapeutic Opportunity" for Anti-Cytokine therapy in patients with coronavirus disease 2019. Front Immunol. 2020;11:2645.
166. Infectious Diseases Society of America Guidelines on the Treatment and Management of Patients with COVID19 (idsociety.org) Published by IDSA on 4/11/2020. Last updated, 12/2/2020 Accessed December 07, 2020.
167. Interim Clinical Guidance for Management of Patients with Confirmed Coronavirus Disease (COVID19) Updated November 03, 2020 https://www.cdc.gov/coronavirus/2019-ncov/hcp/clinical-guidance-management-patients.html Accessed December 07, 2020.
168. Clinical management of COVID19 Interim guidance 27 May 2020 COVID19: Clinical care https://www.who.int/publications/i/item/clinical-management-of-CoViD19. Last accessed December 07, 2020.
169. Coronavirus Disease 2019 (COVID19) Treatment Guidelines. https://www.covid19treatmentguidelines.nih.gov/ Last Updated: July 17, 2020 Accessed December 07, 2020.

170. Moderna's COVID19 Vaccine Candidate Meets its Primary Efficacy Endpoint in the First Interim Analysis of the Phase 3 COVE Study. Moderna. Published on November 16, 2020. https://investors.modernatx.com/news-releases/news-release-details/modernas-CoViD19-vaccine-candidate-meets-its-primary-efficacy Accessed on December 07 2020.
171. O'Callaghan Kevin P, Allison M Blatz, Paul A Offit. Developing a SARS CoV2 vaccine at warp speed. Jama. 2020.
172. Bian Huijie et al. Meplazumab treats COVID19 pneumonia: an open-labelled, concurrent controlled add-on clinical trial. MedRxiv. 2020.

Chapter 6
An Introduction to the Pathogenetic Mechanisms of CoViD19 Complications

Key Questions

- What are the key extracardiac complications in CoViD19?
- Which pathogenetic factors accompany sepsis and multi-organ failure in CoViD19?
- How SARS CoV2 may cause acute pulmonary injury in CoViD19?
- What is the role of immune and hemodynamic regulatory mechanisms in the development of complications in CoViD19?

6.1 Introduction

The CoViD19 is associated with the development of a variety of complications that are associated with high morbidity and mortality burden. These complications may involve multiple body systems, cause organ injury and failure, or cause other systemic complications. (See Fig. 6.1). The development and worsening of sepsis in patients with CoViD19 appear to lead to a critical stage of the evolution of the disease when associated with acute pulmonary injury or acute respiratory distress syndrome (ARDS), critical cardiovascular injuries, and multi-organ failure. The multi-organ injury may involve kidneys, brain, gastrointestinal or central nervous systems, or other systems resulting in serious complications.

U. Mallick, *Cardiovascular Complications of COVID-19*,
https://doi.org/10.1007/978-3-030-90065-6_6

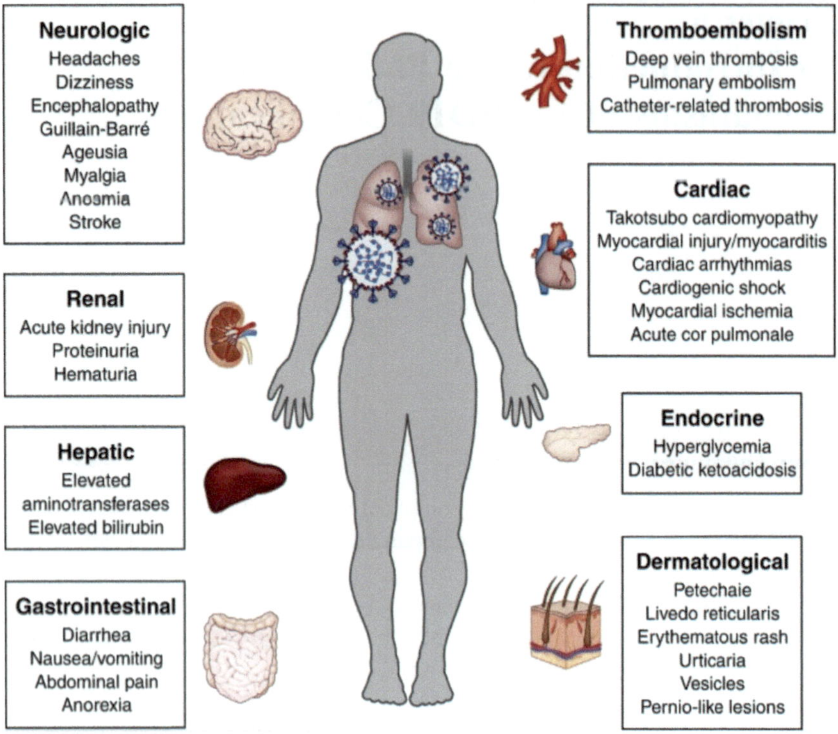

Fig. 6.1 Extrapulmonary manifestations of COVID-19. Common extrapulmonary manifestations of COVID-19. Besides, the pulmonary manifestation of COVID-19 caused by infection with SARS-CoV-2, including pneumonia and ARDS, COVID-19 is associated with deleterious effects on several other body systems. *Source* Figure 2. Gupta, A., Madhavan, M.V., Sehgal, K., Nair, N., Mahajan, S., Sehrawat, T.S., Bikdeli, B., Ahluwalia, N., Ausiello, J.C., Wan, E.Y. and Freedberg, D.E., 2020. Extrapulmonary manifestations of COVID-19. Nature medicine, 26(7), pp. 1017–1032. https://www.nature.com/articles/s41591-020-0968-3. Published by Springer Nature Group

Among several others, the role of inflammatory mechanisms is fundamental in the process of development of these complications. The pathogenetic stages refelct core pulmonary involvement that further leads to activation of other pathogenetic mechanisms and clinical complications. (See Fig. 6.2). The dynamics and interplay of the immune-inflammatory and prothrombotic reactions mark evolution of the disease. The primary inflammatory responses occur during the earlier phase of the viral invasion and may lead to a reduction or even clearance of the viral burden. Although this stage is followed by a decline in the inflammation, a secondary inflammation inflammatory response may develop. This secondary inflammatory response is linked with the development of adaptive immunity and may result in further viral clearance. However, this may be associated with a higher fatality. The CoViD19 complications appear to develop during the later course of the disease, a rapid deterioration of the patients' condition due to the development of acute

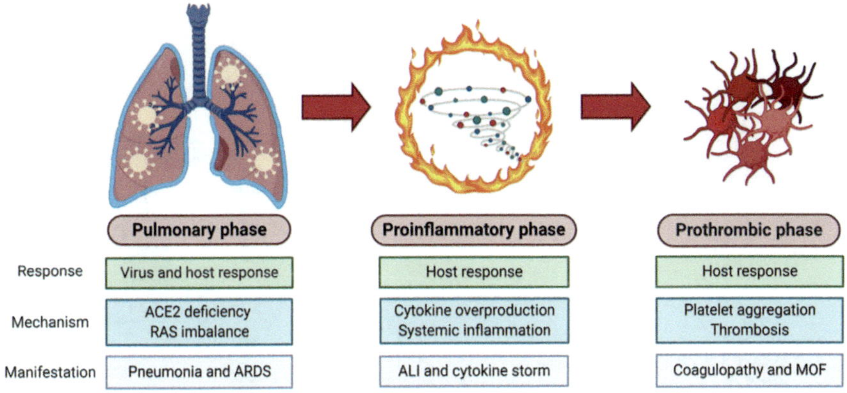

Fig. 6.2 Pathogenesis COVID19. COVID-19 pathogenesis model. The three phases of COVID-19 pathogenesis: pulmonary, proinflammatory, and prothrombic. Response patterns, pathogenic mechanisms, and clinical manifestations for each phase are described. *Source* Figure 1. Lee, C. and Choi, W.J., 2021. Overview of COVID-19 inflammatory pathogenesis from the therapeutic perspective. Archives of pharmacal research, pp. 1–18. https://link.springer.com/article/10.1007/s12272-020-01301-7. Published by Springer Nature

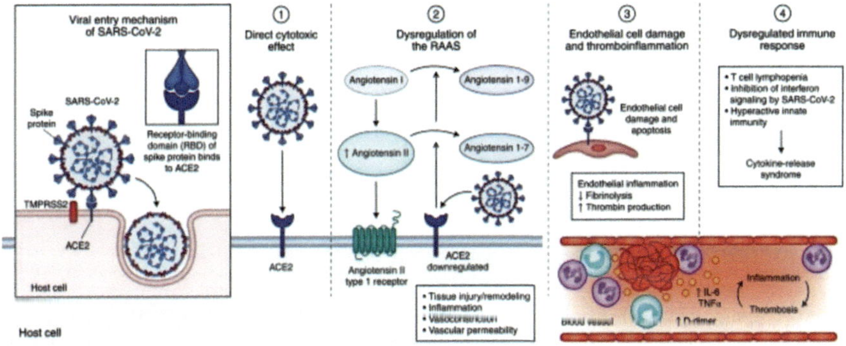

Fig. 6.3 Pathophysiology of CoViD19. SARS-CoV-2 enters host cells through interaction of its spike protein with the entry receptor ACE2 in the presence of TMPRSS2 (far left). Proposed mechanisms for COVID-19 caused by infection with SARS-CoV-2 include (1) direct virus-mediated cell damage; (2) dysregulation of the RAAS as a consequence of downregulation of ACE2 related to viral entry, which leads to decreased cleavage of angiotensin I and angiotensin II; (3) endothelial cell damage and thrombo-inflammation; and (4) dysregulation of the immune response and hyperinflammation caused by inhibition of interferon signaling by the virus, T cell lymphodepletion, and the production of proinflammatory cytokines, particularly IL-6 and TNFα. *Source* Figure 1. Gupta, A., Madhavan, M.V., Sehgal, K., Nair, N., Mahajan, S., Sehrawat, T.S., Bikdeli, B., Ahluwalia, N., Ausiello, J.C., Wan, E.Y. and Freedberg, D.E., 2020. Extrapulmonary manifestations of COVID-19. *Nature medicine*, *26*(7), pp. 1017–1032. https://www.nature.com/articles/s41591-020-0968-3. By Springer Publisher Group

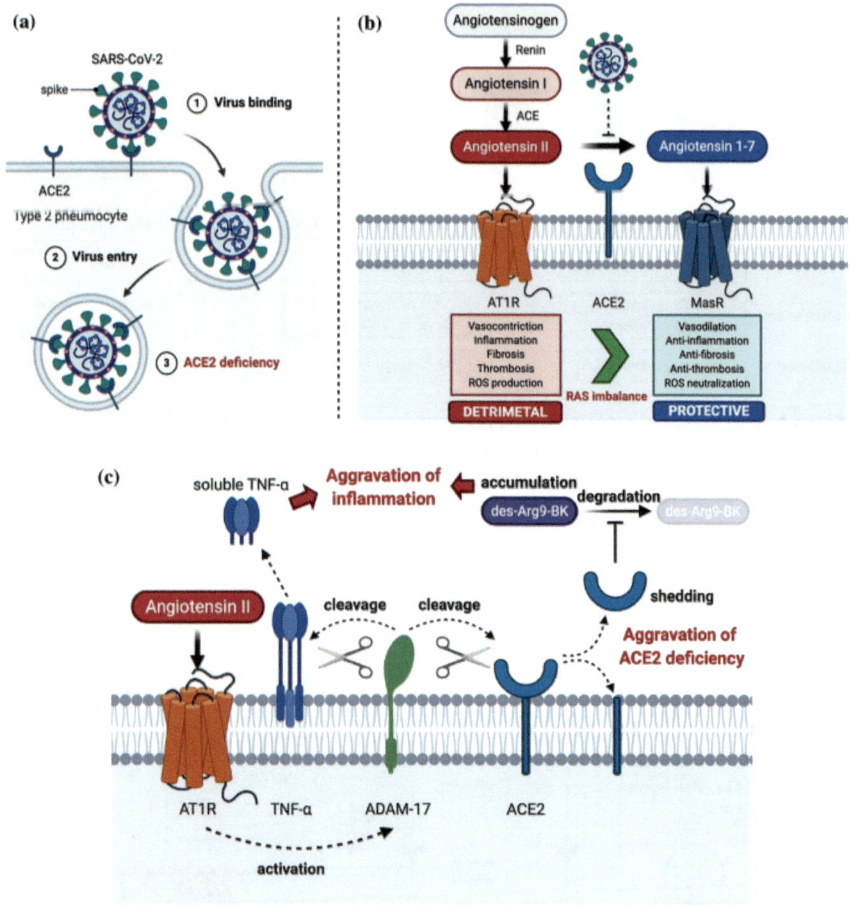

Fig. 6.4 Lung injury mechanism CoViD19. Pulmonary phase of COVID-19 pathogenesis. **a** SARS-CoV-2 enters the type 2 pneumocyte via the host receptor, ACE2. Target cell infection by SARS-CoV-2 induces ACE2 internalization, resulting in ACE2 downregulation and deficiency. **b** SARS-CoV-2-induced ACE2 deficiency decreases the conversion of angiotensin II to angiotensinogen 1–7 and increases angiotensin II availability. Excessive angiotensin II causes AT1R overactivation, resulting in a RAS imbalance. **c** ADAM-17 activation by AT1R promotes cleavage of both membrane-anchored TNF-α and ACE2. ADAM-17 truncates the ACE2 extracellular domain, which enzymatically inactivates ACE2. As a result, des-Arg9-BK degradation by ACE2 is disrupted and its abundancy increases. Liberated soluble TNF-α and accumulated des-Arg9-BK aggravate SARS-CoV-2-induced inflammation. *Source* Figure 2. Lee, C. and Choi, W.J., 2021. Overview of COVID-19 inflammatory pathogenesis from the therapeutic perspective. Archives of pharmacal research, pp. 1–18. https://link.springer.com/article/10.1007/s12272-020-01301-7. Published by Springer Nature

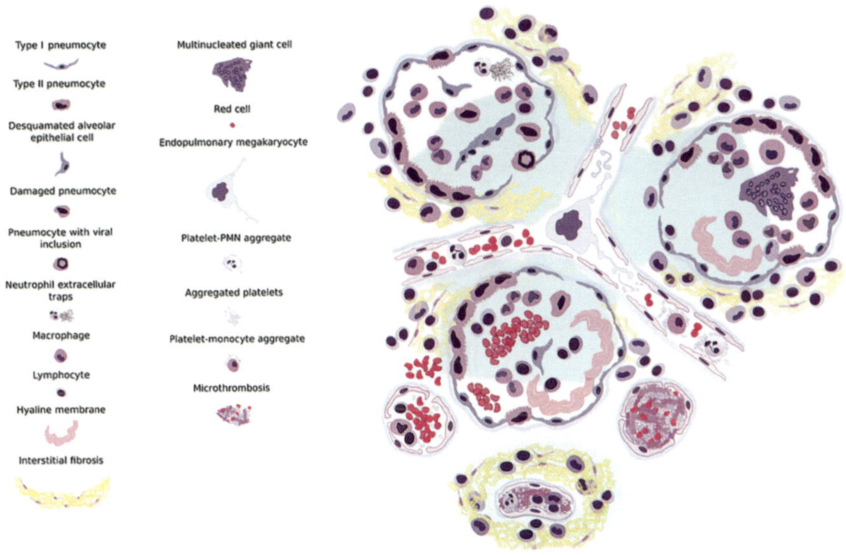

Fig. 6.5 Histopathological changes in lung injury in COVID19. Summary of histopathological features occurring in fatal cases of COVID-19 lung injury. Findings of epithelial, vascular and fibrotic pattern are represented. Note that epithelial damage like viral cytopathic changes, desquamation and reactive hyperplasia of type II pneumocytes, hyaline membrane formation and interstitial inflammatory response have been frequently observed together with findings of vascular damage like capillary congestion, intracapillary micro-thrombosis, alveolar hemorrhage, interstitial and intra-alveolar edema. Furthermore, interstitial fibrous changes, occurring separately or in combination with epithelial and/or vascular injury in a subgroup of patients, are shown. For further details see descriptive text. *Source* Figure 2. Pannone, G., Caponio, V.C.A., De Stefano, I.S., Ramunno, M.A., Meccariello, M., Agostinone, A., Pedicillo, M.C., Troiano, G., Zhurakivska, K., Cassano, T. and Bizzoca, M.E., 2021. Lung histopathological findings in COVID-19 disease–a systematic review. Infectious agents and cancer, 16(1), pp. 1–18. https://link.springer.com/article/10.1186/s13027-021-00369-0. By Springer Nature publishers

respiratory distress syndrome (ARDS) and multi-organ failure (MOF) and may lead to imminent death [1]. The involvement of multiple organs in CoViD19 complications including heart, liver, kidney, brain, and other systems and tissues, strongly correlates with CoViD19 related morbidity and mortality and warrants exploration of the potential pathogenetic factors and mechanisms.

6.2 Acute Pulmonary Injury

The development of ARDS mainly drives the mortality in CoViD19. Acute Respiratory Distress Syndrome (ARDS) is a potentially fatal condition characterized by hypoxia, increased vascular permeability, pulmonary edema, inflammation, and cell destruction that lead to multi-organ failure and death. The ARDS is known

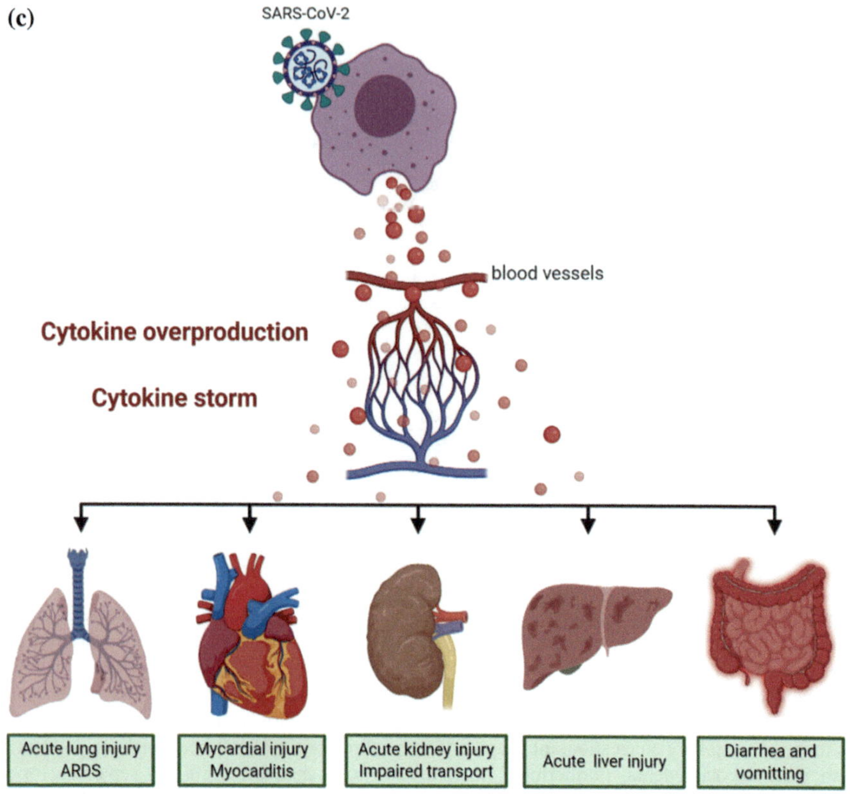

Fig. 6.6 Multi-organ injury and cytokines. Cytokine overproduction and cytokine storm induce clinically relevant extrapulmonary effects on various key organs such as the heart, kidney, liver, and intestines. *Source* Figure 3c. Lee, C. and Choi, W.J., 2021. Overview of COVID-19 inflammatory pathogenesis from the therapeutic perspective. Archives of pharmacal research, pp. 1–18. https://link.springer.com/article/10.1007/s12272-020-01301-7. Published by Springer Nature

to be caused by several factors such as sepsis, trauma, pancreatitis, and others. Hyperinflammatory or cytokine storm appears to be a prominent feature in these conditions, also observed in patients with CoViD19. The core pathology in the ARDS is reflected by pulmonary and interstitial tissue damage caused by non-specific inflammatory cell infiltration [2]. According to the definition "ARDS" is acute hypoxemic respiratory failure following an acute event (such as a respiratory viral infection) that presents as bilateral pulmonary infiltrates on lung imaging in the absence of a purely cardiogenic or hydrostatic etiology [3].

The acute pulmonary injury develops through the extension of the local tissue damage caused by the hyperinflammatory, vasoplegic, and prothrombotic mechanisms that involve several complex systems such as the renin-angiotensin system (RAS), RAS Kallikrein Kinin System (RAS KKS), the immune system involving a range of immune defense cells and proteins, immunomodulatory, and signaling pathways and various vascular structures.

The cytoplasmic viral RNA triggers pro-inflammatory cytokine secretion (interleukin (IL)-1β and IL-18) via several cellular immune signaling mechanisms including Toll-like receptors, mitochondria-associated anti-viral signaling proteins, and the NOD-, LRR- and pyrin domain-containing protein 3 inflammasomes, leading to the recruitment of regulatory and effector cells and upregulation of interferon-stimulated genes and nuclear factor-κB-regulated genes (4-6). This process further involves activation of alveolar macrophages, phagocytosis, and further pro-inflammatory and chemotactic response involving invasion of neutrophils and natural killer (NK) cells and the differentiation of circulating monocytes into monocyte-derived macrophages and dendritic cells [4–6]. In CoViD19, the extreme cytokine reaction is accompanied by infiltration of inflammatory monocytes/macrophages (IMM) into the lung and elevated production of the pro-inflammatory cytokines (IL-1, IL-6, IL-8, CXCL-10, and MCP-1) [7]. These events associated with severe lung damage, accompany profound vascular leakage, and death [8] maybe recognized in patients with ARDS in CoViD19 manifesting massive infiltration of neutrophils and macrophages, diffuse alveolar damage with the formation of hyaline membranes and diffuse thickening of the alveolar wall. The interferon type I [9] and type III responses [10] are impaired in CoViD19 and may contribute to the development of ARDS [11].

The renin-angiotensin system (RAS) is an extremely important player in the development of ARDS. The evidence shows that angiotensin-converting enzyme 2 (ACE2) plays a crucial role in the SARS coronavirus-induced acute lung injury [12–14]. (See Figs. 6.3 and 6.4). The patients with CoViD19 have higher serum ACE2 levels that are in a linear association with the viral load and further with the lung injury [15]. The binding of the virus with ACE 2, results in downregulation of the ACE 2. This further causes an upregulation of the ATII activity that stimulates the ATI/ATII/ATIII/AT1R axis. These reactions increase the vascular permeability, the proinflammatory and profibrotic response, and enhance pulmonary injury [16, 17]. (See Fig. 6.5).

Sepsis acts as the main triggering factor for these mechanisms and may involve direct and indirect actions of the Angiotensin II (AngII). The Angiotensin II may promote expression of the adhesion molecules on vascular endothelial and smooth muscle cells facilitating transendothelial migration of the leukocytes [18, 19]; and may result in ischemic damage through vasoconstriction, microvascular thrombotic mechanisms in association with a reduced blood flow, and local accumulation of the inflammatory cells [20]. Angiotensin II also stimulates the production of inflammatory cytokines and chemokines and result in oxidative stress through the synthesis of the free oxygen radicals via NADPH oxidase-dependent mechanisms [21–24]. Furthermore, these mechanisms may ultimately damage the cells and result in the alveolar epithelial cell apoptosis, and induction of the fibroproliferative responses [25, 26].

ACE2 downregulation also results in increased bradykinin (a potent pro-inflammatory mediator peptide), associated with an increase in systemic inflammatory response [27]. A better understanding of the role of ACE2 in the development of lung injury has prompted researchers to evaluate potential novel therapeutic approaches such as the use of recombinant ACE2 in patients with acute respiratory distress syndrome (ARDS) [28] and pulmonary arterial hypertension.

However, despite confirmed enhanced expression of the angiotensin 1–7 and 1–5, angiotensin II suppression, or reduction in the interleukin 6 levels, these agents have proven to be of a limited clinical value [29].

The prothrombotic and inflammatory mechanisms are interlinked. Endothelial dysfunction acts as a bridge mechanism in the development of injury to the cells. Association of activation of the complement pathway such an MBL (mannose-binding lectin), mannose-binding lectin-associated serine protease -2 (MASP-2), and C3 fragments in CoViD19 patients together with endothelial dysfunction and pro-inflammatory cytokines indicates a poor outcome [30]. Similarly, the presence of inflammasomes (NLRP3) has been indicated as an intermediary mechanism between the viral mechanisms and cytokines [31].

6.3 Sepsis and Multi-organ Failure

Multi-organ failure is a critical complication of CoViD19 that may develop as a complication of sepsis. The complications associated with sepsis, such as cardiac dysfunction or multi-organ failure, may result in adverse outcomes and cause a higher fatality [32, 33]. Various pathogenetic mechanisms associated with sepsis and viral-induced mechanisms and pathways promote the development of complications in patients with CoViD19. The dysregulated immuno-inflammatory factors such as cytokine storm, hypercoagulation, direct viral damage, hypoxia, drug-induced injury particularly play an important role in the development of CoViD19 complications [34–38].

The key features of pathogenetic mechanisms associated with sepsis include circulatory failure with reduced systemic vascular resistance and increased capillary permeability associated with the hyperinflammatory reactions that ultimately lead to multi-organ failure. The sepsis-induced circulatory collapse involves complex intrinsic neuroendocrine response with stimulation of the sympathetic, hypothalamic–pituitary–adrenal axis, activation of the autocrine and paracrine systems such as RAS, endothelin, and vasopressin. Sepsis drives a range of multifactorial cellular stress factors that lead to mitochondrial dysfunction, cell injury, or cell death. The cardiac and vascular dysfunction results from the cellular damage as a result of the accumulation of free radicals, reactive oxygen species (ROS) due to the oxidative and nitro oxidative mechanisms induced by the stress mechanisms [39].

Data show that severe sepsis and septic shock trigger activation and release of several vasoactive substances and neuro-humoral cascades [40, 41]. These pro-inflammatory, immunomodulatory insults cause microcirculatory damage, endothelial dysfunction, ischemic and profibrotic changes, and induce stress mechanisms in other organs that ultimately lead to multi-organ failure. For instance, the development of multi-organ failure and death, and a reduction in the platelet count are closely interrelated. Factors such as platelet activation, the formation of NET traps (through the release of release extracellular traps (ETs), consisting of the DNA and histones), hyperactivity of coagulation factors, resulting in thrombosis.

The platelet aggregation and coagulation factors such as Von Willebrand factor (VWF) in the microvasculature together, lead to endothelial cell activation, impaired vascular integrity, leukocyte recruitment, trans-endothelial migration, tissue inflammation, and target organ injury [42].

The CoViD19 affects kidneys in a variety of clinical and subclinical forms such as acute kidney injury, proteinuria, hematuria, and several others. The renal distribution of the receptors that serve as viral entry mechanisms such as angiotensin-converting enzyme 2 (ACE2), transmembrane serine protease 2 (TMPRSS2), and cathepsin L (CTSL) mediate the development of renal complications in CoViD19. Other mechanisms such as systemic inflammatory reactions together with exaggerated cytokine response induced by the viral disease, hemodynamic dysfunction associated with sepsis as well as direct viral injury, microvascular thrombosis, complement activation, hypoxia, cell death, and several other pathogenetic factors also appear to play a critical role. Similarly, patients with complicated CoViD19 may also present with the hepatic, gastroenterological, central nervous system, and cerebrovascular complications, among several other systemic complications as a result of the viral disease [43, 44].

6.4 Renin Angiotensin System

The renin-angiotensin system serves as a prominent pathogenetic substrate in the complicated CoViD19 and plays a crucial part in the development of the complications. The increased renin-angiotensin system (RAS) activity in sepsis, well documented in the scientific literature, is reflected by the increased plasma renin, angiotensin I, and angiotensin II, and is also recognized in multi-organ failure. The enhanced RAS activity is further associated with the microvascular dysfunction associated with severe sepsis, and septic shock [45]. The enhanced expression of the Ang II is also detected at the plasma and the tissue levels in sepsis [18, 46] and increases significantly during the early and late septic shock in the heart and the aorta [47], possibly suggesting that in sepsis the enhanced Ang II activity in the cardiovascular territory may be associated with the cardiac dysfunction.

Strict regulation of the RAS activity axes is essential for maintaining a homeostatic balance. Data suggest that over-expression of the RAS may cause profound vasoplegia, ischemic damage, and an acute renal impairment, [39] whereas an under-expression may result in refractory shock [48] and multi-organ failure [18, 49]. Furthermore, the ACE 2 offers a protective role in maintaining the homeostatic balance and may play a protective role against the viral invasion in CoViD19. Several protective actions of the ACE2 are mediated through the Ang 1–7/Mas, Ang 1–9/AT2R, Ang II/AT2R pathways. For instance, immune modulation, anti-fibrotic, anti-inflammatory, neuroprotective, neuroregeneration, antihypertensive, anti-apoptotic, and several others [50, 51]. These regulatory proteins also appear to be involved in the immunomodulatory control mechanisms in viral diseases.

Furthermore, interacting mechanisms appear to exist between local and systemic RAS to ensure coordination and synchrony as ACE 2 receptors located in a variety of tissues and macrophages may cross-talk with other cells that express ACE 2 signaling release of interferon to counter the viral invasion [52–54].

In summary, the RAS has an essential role in sepsis and septic shock. However, requires strict regulation to provide a homeostatic balance. The persistent viral insult may induce dysregulation in this system, resulting in organ dysfunction and failure. Since the ACE2 serves as an essential viral entry mechanism for SARS CoV2, dysregulation of the protective cascade may fail to overcome the immunoinflammatory insult, and repair, at the local and systemic levels. The role of the renin-angiotensin system in CoViD19 is not limited to the ACE2 receptors and appears rather more complex. The interrelation between the hyperactivation of the RAS, particularly the Ang II in CoViD19, and the severity of the CoViD19 as well as the rapid deterioration, can be detected in CoViD19 patients. For further reading about the RAS and CoViD19 please refer to Chap. 8.

6.5 Endothelin System

In addition to the RAS, the implication of other peptide systems may also have a role in the settings of the CoViD19 complications. The endothelin 1 (ET1) is a potent vasoconstrictor peptide that may have a role in the development of CoViD19 related complications. Among other peptide systems, the ET 1 is also activated in sepsis. It has pro-inflammatory mechanisms that intersect with cytokine storm, which may contribute towards the development of complications in CoViD19. The evidence suggests that the expression of the ET1 is upregulated in sepsis [55] leading to the activation of the transcriptase factors, or the signaling cascades such as NF-κB, and also stimulates the pro-inflammatory cytokines such as TNF-α, IL-1, and the IL-6 [56]. The transcription factors and the pro-inflammatory cytokines further contribute towards an increase in ET1 production [57]. Furthermore, studies have demonstrated interaction and cross-talk between the ET1 and the RAS. The angiotensin (1–7) may attenuate endothelin 1 induced inflammation and growth or may downregulate ACE-2 expression in the lung epithelial cells [58, 59]. For further reading about the endothelin system and CoViD19 please refer to Chap. 10 Sect. 10.2.2.

6.6 Immune-Inflammation

The bio immunological profile of the patients with CoViD19 exhibits features of the dysregulated cytokine release as a significant characteristic of the complications related to sepsis and multi-organ failure. The proinflammatory cytokines implicated in the development of multi-organ failure and acute respiratory distress syndrome (ARDS) also appear to complicate CoViD19 [60, 61]. (See Fig. 6.6).

In the complicated CoViD19, production of the pro-inflammatory cytokine appears to be poorly controlled at the local and systemic levels. The exaggerated cytokine response is marked by an increase in the interleukin (IL)-2, IL-7, granulocyte-colony stimulating factor (GCS F), interferon-γ inducible protein 10 (IP-10), monocyte chemoattractant protein 1 (MCP-1), macrophage inflammatory protein 1-α (MIP-1α), and tumor necrosis factor-α (TNF-α) [62]. The prolonged hyper inflammation, marked by the TNF-α and IL6, leads to endothelial dysfunction (activation, capillary leak) and circulatory failure.

The cytokines play a critical role in the immune and defense mechanisms, however, may also cause damage to the cells and tissues. Evidence also shows that cytokines are involved in the apoptosis of the T cell lymphocytes, endothelial and epithelial cells of the airways [63–66]. A dysregulated cytokine production is an important feature of the complicated CoViD19 and represents a crucial pathogenetic mechanism. However, physiological (protective) and pathological (harmful) components of the inflammatory response require a careful distinction to understand their clinical implications. In addition to the cytokine-related damage, several factors contribute to the development of organ dysfunction at a local or systemic level, that work in synchrony or interconnection with the uncontrolled systemic inflammatory and immune reactions. Among these hypercoagulability, dysregulated metabolic function, or hypoxia are notable. Such mechanisms may underlie the development of dysfunction in lungs, liver, kidney, gastrointestinal tract and brain, and other tissues, observed in CoViD19,

Another important factor, oxidative stress is among multiple factors that contribute towards the development of inflammation in CoViD19. Oxidative stress appears to be a key feature of CoViD19 and maybe interlinked with several mechanisms involving RAS such as ACE2–Ang-(1–7)–Mas axis, overproduction of NADPH oxidase-2 (NOX-2) [67], production of ROS by the macrophage and neutrophils [68], activation of inflammasome [69] and others. The oxidative stress may induce further inflammatory stress and alter the immune system [70, 71]. Furthermore, pyroptosis an inherently pro-inflammatory process of cell death may also be activated in CoViD19 and sepsis [72, 73].

6.7 Summary

Sepsis, acute lung injury, and multi-organ failure share common pathogenetic factors with lungs central to the pathology in CoViD19. Several body systems including gastrointestinal, renal, neurological, cerebrovascular, endocrine, hematological, immunological systems may share common pathogenetic insult. Among multiple mechanisms and factors implicated in the pathogenesis of complications of CoViD19, hyper inflammation accompanied by the exaggerated immune response, components of the complex renin-angiotensin system, expression and distribution of ACE2, hypercoagulability, and dysregulated metabolism are prominent.

The mechanism of direct viral injury in the complicated CoViD19, interlinking the SARS CoV 2, the viral load, and acute lung injury, is widely acknowledged. The SARS CoV2 tropism in multiple organs and systems such as the central nervous, gastrointestinal, and renal systems, and other tissues has been reported in the literature. The ACE2 receptors, used by the SARS CoV2 to gain entry into the cells, are widely distributed in the human body. The expression and distribution of the SARS CoV2 viral receptors and their dynamics play a pivotal role in the process of direct viral injury. The hyperinflammatory and immune reactions, regulatory mechanisms such as renin-angiotensin system (RAS), endothelin 1 (ET-1), metabolic, and coagulation systems appear to play a significant role in the development of CoViD19 complications. Hyperactivation of the monocytes/macrophages and dysregulated cytokine production results in organ injury with elevated levels of proinflammatory cytokines such as IL-6, IL-10, and TNF-alpha. These mechanisms and pathways demand further exploration, and their complex interactions need to be defined and elaborated to help understand a comprehensive pathogenetic profile of the CoViD19 and its complications.

The pathogenetic mechanisms behind complications of the CoViD19, related to infectivity and pathogeneity of the virus, such as interstitial pneumonia, systemic inflammatory response syndrome, and fatality, strongly intersect with the mechanisms that are also known to determine cardiovascular diseases. A matrix of the grossly dysregulated complex humeral, immune, hemodynamic, and oxidative stress pathways, plays a critical role in this process. These interlinking mechanisms between the CoViD19 and cardiovascular diseases have served as a root to the debate regarding the use of the ACE inhibitors and the Angiotensin Receptor Blockers (ARBs) in patients with CoViD19.

The immune-inflammatory mechanisms, peptide regulatory systems, and other important homeostatic, coagulation as well as hemodynamic systems are interlinked and may cross-talk. The persistent viral load exaggerated immune response, and the associated dysregulated systemic hyperinflammatory reactions may trigger misbalancing of the internal mechanisms and result in organ dysfunction, failure, or death in patients with complicated CoViD19 [74–76]. For further reading about specific pathogenetic mechanisms and CoViD19 please refer to Chaps. 7, 8, 9 and 10.

Summary Box

- Sepsis and multi-organ failure are key features of the complicated CoViD19.
- Sepsis accompanies a myriad of inflammatory, immune, oxidative, and other molecular/cellular stress reactions, as well as turbulences in regulatory peptide systems, such as RAS and endothelin, among others.
- Multi-organ failure may involve several organs and systems such as the heart, lungs, kidney, brain, gastrointestinal system, liver, blood, skin, and other body systems and tissues.

- Notable pathogenetic mechanisms in CoViD19 include viral tropism, hyperinflammatory systemic reactions, renin-angiotensin system, dysregulated immune reactions, pro-thrombotic mechanisms, dysregulated metabolism, and hypoxia.
- Dysregulated immune defense mechanisms, i.e., hyperactivation of the monocytes/macrophages and dysregulated cytokines, may cause multi-organ injury and tissue dysfunction in CoViD19.
- The functioning of the RAS protective arm may be impaired in the presence of a persistent viral load in CoViD19.
- Prothrombotic processes play a critical role in the development of CoViD19 complications.
- The pathogenetic mechanisms behind CoViD19 complications may interact, overlap, and may act synergistically.
- Hemodynamic failure, circulatory collapse, and indicators of vascular and endothelial dysfunction observed in sepsis often lead to organ failure.
- Several therapeutic strategies used in CoViD19 target important pathogenetic mechanisms, related to the immune-inflammatory, prothrombotic mechanisms, and others are under exploration.

References

1. Special Expert Group for Control of the Epidemic of Novel Coronavirus Pneumonia of the Chinese Preventive Medicine Association. An update on the epidemiological characteristics of novel coronavirus pneumonia (COVID-19). Chin J Epidemiol. 2020;41.
2. Force* TADT. Acute Respiratory Distress Syndrome: The Berlin Definition. JAMA. 2012; 307(23):2526–33.
3. Force ADT, Ranieri VM, Rubenfeld GD, Thompson B, Ferguson N, Caldwell E. Acute respiratory distress syndrome. JAMA. 2012;307(23):2526–33.
4. Durbin RK, Kotenko SV, Durbin JE. Interferon induction and function at the mucosal surface. Immunol Rev. 2013;255(1):25–39.
5. Pothlichet J, Meunier I, Davis BK, Ting JP, Skamene E, von Messling V, Vidal SM. Type I IFN triggers RIG-I/TLR3/NLRP3-dependent inflammasome activation in influenza A virus infected cells. PLoS Pathog. 2013; 9(4):e1003256.
6. Acosta MAT. Singer BD. Pathogenesis of COVID-19-induced ARDS: implications for an ageing population. Eur Resp J. 2020; 56(3).
7. Buonaguro FM, Puzanov I, Ascierto PA. Anti-IL6R role in treatment of COVID-19-related ARDS. 2020.
8. Liu L, Wei Q, Lin Q, Fang J, Wang H, Kwok H, Tang H, Nishiura K, Peng J, Tan Z, Wu T. Anti–spike IgG causes severe acute lung injury by skewing macrophage responses during acute SARS-CoV infection. JCI Insight. 2019; 4(4).
9. Li JY, Liao CH, Wang Q, Tan YJ, Luo R, Qiu Y, Ge XY. The ORF6, ORF8 and nucleocapsid proteins of SARS-CoV-2 inhibit type I interferon signaling pathway. Virus Res. 2020; 286:198074.

10. Lokugamage KG, Hage A, Schindewolf C, Rajsbaum R, Menachery VD. SARS-CoV-2 is sensitive to type I interferon pretreatment. BioRxiv. 2020.
11. Broggi A, Ghosh S, Sposito B, Spreafico R, Balzarini F, Cascio AL, Clementi N, De Santis M, Mancini N, Granucci F, Zanoni I. Type III interferons disrupt the lung epithelial barrier upon viral recognition. Science. 2020;369(6504):706–12.
12. Kuba K, Imai Y, Rao S, Gao H, Guo F, Guan B et al. A crucial role of angiotensin converting enzyme 2 (ACE2) in SARS coronavirus-induced lung injury. Nat Med. 2005, August; 11 (8):875–9. doi:https://doi.org/10.1038/nm1267. PMID 16007097.
13. Angiotensin-converting enzyme 2 in lung diseases, Keiji Kuba, Yumiko Imai, Josef M Penninger Current Opinion in Pharmacology. 2006, June; 6(3):271–6.
14. Zhang H, Baker A. Recombinant human ACE2: acing out angiotensin II in ARDS therapy. Crit Care. 2017;21:305.
15. Liu Y, Yang Y, Zhang C, Huang F, Wang F, Yuan J, Wang Z, Li J, Li J, Feng C, et al. Clinical and biochemical indexes from 2019-nCoV infected patients linked to viral loads and lung injury. Sci China Life Sci. 2020. https://doi.org/10.1007/s11427-020-1643-8.
16. Imai Y, Kuba K, Rao S, Huan Y, Guo F, Guan B, Yang P, Sarao R, Wada T, Leong-Poi H et al. Angiotensin-converting enzyme 2 protects from severe acute lung failure. Nature. 2005; 436:112–116. [CrossRef] [PubMed].
17. Liu Y, Yang Y, Zhang C, et al. Clinical and biochemical indexes from 2019-nCoV infected patients linked to viral loads and lung injury. Sci China Life Sci. 2020;63:364–74.
18. Boldt J, Papsdorf M, Kumle B. Influence of angiotensin-converting enzyme inhibitor enalaprilat on endothelial-derived substances in the critically ill. Crit Care Med. 1998;26:1663–70.
19. Pastore L, Tessitore A, Martinotti S. Angiotensin II stimulates intercellular adhesion molecule-1 (ICAM-1) expression by human vascular endothelial cells and increases soluble ICAM-1 release in vivo. Circulation. 1999;100:1646–52.
20. Dielis AW, Smid M, Spronk HM. Changes in fibrinolytic activity after angiotensin II receptor blockade in therapy-resistant hypertensive patients. J Thromb Haemost. 2007;5:1509–15.
21. Miyoshi M, Nagata K, Imoto T. ANG II is involved in the LPS-induced production of proinflammatory cytokines in dehydrated rats. Am J Physiol Regul Integr Comp Physiol. 2003;284:R1092–7.
22. Ruiz-Ortega M, Ruperez M, Lorenzo O. Angiotensin II regulates the synthesis of proinflammatory cytokines and chemokines in the kidney. Kidney Int Suppl. 2002;62:S12-22.
23. Higuchi S, Ohtsu H, Suzuki H. Angiotensin II signal transduction through the AT1 receptor: novel insights into mechanisms and pathophysiology. Clin Sci (Lond). 2007;112:417–28.
24. Lund DD, Brooks RM, Faraci FM, Heistad DD. Role of angiotensin II in endothelial dysfunction induced by lipopolysaccharide in mice. Am J Physiol Heart Circ Physiol. 2007;293:H3726–31.
25. Marshall RP, Webb S, Bellingan GJ, Angiotensin converting enzyme insertion/deletion polymorphism is associated with susceptibility and outcome in acute respiratory distress syndrome. Am J Respir Crit Care Med. 2002; 166:646–50. [Google Scholar].
26. Yao S, Feng D, Wu Q. Losartan attenuates ventilator-induced lung injury. J Surg Res. 2008;145:25–32.
27. Jia H. Pulmonary angiotensin-converting enzyme 2 (ACE2XE “ACE2”) and inflammatory lung disease. Shock. 2016;46(3):239–48.
28. Imai Y, Kuba K, Rao S, Huan Y, Guo F, Guan B, Yang P, Sarao R, Wada T, Leong-Poi H, Crackower MA, Fukamizu A, Hui CC, Hein L, Uhlig S, Slutsky AS, Jiang C, Penninger JM. Angiotensin-converting enzyme 2 protects from severe acute lung failure. Nature. 2005;436:112–6.
29. Haschke M, Schuster M, Poglitsch M, Loibner H, Salzberg M, Bruggisser M, Penninger J, Krähenbühl S. Pharmacokinetics and pharmacodynamics of recombinant human angiotensin-converting enzyme 2 in healthy human subjects. Clin Pharmacokinet. 2013; 52:783–792. ClinicalTrials.gov identifier NCT01597635.

30. Malaquias MAS, Gadotti AC, da Silva Motta-Junior J, Martins APC, Azevedo MLV, Benevides APK, Cézar-Neto P, do Carmo LAP, Zeni RC, Raboni SM, Fonseca AS. The role of the lectin pathway of the complement system in SARS-CoV-2 lung injury. Trans Res. 2021; 231:55–63.
31. Toldo S, Bussani R, Nuzzi V, Bonaventura A, Mauro AG, Cannatà A, Pillappa R, Sinagra G, Nana-Sinkam P, Sime P, Abbate A. Inflammasome formation in the lungs of patients with fatal COVID-19. Inflam Res. 2021; 70(1):7–10.
32. Cardiac dysfunction in severe sepsis and septic shock. Zanotti-Cavazzoni SL, Hollenberg SM. Curr Opin Crit Care. 2009;15(5):392–7.
33. Diastolic dysfunction and mortality in severe sepsis and septic shock. Landesberg G, Gilon D, Meroz Y, Georgieva M, Levin PD, Goodman S, Avidan A, Beeri R, Weissman C, Jaffe AS, Sprung CL. Eur Heart J. 2012;33(7):895–903.
34. Li Y, Xiao SY. Hepatic involvement in COVID-19 patients: Pathology, pathogenesis, and clinical implications. J Med Virol. 2020;92(9):1491–4.
35. Wang D, Hu B, Hu C, Zhu F, Liu X, Zhang J, Wang B, Xiang H, Cheng Z, Xiong Y, Zhao Y. Clinical characteristics of 138 hospitalized patients with 2019 novel coronavirus–infected pneumonia in Wuhan, China. JAMA. 2020;323(11):1061–9.
36. Jin X, Lian JS, Hu JH, Gao J, Zheng L, Zhang YM, Hao SR, Jia HY, Cai H, Zhang XL, Yu GD. Epidemiological, clinical and virological characteristics of 74 cases of coronavirus-infected disease 2019 (COVID-19) with gastrointestinal symptoms. Gut. 2020;69(6):1002–9.
37. Bikdeli B, Madhavan MV, Jimenez D, Chuich T, Dreyfus I, Driggin E, Nigoghossian CD, Ageno W, Madjid M, Guo Y, Tang LV. COVID-19 and thrombotic or thromboembolic disease: implications for prevention, antithrombotic therapy, and follow-up: JACC state-of-the-art review. J Am Coll Cardiol. 2020;75(23):2950–73.
38. Nilsson A, Edner N, Albert J, Ternhag A. Fatal encephalitis associated with coronavirus OC43 in an immunocompromised child. Infect Dis. 2020;52(6):419–22.
39. Doughan AK, Harrison DG, Dikalov SI. Molecular mechanisms of angiotensin II-mediated mitochondrial dysfunction: linking mitochondrial oxidative damage and vascular endothelial dysfunction. Circ Res. 2008;102:488–96.
40. The stress response and critical illness: a review. Cuesta JM, Singer M Crit Care Med. 2012 Dec; 40(12):3283–9.
41. The endocrine response to critical illness. Rolih CA, Ober KP. Med Clin North Am. 1995;79 (1):211–24.
42. Thornton P, McColl BW, Greenhalgh A, Denes A, Allan SM, Rothwell NJ. Platelet interleukin-1alpha drives cerebrovascular inflammation. Blood. 2010;115:3632–9.
43. Yang L, Tu L. Implications of gastrointestinal manifestations of COVID-19. Lancet Gastroent Hepat. 2020;5(7):629–30.
44. Ellul MA, Benjamin L, Singh B, Lant S, Michael BD, Easton A, Kneen R, Defres S, Sejvar J, Solomon T. Neurological associations of COVID-19. Lancet Neurol. 2020.
45. Renin-angiotensin system activation correlates with microvascular dysfunction in a prospective cohort study of clinical sepsis. Doerschug KC, Delsing AS, Schmidt GA, Ashare A Crit Care. 2010; 14(1):R24.
46. Boldt J, Papsdorf M, Kumle B et al. Influence of angiotensin-converting enzyme inhibitor enalaprilat on endothelial-derived substances in the critically ill. Crit Care Med. 1998; 26:1663–70.
47. Bucher M, Hobbhahn J, Kurtz A. Nitric oxide-dependent down-regulation of angiotensin II type 2 receptors during experimental sepsis. Crit Care Med. 2001;29:1750–5.
48. Dong LW, Chang YZ, Tong LJ, et al. Role of regulatory peptide in pathogenesis of shock. Sci China B. 1994;37:162–9.
49. Doughan AK, Harrison DG, Dikalov SI. Molecular mechanisms of angiotensin II-mediated mitochondrial dysfunction: linking mitochondrial oxidative damage and vascular endothelial dysfunction. Circ Res. 2008; 102:488–96.

50. Wray GM, Coakley JH. Severe septic shock unresponsive to noradrenaline. Lancet. 1995;346:1604.
51. Boldt J, Papsdorf M, Kumle B, Influence of angiotensin-converting enzyme inhibitor enalaprilat on endothelial-derived substances in the critically ill. Crit Care Med. 1998; 26:1663–70.
52. Adembri C, Kastamoniti E, Bertolozzi I. Pulmonary injury follows systemic inflammatory reaction in infrarenal aortic surgery. Crit Care Med. 2004;32:1170–7.
53. Namsolleck et al. Namsolleck P, Recarti C, Foulquier S, Steckelings UM, Unger T. AT(2) receptor and tissue injury: therapeutic implications. Curr Hypertens Rep. 2014; 16:416.
54. Steckelings et al. Steckelings UM, Kloet A, Sumners C. Centrally mediated cardiovascular actions of the angiotensin II type 2 receptor. Trends Endocrinol Metab. 2017; 28:684–93.
55. Hansen TH, Bouvier M. MHC class I antigen presentation: learning from viral evasion strategies. Nat Rev Immunol. 2009; 9(7):503e513.
56. Goulder PJ, Watkins DI. Impact of MHC class I diversity on immune control of immunodeficiency virus replication. Nat Rev Immunol. 2008; 8(8):619e630.
57. Qi F, Qian S, Zhang S, Zhang Z. Single cell RNA sequencing of 13 human tissues identify cell types and receptors of human coronaviruses. Biochem Biophys Res Commun. 2020 Mar 18. pii:S0006–291X(20)30523–4. doi: https://doi.org/10.1016/j.bbrc.2020.03.044. [Epub ahead of print].
58. Roth J, De Souza GE. Fever induction pathways: evidence from responses to systemic or local cytokine formation. Braz J Med Biol Res. 2001;34:301–14.
59. Yeager ME, Belchenko DD, Nguyen CM, et al. Endothelin-1, the unfolded protein response, and persistent inflammation: role of pulmonary artery smooth muscle cells. Am J Respir Cell Mol Biol. 2012;46:14–22.
60. Virdis A, Schiffrin EL. Vascular inflammation: a role in vascular disease in hypertension? Curr Opin Nephrol Hypertens. 2003;12:181–7.
61. Zhang H, Li Y, Zeng Y, Wu R, Ou J. Endothelin-1 downregulates angiotensin-converting enzyme-2 expression in human bronchial epithelial cells. Pharmacology. 2013;91(5–6):297–304.
62. Yusuf H, Montezano AC, Callera GE, Nguyen Dinh Cat A, Santos RA, Castro CH, Touyz RM. Angiotensin 1–7 attenuates endothelin-1-induced endothelial cell inflammation and growth through nitric oxide production and activation of Mas and endothelinB receptors. 2012.
63. Wang H, Ma S. The cytokine storm and factors determining the sequence and severity of organ dysfunction in multiple organ dysfunction syndrome. Am J Em Med. 2008; 26(6):711–5. PubMed PMID: 18606328. Eng.
64. Special Expert Group for Control of the Epidemic of Novel Coronavirus Pneumonia of the Chinese Preventive Medicine Association. An update on the epidemiological characteristics of novel coronavirus pneumonia (COVID-19. Chin J Epidemiol. 2020; 41.
65. Huang C, Wang Y, Li X, Ren L, Zhao J, Hu Y, Zhang L, Fan G, Xu J, Gu X, Cheng Z. Clinical features of patients infected with 2019 novel coronavirus in Wuhan, China. The Lancet. 2020;395(10223):497–506.
66. Channappanavar R, Fehr AR, Vijay R, Mack M, Zhao J, Meyerholz DK, et al. Dysregulated type I interferon and inflammatory monocyte-macrophage responses cause lethal pneumonia in SARS-CoV-infected mice. Cell Host Microbe. 2016;19(2):181–93 PubMed PMID: 26867177.
67. Herold S, Steinmueller M, von Wulffen W, Cakarova L, Pinto R, Pleschka S, et al. Lung epithelial apoptosis in influenza virus pneumonia: the role of macrophage-expressed TNF-related apoptosis-inducing ligand. J Exper Med. 2008; 205(13):3065–77. PubMed PMID: 19064696. Epub 2008/12/08.40.
68. Högner K, Wolff T, Pleschka S, Plog S, Gruber AD, Kalinke U, et al. Macrophage-expressed IFN-β contributes to apoptotic alveolar epithelial cell injury in severe influenza virus pneumonia. PLoS Pathogens. 2013; 9(2):e1003188-e. PubMed PMID: 23468627. Epub 2013/02/28.41.

69. Rodrigue-Gervais IG, Labbé K, Dagenais M, Dupaul-Chicoine J, Champagne C, Morizot A, et al. Cellular inhibitor of apoptosis protein cIAP2 protects against pulmonary tissue necrosis during influenza virus infection to promote host survival. Cell Host Microbe. 2014;15(1):23–35 PubMed PMID: 24439895.
70. Violi F, Oliva A, Cangemi R, Ceccarelli G, Pignatelli P, Carnevale R, Cammisotto V, Lichtner M, Alessandri F, De Angelis M, Miele MC. Nox2 activation in Covid-19. Redox Biol. 2020; 36:101655.
71. Merad M, Martin JC. Pathological inflammation in patients with COVID-19: a key role for monocytes and macrophages. Nat Rev Immunol. 2020;20(6):355–62.
72. Derouiche S. Oxidative stress associated with SARS-Cov-2 (COVID-19) increases the severity of the lung disease-a systematic review. J Infect Dis Epidemiol. 2020;6:121.
73. Nagar H, Piao S, Kim CS. Role of mitochondrial oxidative stress in sepsis. Acute Critical Care. 2018;33(2):65.
74. Galley HF. Oxidative stress and mitochondrial dysfunction in sepsis. Br J Anaesth. 2011;107 (1):57–64.
75. Li S, Jiang L, Li X, Lin F, Wang Y, Li B, Jiang T, An W, Liu S, Liu H, Xu P. Clinical and pathological investigation of patients with severe COVID-19. JCI Insight. 2020; 5(12).
76. Yang M. Cell pyroptosis, a potential pathogenic mechanism of 2019-nCoV infection. *Available at SSRN 3527420.* 2020.

Chapter 7
Overview of Cytokines and CoViD19

Key Questions

- What are cytokines and why are they important?
- What role do cytokines play in the development of CoViD19 complications?
- What is cytokine storm?
- How are cytokines linked with the severity of CoViD19?
- Do cytokines play a role in the development of cardiovascular and metabolic diseases?

7.1 Introduction

The CoViD19 has been termed hyperinflammatory viral disease that may lead to a range of complications and result in death. The inflammatory and immune reactions observed in the complicated CoViD19 play a critical role in the pathogenesis of complications. Among CoViD19 complications, the ARDS, cardiovascular diseases, and organ failure are critical. The development of excessive immune response in the CoViD19 has been linked with the hyperinflammatory state as known as "cytokine storm", considered to be responsible for high morbidity and mortality in CoViD19 patients.

The hyper inflammation immune reaction is a complex phenomenon, also observed in association with other viral diseases or drug reactions, and works in conjunction with multiple local and systemic pathophysiological regulatory systems. This dysregulated immune-inflammation results in vascular damage, hyper thrombotic processes, hypoxia, cellular stress, and a variety of other pathogenetic processes that underlie the CoViD19 complications. According to a retrospective,

U. Mallick, *Cardiovascular Complications of COVID-19*,
https://doi.org/10.1007/978-3-030-90065-6_7

multi-center study of 150 confirmed CoViD19 cases in Wuhan, China, the age, presence of underlying diseases, secondary infection, and elevated inflammatory indicators in the blood, were the predictors of a fatal outcome in the CoViD19 cases. The results obtained from this study further suggested that virus-activated "cytokine storm syndrome" or fulminant myocarditis may contribute to the CoViD19 mortality [1].

In this chapter, we examine the cytokines recognized as an essential feature of the hyperimmune inflammatory response observed in CoViD19 and provide an overview of these important constituents of the complex reaction. We also describe the kinetics and the fluctuations of cytokines in relationship with the severity of the disease. We further investigate the association of the immune response with the cardiovascular complications observed in patients with CoViD19. These concepts are not only vital for timely recognition of the CoViD19 in the clinical settings but also form the basis for the development and application of the CoViD19 treatment strategies targetting the immunoinflammatory burden of the disease also currently explored by the researchers worldwide.

7.2 Cytokines

The cytokines are a group of small pleiotropic proteins that form a vital part of the immune and defense mechanisms and bind to the receptors found on most cells aiding inter and intracellular signaling mechanisms. The cytokines coordinate and integrate a panoply of homeostatic responses following a tissue injury. The functional characteristics of the cytokines may help to distinguish, such as their role as a lymphocyte growth factor, pro- or anti-inflammatory, or during the immune response to the antigens. The cytokines may exhibit more than one property, for instance, may primarily be pro-inflammatory yet may also have anti-inflammatory effects (Table 7.1).

Several cytokines such as interferons (INF), interleukins (IL), chemokines, colony-stimulating factors (CSFs), and tumor necrosis factor (TNF), and other distinct profiles of the cytokines are well known. A distinct group of the cytokines "adipokines", produced from the white adipose tissue, plays an important role in the pathophysiology of several metabolic conditions (type 2 diabetes mellitus, obesity).

The cytokines function as a warning mechanism and confer a cytoprotective role, being an important part of the immune system in the fight against infections. Substantial variations in their regulation and dynamics may generate undesirable consequences and induce harm in certain conditions, resulting in hyperinflammatory immune stress (Fig. 7.1).

The physiological (protective) or pathological (harmful) components of the inflammatory process must be distinguished to help understand their clinical implications. Due to the significant biotechnological advancements in the genetic, and cyto-immunological domains, in recent years, a greater understanding of the host defense and immune functions has been acquired, providing further clarity to

Table 7.1 Key cytokines, actions and CoViD19

Cytokine	Examples	Actions	Example in CoViD19
Interferons (IFN)	Type I interferons (IFN-α, IFN-β), type II interferons (IFN-γ), and type III interferons (IFN-λ)	Regulation of innate immunity, activation of antiviral properties, antiproliferative effects, IFN-γ promotes macrophage activation and antigen presentation	IFN-γ elevated in CoViD19[a]
Interleukins (IL)	IL1, IL-6, IL-10, and others	Growth and differentiation of leukocytes; several proinflammatory actions	IL-1β[b], IL-6[b], IL-10[b], IL-17[a,c] elevated with disease and severity
Chemokines	CXCL8 (IL-8), CXCL10 (IP-10), CXCL2 (MIP-2α), CCL2 (MCP-1), CCL3 (MIP-1α)	Control of chemotaxis, leukocyte recruitment; several proinflammatory actions	IP-10 elevated with severity[a]
Colony stimulating factors (CSF)	Granulocyte–macrophage colony-stimulating factor (GM-CSF), Macrophage colony-stimulating factor (M-CSF), and Granulocyte-Colony-Stimulating Factor (G-CSF), and IL3 (multi-CSF)	Stimulate hematopoietic progenitor cell proliferation and maturation; inflammatory processes	GM-CSF elevated in acute phase[a]
Tumor necrosis factor (TNF)	TNF-α, TNF β	Proinflammatory actions, activation of cytotoxic T lymphocytes	TNF-α elevated with disease severity[a]

This table does not give a comprehensive list of cytokines or their actions

Variations in the associations of cytokines with CoViD19 may be reported among CoViD19 reports. For a detailed analysis readers are advised to refer to more comprehensive reports describing dynamics of cytokines and CoViD19

[a]Huang, C., Wang, Y., Li, X., Ren, L., Zhao, J., Hu, Y., Zhang, L., Fan, G., Xu, J., Gu, X. and Cheng, Z., 2020. Clinical features of patients infected with 2019 novel coronavirus in Wuhan, China. The lancet, 395(10,223), pp.497–506

[b]Wan, S., Yi, Q., Fan, S., Lv, J., Zhang, X., Guo, L., Lang, C., Xiao, Q., Xiao, K., Yi, Z. and Qiang, M., 2020. Characteristics of lymphocyte subsets and cytokines in peripheral blood of 123 hospitalized patients with 2019 novel coronavirus pneumonia (NCP). MedRxiv

[c]Liu, Y., Yang, Y., Zhang, C., Huang, F., Wang, F., Yuan, J., Wang, Z., Li, J., Li, J., Feng, C. and Zhang, Z., 2020. Clinical and biochemical indexes from 2019-nCoV infected patients linked to viral loads and lung injury. Science China Life Sciences, 63(3), pp.364–374

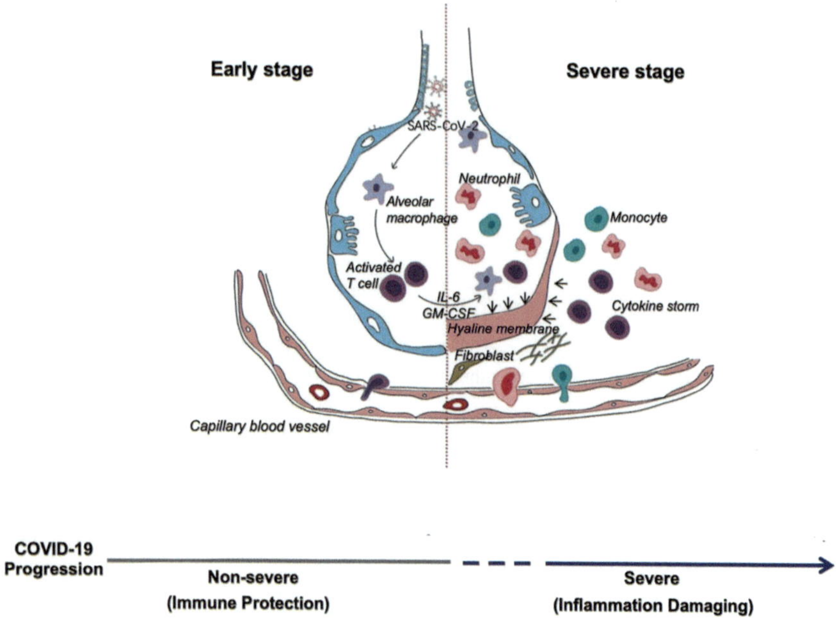

Fig. 7.1 Cytokine storm and progression of CoViD19 *Modified from Source* Figure 1. Shi, Y., Wang, Y., Shao, C., Huang, J., Gan, J., Huang, X., Bucci, E., Piacentini, M., Ippolito, G. and Melino, G., 2020. COVID-19 infection: the perspectives on immune responses. https://www.nature.com/articles/s41418-020-0530-3?fbclid=IwAR1CaaF8eze1pYK8PA1rDBMCy7TejgHITTkIJt6BKpb6NOqbww_3k-7PDmY. Published by Springer Nature

the conundrum of the cytokine function related to the harmful and beneficial effects. This has added excellent value to the diagnostic, therapeutic, and prognostic role of cytokines in immunoinflammatory diseases. The novel coronavirus disease has further challenged the immunological and inflammatory domain. Interpretation of the complex play of the cytokines in CoViD19 and the repercussions on the clinical and prognostic aspects of the disease has emerged as a provocation to clinicians and scientists worldwide. Mitigating the harmful effects of cytokines and inflammation may help to diminish the risk associated with severe CoViD19.

7.2.1 Interferon

The interferons (INF) provide innate immunity to viruses and other pathogens, also carry therapeutic value. Their production is elicited by viral recognition. Three types of interferons I (IFN-α, IFN-β), II (IFN-γ), III (IFNλ) are recognized

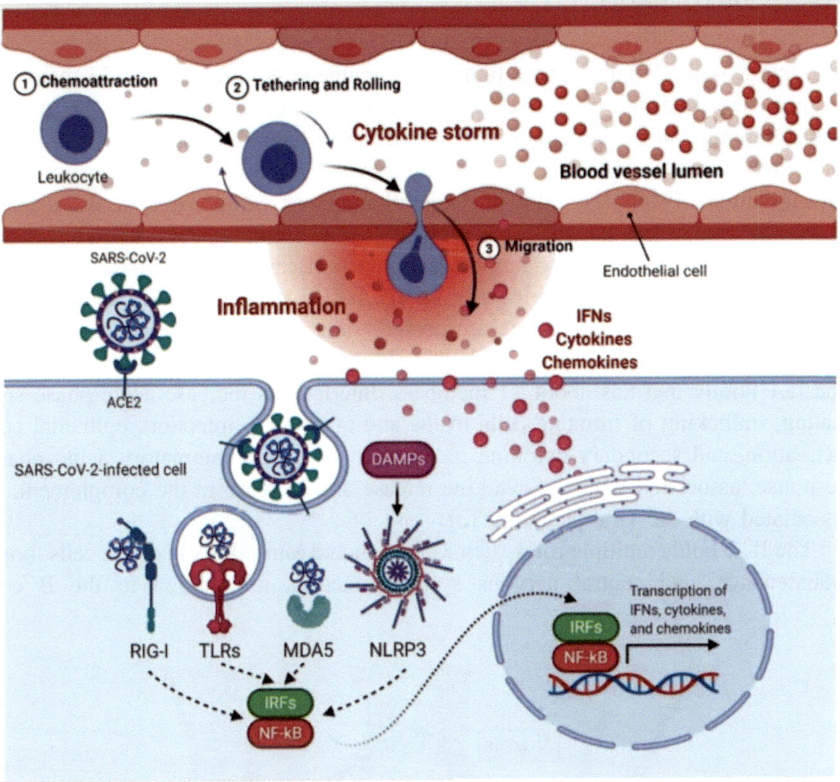

Fig. 7.2 Cytokine production activation. Pro-inflammatory phase of COVID-19 pathogenesis. After target cell entry, innate receptors such as RIG-I, TLRs, and MDA5 recognize SARS-CoV-2 RNA motifs. The NLRP3 inflammasome recognizes DAMPs, which are generated by SARS-CoV-2 infection. This virus-receptor recognition activates transcription factors such as IRFs and NF-kB, activating the transcription of target genes such as IFNs, cytokines, and chemokines. The secretion of these proteins induces endothelial activation by increasing blood vessel permeability. This allows leukocytes to infiltrate the site of infection *Source* Figure 3a (of a, b,c). Lee, C. and Choi, W.J., 2021. Overview of COVID-19 inflammatory pathogenesis from the therapeutic perspective. Archives of pharmacal research, pp.1–18. https://link.springer.com/article/10.1007/s12272-020-01301-7. Published by Springer Nature

according to the type of specific receptors. These are further involved in the activation of transcription factors and the induction of genes that encode protein products with antiviral, antiproliferative, or immunomodulatory properties. Among interferons, IFN type I and III are considered most important in defense against viral disease. The patients with severe COVID19 have altered IFN I response in comparison with mild or moderate cases [2].

7.2.2 *Interleukins*

The interleukins (IL) are a large family of immune system regulators (33 members or more, are produced by the activated leukocytes and are involved in the growth and differentiation of the leukocytes. The ILs may have multiple functional activities, including proinflammatory activities however are also known to have anti inflammatory effects. Immune and inflammatory components of the disease appear to have distinct characteristics. Dysregulated secretion and processing of IL-1β is an important feature of auto-inflammatory diseases. The caspase 1 (inflammasome) is involved in the release of IL-1β, IL-18, and IL-33 in an active form.

The IL-1 alpha and IL-1 beta are proinflammatory cytokines that mediate the host response to infection. The interleukins IL-1α, IL-1β, IL-18, and IL-33 are from the IL1 family that has about 11 members. Interleukins increase acute-phase signaling, trafficking of immune cells to the site of primary infection, epithelial cell activation, and secondary cytokine production. The proinflammatory acute phase response, associated with the cytokine release and increase in the complement, is associated with the viral clearance [3].

The IL-6 holds multiple roles such as growth and inhibition of certain cells, bone maintenance, and central nervous system function, in addition to the B cell

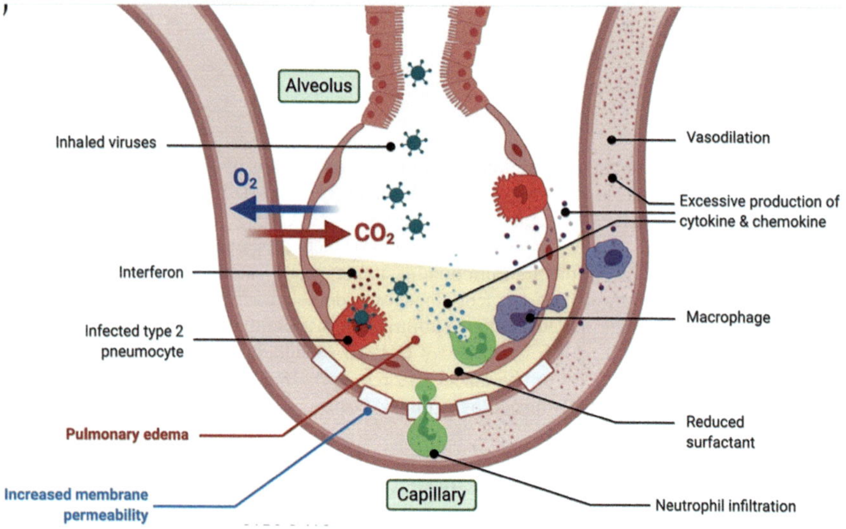

Fig. 7.3 Pneumocyte-SARS CoV2 interaction and cytokine production. SARS-CoV-2 infection of type 2 pneumocytes leads to cytokine overproduction. This increases the membrane permeability of the capillary walls around the infected alveoli, resulting in pulmonary edema. Due to this pulmonary edema, proper gas exchange is impaired in COVID-19 patients. This is clinically manifested by dyspnea, hypoxemia, and ARDS *Source* Figure 3b (of a.b.c) Lee, C. and Choi, W.J., 2021. Overview of COVID-19 inflammatory pathogenesis from the therapeutic perspective. Archives of pharmacal research, pp.1–18. https://link.springer.com/article/10.1007/s12272-020-01301-7. Published by Springer Nature

differentiation. The IL-6 has increased expression in metabolic conditions (obesity, diabetes), inflammatory diseases (infections, autoimmune disorders), cardiovascular diseases, and certain cancers. The IL6 has receptors in the hypothalamus and also contributes to the endocrine function of appetite and energy control, and thermoregulation. An increased expression of the anti inflammatory cytokine IL-10 was reported to induce collagen production and fibrocyte recruitment into the lung [4]. The IL-10 is known to suppress the IFN-γ, IL-1, TNF-α, and IL-6 production, as well as possesses other anti-inflammatory activities and may have a potential role in the process of fibrosis.

The immune profile of patients with severe CoViD19 reveals significantly elevated levels of IL6 with the role of a potential mediator of the critical complications. The SARS CoV2 NSP9 and NSP10 might induce IL-6 and IL-8 production, potentially by inhibition of NKRF, an endogenous NF-kB repressor [5]. The IL6 is also implicated in the pathogenesis of cytokine release syndrome (CRS) that has overlapping characteristics observed in the hyperinflammatory response seen in severe CoViD19 and serves as a potential therapeutic target currently under investigation.

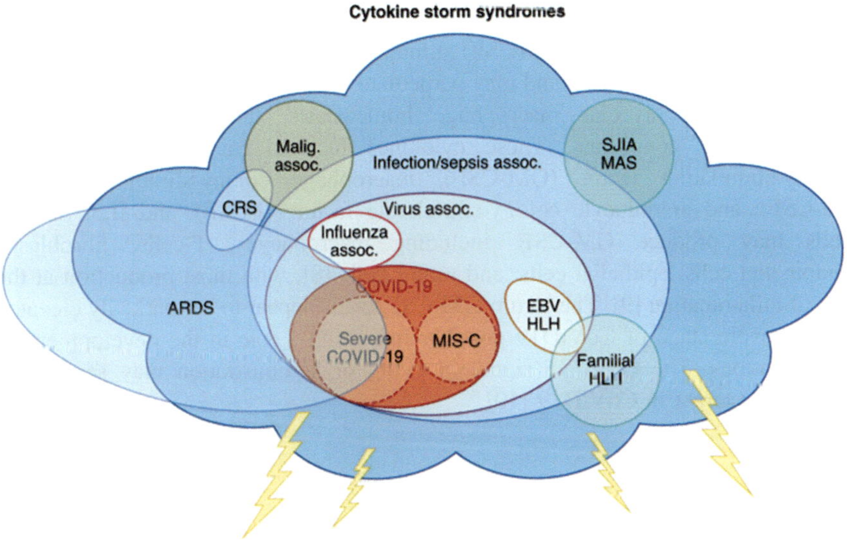

Fig. 7.4 The family of disease states that fall under the umbrella term 'cytokine storm'. The disease phenotype of COVID-19 resembles that of other pathological syndromes that are driven by uncontrolled immune system activation and cause cytokine storm. The consequent inflammation can lead to tissue and organ damage. COVID-19 has overlap with features of acute respiratory distress syndrome (ARDS) and post-viral syndromes. MIS-C has less lung involvement (ARDS) and more features of Kawasaki disease. Assoc., association; CRS, cytokine release syndrome; EBV, Epstein–Barr virus; HLH, hemophagocytic lymphohistiocytosis; Malig., malignancy; MAS, macrophage activation syndrome; SJIA, systemic juvenile idiopathic arthritis. *Source* Figure 1. Buszko, M., Nita-Lazar, A., Park, J.H., Schwartzberg, P.L., Verthelyi, D., Young, H.A. and Rosenberg, A.S., 2021. Lessons learned: new insights on the role of cytokines in COVID-19. https://www.nature.com/articles/s41590-021-00901-9. By Springer Nature Group

7.2.3 Chemokines

The chemokines are the most abundant form of cytokines (with 44 members or more), released by a variety of cells as a response to viral or other microbial infections, and bind to one or more of the 21 G-protein-coupled receptors [6]. The chemokines are mostly pro-inflammatory and help to recruit immune cells (leukocytes) to the site of the infection.

The chemokines appear to have two structural classes such as the CC chemokines and the CXC chemokines and include IL-8, MCP-1, MIP-1α, and others. As chemoattractants, these can be highly specific to certain cells such as CXCL8 (IL-8) for neutrophils, CCL2 (MCP-1) for the monocytes. The chemokines may play a crucial role in the development of hyperinflammatory immune response observed in the complicated CoViD19, with CXCL10 from the CXC family and CXCL2 from the CC family most prominent members [7].

7.2.4 Colony Stimulating Factors

The colony-stimulating factors (CSF) stimulate hematopoietic progenitor cell proliferation and differentiation and may perpetuate inflammatory reactions and plays a critical role in alveolar macrophage homeostasis, lung inflammation, and immunological conditions. These cytokines include granulocyte–macrophage colony-stimulating factor (GM-CSF), macrophage colony-stimulating factor (M-CSF), and granulocyte colony-stimulating factor (G-CSF), and IL3. Several cells may produce GM-CSF, including macrophages, T-cells, fibroblasts, endothelial cells, epithelial cells, and tumor cells [8], with most production at the site of inflammation [9]. The serum GM-CSF levels appear to be markedly elevated in the severe stage of CoViD19 possibly indicating a role in the development of complications. The GM-CSF signal blocking or administration may serve as a therapeutic target in CoViD19 [10].

7.2.5 Tumor Necrosis Factor

The tumor necrosis factor (TNF) is a proinflammatory cytokine and activates cytotoxic T lymphocytes. It plays a central role in acute viral diseases and is associated with chronic inflammatory and autoimmune diseases including atherosclerosis. It is known to be expressed by a variety of immune cells. The superfamily of TNF proteins consists of 19 members that signal through 29 receptors. The TNF alpha levels are elevated in patients with severe CoViD19 and may predict disease severity and death [11]. Several arguments justify the rationale for anti-TNF therapy in patients with CoViD19 [12].

7.3 Cytokine Storm in CoViD19

While the general concept of an excessive or uncontrolled release of proinflammatory cytokines is well known, an actual definition of what constitutes a cytokine storm is lacking [13]. See Fig. 7.4. The SARS CoV2 may produce an excessive immune reaction in the host that results in excessive tissue damage. See Fig. 7.3. In CoViD19, the hyperinflammatory state induced by the SARS CoV2 in its severe form has been profiled as a "cytokine storm".

The tumor necrosis factor (TNF) α, interleukin 1β (IL-1β), IL-6, granulocyte-colony stimulating factor (G CSF), interferon gamma-induced protein-10 (IP 10), monocyte chemoattractant protein-1 (MCP-1), and macrophage inflammatory proteins 1-α (MIP 1-α), were significantly elevated in CoViD19 patients [14, 15]. This excessive cytokine response is characterized by increased interleukin (IL)-2, IL-7, granulocyte colony-stimulating factor (G CSF), interferon (IFN-γ) inducible protein (IP 10), monocyte chemoattractant protein 1 (MCP1), macrophage inflammatory protein 1-α (MIP 1-α), and tumor necrosis factor-α (TNF α).

Multiple factors determine the degree of severity of the cytokine storm, such as dynamics of different cytokines, host susceptibility, genetic factors, pathogen strain, the strength of chemotactic mechanisms, and others. Analysis of a cohort of 41 patients admitted with CoViD19 suggested that the cytokine storm was associated with disease severity. Patients had high serum levels of IL-1β, IFNγ, IP10, and MCP1. However, those with a more severe condition requiring intensive care unit (ICU) admission had higher concentrations of G CSF, IP10, MCP1, MIP1A, and TNFα than did those not requiring ICU admission [16]. In another study three cytokines IP-10, MCP-3, and IL-1ra were closely associated with disease severity and outcome of COVID-19 [16]. An analysis of a large cohort study of 1484 patients admitted with CoViD19 showed high serum IL-6, IL-8 and TNF-α levels at the time of hospitalization were strong and independent predictors of patient survival ($P < 0.0001$, $P = 0.0205$ and $P = 0.0140$, respectively) [11].

7.3.1 *Kinetics of the Cytokine Storm*

A systemic extension of localized acute respiratory infection that results in sepsis, with typical clinical and biochemical features, forms the basis of the cytokine storm in CoViD19. The acute-response cytokines (early minutes to hours after infection) include TNF, IL-1 beta, and the chemotactic cytokines IL-8 and MCP. This is followed by a more sustained increase in interleukin 6 (IL-6). The (IL-6) behaves like a protagonist of the cytokine storm.

At a later stage, the anti inflammatory cytokine IL-10 increases, as a measure to control the acute systemic inflammatory response. The dysregulation of cytokines may also be the result of other mechanisms, such as evasion of innate sensing mechanisms by SARS CoV2, induction of IL-6, and IL-8 production by the SARS-CoV-2 NSP9 and NSP10, potentially by the inhibition of NKRF, (an endogenous NF-kB repressor) in addition to others [5].

According to an analysis, the viral-induced immunosuppression due to the suppression of interferon, lymphopenia, NK cell abnormalities may drive macrophage infiltration and result in hyper cytokinetic picture reflected by overexpression of IL-6, IL-1, IL-18, INFγ, GM-CSF, and others [17]. Following the pro-inflammatory stage, substantial reduction of the peripheral lymphocyte counts, mainly CD4 T and CD8 T cells, is seen in the CoViD19 patients.

7.3.2 The "T" Cell Response

Another important component of the immune system involved in the CoViD19 related hyperimmune response is lymphocytes. The altered lymphocyte count and function in CoViD19 may be a marker of the severity of the disease. Several studies indicate an association of lymphocytopenia with the CoViD19 severity and mortality [18]. The innate immune response involved in the viral recognition through Pathogen Recognition Receptors (PRRs) leads to the initiation of signaling cascades causing the production of cytokines and induction of antiviral programs and adaptive immune response.

A concomitant rise in the inflammatory cytokines may deplete the T cell populations in CoViD19. According to an analysis of a cohort of 123 patients admitted with CoViD19 investigating cytokines and the severity of the disease, low levels of the CD4+T and CD8+ T were common in the severe CoViD19 patients, whereas IL-6 and IL-10 levels were higher in severe patients. Suggesting the possible role of these immune markers as markers of transition from mild to severe disease [19].

The CD4 T helper cells control the adaptive immune response, secret cytokines, and generate a microenvironment that directs the T cell responses. They activate cells in the innate immune system, help B cells in antibody production and with immune response by other cells, produce cytokines and also suppress immune reaction (Th2 cells), while the CD8+T cells eliminate virus-infected cells. The Th1 cells produce cytokines such as IFN γ, IL 2, and TNF beta, and trigger cell-mediated immunity [20]. The Th2 cells produce IL-4, IL-5, IL-6, IL-9, IL-10, and IL-13 to regulate the antibody responses [21].

In patients with CoViD19, the inflammatory cytokines may activate the T-helper type 1 (Th1) cell response [15]. The patients with CoViD19 also have elevated levels of the Th2 cell-secreted cytokines (such as IL-4 and IL-10), which inhibit the inflammatory response [15]. Increased production of the IL10, after the onset of cytokine storm, is associated with counter-anti-inflammatory response or "immunoparalysis". It results in the downregulation of the neutrophil and monocyte function in the systemic circulation and may be a hallmark of a poor outcome as opposed to being seen as an inflammation-controlling mechanism [22–26].

Several mechanisms involving the proinflammatory cytokines, IFN-I and TNF-α, IL-6 [27, 28], as well as the Fas-FasL interactions [29], direct viral T cell infection, and other factors may cause T cell depletion in CoViD19, however exact mechanisms remain unclear. The dysregulated T cell responses may cause immunopathology and contribute to the disease severity and development of complications in patients with CoViD19.

7.3.3 Cytokines and Severity of CoViD19

The prognostic significance of the association of the cytokine storm and CoViD19 has been extensively explored. The cytokine storm is typically associated with acute respiratory distress syndrome (ARDS) and multi-organ failure (MOF) and is known to have a positive correlation with the disease severity. (See Fig. 7.1). In CoViD19, the cytokines appear to play a significant role in the development of sepsis and multi-organ failure. Higher levels of cytokines such as IL6 and IL 1 are associated with higher fatality in these conditions [30–33]. The hyper-immune-inflammatory state may facilitate the development of pathogenetic mechanisms (see Fig. 7.2), thus leading to poor clinical outcomes. Analysis of a retrospective single-center cohort of 138 hospitalized patients with COVID19 indicated that neutrophilia, hypercoagulation, and acute kidney injury associated with the sustained inflammatory response, the cytokine storm, and the viral injury in the CoViD19 patients might contribute to the mortality [34]. The T lymphocytes can activate platelets, which amplify the release of CCL5 (RANTES) a chemokine involved in the inflammation [35]. Other mechanisms may result in damage to cells and tissues. The evidence shows that cytokines may cause the apoptosis of the T cell lymphocytes, endothelial and epithelial cells of the airways [36–39]. The immune thrombotic mechanisms related to the platelets, activation of the extrinsic coagulation cascade, or dysregulated immune myeloid responses [40] are among mechanisms that may explain the damage to the pulmonary, cardiovascular and other systems in the complicated CoViD19.

7.4 Cytokines in Cardiovascular and Metabolic Diseases

Immunopathogenesis is an important mechanism associated with cardiovascular diseases and may be induced by infectious, metabolic, toxic, or autoimmune diseases. The immunoinflammatory stress response in the complicated CoViD19 is responsible for the development of cardiovascular complications frequently associated with the disease, especially in patients with a background of cardiometabolic conditions. Cardiovascular toxicity of cytokines has been previously demonstrated [41]. A large amount of evidence suggests interconnection between the proinflammatory and immune pathogenetic mechanisms, and cardiovascular structures, involved in the development of hypertension and other cardiovascular diseases. Data show that hypertension is a chronic low-grade inflammatory condition and that activation of proinflammatory mechanisms contributes to the pathogenesis of hypertension [42–45]. Both animal and human diseases research models show strong implications of inflammation in hypertension and cardiovascular diseases [46, 47], and confirm the presence of increased proinflammatory cytokines in the heart [48, 49], kidneys [50], and aorta [51]. Exposure of the endothelial surface to stress factors such as infections, inflammation, hyperglycemia, and others results in endothelial injury and expression of surface adhesion molecules such as intercellular adhesion molecule-1 (ICAM-1), vascular cell adhesion molecule-1 (VCAM-1), and P-selectin [52]. These inflammatory molecules (ICAM-1, VCAM-1, monocyte chemoattractant protein-1 (MCP-1), tumor necrosis factor-α (TNF α), and C-reactive protein (CRP) have potential diagnostic and prognostic value in cardiovascular diseases.

Several mechanisms are involved in the generation, mediation, and integration of this complex process. Although the immune response plays a protective role via promotion of viral clearance and induction of repair mechanisms, a dysregulated, exacerbated and persistent response may cause inflammation of the myocardium, microangiopathy, vascular dysfunction, thrombosis, and other harmful reactions, through a variety of mechanisms including the accumulation of dysregulated ER stress, oxidative stress, and other factors.

The interleukins, such as tumor necrosis factor-α, and interferons (IFNs), are major players among the cytokines. Several studies have confirmed the association of myocardial disease, coronary heart disease, and heart failure with an increased expression of several cytokines [41, 52, 53, 77]. Certain pro-inflammatory cytokines interact with the myocardial and vascular cellular structures and induce inflammation and cellular damage through multiple signaling mechanisms and mediators. An important proinflammatory cytokine, the tumor necrosis factor (TNF)-α, produced by the activated macrophages, is involved in the induction of apoptosis. Patients with severe congestive heart failure, or dilated cardiomyopathy, and myocarditis, have raised serum levels of TNF alpha [52, 53]. Evidence strongly suggests that plasma TNF-alpha, IL-1 and IL-6, (that also induce apoptosis), are elevated in congestive heart failure [52–58]. Studies have shown that inhibition of the interleukin (IL-1) reduces cardiovascular events and synthesis of the MMP-9, and may decrease atherosclerotic plaque disruption [59, 60].

The cytokines such as type I (IFN-α and IFN-β) and type II interferons (IFN-γ) are also involved in the mediation of immune response in viral myocarditis. In acute viral coxsackievirus B–induced myocarditis, type I interferons mediate the Th1 response and reduce viral replication, whereas, the IFN-γ regulates monocyte mobilization and fibrosis [61, 62], whereas the Th2 response is associated with an increase in regulatory T cells and anti-inflammatory cytokines that may promote myocarditis. The regulatory mechanisms attempt to diminish such exaggerated pathology. The Tregs downregulate proinflammatory responses and reduce immunopathology, whereas the Th17-mediated immunity worsens the immunopathology.

The pro-inflammatory cytokines may produce cardiac-specific effects such as negative inotropism and left ventricular remodeling. Data show that cytokines and protease enzymes such as ADAM 17, involved in the shedding process of ACE2, may have an important role in the pathogenesis of cardiac remodeling [63, 64]. During the acute inflammatory phase, these cytokines may stimulate matrix metalloproteinases (MMPs) (resulting in collagen degradation and myofibrillar rearrangement) and in the later phase, prolonged stimulation of inflammatory cytokines may cause stimulation of the tissue inhibitors of matrix metalloproteinases (TIMPs) (increasing collagen fibrillar content). After viral infection, enhanced production of the proinflammatory cytokines, such as tumor necrosis factor-α (TNF) 175 [65–68], and interleukin-1 (IL-1) (178 above,179 [69], may increase cardiac damage and result in cardiac dysfunction. Following the acute phase, the development of myocarditis in the subacute phase may be a result of an exaggerated immune response [70].

The cardiac impact of the CoViD19 related inflammatory stress has been demonstrated in several case reports [71]. A case report of the virus-negative lymphocytic myocarditis associated with SARS CoV 2 showed direct evidence of myocardial inflammation in a CoViD19 patient. In this report, acute inflammatory process with diffuse T-lymphocytic inflammatory infiltrates (CD3+ > 7/mm2) with huge interstitial edema and limited foci of necrosis (in the absence of fibrosis) were found in the myocardium [72].

Furthermore, the diabetic patients with CoViD19 appear to have elevated inflammatory markers and cytokine levels as compared to the non-diabetics, and these are also associated with higher mortality. In a single-center, retrospective, observational study of 193 patients with severe CoViD19, patients with diabetes had higher serum levels of the cytokines and markers of inflammation such as hsCRP, procalcitonin, IL-2 receptor, IL-6, IL-8, and TNFα versus non-diabetics. The non-survivor diabetics also had higher levels of leukocyte count, neutrophil count, hsCRP, procalcitonin, ferritin, IL-2 receptor, IL-6, TNFα, and lower levels of lymphocyte count as compared with diabetic who survived. A higher incidence of myocardial injury in diabetics versus non-diabetics and non-survivors was observed [73]. Furthermore, the balance of pro and anti-inflammation may be affected due to dysfunction related to the Th17 and Treg cells in patients with diabetes and obesity that may involve several pathways involving CD4 T cells activation and differentiation through Th1 and Th cells [74–77].

In summary, cytokines play an important role in the development and augmentation of cardiovascular and metabolic diseases and are also associated with the development of cardiovascular complications in patients with severe CoViD19 such as myocarditis, decompensated heart failure, and several others. The viral replication, hypoxia, dysregulated immune cells, and cytokines lead to hyper inflammation and structural damage to the mico and macro vasculature and cardiac cells and tissues, apoptosis, oxidative stress, and ultimately lead to fibrosis and dysfunction through several pathways including ACE2, matrix metalloproteinases (MMP), endothelial injury, dysmetabolism, and others. The important cytokines involved in CoViD19 include IL1, IL6, IL8, TNF alpha, and IFN gamma that are also known to have a role in the immunopathogenesis of chronic cardiovascular diseases. Further investigations are needed to elucidate these mechanisms and signaling pathways involved in the development of CoViD19 cardiovascular complications that could also serve as important therapeutic targets.

7.5 Summary

The cytokines have a multifunctional role in the immune and inflammatory mechanisms in the body with a significant diagnostic and therapeutic value. Although multiple terms are used to describe the hyperinflammatory states such as sHLH (Secondary hemophagocytic lymphohistiocytosis) linked with macrophage activation syndrome (MAS), CRS (cytokines release syndrome), or cytokine storm (CS), observed in the viral diseases or other conditions for instance drugs-related or others. These hyperinflammatory states are frequently associated with an increased risk of complications such as pulmonary (ARDS) and extrapulmonary multi-organ failure. The cytokine storm seen in the CoViD19 exhibits several overlapping features with these conditions such a lymphopenia, elevation of cytokines, markers of inflammation and hypercoagulability as also observed in the CRS. An important association of cytokines and inflammation has been revealed in CoViD19 studies linking several important CoViD19 complications with increased production of cytokines and associated inflammation. Importantly, there appears to be an association between CoViD19 related mortality and dysregulated cytokine release. The cytokine storm observed in CoViD19 patients is marked by increased interleukin (IL)-2, IL-7, granulocyte colony-stimulating factor, interferon-γ inducible protein 10 (IP-10), monocyte chemoattractant protein 1 (MCP-1), macrophage inflammatory protein 1-α (MIP-1α), and tumor necrosis factor-α (TNF-α) [15]. In CoViD19, the increased levels of proinflammatory cytokines (such as IL-1B, IFN-γ, IP-10, and monocyte chemoattractant protein 1 (MCP-1)) may activate Th1 (T helper type 1) response and the Th2 cell-secreted cytokines (such as IL4 and IL10) may inhibit the inflammatory response. The uncontrolled systemic inflammation characterized by excessive concentrations of pro-inflammatory cytokines and chemokines, secreted by the immune effector cells may cause harm in CoViD19 patients. This has given rise to the argument for the use of immunosuppressive therapy in CoViD19 patients with hyperinflammation. Whether the hyper inflammation and hyper cytokinetic state in CoViD19 are related to the systemic activation of the macrophages or a result of pulmonary flare must be further probed.

(cytokine, or cytokine failure. cytokine CoViD19 cytokines inflammation and in the CRS. inflammation CoViD19.

CoViD19 cytokines cytokines inflammation cytokines CoViD19

The cytokines are recognized as an important component of several inflammatory, immune and other chronic diseases including atherosclerosis, diabetes mellitus, obesity, and related metabolic diseases as well as cancer and others. Acute and chronic inflammation both are strongly implicated in the development of cardiovascular complications. The cytokines may induce and augment damage to the cardiac and vascular structures in acute hyperinflammatory settings. Various cytokines including the TNF-alpha, IL-1, and IL-6, are well known for their role in cardiovascular diseases such as myocardial diseases, heart failure, and coronary artery disease. The hyperinflammatory stress may lead to obstructive and non-obstructive cardiovascular diseases and arrhythmias in acute settings of the hyperinflammatory state of the CoViD19.

The myocardial inflammatory disease is a critical process that may lead to decompensated heart failure, shock, or death, in acute settings of the hyperinflammatory state of the CoViD19. Reactivation or exacerbation of the inflammatory processes in patients with pre-existing chronic cardiovascular and metabolic conditions is likely to increase the risk of decompensation or the development of potentially fatal complications when met with CoViD19. Further research is needed to establish exact mechanisms and factors involved in these pathogenetic mechanisms especially concerning cytokines and other inflammatory components of the hyper inflammation that will also help develop well-targeted therapeutic approaches to prevent and treat these complications in patients with the novel coronavirus disease.

Summary Box

- Cytokines are key warning proteins, part of pathogen eliminating mechanisms, and play a crucial role in defense and inflammation.
- Viral conditions, sepsis, drug reactions may result in dysregulated production of cytokines.
- Exaggerated and persistent release of cytokines is frequently associated with multi organ failure.
- CoViD19 patients manifest exaggerated immune response marked by increased production of cytokines and chemokines: IL-1β, IL-2, IL-4, IL-6, IL-8, IL-10, IL-18, CCL2, CCL3, CCL4,), granulocyte colony stimulating factor (GSF), interferon-γ inducible protein 10 (IP-10), monocyte chemoattractant proteins (MCP-1, MCP-3), macrophage inflammatory protein 1-α (MIP-1α), and tumor necrosis factor-α (TNF-α) among others.
- Cytokine storm observed in CoViD19 has several overlapping features of hyperinflammatory states observed in other conditions including the cytokine release syndrome CRS.
- Depletion of the lymphocytes (CD4 and CD8 cells) and altered function is associated with moderate to severe CoViD19.
- Cytokine storm is associated with high risk of ARDS and multi organ failure in CoViD19.
- CoViD19.

- Cytokines are involved in the development of chronic cardiometabolic diseases frequently met in patients with complicated CoViD19.
- The acute hyperinflammatory immune mechanisms in CoViD19 may trigger cardiovascular complications such as myocarditis, decompensated heart failure, among other cardiac complications.
- The hyperinflammatory and immune state associated with CoViD19 may serve as a therapeutic target with immune suppressive and immune modulatory therapies.
- Exact mechanisms related to the hyperinflammatory immune response, specific cellular types and signaling mechanisms, markers of severity, and mechanisms behind individual susceptibility in relationship with CoViD19 complications need further validation.

References

1. Ruan Q, Yang K, Wang W, et al. Clinical predictors of mortality due to COVID-19 based on an analysis of data of 150 patients from Wuhan China. Intensive Care Med. 2020;46:846–8. https://doi.org/10.1007/s00134-020-05991-x.
2. Hadjadj J, Yatim N, Barnabei L, Corneau A, Boussier J, Smith N, Péré H, Charbit B, Bondet V, Chenevier-Gobeaux C, Breillat P. Impaired type I interferon activity and inflammatory responses in severe COVID-19 patients. Science. 2020;369(6504):718–24.
3. Gabay C, Kushner I. Acute-phase proteins and other systemic responses to inflammation. N Engl J Med. 1999;340:448–54.
4. Sun L, et al. New concepts of IL-10-induced lung fibrosis: fibrocyte recruitment and M2 activation in a CCL2/CCR2axis. Am J Physiol Lung Cell Mol Physiol. 2011;300:L341–53.
5. Liang Q, Li J, Guo M, Tian X, Liu C, Wang X, Yang X, Wu P, Xiao Z, Qu Y, Yin Y. Virus-host interactome and proteomic survey of PMBCs from COVID-19 patients reveal potential virulence factors influencing SARS-CoV-2 pathogenesis;2020. BioRxiv.
6. Comerford I, McColl SR. Focus on chemokines. Immunol Cell Biol. 2011;89:183–4.
7. Coperchini F, Chiovato L, Ricci G, Croce L, Magri F, Rotondi M. The Cytokine storm in COVID-19: further advances in our understanding the role of specific chemokines involved. Cytokine Growth Factor Rev. 2021.
8. Griffin JD, Cannistra SA, Demetri GD, Ernst TJ, Kanakura Y, Sullivan R. The biology of GM-CSF: regulation of production and interaction with its receptor. Int J Cell Cloning. 1990;8(S1):35–45.
9. Shiomi A, Usui T. Pivotal roles of GM-CSF in autoimmunity and inflammation. Mediat Inflamm. 2015.
10. Lang FM, Lee KMC, Teijaro JR, Becher B, Hamilton JA. GM-CSF-based treatments in COVID-19: reconciling opposing therapeutic approaches. Nat Rev Immunol. 2020:1–8.
11. Del Valle DM, Kim-Schulze S, Huang HH, Beckmann ND, Nirenberg S, Wang B, Lavin Y, Swartz TH, Madduri D, Stock A, Marron TU. An inflammatory cytokine signature predicts COVID-19 severity and survival. Nat Med. 2020;26(10):1636–43.
12. Robinson PC, Richards D, Tanner HL, Feldmann M. Accumulating evidence suggests anti-TNF therapy needs to be given trial priority in COVID-19 treatment. Lancet Rheumatol. 2020;2(11):e653–5.

13. Tisoncik JR, Korth MJ, Simmons CP, Farrar J, Martin TR, Katze MG. Into the eye of the cytokine storm. Microbiol Mol Biol Rev. 2012;76(1):16–32. https://doi.org/10.1128/MMBR.05015-11.
14. Liu J, Li S, Liu J. Longitudinal characteristics of lymphocyte responses and cytokine profiles in the peripheral blood of SARS-CoV-2 infected patients;2020. medRxiv. https://doi.org/10.1101/2020.02.16.20023671. Published online Feb 22 (preprint).
15. Huang C, Wang Y, Li X. Clinical features of patients infected with 2019 novel coronavirus in Wuhan China. Lancet. 2020;395:497–506.
16. Yang Y, Shen C, Li J, Yuan J, Yang M, Wang F, Li G, Li Y, Xing L, Peng L, Wei J. Exuberant elevation of IP-10, MCP-3 and IL-1ra during SARS-CoV-2 infection is associated with disease severity and fatal outcome;2020. MedRxiv.
17. McGonagle D, Sharif K, O'Regan A, Bridgewood C. The role of cytokines including Interleukin-6 in COVID-19 induced Pneumonia and Macrophage Activation Syndrome-like disease. Autoimmun Rev. 2020:102537. https://doi.org/10.1016/j.autrev.2020.102537. [Epub ahead of print] Review. PubMed PMID: 32251717.
18. Vabret N, Britton GJ, Gruber C, Hegde S, Kim J, Kuksin M, Levantovsky R, Malle L, Moreira A, Park MD, Pia L. Immunology of COVID-19: current state of the science. Immunity. 2020.
19. WanS, Yi Q, Fan S, Lv J, Zhang X, Guo L, et al. Characteristics of lymphocyte subsets and cytokines in peripheral blood of 123 hospitalized patients with 2019 novel coronavirus pneumonia (NCP);2020. medRxiv 2020.02.10.20021832.
20. Raphael I, Nalawade S, Eagar TN, Forsthuber TG. T cell subsets and their signature cytokines in autoimmune and inflammatory diseases. Cytokine. 2015;74(1):5–17.
21. Kahn SE, Hull RL, Utzschneider KM. Mechanisms linking obesity to insulin resistance and type 2 diabetes. Nature. 2006;444(7121):840–6.
22. Cohen J. The immunopathogenesis of sepsis. Nature. 2002;420:885–91.
23. Docke WD, et al. Monocyte deactivation in septic patients: restoration by IFN-gamma treatment. Nat Med. 1997;3:678–81.
24. Fowler AA, Fisher BJ, Centor RM, Carchman RA. Development of the adult respiratory distress syndrome: progressive alteration of neutrophil chemotactic and secretory processes. Am J Pathol. 1984;116:427–35.
25. Monneret G, et al. Persisting low monocyte human leukocyte antigen-DR expression predicts mortality in septic shock. Intensive Care Med. 2006;32:1175–83.
26. Munford RS, Pugin J. Normal responses to injury prevent systemic inflammation and can be immunosuppressive. Am J Respir Crit Care Med. 2001;163:316–21.
27. Diao B, Wang C, Tan Y, Chen X, Liu Y, Ning L, Chen L, Li M, Liu Y, Wang G, Yuan Z. Reduction and functional exhaustion of T cells in patients with coronavirus disease 2019 (COVID-19). Front Immunol. 2020;11:827.
28. Kamphuis E, Junt T, Waibler Z, Forster R, Kalinke U. Type I interferons directly regulate lymphocyte recirculation and cause transient blood lymphopenia. Blood. 2006;108(10):3253–61.
29. Feng Z, Diao B, Wang R, Wang G, Wang C, Tan Y, Liu L, Wang C, Liu Y, Liu Y, Yuan Z. The novel severe acute respiratory syndrome coronavirus 2 (SARS-CoV-2) directly decimates human spleens and lymph nodes;2020. MedRxiv.
30. Chousterman BG, Swirski FK, Weber GF. Cytokine storm and sepsis disease pathogenesis. Semin Immunopathol. 2017;39(5):517–28.
31. Chen L, Liu H-G, Liu W, Liu J, Liu K, Shang J, et al. Analysis of clinical features of 29 patients with 2019 novel coronavirus pneumonia. Chin J Tuberc Respir Dis. 2020;43.
32. Parsons PE, Eisner MD, Thompson BT, Matthay MA, Ancukiewicz M, Bernard GR, et al. Lower tidal volume ventilation and plasma cytokine markers of inflammation in patients with acute lung injury. Critical Care Med. 2005;33(1):1 232. PubMed PMID: 15644641.
33. Wang H, Ma S. The cytokine storm and factors determining the sequence and severity of organ dysfunction in multiple organ dysfunction syndrome. Am J Emerg Med. 2008;26 (6):711–5. PubMed PMID: 18606328.

34. Wang D, Hu B, Hu C, et al. Clinical characteristics of 138 hospitalized patients with 2019 novel coronavirus-infected pneumonia in Wuhan China. JAMA. 2020;323:1061.
35. Danese S, de la Motte C, Reyes BM, Sans M, Levine AD, Fiocchi C.Cutting edge: T cells trigger CD40-dependent platelet activation and granular RANTES release: a novel pathway for immune response amplification. J Immunol. 2004;172(4):2011–5. [PubMed] [Ref list].
36. Channappanavar R, Fehr AR, Vijay R, Mack M, Zhao J, Meyerholz DK, et al. Dysregulated type I interferon and inflammatory monocyte-macrophage responses cause lethal pneumonia in SARS-CoV-infected mice. Cell Host Microbe. 2016;19(2):181–93 PubMed PMID: 26867177.
37. Herold S, Steinmueller M, von Wulffen W, Cakarova L, Pinto R, Pleschka S, et al. Lung epithelial apoptosis in influenza virus pneumonia: the role of macrophage-expressed TNF-related apoptosis-inducing ligand. J Exp Med. 2008;205(13):3065–77. PubMed PMID: 19064696. Epub 2008/12/08.
38. Högner K, Wolff T, Pleschka S, Plog S, Gruber AD, Kalinke U, et al. Macrophage-expressed IFN-β contributes to apoptotic alveolar epithelial cell injury in severe influenza virus pneumonia. PLoS Pathog. 2013;9(2):e1003188-e. PubMed PMID: 23468627. Epub 2013/02/28.
39. Rodrigue-Gervais IG, Labbé K, Dagenais M, Dupaul-Chicoine J, Champagne C, Morizot A, et al. Cellular inhibitor of apoptosis protein cIAP2 protects against pulmonary tissue necrosis during influenza virus infection to promote host survival. Cell Host Microbe. 2014;15(1):23–35 PubMed PMID: 24439895.
40. Mehta P, McAuley DF, Brown M, Sanchez E, Tattersall RS, Manson JJ. COVID-19: consider cytokine storm syndromes and immunosuppression. The Lancet. 2020;395(10229):1033–34.
41. Jamal FA, Khaled SK. The cardiovascular complications of chimeric antigen receptor T cell therapy. Curr Hematol Malig Rep. 2020;15(2):130–2.
42. Sriramula S, Cardinale JP, Lazartigues E, Francis J. ACE2 overexpression in the paraventricular nucleus attenuates angiotensin II-induced hypertension. Cardiovasc Res. 2011;92:401–8.
43. Marvar PJ, Thabet SR, Guzik TJ, Lob HE, McCann LA, Weyand C, Gordon FJ, Harrison DG. Central and peripheral mechanisms of T-lymphocyte activation and vascular inflammation produced by angiotensin II-induced hypertension. Circ Res. 2010;107:263–70.
44. Lu Y, Chen J, Yin X, Zhao H. Angiotensin II receptor 1 involved in the central pressor response induced by interleukin-1 beta in the paraventricular nucleus. Neurol Res. 2009;31:420–24.
45. Shi P, Diez-Freire C, Jun JY, Qi Y, Katovich MJ, Li Q, Sriramula S, Francis J, Sumners C, Raizada MK. Brain microglial cytokinesXE "Cytokines" in neurogenic hypertension. Hypertension. 2010;56:297–330.
46. Ferrario CM, Strawn WB. Role of the renin-angiotensin-aldosterone system and proinflammatory mediators in cardiovascular disease. Am J Cardiol. 2006;98:121–8.
47. Shi P, Raizada MK, Sumners C. Brain cytokines as neuromodulators in cardiovascular control. Clin Exp Pharmacol Physiol. 2010;37:e52–7.
48. Kagitani S, Ueno H, Hirade S, Takahashi T, Takata M, Inoue H. Tranilast attenuates myocardial fibrosis in association with suppression of monocyte/macrophage infiltration in DOCA/salt hypertensive rats. J Hypertens. 2004;22:1007–15.
49. Francis J, Weiss RM, Johnson AK, Felder RB. Central mineralocorticoid receptor blockade decreases plasma TNF-alpha after coronary artery ligation in rats. Am J Physiol Regul Integr Comp Physiol. 2003;284:R328–35.
50. Wang Y, Wang DH. Aggravated renal inflammatory responses in TRPV1 gene knockout mice subjected to DOCA-salt hypertension. Am J Physiol Renal Physiol. 2009;297:F1550–9.
51. Seifi B, Kadkhodaee M, Xu J, Soleimani M. Pro-inflammatory cytokines of rat vasculature in DOCA-salt treatment. Mol Biol Rep. 2010;37:2111–15.
52. Ross R. Atherosclerosis—an inflammatory disease. N Engl J Med. 1999;340:115–26.
53. Levine B, Kalman J, Mayer L, Fillit HM, Packer M. Elevated circulating levels of tumor necrosis factor in severe chronic heart failure. N Engl J Med. 1990;323(4):236–41.

54. Matsumori A, Yamada T, Suzuki H, et al. Increased circulating cytokines in patients with myocarditis and cardiomyopathy. Br Heart J. 1994;72:561–6.
55. McMurray J, Abdullah I, Dargie HJ, Shapiro D. Increased concentrations of tumor necrosis factor in cachectic patients with severe chronic heart failure. Br Heart J. 1991;66:356–8.
56. Katz SD, Rao R, Berman JW, et al. Pathophysiological correlation of increased serum tumor necrosis factor in patients with congestive heart failure: relation to nitric oxide-dependent vasodilation in the forearm circulation. Circulation. 1994;90:12–6.
57. Ferrari R, Bachetti T, Confortini R, et al. Tumor necrosis factor soluble receptors in patients with various degrees of congestive heart failure. Circulation. 1995;92:1479–86.
58. Ali M, Girgis S, Hassan A, Rudick S, Becker RC. Inflammation and coronary artery disease: from pathophysiology to Canakinumab anti-inflammatory thrombosis outcomes study (CANTOS). Coron Artery Dis. 2018;29:429–37.
59. Newby AC. Metalloproteinases promote plaque rupture and myocardial infarction: a persuasive concept waiting for clinical translation. Matrix Biol. 2015;44–46:157–66.
60. Burke JD, Sonenberg N, Platanias LC, Fish EN. Antiviral effects of interferon-β are enhanced in the absence of the translational suppressor 4E-BP1 in myocarditis induced by Coxsackievirus B3. Antivir Ther. 2011;16:577–84. https://doi.org/10.3851/IMP1752.
61. Fairweather D, Frisancho-Kiss S, Yusung SA, Barrett MA, Davis SE, Steele RA, Gatewood SJ, Rose NR. IL-12 protects against coxsackievirus B3-induced myocarditis by increasing IFN-gamma and macrophage and neutrophil populations in the heart. J Immunol. 2005;174:261–9.
62. Fedak PW, Moravec CS, McCarthy PM, et al. Altered expression of disintegrin metalloproteinases and their inhibitor in human dilated cardiomyopathy. Circulation. 2006;113:238–45.
63. Rutschow S, Li J, Schultheiss HP, Pauschinger M. Myocardial proteases and matrix remodeling in inflammatory heart disease. Cardiovasc Res. 2006;69:646–56.
64. Bachmaier K, Pummerer C, Kozieradzki I, Pfeffer K, Mak TW, Neu N, Penninger JM. Low-molecular-weight tumor necrosis factor receptor p55 controls induction of autoimmune heart disease. Circulation. 1997;95:655–61.
65. Huber SA, Sartini D. Roles of tumor necrosis factor alpha (TNFalpha) and the p55 TNF receptor in CD1d induction and coxsackievirus B3-induced myocarditis. J Virol. 2005;79:2659–65. https://doi.org/10.1128/JVI.79.5.2659-2665.2005.
66. Kim JM, Lim BK, Ho SH, Yun SH, Shin JO, Park EM, Kim DK, Kim S, Jeon ES. TNFR-Fc fusion protein expressed by in vivo electroporation improves survival rates and myocardial injury in coxsackievirus induced murine myocarditis. Biochem Biophys Res Commun. 2006;344:765–71. https://doi.org/10.1016/j.bbrc.2006.03.170.
67. Lane JR, Neumann DA, Lafond-Walker A, Herskowitz A, Rose NR. Interleukin 1 or tumor necrosis factor can promote coxsackie B3-induced myocarditis in resistant B10.A mice. J Exp Med. 1992;175:1123–29.
68. Lim BK, Choe SC, Shin JO, Ho SH, Kim JM, Yu SS, Kim S, Jeon ES. Local expression of interleukin-1 receptor antagonist by plasmid DNA improves mortality and decreases myocardial inflammation in experimental coxsackieviral myocarditis. Circulation. 2002;105:1278–81.
69. Kindermann I, Barth C, Mahfoud F, Ukena C, Lenski M, Yilmaz A, Klingel K, Kandolf R, Sechtem U, Cooper LT, Böhm M. Update on myocarditis. J Am Coll Cardiol. 2012;59:779–92. https://doi.org/10.1016/j.jacc.2011.09.074.
70. Inciardi RM, Lupi L, Zaccone G, et al. Cardiac involvement in a patient with coronavirus disease 2019 (COVID-19). JAMA Cardiol. Published online March 27, 2020. https://doi.org/10.1001/jamacardio.2020.1096.
71. Sala S, Peretto G, Gramegna M, Palmisano A, Villatore A, Vignale D, De Cobelli F, Tresoldi M, Cappelletti AM, Basso C, Godino C, Esposito A. Acute myocarditis presenting as a reverse Tako-Tsubo syndrome in a patient with SARS-CoV-2 respiratory infection. Eur Heart J. 2020;41(19):1861–62. https://doi.org/10.1093/eurheartj/ehaa286.

72. Yan Y, Yang Y, Wang F, et al. Clinical characteristics and outcomes of patients with severe covid-19 with diabetes. BMJ Open Diab Res Care. 2020;8:e001343. https://doi.org/10.1136/bmjdrc-2020-001343.
73. Xia C, Rao X, Zhong J. Role of T lymphocytes in type 2 diabetes and diabetes-associated inflammation. J Diabetes Res. 2017;2017:1–6.
74. Shirakawa K, Yan X, Shinmura K, et al. Obesity accelerates T cell senescence in murine visceral adipose tissue. J Clin Invest. 2016;126:4626–39.
75. Zhang C, Xiao C, Wang P, et al. The alteration of Th1/Th2/Th17/Treg paradigm in patients with type 2 diabetes mellitus: relationship with diabetic nephropathy. Hum Immunol. 2014;75:289–96.
76. Jagannathan- Bogdan M, McDonnell ME, Shin H, et al. Elevated proinflammatory cytokine production by a skewed T cell compartment requires monocytes and promotes inflammation in type 2 diabetes. J Immunol. 2011;186:1162–72.
77. Armstrong EJ, Morrow DA, Sabatine MS. Inflammatory biomarkers in acute coronary syndromes: part I: introduction and cytokines. Circulation. 2006;113(6):e72–e75.

Chapter 8
The Renin-Angiotensin System in COVID19

Key Questions

- What is renin-angiotensin aldosterone system (RAAS)?
- What is the significance of RAAS in CoViD19?
- What are the key characteristics of the ACE2?
- What are the implications of ACE2 in cardiovascular diseases?
- What are the dynamics of various components of RAAS?
- What is the importance of ACE2 dynamics in relation to CoViD19 complications?
- How gender variations in ACE2 interlink with CoViD19?

8.1 Introduction

The renin angiotensin" aldosterone system (RAAS) is one of the most widely explored homeostatic mechanisms known to have a pivotal role in the maintenance of blood pressure and fluid balance in the body. The pathogenetic and therapeutic value of the RAAS in cardiovascular and renal diseases is well documented. This complex peptide system has also emerged as an important pathogenetic substrate interlinked with the induction and propagation of the mechanisms involved in the development of complications of CoViD19. Several immuno-inflammatory, humoral, metabolic, and other factors, known to play an important role in this process, are triggered under the stressful conditions of viral sepsis. In CoViD19, a dysregulated RAAS may result in destructive mechanisms that ultimately contribute to tissue damage, organ dysfunction, and failure, making it a potential therapeutic target.

U. Mallick, *Cardiovascular Complications of COVID-19*,
https://doi.org/10.1007/978-3-030-90065-6_8

The therapeutic value of the RAAS is widely established in the context of cardiovascular, metabolic, and renal diseases. Due to overlapping mechanisms in the pathogenesis of complications of CoViD19 and cardiovascular diseases, the usefulness of inhibition of the RAAS pathways in subjects with CoViD19 has been widely debated. The RAAS mechanism is currently being explored as a valuable therapeutic target in patients with CoViD19.

In this chapter, we outline the key features of the RAAS machinery and how this system is affected in CoViD19. We explain possible mechanisms through which dysregulated RAAS may facilitate the development of CoViD19 complications. We specifically focus on the complex dynamics of the ACE2, a crucial viral entry mechanism for the SARS CoV2, and describe physiological and pathological variability of the ACE2 in relationship with the cardiometabolic conditions, closely associated with CoVID19 as well as the gender variations.

8.2 The Renin Angiotensin System

The renin-angiotensin system (RAAS) cascade has several components, among which major elements include renin, angiotensin, and aldosterone. The "renin" was discovered by Robert Tigerstedt and Per Gunnar Bergman in 1898 [1], whereas the classical renin-angiotensin system (RAAS) was described in the 1960 and 70s [2]. The main functions of the RAAS include regulation of the hemodynamics, vascular tone, electrolyte balance, and volemia. The expression of the RAAS in the adipose tissue reflects its role in the metabolic pathways.

The RAAS appears to have several autocrine and paracrine functions through the local, systemic, and intracellular presence, and plays a critical role in vascular, renal, and myocardial physiology, with notable therapeutic value. The inhibition of the ACE pathway reduces blood pressure, reverses cardiomyocyte hypertrophy and fibrosis, as well as protects against renal vascular disease. Inhibition of the RAAS mechanisms in the treatment of cardiovascular and renal disease as well as lung injury are important therapeutic developments involving this system (3 Ref H,K, 45; [3]. Upregulation of the ACE2 expression and function is increasingly recognized as a potential therapeutic strategy in hypertension and cardiovascular disease, diabetes, lung injury, and fibrotic disorders. Due to its crucial role ACE2, its auxiliary co proteins, and associated pathways may serve as a therapeutic target in CoViD19. Angiotensin II is used in shock therapy as a potent vasoconstrictor [4].

The "renin" is secreted in the kidneys and converts the "angiotensinogen (AGT)" (mainly produced in the liver) into "angiotensin I (Ang I)". This is then converted into the "angiotensin II (Ang II)" by the "endothelial angiotensin-converting-enzyme (ACE)", a non-specific enzyme (mostly in the lungs), recognized as one of the two principal arms of the RAAS. The "Ang II" binds to the "angiotensin II Type 1 Receptor (AT1R)" and the "angiotensin II Type

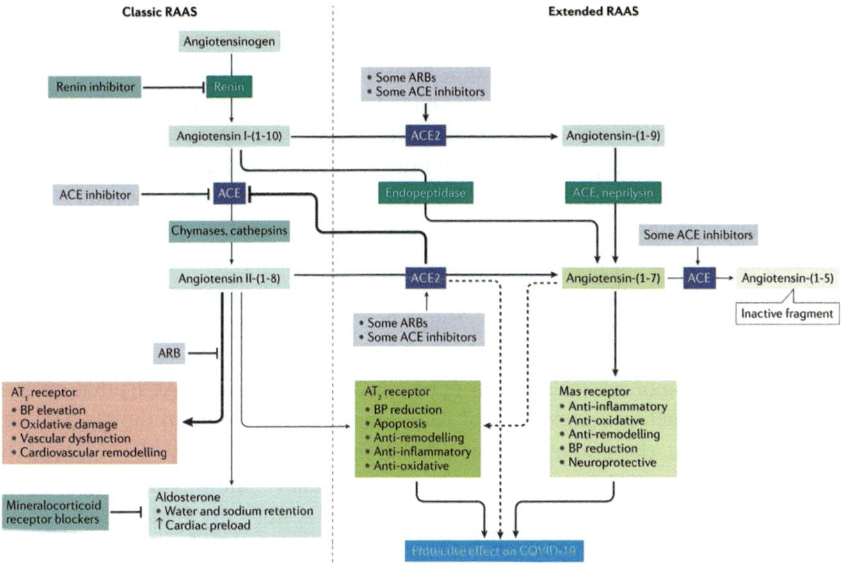

Fig. 8.1 Renin Angiotensin System. Because angiotensin-converting enzyme 2 (ACE2) is considered an important severe acute respiratory syndrome coronavirus 2 (SARS-CoV-2) receptor facilitating infection of relevant cells, such as pneumocytes, it is important to understand its normal physiological function. Inhibition of ACE blocks metabolism of angiotensin-(1–7) to angiotensin-(1–5) and can lead to elevation of angiotensin-(1–7) levels in plasma and tissues (258). In animal models, angiotensin-(1–7) enhances vasodilation and inhibits vascular contractions to angiotensin II258. An ex vivo study using human internal mammary arteries showed that angiotensin-(1–7) blocks angiotensin II-induced vasoconstriction and inhibits ACE in human cardiovascular tissues (258). In an ex vivo study, angiotensin-(1–7) and some ACE inhibitors, such as quinaprilat and captopril, potentiated bradykinin, resulting in blood pressure reduction by inhibiting ACE (259). Thus, angiotensin-(1–7) acts as an ACE inhibitor and might stimulate bradykinin release (259). These results show that angiotensin-(1–7) might be an important modulator of the human renin–angiotensin–aldosterone system (RAAS). ARB, angiotensin receptor blocker; AT1, angiotensin type 1; AT2, angiotensin type 2; BP, blood pressure. *Source* Figure 2, Lim, S., Bae, J.H., Kwon, H.S. and Nauck, M.A., 2021. COVID-19 and diabetes mellitus: from pathophysiology to clinical management. Nature Reviews Endocrinology, 17(1), pp. 11–30. https://www.nature.com/articles/s41574-020-00435-4. By Springer Nature Group

2 Receptor (AT2R)". The "Ang II" mediates the vasoconstriction and aldosterone secretion from the adrenal gland, besides having profibrotic and pro-inflammatory actions through the "AT1 Receptors" (Fig. 8.1).

8.2.1 ACE2 Synthesis and Distribution

The angiotensin-converting enzyme 2 (ACE2) is a membrane-associated protein and secreted enzyme, also expressed in the circulation, was first identified in the year 2000 [5]. The ACE2 is a carboxypeptidase, a homolog to the angiotensin-converting enzyme (ACE) that carries about 40% similarity to the ACE with its gene mapped to the X chromosome. There are two forms of the ACE2. The full-length ACE2 contains a structural transmembrane domain, which anchors its extracellular domain to the plasma membrane. The soluble form of the ACE2 lacks the membrane anchor and circulates in small amounts in the blood [6].

The ACE2 is regulated at multiple levels including transcriptional, post-transcriptional (miRNA and epigenetic), and post-translational. Many cell-surface proteins such as enzymes, cytokines, adhesion molecules go through proteolytic cleavage important for their expression and function. The ACE2 expression is linked with a process of cleavage of the cell membrane protein in the extracellular environment known as "shedding". The ACE2 shedding is mediated by ADAM 17 TACE, a disintegrin and metalloproteinase proteinase ADAM17, also known as tumor necrosis factor-alpha converting enzyme (TACE) that releases the catalytically active ectodomain of ACE2 through cleavage into the extracellular milieu making it detectable in the circulation [7–9]. ACE2 is also cleaved by TMPRSS2 protease, however, appears to be mainly intra-cytoplasmatic [10]. Although regulation of ADAM 17 TACE activity is not fully understood, several factors may impact its activity including apoptosis, protein kinase C, and others [11]. A study investigating the ability of ACE2 to undergo proteolytic shedding and mechanisms responsible for shedding showed that ablation of ADAM17 expression using specific small interfering RNA duplexes reduced regulated ACE2 shedding, whereas overexpression of ADAM17 significantly increased shedding [7] Studies have also shown that Ang-II–mediated upregulation of ADAM17 contributes to ACE2 shedding, thus reducing the membrane-bound carboxypeptidase levels and increasing its soluble form [12]. Furthermore, the ADAM17 also mediates the release of membrane-bound precursors of TNFα, IFN-γ, and IL-4 pro-inflammatory cytokines, into the circulation, hence named as tumor necrosis factor converting enzyme (TACE). Downregulation of the cell surface expression of the ACE2 and reduction in the ACE2 mRNA levels due to the IL-4 and IFN-γ [13] may also be induced by the CoViD19 associated systemic and tissue inflammation and may suggest an alternative route for the loss of mACE2 seen with SARS CoV 2.

The impact of the use of the pharmaceutical interventions interfering with the RAAS, on the ACE2 expression has also been explored amidst the controversy related to the adverse impact of using the ACEi/ARBs in patients with CoViD19 [14]. In contrast, the use of angiotensin-receptor blockers in the repair of lung injury has been shown beneficial [15], and may also be positive in CoViD19 [16]. According to a large multi-center study, the researchers reported that ACE inhibitors ($P = 0.002$) and ARBs ($P = 0.003$) were independent predictors of lower plasma ACE2 in the validation cohort of 1123 men and 575 women with heart failure, while the use of MRA (Mineralo Receptor Antagonists) was a predictor of higher plasma ACE2 concentrations ($P = 0.04$). The use of ACE inhibitor or ARB was not associated with higher plasma ACE2 concentrations [17].

8.2.2 ACE2 Expression

The ACE2 is expressed in the circulatory (soluble form) as well as in the tissue forms. The degree of expression of the ACE2 varies across the tissues and the circulation. The ACE2 can be found in numerous body tissues such as cardiac, vascular, lungs, liver, kidneys, adrenal glands, brain, testes, and the gastrointestinal tract (esophagus, stomach, ileum, colon, and the pancreas) [18].

Several studies demonstrate variations in the distribution of the ACE2 across a range of organs and tissues in the human body. Data shave shown an increased expression of ACE2 in the lung tissue and the cardiovascular system [19–21]. Studies also show that ACE2 is highly expressed in the renal tubular cells, Leydig cells, and cells in seminiferous ducts in testicular tissue in the male subjects [22].

A variety of specialized cells harbor ACE2 across the tissues. Studies demonstrate that ACE2 is abundantly present in humans in the epithelia of the lungs and the small intestine [21]. In the lungs, the ACE2 is expressed in the airways and type 2 pneumocytes and the capillaries of lung vasculature, and in the heart in the cardiomyocytes [15, 23, 24]. According to a study, 83% of the ACE2-expressing cells were alveolar epithelial type II cells [20].

In the cardiovascular system, the ACE2 is found on the endothelial cells, smooth muscle cells, cardiomyocytes, and macrophages [25]. The ACE2 is located on the cell surface membrane and is predominantly expressed in the endothelium of the coronary artery, coronary smooth muscle, intra-renal vasculature, and renal tubular epithelium.

Data from a study investigating ACE2 expression in the adult human hearts from healthy and diseased individuals explored the potential capacity of heart infection by SARS-CoV-2, revealed that ACE2 is highly expressed in the pericytes of the adult human hearts, which indicated an intrinsic susceptibility of the heart to SARS CoV2 infection [26].

8.2.3 ACE2 Detection

The angiotensin-converting enzyme 2 (ACE2) is detectable in both blood and urine, although the detection of the soluble ACE2 in urine and blood may not be a reliable indicator of the activity of the membranous ACE2 [16]. Studies show that ACE2 is released from the renal proximal tubules and can be detected in the urine [27, 28]. The concentration of different components of the renin–angiotensin–aldosterone system (RAAS) fluctuates in tissues. Specialized cells across various tissues produce components of the RAAS, once released may be redistributed. The variability in the concentrations depends upon several local and systemic factors, volumes produced and redistributed. The ACE2 is expressed in the renal and cardiovascular systems in different concentrations, and variations in the detection of ACE2 in the circulation are associated with the concentrations of the ACE2 expressed and redistributed in the circulation.

Furthermore, data suggest that the concentrations of the components of the RAAS detected in different systems, such as cardiovascular and renal, vary in relationship with the plasma concentrations. The cardiac interstitial fluid carries high concentrations (100-fold those of plasma) of the "Ang I and Ang II", while the "renin" and "angiotensinogen" in the myocardium are 1–4% of the plasma [29, 30]. In the renal interstitium, the "Ang II" levels are 1000-fold higher than those in the plasma [31].

The differences in the detection of various components of the RAAS in specific tissues are crucial to maintaining homeostasis and functioning of the local systems and have clinical implications. The expression of the ACE2 has been shown to have prognostic implications in cardiovascular diseases. The relationship of the ACE2 with gender and age-related variations, observed in cardiovascular diseases, as previously investigated, appears to be reflected in the cardiovascular complications seen in the severe CoViD19. The therapeutic value of the ACE2 is also currently being further explored in CoViD19 being an important viral entry mechanism for SARS CoV2 [32].

8.3 The Dynamics of ACE2 Expression in CoViD19

The ACE2 is located in a variety of tissues, found both as a structural entity in the cell membrane, and the circulatory form plays a crucial role in CoViD19 (Fig. 8.2). The dynamics or ACE2 distribution and expression may determine variations in disease incidence and severity, as well as associated bias related to the gender and age or other traits in patients with CoViD19. Such factors may also be associated with the risk of developing CoViD19 or complications. The expression of ACE2 is low in healthy individuals [33]. Studies show that subjects with higher risk for severe COVID19 had a higher sACE2 (adults>children and men>women) [32]. Furthermore, the pathogenetic implications of the dynamics of ACE2 expression in different tissues may determine individual susceptibility and risk of complications in CoViD19. Single-cell RNA-seq data analysis on the receptor ACE2 expression reveals the potential risk of different human organs vulnerable to the SARS CoV 2 infection [34].

The critical anti-inflammatory role of the ACE2 may be compromised in CoViD19 due to its role as a viral entry mechanism in conjunction with dysregulated RAAS processes. The ACE2 serves as a principal viral entry machine in addition to the cathepsin B and L, assisted by the co-protein TMPRSS2 [35–41], and also serves as principal viral entry mechanisms for SARS CoV2 [42, 43].

The ACE2 soluble form (sACE2) may be increased by the SARS CoV2, as surface cell-bound, membranous ACE2 is down-regulated by the virus (Fig. 8.3). A proposed valid mechanism through which membrane ACE2 is downregulated by the SARS CoV 2 in CoViD19, involves the process of endocytosis, through which interaction between viral spike protein with membranous ACE2 is internalized. Endocytosis upregulates ADAM 17 activity that increases ACE2 shedding in the

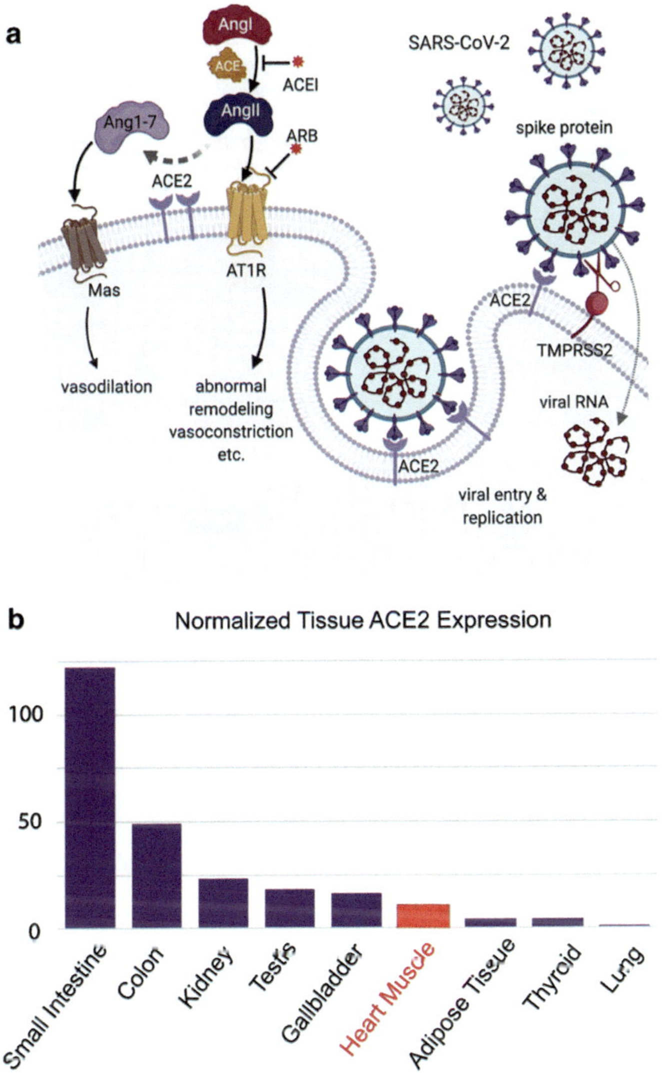

Fig. 8.2 The role of ACE2 in CoViD19. **a** The spike protein of SARS-CoV-2 binds ACE2 on a cellular membrane, which triggers 1) endocytosis of the virus and subsequent sequestration of ACE2 or 2) cleavage of the viral spike protein via an enzyme TMPRSS2 leading to the entry of viral contents into the cytoplasm. **b** Normalized RNA expression of different tissue types from three transcriptomics datasets (HPA, GTEx, and FANTOM5) shows significant ACE2 expression in GI organs, the kidney, and the heart. *Source* Figure 1. Cheng, P., Zhu, H., Witteles, R.M., Wu, J.C., Quertermous, T., Wu, S.M. and Rhee, J.W., 2020. Cardiovascular risks in patients with COVID-19: potential mechanisms and areas of uncertainty. Current cardiology reports, 22(5), pp. 1–6. https://link.springer.com/article/https://doi.org/10.1007/s11886-020-01293-2. Published by Springer Nature

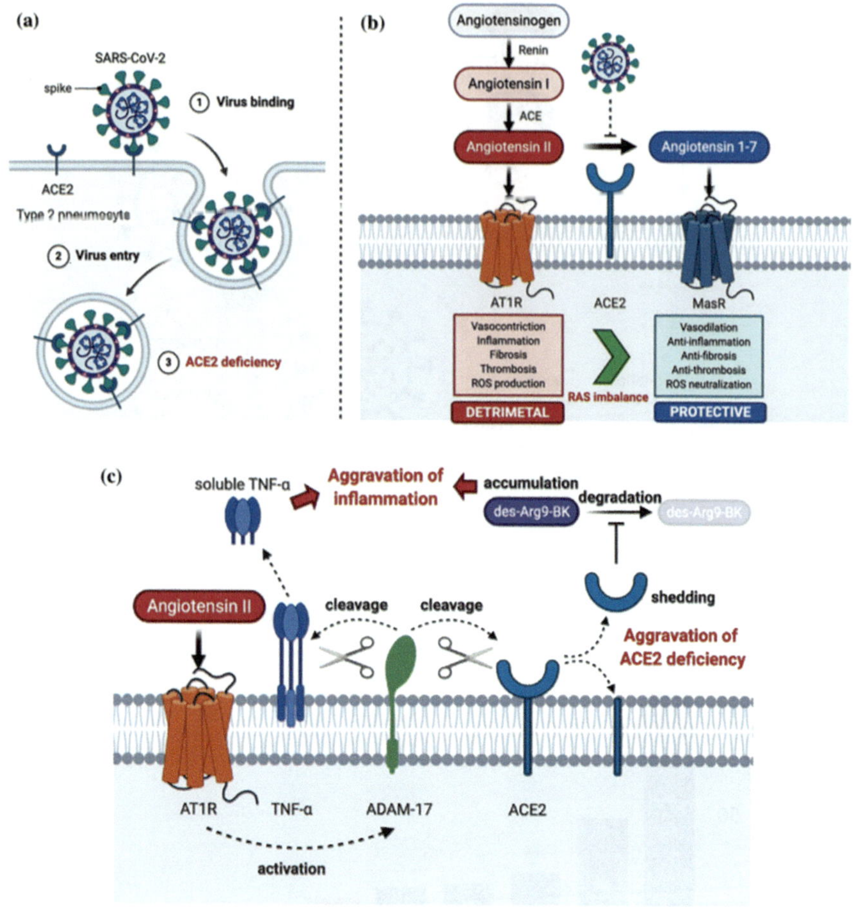

Fig. 8.3 SARS CoV2 and RAS interaction. Pulmonary phase of COVID-19 pathogenesis: **a** SARS-CoV-2 enters the type 2 pneumocyte via the host receptor, ACE2. Target cell infection by SARS-CoV-2 induces ACE2 internalization, resulting in ACE2 downregulation and deficiency. **b** SARS-CoV-2-induced ACE2 deficiency decreases the conversion of angiotensin II to angiotensinogen 1–7 and increases angiotensin II availability. Excessive angiotensin II causes AT1R overactivation, resulting in a RAS imbalance. **c** ADAM-17 activation by AT1R promotes cleavage of both membrane-anchored TNF-? and ACE2. ADAM-17 truncates the ACE2 extracellular domain, which enzymatically inactivates ACE2. As a result, des-Arg9-BK degradation by ACE2 is disrupted and its abundancy increases. Liberated soluble TNF-? and accumulated des-Arg9-BK aggravate SARS-CoV-2-induced inflammation. *Source* Figure 2. Lee, C. and Choi, W.J., 2021. Overview of COVID-19 inflammatory pathogenesis from the therapeutic perspective. Archives of pharmacal research, pp. 1–18. https://link.springer.com/article/https://doi.org/10.1007/s12272-020-01301-7. Published by Springer Nature

circulation resulting in loss of ACE2 from the tissue RAAS. This leads to the accumulation of Ang II that upregulates ADAM17 through AT1 receptors, thereby resulting in further loss of ACE2 from tissue RAAS [44]. This process results in accelerating the RAAS-mediated injury including severe lung damage [45–47]. However, an increase in the soluble ACE2 may counter the deleterious Ang II actions by inducing protective pathways. Since the elevated sACE2 levels reflect a high mACE2 and/or high ADAM-17 activity, the sACE2 may be a marker of both the susceptibility and the severity of the CoViD19.

8.3.1 ACE2 Expression in Cardiovascular and Metabolic Conditions

The pathogenetic and clinical significance of ACE2 in cardiovascular diseases has been extensively explored. An enhanced expression of ACE and ACE2 in hypertension, myocardial infarction, heart failure, and diabetes mellitus, has led to establishing the role of these circulatory proteins as biomarkers in hypertension, coronary heart disease, and heart failure [48, 49]. Studies have shown serum ACE2 levels are lower in healthy individuals and increased in the subjects with hypertension, heart failure, and myocardial infarction[46, 49–51]. According to a large multi-center prospective study in 11 European countries, in which the ACE2 concentrations were measured in 1485 men and 537 women with heart failure, the plasma concentrations of the ACE2 were higher in men, than in women in the two independent cohorts of patients with heart failure, and male sex appeared to be the strongest predictor of the elevated concentrations of ACE2 in both cohorts (estimate = 0.26, $P < 0.001$; and 0.19, $P < 0.001$, respectively) [17]. Studies further indicate the role of these proteins as markers of the severity of cardiovascular diseases. An association of enhanced ACE2 expression with risk of development of heart failure in the hypertensive subjects as well as a positive correlation with the severity of heart failure has been demonstrated [46, 52]. Subjects with type 1 diabetics have increased circulating ACE2 activity especially higher in those with a history of coronary heart disease [53]. Multiple factors such as dysglycemia, insulin resistance, and pro-inflammatory factors associated with metabolic conditions such as diabetes mellitus, accompany inflammatory stress, and prothrombotic mechanisms that result in further complications. Dysregulated RAAS in the diabetics and other metabolic conditions, may augment the harmful impact of the underlying cardiometabolic pathogenetic states associated with CoViD19.

A variety of specific ACE2 harboring cells in the cardiovascular tissues appear to be implicated in the pathogenesis, and severity of cardiovascular diseases, through regulation of the ACE2 activity. Besides the endothelial cells, the ACE2 protein has been detected in the macrophages, smooth muscle cells, and cardiac myocytes in myocardial infarction, with significantly increased levels seen in heart failure, and could predict adverse cardiac events [25, 54, 55].

The ACE2 shedding and AngII/ADAM17 activity, linked with the regulation of ACE2 activity, are affected in cardiovascular diseases. The increased activity of ADAM17 may be associated with cardiovascular diseases [56, 57]. Under the stressful conditions, membrane-bound ACE2 protein is cleaved by the transmembrane disintegrin, and metalloproteinase 17 ADAM17, thereby releasing ACE2 into the interstitium, or circulation, without depleting intracellular ACE2 levels [58]. Pro-inflammatory conditions, prothrombotic oxidative and metabolic stress play an important role in the dynamics of RAAS components.

8.3.2 The Dynamics of ACE2 Expression and Cardiovascular Risk in CoViD19

The ACE2 expressing cardiovascular structures serve as fertile ground for cardiovascular complications in CoViD19. The dynamics of expression of the ACE2 and its forms (serum ACE2 (sACE2) and membranous (mACE2)), in various cardiovascular structures may influence the associations of CoViD19 with several cardiovascular conditions including hypertension, heart failure, coronary heart disease, and metabolic diseases such as diabetes mellitus. These factors are further impacted by gender, age, and several other associated mechanisms that require further exploration. According to a study higher levels of ACE2 were observed in the females with coronary heart disease (CHD), independently predicting the CHD in the female subjects, especially those with multivessel disease [59], indicating the predictive value of ACE2 expression for coronary risk in females.

The analysis exploring the expression of ACE2 in adult heart tissue has shown a high expression of ACE2 in the pericytes that might act as the target cardiac cell of SARS CoV2 [26]. The pericytes are vascular cells on the abluminal surface of the micro-vessels based in the basement membrane and communicate with the endothelial cells through the Gap junctions, to help with the exchange of the molecules, proteins, ions, vital for vascular structural and functional maintenance [60]. The pericytes play an important role in vascular repair, regulation of the vascular tone, and play a major role in vascular homeostasis, most importantly in the states of inflammation, where they cover gap junctions [61]. The susceptibility of the pericytes towards SARS CoV2, may promote viral-cardiovascular direct interactions, and play a role in the development of viral-induced capillary endothelial cell and microvascular dysfunction, however, these interlinks remain largely unconfirmed.

An increased ACE2 expression at both the mRNA and protein levels is also seen in the patients with heart failure that further increases the risk of cardiac complications, and or of development of severe disease if infected with the virus. Furthermore, the increased Ang II activity due to dysregulated RAAS in CoViD19, in association with the increased ADAM17 activity, may lead to inflammation, and an increased risk of cardiovascular complications, including hypertension, and heart failure. Increased ADAM17 activity is known to be involved in the shedding of inflammatory cytokines (including INF -Î³ and IL-4) and inflammation-mediated hypertension [62–64], may lead to an uncontrolled inflammatory response [65].

A decline in the membranous ACE2 as a result of the increased activity of ADAM 17 leads to a decreased tissue protection, due to the decline in the membranous ACE2. Data show that protease enzymes such as ADAM 17 and cytokines, play important role in the pathogenesis of cardiac remodeling [66, 67], possibly indicating the compensatory role of these mechanisms in cardiovascular diseases.

The impact of age and gender may alter cardiovascular risk in CoViD19. Analyses indicate that the male gender may exhibit a decreased cardiac ACE2 expression with age-related decline in the expression of ACE2, which may determine enhanced cardiovascular risk in the male subjects. According to a study, cells in the male adult heart showed a lower ACE2+ rate than in females (5.93% vs. 9.32%, $P < 0.01$), and ACE2Â expression in the cardiac cells seems to be lower with older age, and TMPRSS2 is rarely expressed in the human adult heart [68]. The absence of TMPRSS2 may offer protection against the SARS CoV2. These associations however demand further exploration. The gender-related variations in ACE2 expression have a significant link with heart failure, an important complication, and comorbidity in CoViD19. According to an analysis, higher circulating ACE2 plasma concentration in male subjects are significantly linked with heart failure [17].

8.3.3 Age and Gender Variations of ACE2 and CoViD19

Several clinical and experimental models have explored variations in the expression of various elements of the RAAS, according to gender and age that may have significant implications in CoViD19. Multiple factors account for the age and gender variations observed in CoViD19, and possibly, increased severity of the diseases in male subjects, therefore, indicating that the degree and pattern of the expression of ACE2 may influence the susceptibility and outcome in CoViD19.

Data indicate that expression of ACE2 concentrations may be higher in male subjects [17, 33, 69], although reports also suggest elevated ACE2 expression in females [70]. Although genetic mechanisms favor the elevated ACE2 expression in females due to the location of the ACE2 gene on the X chromosome [71], emerging data from larger studies favor the argument that male subjects have higher serum ACE2 levels as compared to the females and have gained better recognition. According to an analysis, the increased expression of the ACE2 in the testes, may account for a higher ACE2 expression in males, justifying the ACE2 related gender dichotomy [17].

ACE2 polymorphism observed in the different population or ethnic groups has been shown to have an impact on CoViD19 [72, 73] and has gender-based implications. Several variants of ACE2 have been identified that may have gender implications. A study exploring the expression and polymorphism of the ACE2 in different population groups showed that ACE2 variants that boost viral ACE2 binding can be more substantial in males than females. The ACE2 variants impact viral-receptor binding interaction differently, with a higher expression of the viral binding booster variants in the males [74]. Accordingly, the hemizygous viral-entry interaction booster variants of ACE2 can explain the gender bias towards a higher mortality rate caused by the SARS CoV2 in males. More than half of the ACE2 rare variants were found in males due to the ACE2 location on the "X" chromosome. The authors suggest investigating the enrichment of the rare variants among the SARS CoV2 infected cases with severe symptoms.

The expression of ACE2 is low in healthy individuals [33] and decreases with age [75, 81]. The higher ACE2 levels in the younger individuals are linked with a greater predisposition to incur the disease [76], whereas the higher risk for severity of CoViD19, has been linked with higher sACE2 expression (adults > children and men > women) [32, 77].

Data show that estrogens may offer a protective role against CVD in females through upregulation of ADAM17 and ADAM10 expression involved in ectodomain cleavages in atherosclerosis [78]. Although the above arguments strongly implicate ACE2 as a major contributing factor to the gender variations in CoViD19 and disease severity and complications, further research is needed to elaborate these mechanisms and identify other factors that determine inter-individual variations in the susceptibility towards the disease and severity. For further reading about age and gender dynamics and CoViD19 please refer to Chaps. 18 and 19, respectively.

8.4 ACE2 is a Marker of Severity or a Compensatory Mechanism?

In the renin-angiotensin-aldosteroe system (RAAS), the ACE2 forms part of the ATI/ATII/AT2R axis acting as a protective regulator (Table 8.1). The ACE2 controls RAAS regulatory balance by converting angiotensin I to angiotensin 1–9 (Ang 1–9) (restricting substrate availability for angiotensin II (Ang II) generation), by converting Ang II to angiotensin 1–7 (Ang 1–7) (limiting angiotensin II stimulation of the AT1 receptor), and by generating Ang 1–7 that may bind to its receptor, the Mas receptor or the AT2 receptor (to counter negative actions of the AT1 receptor. These protective actions of the ACE2 counter the negative balance induced by the Ang II in the equation through its molecular and cellular reactions, through degradation of the Ang I to 1–9 and of Ang II, and generation of angiotensin 1–7.

The dysregulation of the RAAS associated with CoViD19 leading to the decreased expression of ACE2 results in overactivation of the AngII/AT1R axis may induce the deleterious effects of Ang II that include pro-inflammatory, prothrombotic activities including macrophage activation syndrome (MAS) [79] (See Table 8.2). The damaging effects of Ang II are countered by the increase in the process of mACE2 shedding as Ang II may induce ADAM17 TACE activity inducing the shedding process of mACE2. Data show that Ang II induces the

Table 8.1 Actions of ACE2 Ang 1-7/Ang 1-9 AT2/Mas-Receptors leading to cell protection

Decreases inflammation
Anti-oxidant
Anti-thrombotic
Anti-proliferation
Anti-fibrotic
Promotes

Table 8.2 Action of angiotensin II/AT1R pathway leading to cell injury

Pro-inflammatory
Oxidative stress
Pro-thrombotic
Anti-fibrinolytic
Cell proliferation
Pro-fibrotic
Vasoconstriction
Na and H2O absorption
Pro apoptosis

mACE2 shedding by promoting the TACE activity as a positive feedback mechanism whereby the Ang II facilitates loss of its negative regulator, suggesting elevated plasma ACE2 activity (sACE2) in the heart failure may reflect the loss of the protective effects of ACE2 in the heart [80]. The circulatory increase in the sACE2 may reflect the loss of tissue protection offered by the mACE2 in the heart, hence reflecting the severity of the disease.

The elevated levels of Ang II have been shown in CoViD19 patients and may be directly associated with the severity of viral disease [81]. Several potentially negative actions of Ang II may facilitate the development of cardiovascular complications, also observed in CoViD19. The important mediators of the pro-inflammatory impact of Ang II on the leucocytes, endothelial cells, and vascular smooth muscle cells involve intracellular and vascular adhesion molecules (ICAM/VCAM), reactive oxygen species (ROS), nuclear factor-kB (NFLB), and superoxide. Angiotensin II stimulates the NADPH oxidase and results in the acceleration of oxidative stress [82], and induces mitochondrial dysfunction resulting in endothelial dysfunction. Mitochondrial dysfunction is induced by a protein kinase C–dependent pathway by the activation of the endothelial cell NADPH oxidase and formation of peroxynitrite [83, 84]. Furthermore, Ang II is also known to promote metabolic dysregulation, prostacyclin synthesis, differentiation of the adipocytes, and lipogenesis.

Whether the expression of sACE2, as a marker of severity of disease process, is a compensatory mechanism or is a marker of the decompensation, is subject to debate. Human and animal models investigating the association of serum ACE2/ Angiotensin 1–7 expression with cardiovascular disease as a disease marker may reflect a counter-regulatory effect or a compensatory regulatory mechanism, mainly show the protective role of ACE2 reflecting a compensatory mechanism that facilitates balancing peripheral ACE/ACE2 concentration via release from the vascular endothelium. Since angiotensin 1–7 has a very short half-life (less than 9Â s) the expression of ACE2 facilitates the compensatory mechanism. The exact role of increase in circulating soluble ACE2 needs to be better understood, although it might reflect a pathological shift of the ACE2 from the tissue membrane or perhaps signifies the activation of counter-regulatory mechanisms. The balance of these two forms of ACE2 may have significant implications in CoViD19. In the animal models an overexpression of both ACE2, as well as Angiotensin 1–7, has been shown to confer protective action against atherosclerosis ie attenuation of progression of atherosclerotic lesions, stabilizing plaques [85, 86].

8.5 Summary

A strict balance between the negative and protective arms of the complex regulatory peptide system renin-angiotensin-aldosterone system (RAAS), widely distributed in the body, is essential for the maintenance of homeostatic control. The mechanisms involving ACE2 in RAAS have been well elucidated in the process of blood pressure control, the pathophysiology of hypertension, cardiovascular diseases including heart failure, and renal disease. This regulatory system serves as an important therapeutic target in various cardiovascular, renal, and metabolic diseases. The therapeutic role of ACE inhibitors or ARBs and other drugs interfering in RAAS mechanisms is already well established. The ARBs have potential therapeutic value in lung injury, are currently being investigated in CoViD19 [88].

The ACE2 found insoluble (circulatory) and membranous form (a structural protein), is an essential part of RAAS, plays a crucial role in CoViD19. Although the ACE2 has a protective role against lung injury, it also serves as a gateway for the viral cell entry playing a dual role. The ACE2 soluble form (sACE2) may be increased by the SARS CoV2 as the surface cell-bound membranous ACE2 is down-regulated by the virus. A decline in the mACE2 may signify the loss of tissue protection whereas the increase in sACE2 levels may reflect the vulnerability of the tissue and sign of the severity of the condition. The decline in mACE2 induces damaging activation of the harmful Ang II–AT1R axis. At the same time, an increase in sACE2 through other signaling mechanisms in the regulatory system may be considered compensatory, offering protection and repair to the tissues through MasR and AT2R signaling cascade and other indirect mechanisms. A soluble form of human ACE2 (rhACE2) is currently considered as a therapeutic approach that halts the interaction between SARS CoV2 and ACE2 impeding viral entry [87].

The viral invasion leads to the dysregulation of RAAS mechanisms in CoViD19 and constitutes a major pathogenetic route towards critical complications associated with the viral disease involving the lungs, heart, kidneys, and vasculature. The downregulation of ACE2 increases Ang II–AT1R axis activation causing damage through proinflammatory, prothrombotic, vasoplegic, and other toxic mechanisms. The complex dynamics related to the distribution of ACE2 in various tissues and other RAAS components play a trivial role in this process and may determine individual susceptibility and impact the outcome of the disease. The single-cell RNA-seq data analysis on the receptor ACE2 expression reveals the potential risk of different human organs vulnerable to the SARS CoV 2 infection [34]. The patients with diabetes mellitus and other metabolic diseases have elevated underlying metabolic proinflammatory, prothrombotic, and other forms of stress mechanisms that may increase the risk of complications when met with dysregulated RAAS induced by CoViD19.

Various studies reveal the role of specialized cells in the cardiac tissues that take part in the synthesis and regulation of the ACE2 such as endothelial cells, pericytes, myocytes, macrophages, and others. The shedding process of the ACE2 is regulated by ADAM 17 TACE and is influenced by several factors including inflammatory processes, circulating volumes of the ACE2, Ang II, and others. Under stressful conditions, these factors trigger mechanisms that may induce a compensatory increase in the ACE2 levels that also mark the severity of the disease. These changes might be adaptive or maladaptive. The interplay of sACE2 and mACE2 dynamics, and associated factors that influence the shedding process needs to be better understood. Sound evidence indicates the role of ACE2 in cardiovascular diseases. An increase in soluble ACE2 has been associated with advanced heart failure [46]. Various cardiovascular conditions including hypertension, heart failure frequently associated with complicated CoViD19, exhibit variations in ACE2 expression validating the use of ACE2 expression as a biochemical marker of disease severity. The increased ACE2 activity in hypertension, and its value as a predictor of its complications, further strengthens the argument defining its value as a predictor of cardiovascular complications in CoViD19. The variations in ACE2 expression with the age (older age) and gender (male sex) are linked with the individual susceptibility to develop CoViD19 or the complications, has been a focus of research [76]. Various factors such as ACE2 polymorphism, tissue distribution, the protective role of estrogen, and others may account for these differences. The evidence shows ACE2 polymorphism among different population groups and links the ACE2 variants with the individual competence in the fight against SARS CoV 2. Specific rare variants may play a decisive role in viral recognition or susceptibility towards severe disease. Further research is needed to better validate these findings and develop strategies to early identify individuals and population groups at a higher risk of developing CoViD19 or those at risk of complications and death and develop precautionary measures.

Summary Box

- The CoViD19 results in dysregulation of the renin-angiotensin-aldosterone system.
- Local and systemic RAAS are both affected in CoViD19.
- ACE2 is a viral entry mechanism while also has a protective role.
- Excessive Ang II levels lead to damage to tissues though pro inflammatory, prothrombotic, vasoplegic and other actions.
- Ang II may also stimulate ACE2 expression by inducing ADAM 17 TACE.
- Enhanced ACE2 expression is associated with an increased risk of cardiovascular diseases.
- ACE2 soluble form (sACE2) may be increased by SARS CoV 2 as surface cell-bound membranous ACE2 is down-regulated by the virus.
- A low membranous ACE2 (mACE2), increased ADAM 17 activity, inflammatory cytokines INF -γ and IL-4, may contribute to a higher risk of cardiovascular complications in CoViD19.
- The distribution of ACE2 across different tissues represents an important route to multi-organ failure in complicated CoViD19.
- Gender and age risk in CoViD19 may be facilitated by the differences in the ACE2 expression.
- ACE2 protein and gene polymorphism and ACE2 mRNA expression may determine inter-individual susceptibility for CoViD19 and the disease severity.
- Further research is needed to confirm the interplay of the dynamics of sACE2 expression and affiliated factors and mechanisms in relationship with CoViD19 and complications.

References

1. Paul M, Poyan Mehr A, Kreutz R. Physiology of local renin-angiotensin systems. Physiol Rev. 2006;86(3):747–803. Review. PubMed PMID: 16816138.
2. Skrbic R, Igic R. Seven decades of angiotensin (1939–2009). Peptides. 2009;30(10):1945–50.
3. Morrell NW, Higham MA, Phillips PG, Shakur BH, Robinson PJ, Beddoes RJ. Pilot study of losartan for pulmonary hypertension in chronic obstructive pulmonary disease. Respir Res. 2005;6:88.
4. Khanna A, English SW, Wang XS, Ham K, Tumlin J, Szerlip H, Busse LW, Altaweel L, Albertson TE, Mackey C, McCurdy MT. Angiotensin II for the treatment of vasodilatory shock. N Engl J Med. 2017;377(5):419–30.
5. Tipnis SR, Hooper NM, Hyde R, Karran E, Christie G, Turner AJ. A human homolog of angiotensin-converting enzyme. Cloning and functional expression as a captopril-insensitive carboxypeptidase. J Biol Chem. 2000;275:33238–43.

6. Wysocki J, Ye M, Rodriguez E, Gonzalez-Pacheco FR, Barrios C, Evora K, et al. Targeting the degradation of Angiotensin II with recombinant angiotensin-converting enzyme 2: prevention of Angiotensin II-dependent hypertension. Hypertension. 2010;55:90–8. https://doi.org/10.1161/HYPERTENSIONAHA.109.138420[PubMed].
7. Lambert DW, Yarski M, Warner FJ, et al. Tumor necrosis factor-alpha convertase (ADAM17) mediates regulated ectodomain shedding of the severe-acute respiratory syndrome-coronavirus (SARS-CoV) receptor, angiotensin-converting enzyme-2 (ACE2). J Biol Chem. 2005;280(34):30113–9.
8. Lambert DW, Clarke NE, Hooper NM, Turner AJ. Calmodulin interacts with angiotensin-converting enzyme-2 (ACE2) and inhibits shedding of its ectodomain. FEBS Lett. 2008;582:385–90.
9. Lew RA, Warner FJ, Hanchapola I, et al. Angiotensin-converting enzyme 2 catalytic activity in human plasma is masked by an endogenous inhibitor. Exp Physiol. 2008;93:685–93.
10. Heurich A, Hofmann-Winkler H, Gierer S, Liepold T, Jahn O, PÃ¶hlmann S. TMPRSS2 and ADAM17 cleave ACE2 differentially and only proteolysis by TMPRSS2 augments entry driven by the severe acute respiratory syndrome coronavirus spike protein. J Virol. 2014;88 (2):1293–307.
11. Chalaris A, Rabe B, Paliga K, Lange H, Laskay T, Fielding CA, Jones SA, Rose-John S, Scheller J. Apoptosis is a natural stimulus of IL6R shedding and contributes to the proinflammatory trans-signaling function of neutrophils. Blood, The J Am Soc Hematol. 2007;110(6):1748–55.
12. Xia H, Sriramula S, Chhabra KH, Lazartigues E. Brain angiotensin-converting enzyme type 2 shedding contributes to the development of neurogenic hypertension. Circ Res. 2013;113 (9):1087–96. https://doi.org/10.1161/CIRCRESAHA.113.301811.
13. de Lang A, Osterhaus AD, Haagmans BL. Interferon-Î³ and interleukin-4 downregulate expression of the SARS coronavirus receptor ACE2 in Vero E6 cells. Virology. 2006;353 (2):474–81.
14. Sommerstein R, GrÃ¤ni C. Preventing a COVID-19 pandemic: ACE inhibitors as a potential risk factor for fatal COVID-19.Â BMJ. 2020;368, p.m810.
15. Imai Y, Kuba K, Rao S, Huan Y, Guo F, Guan B, Yang P, Sarao R, Wada T, Leong-Poi H, Crackower MA. Angiotensin-converting enzyme 2 protects from severe acute lung failure. Nature. 2005;436(7047):112–6.
16. Vaduganathan M, Vardeny O, Michel T, McMurray JJ, Pfeffer MA, Solomon SD. Renin-angiotensin-aldosterone system inhibitors in patients with Covid-19. N Engl J Med. 2020;382(17):1653–9.
17. Sama IE, Ravera A, Santema BT, van Goor H, Ter Maaten JM, Cleland JGF, Rienstra M, Friedrich AW, Samani NJ, Ng LL, Dickstein K, Lang CC, Filippatos G, Anker SD, Ponikowski P, Metra M, van Veldhuisen DJ, Voors AA. Circulating plasma concentrations of angiotensin-converting enzyme 2 in men and women with heart failure and effects of renin angiotensin-aldosterone inhibitors. Eur Heart J. 2020;41(19):1810–7. https://doi.org/10.1093/eurheartj/ehaa373.
18. Harmer D, Gilbert M, Borman R, Clark KL. Quantitative mRNA expression profiling of ACE2, a novel homologue of angiotensin converting enzyme. FEBS Lett. 2002;532:107–10.
19. Turner AJ, Hiscox JA, Hooper NM. ACE2: from vasopeptidase to SARS virus receptor. Trends Pharmacol Sci. 2004;25:291–4.
20. Zhao Y, Zhao Z, Wang Y, Zhou Y, Ma Y, Zuo W. Single-cell RNA expression profiling of ACE2, the putative receptor of Wuhan COVID-19. 2020. https://doi.org/10.1101/2020.01.26.919985.
21. Hamming I, Timens W, Bulthuis M, Lely A, Navis G, van Goor H. Tissue distribution of ACE2 protein, the functional receptor for SARS coronavirus. A first step in understanding SARS pathogenesis. J Pathol. 2004;203:631–7. https://doi.org/10.1002/path.1570.
22. Fan C, Li K, Ding Y, Lu WL, Wang J. ACE2 expression in kidney and testis may cause kidney and testis damage after 2019-nCoV infection. MedRxiv. 2020. https://doi.org/10.1101/2020.02.12.20022418.

23. Gallagher PE, Ferrario CM, Tallant EA. Regulation of ACE2 in cardiac myocytes and fibroblasts. Am J Physiol Heart Circ Physiol. 2008;295(6):H2373–9.
24. Studdy PR, Lapworth R, Bird R. Angiotensin-converting enzyme and its clinical significanceâ €"a review. J Clin Pathol. 1983;36:938–47.
25. Burrell LM, Risvanis J, Kubota E, et al. Myocardial infarction increases ACE2 expression in rat and humans. Eur Heart J. 2005;26: 369–75. First published on January 24, 2005. https://doi.org/10.1093/eurheartj/ehi114.
26. Chen L, Li X, Chen M, Feng Y, Xiong C. The ACE2 expression in human heart indicates new potential mechanism of heart injury among patients infected with SARS-CoV-2, Cardiovasc Res. 2020;116(6):1097–100.https://doi.org/10.1093/cvr/cvaa078.
27. Shaltout HA, Westwood BM, Averill DB, Ferrario CM, Figueroa JP, Diz DI, Rose JC, Chappell MC. Angiotensin metabolism in renal proximal tubules, urine, and serum of sheep: evidence for ACE2-dependent processing of Angiotensin II. Am J Physiol Renal Physiol. 2007;292:F82–91.
28. Warner FJ, Lew RA, Smith AI, Lambert DW, Hooper NM, Turner AJ. Angiotensin-converting enzyme 2 (ACE2), but not ACE, is preferentially localized to the apical surface of polarized kidney cells. J Biol Chem. 2005;280:39353–62.
29. Danser AHJ, van Kesteren CAM, Bax WA, Tavenier M, Derkx FHM, Saxena PR, Schalekamp MADH. Prorenin, renin, angiotensin, and angiotensin converting enzyme in normal and failing hearts: evidence for renin binding. Circulation. 1997;96:220–6.
30. Danser AHJ, van Kats JP, Admiraal PJ, Derkx FH, Lamers JM. Cardiac renin and angiotensins: uptake from plasma versus in situ synthesis. Hypertension. 1994;24:37–48.
31. Nishiyama A, Seth DM, Navar LG. Renal interstitial fluid concentrations of angiotensins I and II in anesthetized rats. Hypertension. 2002;39:129–34.
32. Batlle D, Wysocki J, Satchell K. Soluble angiotensin-converting enzyme 2: a potential approach for coronavirus infection therapy? Clin Sci (Lond). 2020;134(5):543–5. https://doi.org/10.1042/CS20200163.
33. Patel SK, Velkoska E, Burrell LM. Emerging markers in cardiovascular disease: where does angiotensin-converting enzyme 2 fit in? Clin Exp Pharmacol Physiol. 2013;40(8):551–9.
34. Zou X, Chen K, Zou J, Han P, Hao J, Han Z. Single-cell RNA-seq data analysis on the receptor ACE2 expression reveals the potential risk of different human organs vulnerable to 2019-nCoV infection. Front Med. 2020;14(2):185–92.
35. Kuba K, Imai Y, Rao S, Gao H, Guo F, Guan B, et al. A crucial role of angiotensin converting enzyme 2 (ACE2) in SARS coronavirus-induced lung injury. Nat Med. 2005;11(8):875–9. https://doi.org/10.1038/nm1267.PMID16007097.
36. Kuba K, Imai Y, Penninger JM. Angiotensin-converting enzyme 2 in lung diseases. Curr Opin Pharmacol. 2006;6(3):271–6.
37. Zhang H, Baker A. Recombinant human ACE2: acing out Angiotensin II in ARDS therapy. Crit Care. 2017;21:305.
38. Simmons G, Gosalia DN, Rennekamp AJ, Reeves JD, Diamond SL, Bates P. Inhibitors of cathepsin L prevent severe acute respiratory syndrome coronavirus entry. Proc Natl Acad Sci U S A. 2005;102(33):11876–81. Epub 2005 Aug 4. PubMed PMID: 16081529; PubMed Central PMCID: PMC1188015.
39. Shulla A, Heald-Sargent T, Subramanya G, Zhao J, Perlman S, Gallagher T. A transmembrane serine protease is linked to the severe acute respiratory syndrome coronavirus receptor and activates virus entry. J Virol. 2011;85:873–82.
40. Glowacka I, Bertram S, MÃ¼ller MA, Allen P, Soilleux E, Pfefferle S, Steffen I, Tsegaye TS, He Y, Gnirss K, et al. Evidence that TMPRSS2 activates the severe acute respiratory syndrome coronavirus spike protein for membrane fusion and reduces viral control by the humoral immune response. J Virol. 2011;85:4122–34.
41. Matsuyama S, Nagata N, Shirato K, Kawase M, Takeda M, Taguchi F. Efficient activation of the severe acute respiratory syndrome coronavirus spike protein by the transmembrane protease TMPRSS2. J Virol. 2010;84:12658–64. [PMC free article] [PubMed] [Google Scholar].

42. Hoffmann M, Kleine-Weber H, Schroeder S, KrÃ¼ger N, Herrler T, Erichsen S, Schiergens TS, Herrler G, Wu NH, Nitsche A, MÃ¼ller MA. SARS CoV2cell entry depends on ACE2 and TMPRSS2 and is blocked by a clinically proven protease inhibitor. Cell. 2020;181(2):271–80.
43. Yan R, Zhang Y, Li Y, Xia L, Guo Y, Zhou Q. Structural basis for the recognition of SARS CoV2 by full-length human ACE2. Science. 2020;367(6485):1444–8.
44. Wang K, Gheblawi M, Oudit GY. Angiotensin converting enzyme 2: a double-edged sword [published online ahead of print, 2020a Mar 26]. Circulation. 2020. https://doi.org/10.1161/CIRCULATIONAHA.120.047049.
45. Gheblawi M, Wang K, Viveiros A, Nguyen Q, Zhong JC, Turner AJ, Raizada MK, Grant MB, Oudit GY. Angiotensin converting enzyme 2: SARS CoV2receptor and regulator of the renin-angiotensin system. Circ Res. 2020. https://doi.org/10.1161/CIRCRESAHA.120.317015.
46. Epelman S, Tang WH, Chen SY, Van Lente F, Francis GS, Sen S. Detection of soluble angiotensin-converting enzyme 2 in heart failure: insights into the endogenous counter-regulatory pathway of the renin-angiotensin-aldosterone system. J Am Coll Cardiol. 2008;52(9):750–4.
47. Basu R, Poglitsch M, Yogasundaram H, Thomas J, Rowe BH, Oudit GY. Roles of angiotensin peptides and recombinant human ACE2 in heart failure. J Am Coll Cardiol. 2017;69:805–19.
48. Fagyas M, Uri K, Siket IM, Fulop GA, Csato V, Darago A, Boczan J, Banyai E, Szentkiralyi IE, Maros TM, Szerafin T, Edes I, Papp Z, Toth A. New perspectives in the renin-angiotensin-aldosterone system (RAAS) II: albumin suppresses angiotensin converting enzyme (ACE) activity in human. PLoS One. 2014;9:e87844.
49. Uri K, Fagyas M, Manyine Siket I, Kertesz A, Csanadi Z, Sandorfi G, Clemens M, Fedor R, Papp Z, Edes I, Toth A, Lizanecz E. New perspectives in the renin-angiotensinaldosterone system (RAAS) IV: circulating ACE2 as a biomarker of systolic dysfunction in human hypertension and heart failure. PLoS One. 2014;9(4):e87845.
50. Zisman LS, Keller RS, Weaver B, Lin Q, Speth R, Bristow MR, Canver CC. Increased angiotensin-(1-7)-forming activity in failing human heart ventricles: evidence for upregulation of the angiotensin-converting enzyme Homologue ACE2. Circulation. 2003;108(14):1707–12. Epub 2003 Sep 22. PubMed PMID: 14504186.
51. Ocaranza MP, Godoy I, Jalil JE, Varas M, Collantes P, Pinto M, Roman M, Ramirez C, Copaja M, Diaz-Araya G, Castro P, Lavandero S. Enalapril attenuates downregulation of Angiotensin-converting enzyme 2 in the late phase of ventricular dysfunction in myocardial infarcted rat. Hypertension. 2006;48(4):572–8.
52. Ãšri K, Fagyas M, MÃ¡nyinÃ© Siket I, KertÃ©sz A, CsanÃ¡di Z, SÃ¡ndorfi G, Clemens M, Fedor R, Papp Z, Ã‰des I, TÃ³th A, Lizanecz E. New perspectives in the renin-angiotensin-aldosterone system (RAAS) IV: circulating ACE2 as a biomarker of systolic dysfunction in human hypertension and heart failure. PLoS One. 2014;9(4):e87845. https://doi.org/10.1371/journal.pone.0087845.eCollection2014 PubMedPMID:24691269; PubMedCentralPMCID:PMC3972189).
53. Soro-Paavonen A, Gordin D, Forsblom C, Rosengard-Barlund M, Waden J, Thorn L, Sandholm N, Thomas MC, Groop PH, FinnDiane Study G. Circulating ACE2 activity is increased in patients with type 1 diabetes and vascular complications. J Hypertens. 2012;30:375–83.
54. Lin Q, Keller RS, Weaver B, Zisman LS. Interaction of ACE2 and integrin beta1 in failing human heart. Biochim Biophys Acta. 2004;1689:175–8.
55. Epelman S, Shrestha K, Troughton RW, Francis GS, Sen S, Klein AL, Tang WH. Soluble angiotensin-converting enzyme 2 in human heart failure: relation with myocardial function and clinical outcomes. J Card Fail. 2009;15(7):565–71.
56. Chemaly M, McGilligan V, Gibson M, Clauss M, Watterson S, Alexander HD, Bjourson AJ, Peace A. Role of tumour necrosis factor alpha converting enzyme (TACE/ADAM17 and

associated proteins in coronary artery disease and cardiac events. Arch Cardiovasc Dis. 2017;110(12):700–11.
57. Kawai T, Elliott KJ, Scalia R, Eguchi S. Contribution of ADAM17 and related ADAMs in cardiovascular diseases. Cell Mol Life Sci. 2021:1–27.
58. Pedersen KB, Chodavarapu H, Porretta C, Robinson LK, Lazartigues E. Dynamics of ADAM17-mediated shedding of ACE2 applied to pancreatic islets of male db/db mice. Endocrinology. 2015;156:4411–25.
59. Zhou X, Zhang P, Liang T, Chen Y, Liu D, Yu H. Relationship between circulating levels of angiotensin-converting enzyme 2-angiotensin-(1–7)-MAS axis and coronary heart disease. Heart Vessels. 2020;35(2):153–61.
60. Hirschi KK, Dâ€™Amore PA. Pericytes in the microvasculature. Cardiovasc Res. 1996;32:687–98.
61. Sims DE. Diversity within pericytes. Clin Exp Pharmacol Physiol. 2000;27:842–6.
62. de Queiroz TM, Lakkappa N, Lazartigues E. ADAM17-mediated shedding of inflammatory cytokines in hypertension. Front Pharmacol. 2020;11:1154.
63. Seals DF, Courtneidge SA. The ADAMs family of metalloproteases: multidomain proteins with multiple functions. Genes Dev. 2003;17(1):7–30.
64. Liu H, Wang H, Cheng D, Wang Q, Pei Z, Zhu N, Fang W, Yu Q. Potential role of a disintegrin and metalloproteinase-17 (ADAM17) in age-associated ventricular remodeling of rats. RSC Adv. 2019;9(25):14321–30.
65. Wang K, Gheblawi M, Oudit GY. Angiotensin converting enzyme 2: a double-edged sword. Circulation. 2020;142(5):426–8.
66. Fedak PW, Moravec CS, McCarthy PM, et al. Altered expression of disintegrin metalloproteinases and their inhibitor in human dilated cardiomyopathy. Circulation. 2006;113:238–45.
67. Rutschow S, Li J, Schultheiss HP, Pauschinger M. Myocardial proteases and matrix remodeling in inflammatory heart disease. Cardiovasc Res. 2006;69:646–56.
68. Liu H, Gai S, Wang X, Zeng J, Sun C, Zhao Y, Zheng Z. Single-cell analysis of SARS CoV2 receptor ACE2 and spike protein priming expression of proteases in the human heart. Cardiovasc Res. 2020;116(10):1733–41.
69. SwÃ¤rd P, Edsfeldt A, Reepalu A, Jehpsson L, Rosengren BE, Karlsson MK. Age and sex differences in soluble ACE2 may give insights for COVID-19. Crit Care. 2020;24(1):221. Published 2020 May 14. https://doi.org/10.1186/s13054-020-02942-2.
70. Ciaglia E, Vecchione C, Puca AA. COVID-19 infection and circulating ACE2 levels: protective role in women and children. Front Pediatr. 2020;8:206.
71. Bhatia K, Zimmerman MA, Sullivan JC. Sex differences in angiotensin-converting enzyme modulation of Ang (1–7) levels in normotensive WKY rats. Am J Hypertens. 2013;26:591–8.
72. Cao Y, Li L, Feng Z, Wan S, Huang P, Sun X, Wen F, Huang X, Ning G, Wang W. Comparative genetic analysis of the novel coronavirus (2019-nCoV/SARS-CoV-2) receptor ACE2 in different populations. Cell Discov. 2020;6(1):1–4.
73. Wu C, Zheng S, Chen Y, Zheng M. Single-cell RNA expression profiling of ACE2, the putative receptor of Wuhan 2019-nCoV, in the nasal tissue.Â MedRxiv. 2020.
74. Darbani B. The expression and polymorphism of entry machinery for COVID-19 in human: juxtaposing population groups, gender, and different tissues. Int J Environ Res Public Health. 2020;17:3433.
75. Xudong X, Junzhu C, Xingxiang W, Furong Z, Yanrong L. Age-and gender-related difference of ACE2 expression in rat lung. Life Sci. 2006;78(19):2166–71.
76. AlGhatrif M, Cingolani O, Lakatta EG. The dilemma of coronavirus disease 2019, aging, and cardiovascular disease: insights from cardiovascular aging science. JAMA Cardiol. 2020;5 (7):747–8.
77. Devaux CA, Rolain JM, Raoult D. ACE2 receptor polymorphism: Susceptibility to SARS-CoV-2, hypertension, multi-organ failure, and COVID-19 disease outcome.Â J Microbiol, Immunol Infect. 2020.

78. Zhou M, Dai W, Cui Y, Li Y. Estrogen downregulates gp130 expression in HUVECs by regulating ADAM10 and ADAM17 via the estrogen receptor. Biochem Biophys Res Commun. 2020;523:753–8.
79. Banu N, Panikar SS, Leal LR, Leal AR. Protective role of ACE2 and its downregulation in SARS CoV2 infection leading to macrophage activation syndrome: therapeutic implications. Life Sci. 2020:117905.
80. Patel VB, Clarke N, Wang Z, et al. Angiotensin II induced proteolytic cleavage of myocardial ACE2 is mediated by TACE/ADAM-17: a positive feedback mechanism in the RAS. J Mol Cell Cardiol. 2014;66:167–76. https://doi.org/10.1016/j.yjmcc.2013.11.017.
81. Liu Y, Yang Y, Zhang C, Huang F, Wang F, Yuan J, Wang Z, Li J, Li J, Feng C, Zhang Z. Clinical and biochemical indexes from 2019-nCoV infected patients linked to viral loads and lung injury. Sci China Life Sci. 2020;63(3):364–74.
82. Dikalov SI, Ungvari Z. Role of mitochondrial oxidative stress in hypertension. Am J Physiol Heart Circ Physiol. 2013;305:H1417–27.
83. Doughan AK, Harrison DG, Dikalov SI. Molecular mechanisms of Angiotensin II-mediated mitochondrial dysfunction: linking mitochondrial oxidative damage and vascular endothelial dysfunction. Circ Res. 2008;102:488–96.
84. Kimura S, Zhang GX, Nishiyama A, Shokoji T, Yao L, Fan YY, Rahman M, Abe Y. Mitochondria-derived reactive oxygen species and vascular MAP kinases: comparison of Angiotensin II and diazoxide. Hypertension. 2005;45(3):438–44.
85. Zhang C, Zhao YX, Zhang YH, Zhu L, Deng BP, Zhou ZL, Li SY, Lu XT, Song LL, Lei XM, Tang WB, Wang N, Pan CM, Song HD, Liu CX, Dong B, Zhang Y, Cao Y. Angiotensin-converting enzyme 2 attenuates atherosclerotic lesions by targeting vascular cells. Proc Natl Acad Sci USA. 2010;107(36):15886–91.
86. Dong B, Zhang C, Feng JB, Zhao YX, Li SY, Yang YP, Dong QL, Deng BP, Zhu L, Yu QT, Liu CX, Liu B, Pan CM, Song HD, Zhang MX, Zhang Y. Overexpression of ACE2 enhances plaque stability in a rabbit model of atherosclerosis. Arterioscler Thromb Vasc Biol. 2008;28 (7):1270–6.
87. Zhang H, Penninger JM, Li Y, Zhong N, Slutsky AS. Angiotensin-converting enzyme 2 (ACE2) as a SARS CoV2 receptor: molecular mechanisms and potential therapeutic target. Intensive Care Med. 2020;46(4):586–90.
88. Host Response Mediators in Coronavirus (COVID-19). Infection - Is There a Protective Effect of Losartan on Outcomes of Coronavirus Infection? (ARBs CORONA II). Available on: https://clinicaltrials.gov/ct2/show/NCT04606563?term=Angiotensin+receptor+blockers+and+lung+injury&cond=COVID-19&draw=2&rank=3. ClinicalTrials.gov. Identifier: NCT04606563. Last Updated: October 28, 2020. Accessed on 27 December 2021.

Chapter 9
Thrombosis in CoViD19

Key Questions

- What is the occurrence of vascular thrombosis in CoViD19?
- Which thrombotic complications are associated with CoViD19?
- Which mechanisms promote the development of thrombotic complications in CoViD19?
- Does the renin-angiotensin system play part in thrombosis in CoViD19?
- How inflammatory and immune mechanisms are linked with hypercoagulation in CoViD19?
- What is the role of platelets and D Dimers in thrombotic complications in CoViD19?
- What is the connection between hypoxia and hypercoagulation in CoViD19?
- What is the importance of ethnic and demographic factors in thrombotic complications in CoViD19?

9.1 Epidemiology

Vascular and coagulation disorders are recognized complications of sepsis. The novel coronavirus disease CoViD19 has been referred to as an inflammatory thrombotic disease, witnessed across a range of demographic diversities throughout the globe. The vast scale of epidemiological boundaries of CoViD19 has resulted in unprecedented health and economic implications. The thrombotic complications in CoViD19 appear to affect multiple organs and tissues and constitute a significant proportion of the associated morbidity and mortality. Multiple macrovascular and microvascular territories may be affected resulting in a variety of peripheral and

U. Mallick, *Cardiovascular Complications of COVID-19*,
https://doi.org/10.1007/978-3-030-90065-6_9

organic thrombotic events. The coronary, cerebrovascular, mesenteric, peripheral arterial, and venous structures may be involved resulting in serious life-threatening complications such as myocardial infarction (MI), stroke, pulmonary embolism (PE), and mesenteric thrombosis, among others.

The burden of vascular and thrombotic disease in CoViD19 appears to be particularly high among the critical patients, although variations in the incidence and mortality exist. An observational study of 3334 consecutive hospitalized CoViD19 patients investigating the incidence of, and risk factors for, venous and arterial thrombotic events in all hospitalized patients, reported a 16% incidence of thrombotic events (207 (6.2%) were venous (3.2% PE and 3.9% DVT) and 365 (11.1%) were arterial (1.6% ischemic stroke, 8.9% MI, and 1.0% systemic thromboembolism). A thrombotic event was independently associated with mortality (adjusted hazard ratio, 1.82; 95% CI, 1.54–2.15; $P < 0.001$) (venous thrombosis (adjusted hazard ratio, 1.37; 95% CI, 1.02–1.86; $P = 0.04$) and arterial thrombosis (adjusted hazard ratio, 1.99; 95% CI, 1.65–2.40; $P < 0.001$) were associated for mortality $P = 0.25$ for interaction). Among 829 critical ICU patients, 29.4% had a thrombotic event (13.6% venous and 18.6% arterial), whereas, among 2505 non-ICU patients, 11.5% had a thrombotic event (3.6% venous and 8.4% arterial) [1].

Similarly, other large cohorts also describe a high incidence of thromboembolic events in CoViD19 and significantly high mortality, especially among critical patients. In an observational study of 3678 patients with confirmed CoViD19, 892 (24.3%) were hospitalized of which 296 (8.0%) were admitted to the intensive care unit. Among the hospitalized patients, 46 (5.2%) patients had acute thrombotic events, 24 (2.7%) patients had venous thromboembolism, 11 (1.2%) patients had an acute ischemic stroke, and 11 (1.2%) patients had acute myocardial infarction). The incidence of thrombotic events was much higher among the critical patients admitted in the intensive care unit: 26 (8.8%) patients had acute thrombotic events 15 (5.1%) patients had venous thromboembolism, 5 (1.7%) patients had acute ischemic stroke and 7 (2.4%) patients had acute myocardial infarction) (MI). The in-hospital all-cause mortality was 12.2% and numerically higher for those with thrombotic events versus not (17.5% versus 12.0%, $P = 0.21$) [2].

The lungs appear to be central to the microvascular thrombotic disease in CoViD19. This is due to the highly sophisticated matrix of the immune-secretory and modulatory structural cells that face the viral invasion. Pulmonary embolism and microvascular disease appear to be prominent pulmonary vascular pathology associated with severe CoViD19. Significantly higher rates of venous thromboembolism (31%) have been described in an analysis of data of a cohort of 184 patients with proven CoViD19 pneumonia admitted in the intensive care unit (ICU). In this study, the cumulative incidence of the composite outcome (symptomatic acute pulmonary embolism (PE), deep-vein thrombosis (DVT), ischemic stroke, myocardial infarction (MI), or systemic arterial embolism) was 31% (95% CI 20–41), confirmed VTE in 27% (95%CI 17–37%) and arterial thrombotic events in 3.7% (95% CI 0–8.2%), with PE was the most frequent thrombotic complication ($n = 25$, 81%) [3]. Similarly, other studies describe a high incidence of venous thromboembolism at 25% (20/81) among the critical CoViD19 patients in ICU [4].

In a prospective cohort study of 150 patients hospitalized with severe CoViD19, propensity score matching was performed to analyze the occurrence of thromboembolic events. The incidence of thromboembolic complications was 11.7% (9/77), odds ratio (1.1–6.1) p. 004 [5].

Several studies report the incidence of stroke in CoViD19 patients. A retrospective study analyzing data of the CoViD19 patients showed that the incidence of stroke among the hospitalized patients was approximately 5% [6]. Furthermore, the association of large vessel stroke with CoViD19 was also reported in a case series in patients younger than age 50 years, indicating the occurring of stroke in younger patients in CoViD19 [7].

Differences in the incidence and risks of thromboembolism have been observed in different populations and across ethnicities in various countries [8, 9]. According to analyses, the burden of CoViD19 appears high in the ethnic groups [10] and incidence of death varies among different ethnic groups with 5.38-fold disparity for non-Hispanic Black, relative to white, communities with CoViD19 [11]. In the UK, age-sex adjusted hospital death rates for CoViD19 were found 2·17-times higher for people with ethnicity recorded as Black compared to those recorded as White, and 1·95 higher for those recorded as Asia [12].

Several complex pathogenetic factors determine these variations and are currently under exploration. A wide range of variabilities may be observed in the incidence of VTE in CoViD19, and the rates appear to be much higher among the critical CoViD19 patients. For instance in France, in the inpatient settings, the incidence of VTE in CoViD19 patients varied between 3 to 85% [13]. In another French study the overall reported rate of VTE in critical CoViD19 patients was 69% [14]. According to a study, in Italy VTE occurred in 8% of hospitalized CoViD19 patients [15]. Overall, the reported rates of VTE CoViD19 appear much elevated among critical CoViD19 patients. Data from a Chinese cohort of ICU admitted CoViD19 patients further reveal, an extremely high incidence of VTE, varying between 46 to 85.4%, in this patient subgroup [16].

Moreover, the laboratory characteristics of the complicated CoViD19 patients have been highlighted in several studies internationally. The hematological profile of the complicated CoViD19 commonly shows lymphopenia, thrombocytopenia, increased Fibrinogen Degradation Products (FDP), D dimers, ferritin, PTT (Partial Thromboplastin Time) and a PTT (activated Partial Thromboplastin Time), and several other specific immunoglobulins, antibodies such as Antiphospholipid antibodies [17, 18].

The pathology reports from CoViD19 studies across the globe further indicate the presence of a range of mechanisms that may promote thrombotic complications in the CoViD19 patients. The data suggest that the development of the coagulation abnormalities may be triggered by multiple dysregulated homeostatic mechanisms as a result of the viral disease (Figs. 9.8 and 9.9). The pathogenetic mechanisms related to the viral and immunopathological complications, and associated inflammatory and complex regulatory mechanisms affecting the vasculature and coagulation mechanisms, may lead to a variety of vascular and coagulation abnormalities observed in CoViD19 [19] (Fig. 9.7).

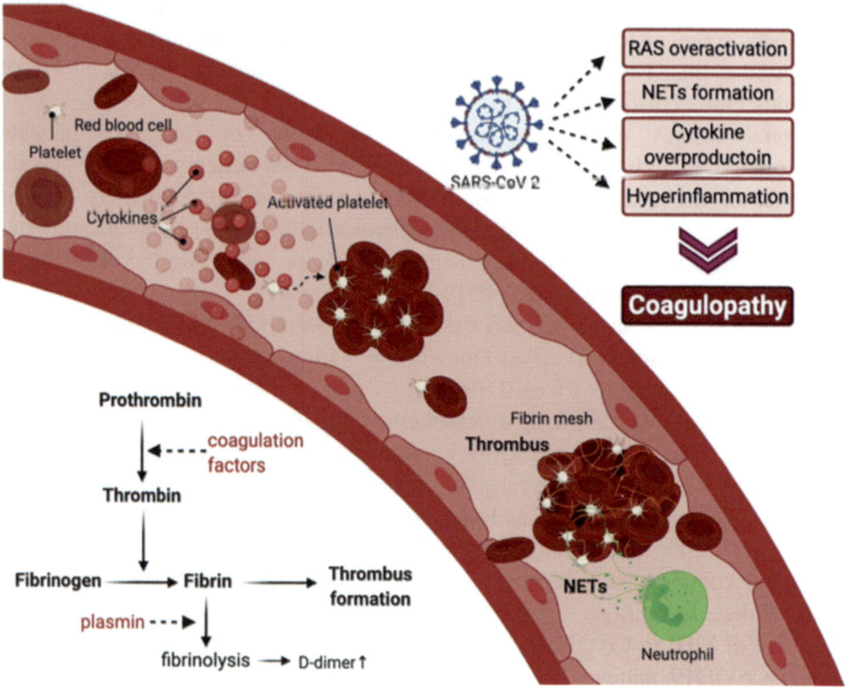

Fig. 9.1 Coagulopathy in COVID19. Prothrombotic phase of COVID-19 pathogenesis. SARS-CoV-2 infection induces RAS overactivation, NETs formation, cytokine overproduction, and hyperinflammation. These effects translate into increased risk for coagulation disorder. *Source* Fig. 4. Lee, C. and Choi, W.J., 2021. Overview of COVID-19 inflammatory pathogenesis from the therapeutic perspective. Archives of pharmacal research, pp. 1–18. https://link.springer.com/article/10.1007/s12272-020-01301-7. Published by Springer Nature Group

Although the current data divulge several important clues to the pathogenesis of the prothrombotic complications associated with CoViD19, the exact mechanisms related to vascular injury and hypercoagulability need to be established. Further research is required to fully recognize the pathogenetic factors that may be used as the potential therapeutic targets and define the effective diagnostic and treatment strategies in patients with the novel coronavirus disease.

9.2 Mechanisms Promoting Thrombosis in CoViD19

A myriad of complex mechanisms appears to be responsible for the thrombotic complications and vasoplegic insults in CoViD19. (Figs. 9.1 and 9.6). The infectious and hyper-immune-inflammatory nature of the viral disease may lead to dysregulation of important homeostatic systems, causing injury to a variety of

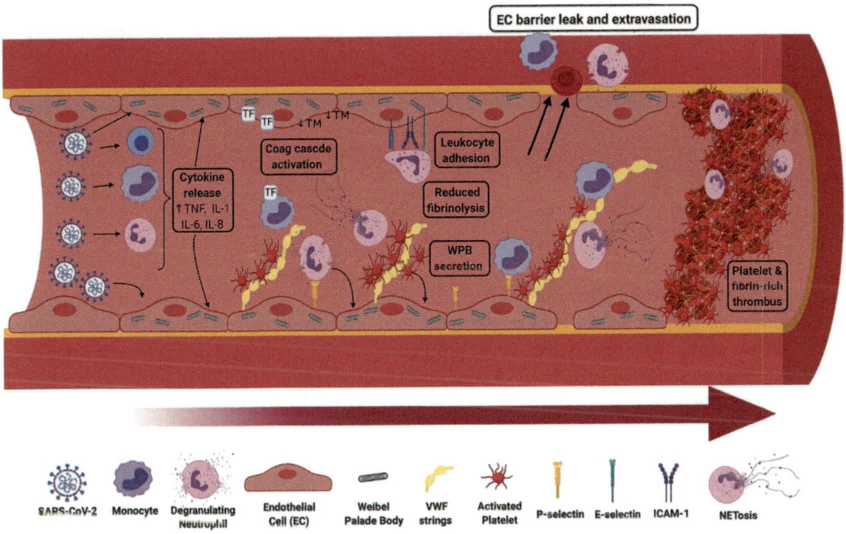

Fig. 9.2 Pulmonary immune-thrombosis and endotheliopathy in COVID-19 pathogenesis. COVID-19 is associated with a pulmonary-centric vasculopathy. The SARS-CoV-2 virus causes activation of monocytes and platelets, as well as neutrophil degranulation. The virus can also activate and gain entry into endothelial cells lining the blood vessel wall. In severe COVID-19, EC activation is further activated by pro-inflammatory cytokines. Acute EC activation and damage triggers secretion of high molecular weight von Willebrand factor (VWF) multimers normally stored within Weibel Palade bodies. This results in high local concentrations of VWF. Large VWF strings anchored on the EC surface can then tether circulating platelets and recruit neutrophils and monocytes. In addition, WPB secretion results in externalization of P-selectin to the EC surface where it facilitates leukocyte and platelet adherence. Enhanced expression of other adhesion molecules, including VCAM-1, ICAM-1, and E-selectin, further promote neutrophil and monocyte recruitment. TF expression on EC and monocytes, coupled with NETosis, leads to coagulation cascade activation. Moreover, normal anti-coagulant pathways on the EC surface are down-regulated. Additionally, inflammation affects fibrinolysis by promoting local release of tPA and PAI-1 from EC. Significant amounts of PAI-1 are also secreted from activated platelets, and TAFI and α2-antiplasmin levels are both increased. Consequently, fibrinolysis is attenuated in severe COVID-19. Furthermore, EC tight-barrier junctions become disrupted leading to enhanced permeability and extravasation. The net effect of this dysregulated immune-thrombosis is the generation of platelet- and fibrin-rich thrombi and pulmonary vaso-occlusion. *Source* Fig. 1. O'Donnell, J.S., Peyvandi, F. and Martin-Loeches, I., 2021. Pulmonary immuno-thrombosis in COVID-19 ARDS pathogenesis. Intensive Care Medicine, pp. 1–4. https://link.springer.com/article/10.1007/s00134-021-06419-w

cellular structures and tissues. The invasion of SARS CoV2 leads to the activation of several hyperimmune, dysmetabolic, and prothrombotic processes adding to the pathological state. Various macro and microvascular structures may be damaged in this process and cause macro and microangiopathy and thrombosis. The systemic complications associated with the CoViD19 may accompany the arterial and venous territories in various organs, resulting in multi-organ failure. In a prospective cohort observational, cross-sectional study of hospitalized moderate to

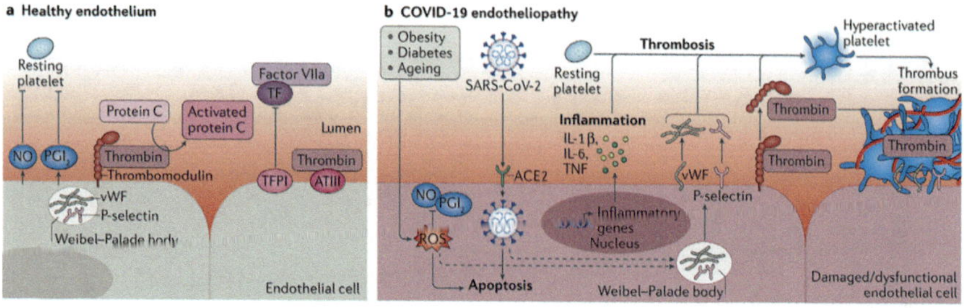

Fig. 9.3 CoViD19 associated endotheliopathy. The normal resting endothelium is crucial for maintaining vascular homeostasis through production of several anti-inflammatory and antithrombotic factors, including nitric oxide (NO), prostaglandin I2 (PGI2; also known as prostacyclin), thrombomodulin, activated protein C, tissue factor pathway inhibitor (TFPI) and antithrombin III (ATIII). **b** In disease states, such as obesity and diabetes mellitus, increased oxidative stress with elevated intracellular levels of reactive oxygen species (ROS) can promote the production of pro-inflammatory cytokines (such as IL-1β, IL-6 and TNF), decrease the bioavailability of NO and PGI2 and induce endothelial cell apoptosis, leading to endothelial damage and dysfunction. Furthermore, the release of pro-inflammatory and prothrombotic factors (such as von Willebrand factor (vWF) and thrombin) can lead to vascular inflammation, platelet aggregation and thrombosis. Simultaneous invasion of the endothelium by severe acute respiratory syndrome coronavirus 2 (SARS-CoV-2)—the virus that causes coronavirus disease 2019 (COVID-19)—via the angiotensin-converting enzyme 2 (ACE2) receptor can exacerbate endothelial dysfunction and damage, further promoting vascular inflammation and thrombosis. The dashed arrows represent complex molecular signalling mechanisms that remain to be defined in the context of COVID-19. TF, tissue factor. *Source* Fig. 4. Gu, S.X., Tyagi, T., Jain, K., Gu, V.W., Lee, S.H., Hwa, J.M., Kwan, J.M., Krause, D.S., Lee, A.I., Halene, S. and Martin, K.A., 2020. Thrombocytopathy and endotheliopathy: crucial contributors to COVID-19 thromboinflammation. Nature Reviews Cardiology, pp. 1–16. https://www.nature.com/articles/s41569-9.020-9.00469-9.1#Fig4. Published by Springer Nature Group

severe 23 CoViD19 non-consecutive patients (mostly male 20/23) analyzing microvascular alterations, severe alterations of the microcirculation and the endothelial glycocalyx were observed [20].

Furthermore, the variations in systemic vascular resistance and hemodynamic failure are important features of vascular complications in sepsis may play a pivotal role in complicated CoViD19. Vasoconstriction, poor organ perfusion result in micro vasculopathies, hypercoagulability, and prothrombotic reactions ultimately lead to ischemic injury in the organs. In this pathological state the dysregulation of the clotting factors results in thrombotic phenomena accompanied by an increase in prothrombotic coagulation factors, vascular damage, and platelet hyperactivity, among other important mechanisms. The presence of autoimmune components related to thrombosis has also been indicated in CoViD19, however, further links need to be established [21].

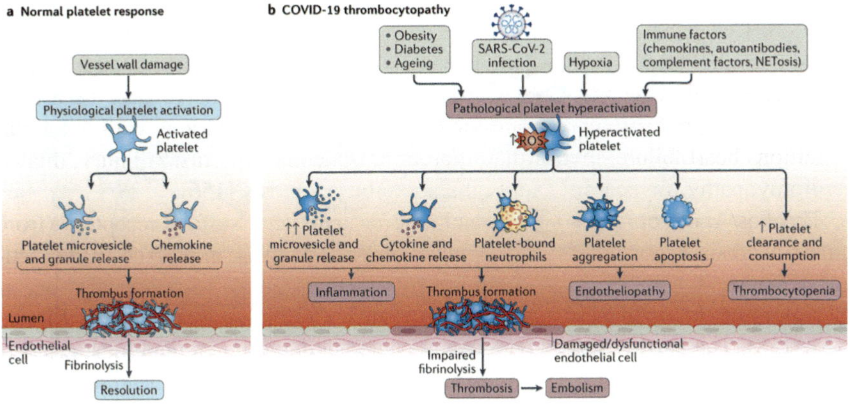

Fig. 9.4 CoViD19 associated thrombocytopathy. Schematic diagram summarizing the normal physiological platelet response to vessel wall damage, that is, haemostasis (panel a) and the thrombocytopathy associated with coronavirus disease 2019 (COVID-19; panel b). Possible additional inducers of pathological platelet hyperactivation include cardiovascular risk factors such as old age, diabetes mellitus, obesity and hypoxia from lung disease, and immune factors leading to increased intracellular levels of reactive oxygen species (ROS). The consequences of pathological platelet hyperactivation include increased platelet microvesicle and granule release that contribute to increased thrombosis and cytokine storm (local and circulating). Increased platelet activation can result in platelet–leukocyte conjugates (primarily neutrophils) and platelet apoptosis and/or aggregation, which in turn can further lead to increased thrombosis and inflammation. The presence of impaired fibrinolysis and endotheliopathy can contribute to increased thrombosis and can lead to life-threatening thrombosis and thromboembolism. The lungs are the most susceptible organ to thrombosis but these events can occur in many organs, including the heart, kidneys and liver. With platelet hyperactivation, apoptosis and increased thrombus formation, platelet clearance and consumption are higher, leading to thrombocytopenia. Thrombocytopenia occurs only if megakaryocytes are unable to produce sufficient platelets to compensate for the platelet loss. SARS-CoV-2, severe acute respiratory syndrome coronavirus 2. *Source* Fig. 3. Gu, S.X., Tyagi, T., Jain, K., Gu, V.W., Lee, S.H., Hwa, J.M., Kwan, J.M., Krause, D.S., Lee, A.I., Halene, S. and Martin, K.A., 2020. Thrombocytopathy and endotheliopathy: crucial contributors to COVID-19 thromboinflammation. Nature Reviews Cardiology, pp. 1–16. https://www.nature.com/articles/s41569-9.020-9.00469-9.1#Fig4. Published by Springer Nature Group

9.2.1 Renin Angiotensin System and Thrombosis

Dysregulation of the renin-angiotensin system (RAS) related mechanisms such as enhanced expression of the angiotensin II (Ang II) may severely impact endothelial cells and cause vascular injury and dysfunction. Ang II induces vasoconstriction and promotes pro-inflammatory/prothrombotic mechanisms. The downregulation of ACE2 due to SARS CoV2 results in dysregulated the RAS through imbalance between the ACE/AngII/AT1 Receptor axis and the ACE2/Ang 1–7/Mas Receptor axis [22]. A diminished degradation of the Ang II into angiotensin 1–7, a protective axis in opposition to the Ang II, promotes the harmful impact of the ACE/Ang II/AT1 Receptor axis.

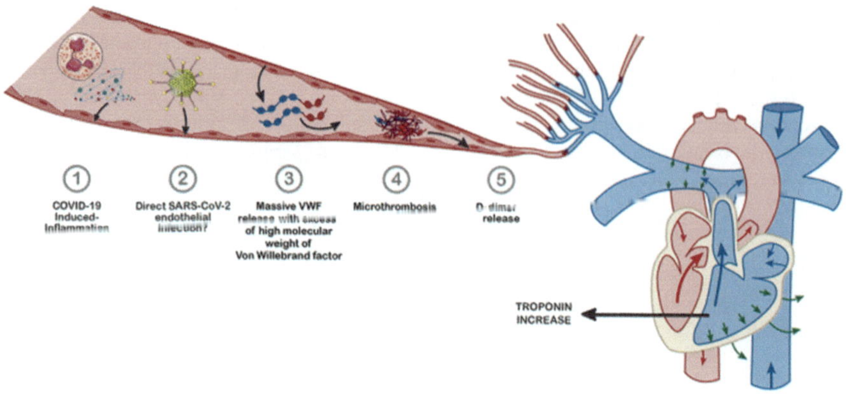

Fig. 9.5 Pathophysiology for microthrombosis in patients with COVID-19. The figure summarizes hypothetical steps of the thrombotic sequence from direct or indirect of SARS-CoV-2 effects on endothelial cells inducing an endotheliopathy and a coagulopathy leading to lung obstruction and potential consequences on the right heart ventricle. *Source* Fig. 1. Smadja, D.M., Mentzer, S.J., Fontenay, M. et al. COVID-19 is a systemic vascular hemopathy: insight for mechanistic and clinical aspects. Angiogenesis (2021). https://doi.org/10.1007/s10456-021-09805-6. Published by Springer Nature Group

Moreover, the ACE2 expression on vascular endothelium offers direct viral-ACE2 interaction, thereby another route to the endothelial cell injury in CoViD19. Animal studies have shown antithrombotic and antiplatelet aggregatory activity of ACE2 [23]. The development of acute ischemic stroke has been linked with the RAS-related mechanisms with vasoplegic actions. Upregulation of the ACE/Ang II/AT1R axis may result in vasoconstriction of the cerebral vessels, in addition to pro-fibrotic, pro-inflammatory, and increased oxidative stress impact upon the brain parenchyma [24]. The angiotensin receptors are expressed on the surface of platelets, and inhibition of the RAS may diminish platelet activation [25, 26].

A dysregulation of other hemodynamic peptide systems such as RAS and Kallikrein–Kinin System (KKS) may contribute to the prothrombotic state observed in CoViD19 directly and through interactions, although these interactions need to be further defined. The RAS and KKS may cross-talk at several levels [27, 28]. The functional activities of angiotensin 1–7 (on MAS receptor and AT1R) and bradykinin (on B2R) may depend on each other [29]. The ACE2 is known to down-regulate the KKS. ACE2 plays a role in the degradation of Des-Arg^9-Kallidin and Des-Arg^9-Bradykinin [30]. A decrease in ACE2 in CoViD19 may be associated with hyperactivation of the KKS and an increase in local and systemic clotting mechanisms [31]. Through regulation of vessel wall tissue factor, the B2R, AT2R, and Mas work in concert to counterbalance the prothrombotic impact of the AT1R [32, 33]. The KKS has a key function in tissue repair, inflammation, cell proliferation and platelet aggregation and may also be involved in the prothrombotic mechanisms through Factor XII and activation of complement C3 [34]. These mechanisms may represent important links reflecting cross-talk between regulatory mechanisms that result in the prothrombotic state associated with CoViD19.

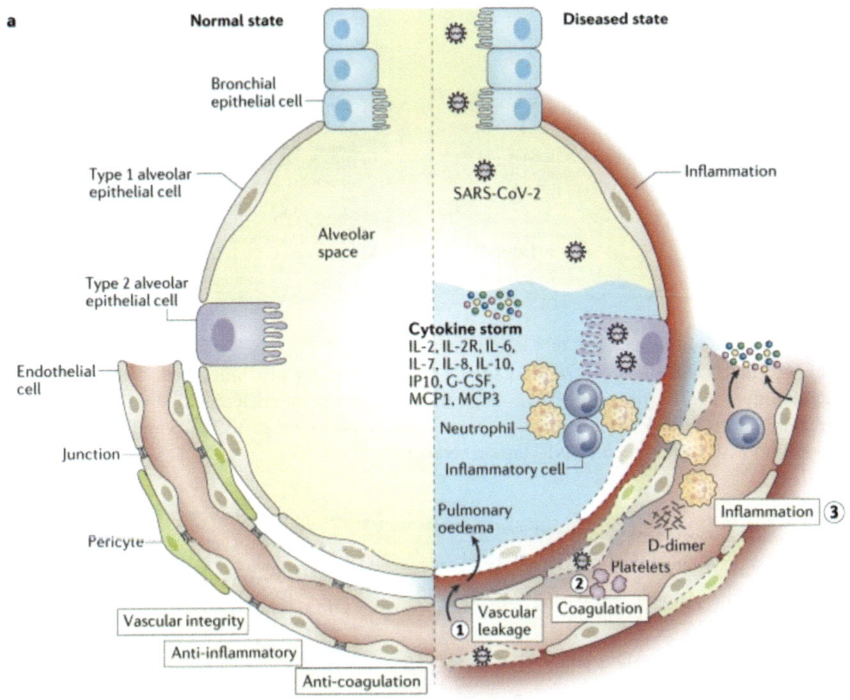

Fig. 9.6 Proposed vessel–lung tissue interface in normal state and in COVID-19 disease. On the left, the normal interface between the alveolar space and endothelial cells is depicted; the right side highlights pathophysiological features of coronavirus disease 2019 (COVID-19) in the lung, including loss of vascular integrity (1), activation of the coagulation pathway (2) and inflammation (3). *Source* Fig. 1. Teuwen, L.A., Geldhof, V., Pasut, A. and Carmeliet, P., 2020. COVID-19: the vasculature unleashed. Nature Reviews Immunology, 20(7), pp. 389–391. https://www.nature.com/articles/s41577-020-0343-0. By Springer Nature Group

9.2.2 *Endothelial Cell Damage and Thrombosis*

The endothelial cells that cover the entire vascular bed have a multifunctional role in vascular hemodynamics, maintenance of blood fluidity, immune function, coagulability, inflammation, and repair mechanisms, and carry vessel and tissue-specific functions. The hemostatic function of the endothelial cells is dependent on several factors including the control of coagulation, platelet adhesion, activation, and disintegration, as well as vasoregulation. The anticoagulant properties of the endothelial cells countering the platelet activation and aggregation are important mechanisms in hemostasis. The mechanisms causing endothelial injury may perturb these functions. Another important factor, vasoconstriction associated with endothelial damage, results from circumvention of the vasodilatory actions of the endothelial cells by the local vasoactive agents that directly impact smooth muscle cells.

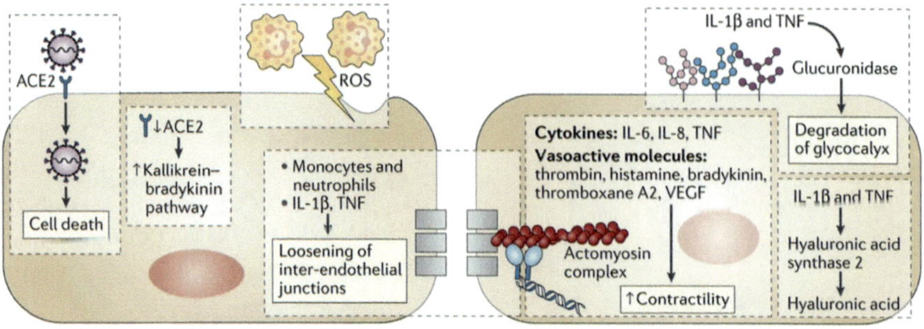

Fig. 9.7 Proposed mechanisms of vascular leakage. *Source* Fig. 1b. Teuwen, L.A., Geldhof, V., Pasut, A. and Carmeliet, P., 2020. COVID-19: the vasculature unleashed. Nature Reviews Immunology, 20(7), pp. 389–391. https://www.nature.com/articles/s41577-020-0343-0. By Springer Nature Group. ACE2, angiotensin-converting enzyme-2; VEFG, vascular endothelial growth factor; IL, interleukin; TNF, tumor necrosis factor

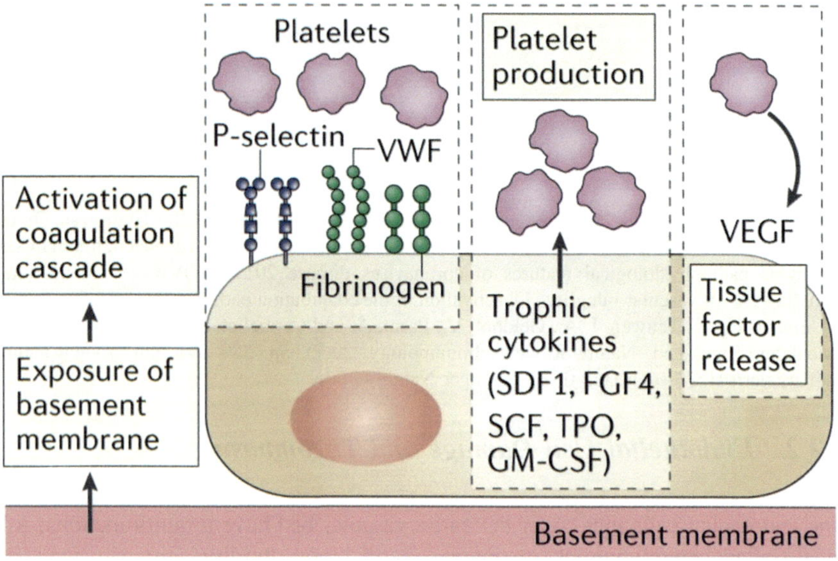

Fig. 9.8 Proposed mechanism of coagulation initiation. VWF, von Willebrand factor; SDF1, stroma cell-derived factor 1; FGF, fibroblast growth factor; SCF, stem cell factor; TPO, thrombopoietin; GM-CSF, granulocyte macrophage-colony-stimulating factor; VEGF, vascular endothelial growth factor. *Source* Fig. 1c. Teuwen, L.A., Geldhof, V., Pasut, A. and Carmeliet, P., 2020. COVID-19: the vasculature unleashed. Nature Reviews Immunology, 20(7), pp. 389–391. https://www.nature.com/articles/s41577-020-0343-0. By Springer Nature Group

The CoViD19 may result in endotheliopathy. (Fig. 9.3). The direct endothelial damage and indirect consequence of the viral insult causing dysregulated immunomodulatory impact of the CoViD19 or cytokine storm, adversely influence

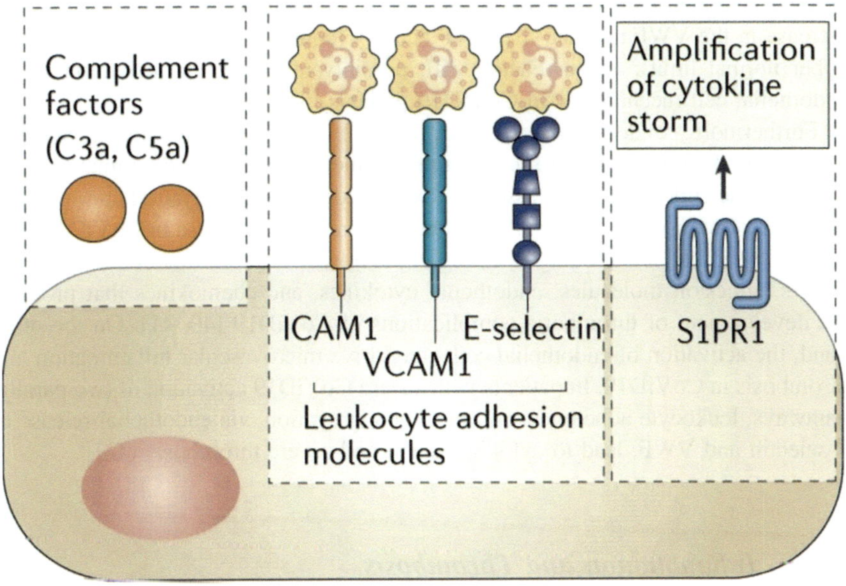

Fig. 9.9 Proposed mechanism of promotion of inflammation. S1PR1, sphingosine 1 phosphate receptor 1; ICAM1, intercellular adhesion molecule-1; VCAM1, vascular cell adhesion molecule-1. *Source* Fig. 1d. Teuwen, L.A., Geldhof, V., Pasut, A. and Carmeliet, P., 2020. COVID-19: the vasculature unleashed. Nature Reviews Immunology, 20(7), pp. 389–391. https://www.nature.com/articles/s41577-020-0343-0. By Springer Nature Group

the cardiovascular endothelial bed. These mechanisms are further linked with the intracellular stress mechanisms that have a deleterious impact on vascular health. The evidence shows the involvement of endothelial cells across vascular beds such as the heart, small bowel, kidneys, and lungs in CoViD19 with diffuse lymphocytic endotheliitis and apoptotic bodies [35, 36]. The induction of apoptosis and pyroptosis may have an important role in the endothelial cell injury in patients with CoViD19 [37], and may promote the development of vascular and thrombotic complications in CoViD19.

The endothelial cells secrete endothelium-derived glycoproteins including von Willebrand factor (vWF), tissue-type plasminogen activator, and urokinase-type plasminogen activator, as well as soluble thrombomodulin a marker of endothelial cell injury. The elevated serum levels of the vWF:Ag and FVIII, and high tissue factor (TF), and intercellular adhesion molecule (ICAM-1), are known markers of endothelial dysfunction. In a multi-center prospective study investigating the risk of thromboembolism in 150 severe CoViD19 patients, the Factor VIII (*normal range: 60–150%*) 341% (258; 416), the Von Willebrand factor (vWF) activity 328% (212; 342), and the vWF antigen (vWF:Ag) (*normal range: 50–150%*) 455 (350; 521), were considerably increased [38]. The hemato-immunological profile of a patient with CoViD19 pneumonia and ARDS showed elevated serum levels of the

D-dimer, the anti-cardiolipin antibodies (IgM), and the IgM anti-β2-GPI, a marked increase in the VWF antigen, the VWF activity (approximately fourfold above the upper normal limit), and in Factor VIII, possibly reflecting the activation of the endothelial cell mechanisms in CoViD19 patients [39].

Furthermore, endothelial cells act as a bridge between thrombosis and inflammation. (Fig. 9.2) The intense immune mechanisms and inflammatory activation of the endothelium are associated with endothelial cell dysfunction in sepsis and related multi-organ failure. A dysregulated immune response in CoViD19 may result in endothelial cell injury resulting in the release of prothrombotic coagulation factors, adhesion molecules, endothelial cytokines, and chemokines that promote the development of thrombotic complications of CoViD19 [40, 41]. On the other hand, the activation of endothelial cells may drive microvascular inflammation and thrombosis in CoViD19. In patients with severe CoViD19 activation of two parallel pathways, leukocyte adherence, and platelet aggregation, via endothelial release of P-selectin and VWF, lead to cytokine storm and severe thrombosis [42].

9.2.3 Inflammation and Thrombosis

Inflammation promotes thrombosis by influencing hemostasis through augmenting pro-coagulation factors, decreasing anticoagulation, and blocking fibrinolytic pathways. Inflammation is a repair mechanism, however persistent and intense leads to tissue injury. Several structures such as the leukocytes, platelets, smooth muscle cells, and endothelial cells are involved in the obscure interface between inflammation and thrombosis and contribute to inflammation in the complex vascular environment. While inflammation promotes thrombosis, the thrombosis can also induce inflammation through multiple mechanisms, such as stimulation of smooth muscle cells to produce IL-6, by thrombin generation or release of Platelet-Derived Growth Factor from the platelet alpha granules during thrombosis [43, 44].

Production of several pro-inflammatory cytokines, chemokines (IL-6, IL-8, PAF (platelet-activating factor), and MCP-1), and pro adhesive molecules (ICAM-1, E- and P-selectin) may be activated by thrombin-induced endothelial activation via PAR1 [45–47].

In CoViD19, inflammation and cytokine storm play an important role in the development of thrombosis. Multi-organ failure and ARDS are among serious complications in CoViD19 patients. The IL-6 derived from the lungs induces hematopoiesis, specifically the production of platelets by stimulating hepatocytes to produce the acute phase proteins, such as CRP, fibrinogen, and antiproteases [48]. Patients with cardiovascular diseases have a higher risk of severity of disease and complications in CoViD19. Elevated inflammatory burden including with associated lung injury may precipitate cardiac thrombotic complicatons. Inflammation may promote formation of an occlusive thrombus over a ruptured coronary plaque through endothelial dysfunction and procoagulant activity of the blood [49]. Data from a cohort analysis of 416 patients admitted with CoViD19 showed that 2.9% (12) of the overall cohort had coagulation disorders and were more common 7.3% (6 of 82) in patients with cardiac injury versus 1.8% (6 of 334) P = 0.02) [50].

Hyper inflammatory impact of sepsis is a recognized mechanism that results in micro and macrovascular injury in multiple organs resulting in organ failure. The interplay of cytokine storm marked by an increase in pro-inflammatory cytokines such as IL-6, elevated C reactive protein (CRP), ferritin, and D Dimers, important pathogenetic markers of hyper inflammation in the complicated CoViD19, may result in vascular injury and prothrombotic abnormalities. The CRP has been reported to induce expression of the leukocyte adhesion molecules, tissue factors, monocyte recruitment to the arterial wall with the induction of MCP-1, and increased complement activation play a significant role in the development of these complications.

Other mechanisms such as Neutrophil Extracellular Traps (NETs) consisting of circulating free DNA and histones are linked with inflammation, coagulation and thrombosis both locally and systemically in a variety of conditions [51]. Viruses can stimulate neutrophils to produce Neutrophil Extracellular Traps (NETs), a network structure formed by freely circulating DNA expelled by neutrophils, and a variety of proteins. This process leads to cell death that is characterized by the destruction of the nuclear membrane before the plasmatic membrane that is apart from necrosis or apoptosis. In dysregulated forms, this process generates an extreme systemic response with the production of cytokines, interferon I, and immune complexes, and may result in local and systemic damage. Patients with CoViD19 have high levels of circulating free (cf-DNA) and DNA-myeloperoxidase complexes [52]. Elevated levels of these freely circulating complexes correlated with the acuity of illness, inflammatory response, and severe disease. Studies have shown that elevated NETs are correlated with the severity of CoViD19 [53]. The circulating free RNA (cf-RNA) from SARS CoV 2 may trigger a coagulation cascade. Evidence shows that cf-RNA serves as a cofactor for auto-activation of Factor VII-activating protease, thereby initiating coagulation [54]. The prothrombotic activity of NETs involves multiple mechanisms such as enhancement of tissue factor activity and thrombin generation via anticoagulant protein degradation [55], and via platelet-dependent mechanisms [56]. The potential role of these novel mechanisms NETosis, the association between NETs activity and mortality from CoViD19, and markers of NETosis, and serum markers of inflammation and thrombosis in CoViD19, are currently being explored [57].

9.2.4 Microangiopathy and Thrombosis in CoViD19

Microangiopathy is a prominent pathogenetic feature of ARDS observed in severe CoViD19. Data indicate that the microscopic platelet–fibrin thrombi are commonly found in the small vasculature of lungs of the deceased CoViD19 patients [58–60]. (Fig. 9.5). According to a study, the prevalence of alveolar-capillary microthrombi was 9 times higher in CoViD19 related respiratory failure as compared to influenza [61].

Conditions including thrombotic microangiopathy (TMA), thrombotic thrombocytopenic purpura (TTP), and hemolytic uremic syndrome (HUS) are recognized complications of sepsis. COVID19 infection appears to have pathogenetic features of complement-mediated thrombotic microangiopathies (TMA). The hypercoagulation or hypofibrinolytic form of disseminated intravascular coagulation (DIC) with a prominent feature of organ failure is observed in infections or sepsis.

The development of pathogenetic features of disseminated intravascular coagulation (DIC) is seen among severely ill patients with CoViD19. The DIC is also regarded as a marker of poor prognosis in CoViD19. In a retrospective cohort study of 799 patients, analysis of 113 deceased patients and 161 recovered patients showed the incidence of Disseminated Intravascular Coagulation in overall 8% (21), died 17% (19) and recovered patients 1% (2) [62]. A meta-analysis of 14 CoViD19 studies investigating the association of DIC with the severity and prognosis of COVID-19 indicated the incidence of DIC was 3% (95%: 1–5%, $P < 0.001$). A significant correlation between DIC and CoViD19 severity and poor prognosis was seen (Log OR = 2.46, 95% CI: 0.94–3.99, $P < 0.001$) [63].

The laboratory characteristics pointing to such complications in CoViD19 patients are anemia, thrombocytopenia, and microvascular platelet thrombi, and organ dysfunction. The main features of the DIC include activation of the fibrinolytic system, reduced endothelial cell surface proteases (antithrombin, protein C), and thrombocytopenia. The advanced phase of DIC may be associated with thrombocytopenia, increased PT and PTT, elevated fibrin (ogen) degradation products, and decreased protease inhibition. Endothelial cell and platelet dysfunction, and tissue injury are the main pathogenetic features of DIC also observed in complicated CoViD19 marked by hypercytokinetic state. Increased cytokines may determine hypofibrinolysis through activation of plasminogen activator inhibitor-1 (PAI 1) [64, 65].

The complement system is part of innate immunity activated by antigen–antibody complexes (classic pathway), specific surface antigens (alternative pathway), and mannose on the pathogen surface (lectin pathway) as a protective mechanism against bacterial or viral invasion and promotes inflammation. These pathways lead to a common pathway (production of C3a and C5a inflammatory mediators and C3b-initiated pathogen opsonization) and end in the formation of the C5b-9 membrane attack complex that kills the target cells. Complement activates cytokine production important in the fight against the virus. The complement system is overactivated in the lungs of CoViD19 patients [66]. Dysregulated complement activation and dysregulated cytokine release in CoViD19 may lead to excessive inflammation and end-organ dysfunction.

Elevated complement activity is associated with CoViD19 disease severity, and increased activation of the complement system leads to consumption of C3 and decreased complement activity increases the risk of death in CoViD19 patients [67]. The activation of the complement system and microvascular deposits are linked with microangiopathies. The complement components (C5b-9 and C4d), MASP-2 (mannose-binding lectin-associated serine protease), SARS CoV2 viral spike glycoproteins, and microvascular thrombi were found on the histological examination of the biopsies obtained from CoViD19 patients [66, 68]. Furthermore, thrombomodulin a product of endothelial cells inactivates complement factor C5a through tissue-associated fibrinolysis inhibitor activation [69, 70]. These findings suggest complement activation possibly leading to the hypercoagulability state observed in CoViD19 patients. The complement activation has also been linked with elevated CRP levels that are also found in severe CoViD19 patients [71]. Furthermore, the kallikrein (part of the kallikrein kinin system KKS) that plays an important role in vascular regulation and mediates inflammation, may activate the complement system [34].

Excessive complement activation may lead to thrombotic micro-angiopathy (TMA) and organ dysfunction such as cardiac or renal dysfunction. Pathogenic complement activation may cause endothelial dysfunction a marker of CoViD19. The DIC and related microangiopathies in CoViD19 might represent an intermediary process towards the severity of the disease. Pathogenetic processes involving complement activation and mechanisms related to the TMA in CoViD19 patients need to be further investigated. Complement inhibition may serve as a therapeutic route in severe CoViD19 patients. Trials are underway investigating complement inhibition in CoViD19 patients [110, 111].

9.2.5 *Platelets and Thrombosis in CoViD19*

The platelets play an important role in the pathogenesis of CoViD19 and contribute to inflammation and thrombosis. (Fig. 9.4). Association of thrombocytopenia in CoViD19 is associated with complicated disease. A multi-center cohort analysis of 1099 patients admitted with CoViD19 indicated an incidence of thrombocytopenia in 36.2% on admission (defined as a platelet count less than 150,000 per cubic millimeter) [72]. In another retrospective study of 799 patients admitted with CoViD19, data of 113 deceased and 161 survivors were analyzed. The incidence of thrombocytopenia was much higher in the deceased 156.0 (111.8–219.3) as compared to the survivors 198.0 (160.0–256.0) (Median (IQR) platelet count, ×109/L (125–350)) [62]. Positive relation of thrombocytopenia with mortality was also shown in a retrospective cohort study of 449 patients with severe CoViD19 investigating sepsis-induced coagulopathy [73]. According to a meta-analysis, thrombocytopenia may increase the risk of severe CoViD19 about 5 times [74, 75].

The platelets have a multifunctional role in hemostasis, inflammation, and immune defense mechanisms. The immune defense role in pathogen clearance involves neutrophil migration, pathogens sequestration/clearance, via the release of microbicide proteins and chemokines, or direct or indirect binding with a pathogen. Platelets facilitate interaction between endothelial cells and leukocytes and may contribute to pulmonary vascular repair with thrombocytopenia possibly leading to leakiness of the vessels [76]. Association of thrombocytopenia with complications of CoVID19 is a marker of poor outcome.

Several mechanisms in CoViD19 result in platelet reactivity leading to inflammation and thrombosis. These include dysregulated RAAS, endothelial cell dysfunction, or direct interaction with the virus via “Toll-like receptors” (TLR 7), FcγRIIa, and CXC/CCL receptors. The TLRs are involved in platelet degranulation, formation of leukocyte aggregates, and release of platelet C3 that stimulates NETosis [77–79], and play an important role in inflammation and prothrombotic activities. Furthermore, platelets may contribute to the increased cytokine load in CoViD19 patients [80], reaffirming the pro-inflammatory role of these cells in the severe disease.

9.2.6 D Dimers in CoViD19

The biochemical and hematological profile of patients with CoViD19 reveals markers of active coagulation and several inflammatory markers that are elevated and may be interconnected. The D Dimer, a fibrin degradation product, is an important marker of activation of coagulation, result of the cleavage of cross-linked fibrin by plasmin. The role of D dimers as a prognostic maker in CoViD19 has been advocated in several studies. In a retrospective cohort of 449 patients with severe CoViD19, significantly raised D Dimers and prothrombin time were associated with higher 28 day mortality [73]. Another retrospective cohort of 138 patients admitted with CoViD19 had higher D dimer levels reported in the non-survivors and much higher in those who received ICU care 414 mg/L (191–1324) verses overall cohort 203 mg/L (121–403) or non ICU patients 166 mg/L (101–285) (Ref range 0–500 mg/L) [81]. Similarly, another multi-center retrospective cohort of 191 patients admitted with CoViD19 showed an association of elevated serum levels of D dimers with poor prognosis with D Dimer levels of 0·8 μg/mL (0.4–3.2) in the overall cohort, 5·2 μg/mL (1.5–21.1) in non-survivors and 0·6 μg/mL (0.3–1.0) in the survivors ($P < 0{\cdot}0001$) [82].

Furthermore, high D dimer levels are also found in association with markers of cardiac injury in complicated CoViD19 suggesting a correlation of coagulopathy and cardiac injury CoViD19 with a high thrombo-inflammatory burden. Analysis of a retrospective case series in a cohort of 187 patients admitted with CoViD19 revealed that D dimer levels were high in patients with elevated troponin and BNP levels. In the overall cohort D-dimer levels were 0.43 μg/mL (0.19–2.66), in the normal troponin group were 0.29 μg/mL (0.17–0.60) and in elevated troponin group were recorded at 3.85 μg/mL (0.51–25.58) $P < 0.001$. In this cohort, overall mortality was 23% (43/187). A high incidence of ARDS was recorded in this study, 24.6% (46) in the overall cohort, especially in patients with elevated troponin 57.7% (30) compared to 11.9% (16) with normal troponin values $p < 0.001$. Therefore, implicating an important pathogenetic role of inflammation in these complications [83].

9.2.7 Hypoxia and Thrombosis

Hypoxia is a recognized cause of inflammation and is commonly associated with obesity especially when complicated with conditions like obstructive sleep apnoea [84–86]. Several mechanisms are involved in hypoxia-induced thrombotic complications. Severe hypoxia in pulmonary microvasculature causes vasoconstriction results in vascular occlusion [87]. Hypoxia-inducible factor (HIF)-1 is regarded as the master regulator of O2 homeostasis. Target genes of hypoxia-inducible transcription factors (HIFs) regulated mechanisms may control thrombus formation. Hypoxia-induced factors upregulate endothelial expression of tissue factor linked with thrombin formation., and are negatively correlated with anticoagulants such as Protein S and Tissue Factor Plasmin Inhibitor (TFPI) this creating a procoagulant endothelial phenotype [88]. Hypoxia found in severe CoViD19 may stimulate thrombosis through not only increasing blood viscosity but also a hypoxia-inducible transcription factor-dependent signaling pathway [88]. A role of the nucleotide-binding domain, leucine-rich-containing family, pyrin domain containing 3 (NLRP3) inflammasome and IL-1β during hypoxia-induced venous thrombosis has been implicated in this process [89]. Obesity in CoViD19 is associated with poor outcomes. Pathogenetic mechanisms and signaling pathways involving HIF in obesity and metabolic diseases have been explored [90]. These mechanisms may suggest a possible high incidence of thrombotic complications in obese patients with CoViD19, warranting further exploration.

9.2.8 Ethnic Disparities, High-Risk Subgroups and Coagulation

Ethnic disparities have been observed in CoViD19 [91]. An increases mortality has been observed in the ethnic groups affected by CoViD19 [92], especially in the black population [12]. Data further demonstrate a higher incidence of venous thromboembolism (VTE) in the black population as compared to whites or Asians [93–95]. Polymorphisms in the PAR (protease-activated receptor)-4, resulting in increased platelet aggregation response to thrombin in the black population may account for the difference [96]. The risk of thrombotic complications in CoViD19 has been investigated concerning racial and ethnic differences [97], however, no biological differences have been observed. According to a study, a greater burden of mortality and morbidity was observed in black and Hispanic patients. However, this was attributed to the disproportionate representation among CoViD19 hospitalizations. No difference in in-hospital mortality was found among 7,868 patients admitted with CoViD19 in the retrospective observation registry [98]. In this study, the higher burden of morbidity and mortality in CoViD19 patients was mainly due to the disproportionate representation of the ethnic groups.

Patients with demographics including advanced age, male gender, increased body mass index (BMI), and cardiovascular, and metabolic risk factors exhibit a higher risk of vascular and coagulation complications and appear to have a poor outcome and more often require critical care in CoViD19. The interplay and dynamics of several mechanisms related to endothelial dysfunction, increased inflammatory activity, immune-thrombotic and thrombo-inflammation in relation to these factors may play an important role in the development of vascular and thrombotic complications in CoViD19. Furthermore, an interlink between plasmin (ogen) activity (a marker of cardiovascular risk) and CoViD19 susceptibility may exist. Plasmin is an enzyme responsible for fibrinolysis [112]. Patients with cardiovascular and metabolic diseases have elevated plasmin levels that may increase virulence and infectivity of the SARS-CoV-2 virus by cleaving its spike proteins. Increased plasmin levels have been regarded as a risk factor for CoViD19 susceptibility [99]. A higher immune-inflammatory burden among high risk individuals may precipitate increased thrombotic acitvity.

Data show that macrophage release of proinflammatory cytokines such as tumor necrosis factor-α (TNF-α) and interleukin-1β (IL-1β) results in the conversion of the endothelium over the plaque from an anticoagulant to a prothrombotic state [100–102]. Subjects with cardiovascular risk factors and obesity have altered levels of transcripts for some NF-κB pathway members and TLR2 in platelets [103]. Increased incidence of coagulation abnormalities is seen in patient subgroups with poor disease outcomes who frequently have a high burden of background risk factors [62, 82, 83]. For further reading about high risk subgroups and CoViD19 please refer to Chaps. 16, 17, 18, and 19 in this book.

9.3 Summary

Evidence confirms that thrombotic complications are commonly associated with severe CoViD19 and significantly increase the risk of mortality, especially among critically ill patients. Venous thromboembolism appears to be the most common form of thrombotic complication that often involves the lungs. Lungs are central to the CoViD19 pathology and pulmonary vasculature appears to be significantly affected. Pulmonary microangiopathy and micro thrombosis are important features of CoViD19 related pulmonary disease that may be associated with hemorrhagic complications. The incidence of venous thromboembolism varies in different populations and may be related to a variety of factors related to the burden of risk factors such as diabetes, obesity, or other cardiovascular conditions, or maybe determined by the differences in genetic, lifestyle, demographics, socio-economic or the healthcare systems. Further exploration is needed to determine these associations and unique thrombotic risk profiles of CoViD19 patients in different populations. Variations in biological risk factors such as coagulation proteins are well recognized, as observed in the African Americans, reported to have higher circulating levels of VWF, Factor VIII, and fibrinogen [104] or other differences such as in BMI, hypertension, kidney disease or socio-economic factors [105–107] that may be responsible for the differences in such complications associated with severe CoViD19.

Several research studies reveal the laboratory characteristics of various severities of CoViD19. The autopsy series and pathology reports of patients with severe CoViD19 further confirm the presence of clots in a variety of vascular territories involving different organs and tissues. Studies also demonstrate the nature and behavior of several important biomarkers of the prothrombotic and inflammatory activities observed in the complicated CoViD19 patients. These biomarkers may reflect the risk or severity of the disease and may help guide early therapeutic interventions. Attempts have been made to better characterize these biomarkers, however, important details are still lacking. The threshold values of the specific biomarkers and strategies for judicious use of the appropriate diagnostic methods, in conjunction with these markers in patients with CoViD19, yet remain to be clearly defined.

Several factors may facilitate the higher incidence and mortality related to thrombosis in CoViD19. These include important regulatory mechanisms that appear to be affected in CoViD19 patients and may promote thrombosis and vascular injury. Hyper inflammation, excessive cytokine release, dysregulated renin-angiotensin system that contribute to hypercoagulation, are notable (Table 9.1). These mechanisms may intersect each other, and exert a synergistic impact. For insatance, the excessive Ang II due to SARS CoV2 induced RAS dysregulation, may lead to endothelial dysfunction, inducing platelet activation, release of superoxide radicals, expression of tissue factor, and several proinflammatory and prothrombotic mechanisms related to the coagulation cascade. Persistent and exaggerated cytokine release in CoViD19 and inflammation augment damage to the vascular cells and coagulation pathways. The proinflammatory cytokines such as IL-6 may also induce hematopoiesis and generation of acute-phase proteins in the complicated CoViD19 involving ARDS.

Among other mechanisms, NETosis and features of microangiopathy appear to have gained particular attention in CoViD19 research and are currently under exploration (55). The formation of NETs induced by the virus is associated with the severity of CoViD19 facilitates a hyperthrombotic state. Several biochemical and hematological features in CoViD19 overlap with features of TMA. The endothelial

Table 9.1 Key features of thrombosis in CoViD19

Hypercoagulation
Impaired fibrinolytic function
Profound hypoxemia
Raised proinflammatory cytokines
Endothelial injury
Platelet activation
Other factors. Immobilization, mechanical ventilation and the use of central venous catheters and other invasive procedures

and platelet dysfunction and complement activation lead to microthrombi formation and organ dysfunction. The development of the hypercoagulatory form of DIC known to be associated with sepsis and infections is observed in CoViD19. The DIC appears to be an intermediary process indicating the course of the severity of the disease. The thrombocytopenia in CoViD19 is closely related to inflammation, immune mechanisms, and endothelial dysfunction, and marks the severity of CoViD19. The rise in D Dimers in CoViD19 marks inflammatory and thrombotic association of the disease, and together with prothrombin time and partial prothrombin time, may be used as a guide for anticoagulation. The elevation of D Dimers and thrombocytopenia indicate the severity of the disease in CoViD19 patients.

Elevated prothrombotic activity is associated with cardiovascular diseases in CoViD19 patients. Patients with cardiovascular and metabolic diseases have high plasmin levels and this may increase virulence and infectivity of the SARS-CoV-2 virus by cleaving its spike proteins. The widespread dysfunction of the vascular endothelial bed along with the increased cellular stress, elevated ROS and reduced NO, platelet dysfunction, and several other mechanisms including the complement activation, and others involving coagulation factors in conjunction with inflammatory immune-mediated prothrombotic processes, may lead to increased prothrombotic micro and macrovascular cardiac complications and stroke. The activated complement system may induce cytokine production via endothelial cells and upregulation of endothelial adhesion molecules (P Selectin and VWF) [108, 109], may represent an important prothrombotic mechanism in CoViD19 patients. An increased incidence of CoViD19 complications in the black population and ethnic groups, such as Hispanics, Asians, has been observed in the literature. Although a higher incidence of prothrombotic complications is a feature of complicated CoViD19 across ethnicities and demographic characteristics, no significant prothrombotic biological traits appear to be related to the increased susceptibility of CoViD19 complications observed in the black population groups.

Multiple dysregulated mechanisms appear to intersect in the development of thrombotic complications in CoViD19. The close association and interplay of prothrombotic and inflammatory mechanisms, lead to hypercoagulability in CoViD19. (Table 9.2). The anticoagulation treatment especially in prophylactic form has gained significant value in the prevention of prothrombotic CoViD19 complications. However, the specific utility of these drugs according to the stage of CoViD19 disease remains uncertain. Furthermore, the exact nature of the viral and

Table 9.2 Key markers reflecting pathogenesis of hyper-thromboses in CoViD19. (This is not a comprehensive list of markers of thrombosis in CoViD19. For details please refer to analyses reflecting on pathogenesis of thrombotic complications in CoViD19)

Increased pro-inflammatory interleukins (IL)-1β and IL-6
Increased TF expression
Increased Von Willebrand factor (VWF)
Increased D dimer

related immune mechanisms, the signaling transduction and cellular activation mechanisms that are involved in inducing abnormalities in the complement pathways, and the imbalance between pro and anticoagulation proteins, need to be further investigated. A better understanding of the mechanisms leading to endothelial dysfunction may help develop interventions that might prevent series of destructive mechanisms impacting platelets, vascular leak, the release of prothrombotic proteins, and an intense proinflammatory tune observed in CoViD19.

Summary Box

- Thrombotic complications are frequent and potentially fatal in CoVi19.
- Critical CoViD19 patients have a significantly elevated burden of thrombotic complications and higher mortality.
- The incidence of thrombotic complications varies in different populations and ethnic groups.
- Both venous and arterial territories may be affected in CoViD19.
- Microvascular injury and microthrombotic reactions are associated with CoViD19 related multi-organ failure.
- Prothrombotic processes in micro and macrovasculature are the main pathogenetic feature of complicated CoViD19.
- Endotheliopathy is a crucial pathogenetic mechanism induced directly by the virus or immune mechanisms in CoViD19 that leads to prothrombotic complications.
- Immuno-inflammation and thrombosis interlink lead the pathogenetic drive in CoViD19 associated with the thrombogenic impact of hypercytokinesis.
- A bidirectional interlink can be found between endothelial dysfunction and inflammation in CoViD19 patients.
- Complement activation may lead to disturbance of pro and antithrombotic mechanisms.
- Thrombocytopenia is associated with poor prognosis in CoViD19.
- An increase in D dimers marks the severity of the disease, is an important hematological marker in CoViD19.
- NETosis is an important marker of inflammation and thrombosis in CoViD19.
- Further research is needed to establish the interplay of multiple prothrombotic mechanisms and best strategies to counter the immune, inflammatory stress to reduce the thrombotic impact of the disease.

References

1. Bilaloglu S, Aphinyanaphongs Y, Jones S, Iturrate E, Hochman J, Berger JS. Thrombosis in hospitalized patients with COVID-19 in a New York City health system. JAMA. 2020;324 (8):799–801.
2. Elbadawi A, Elgendy IY, Sahai A, Bhandari R, McCarthy M, Gomes M, Bishop GJ, Bartholomew JR, Kapadia S, Cameron SJ. Incidence and outcomes of thrombotic events in symptomatic patients with COVID-19. Arterioscler Thromb Vasc Biol. 2021;41(1):545–7.
3. Klok FA, Kruip MJHA, Van der Meer NJM, Arbous MS, Gommers DAMPJ, Kant KM, Kaptein FHJ, van Paassen J, Stals MAM, Huisman MV, Endeman H. Incidence of thrombotic complications in critically ill ICU patients with COVID-19. Thromb Res. 2020;191:145–7.
4. Cui S, Chen S, Li X, Liu S, Wang F. Prevalence of venous thromboembolism in patients with severe novel coronavirus pneumonia. J Thromb Haemost. 2020;18(6):1421–4.
5. Helms J. High risk of thrombosis in patients in severe SARS-CoV-2 infection: a multicenter propspective cohort study. J Intensive Care Med. 2020. https://doi.org/10.1007/s0013-4-020-06062.
6. Li Y, Wang M, Zhou Y, et al. Acute cerebrovascular disease following COVID-19: a single center, retrospective, observational study. 2020. https://papers.ssrn.com/sol3/papers.cfm?abstract_id=3550025.
7. Oxley TJ, Mocco J, Majidi S, Kellner CP, Shoirah H, Singh IP, De Leacy RA, Shigematsu T, Ladner TR, Yaeger KA, Skliut M, Weinberger J, Dangayach NS, Bederson JB, Tuhrim S, Fifi JT. Large-vessel stroke as a presenting feature of Covid-19 in the young. New Engl J Med. 2020. https://doi.org/10.1056/NEJMc-20097-87.
8. Fogarty H, Townsend L, Ni Cheallaigh C, Bergin C, Martin-Loeches I, Browne P, Bacon CL, Gaule R, Gillett A, Byrne M, Ryan K. COVID19 coagulopathy in Caucasian patients. Br J Haematol. 2020;189(6):1044–9.
9. Iba T, Connors JM, Spyropoulos AC, Wada H, Levy JH. Ethnic differences in thromboprophylaxis for COVID-19 patients: should they be considered? Int J Hematol. 2021:1–7.
10. Rentsch CT, Kidwai-Khan F, Tate JP, Park LS, King Jr JT, Skanderson M, Hauser RG, Schultze A, Jarvis CI, Holodniy M, Re III VL. Covid-19 by race and ethnicity: a national cohort study of 6 million United States veterans. MedRxiv. 2020.
11. Holtgrave DR, Barranco MA, Tesoriero JM, Blog DS, Rosenberg ES. Assessing racial and ethnic disparities using a COVID-19 outcomes continuum for New York State. Ann Epidemiol. 2020;48:9–14.
12. Williamson E, Walker AJ, Bhaskaran K, Bacon S, Bates C, Morton CE, Curtis HJ, Mehrkar A, Evans D, Inglesby P, Cockburn J. OpenSAFELY: factors associated with COVID-19-related hospital death in the linked electronic health records of 17 million adult NHS patients. MedRxiv. 2020.
13. Marchandot B, Trimaille A, Curtiaud A, Matsushita K, Jesel L, Morel O. Thromboprophylaxis: balancing evidence and experience during the COVID-19 pandemic. J Thromb Thrombolysis. 2020;50(4):799–808.
14. Llitjos JF, Leclerc M, Chochois C, Monsallier JM, Ramakers M, Auvray M, Merouani K. High incidence of venous thromboembolic events in anticoagulated severe COVID-19 patients. J Thromb Haemost. 2020;18(7):1743–6.
15. Lodigiani C, Iapichino G, Carenzo L, Cecconi M, Ferrazzi P, Sebastian T, Kucher N, Studt JD, Sacco C, Alexia B, Sandri MT. Venous and arterial thromboembolic complications in COVID-19 patients admitted to an academic hospital in Milan, Italy. Thromb Res. 2020; 191:9–14.
16. Ren B, Yan F, Deng Z, Zhang S, Xiao L, Wu M, Cai L. Extremely high incidence of lower extremity deep venous thrombosis in 48 patients with severe COVID-19 in Wuhan. Circulation. 2020;142(2):181–3.

17. Zhang et al. Coagulopathy and antiphospholipid antibodies in patients with Covid-19. N Engl J Med. 2020; 382:e38. https://doi.org/10.1056/NEJMc2007575.
18. Chen N, Zhou M, Dong X, Qu J, Gong F, Han Y, Qiu Y, Wang J, Liu Y, Wei Y, Yu T. Epidemiological and clinical characteristics of 99 cases of 2019 novel coronavirus pneumonia in Wuhan, China: a descriptive study. Lancet. 2020;395(10223):507–13.
19. Giannis D, Ziogas IA, Gianni P. Coagulation disorders in coronavirus infected patients: COVID-19, SARS-CoV-1, MERS-CoV and lessons from the past. J Clin Virol. 2020; 127:104362.
20. Rovas A, Osiaevi I, Buscher K, Sackarnd J, Tepasse PR, Fobker M, Kühn J, Braune S, Göbel U, Thölking G, Gröschel A. Microvascular dysfunction in COVID-19: the MYSTIC study. Angiogenesis. 2021;24(1):145–57.
21. Ehrenfeld M, Tincani A, Andreoli L, Cattalini M, Greenbaum A, Kanduc D, Alijotas-Reig J, Zinserling V, Semenova N, Amital H, Shoenfeld Y. Covid-19 and autoimmunity. Autoimmun Rev. 2020.
22. Verdecchia P, Cavallini C, Spanevello A, Angeli F. The pivotal link between ACE2 deficiency and SARS-CoV-2 infection. Eur J Intern Med. 2020.
23. Fraga-Silva RA, Sorg BS, Wankhede M. ACE2 activation promotes antithrombotic activity. Mol Med. 2010;16:210–5. https://doi.org/10.2119/molmed.2009.00160.
24. Wright JW, Harding JW. The brain renin-angiotensin system: a diversity of functions and implications for CNS diseases. Pflugers Arch. 2013;465:133–51. https://doi.org/10.1007/s00424-012-1102-2.
25. Li P, Fukuhara M, Diz DI, Ferrario CM, Brosnihan KB. Novel angiotensin IIXE "Angiotensin II" AT1 receptor antagonist irbesartan prevents thromboxane A2-induced vasoconstriction in canine coronary arteries and human platelet aggregation. J Pharmacol Exp Ther. 2000;292(1):238–46.
26. Kalinowski L, Matys T, Chabielska E, Buczko W, Malinski T. Angiotensin IIXE "Angiotensin II" AT1 receptor antagonists inhibit platelet adhesion and aggregation by nitric oxide release. Hypertension. 2002;40(4):521–7.
27. Schmaier AH. The kallikrein-kinin and the renin-angiotensin systems have a multilayered interaction. Am J Physiol Regul Integr Comp Physiol. 2003;285(1):R1-13.
28. Stoka V, Turk V. A structural network associated with the kallikrein-kinin and renin-angiotensin systems. Biol Chem. 2010;391(4):443–54. https://doi.org/10.1515/BC.2010.046.
29. Gouda AS, Mégarbane B. Snake venom-derived bradykinin-potentiating peptides: A promising therapy for COVID-19?. Drug Development Research. 2021;82(1):38–48.
30. Cooper SL, Boyle E, Jefferson SR, Heslop CR, Mohan P, Mohanraj GG, Sidow HA, Tan RC, Hill SJ, Woolard J. Role of the renin–angiotensin–aldosterone and kinin kallikrein systems in the cardiovascular complications of COVID-19 and long COVID. International Journal of Molecular Sciences. 2021;22(15):8255.
31. Tolouian R, Vahed SZ, Ghiyasvand S, Tolouian A, Ardalan M. COVID-19 interactions with angiotensin-converting enzyme 2 (ACE2) and the kinin system; looking at a potential treatment. J Renal Inj Prev. 2020; 9(2):e19.
32. Fang C, Stavrou E, Schmaier AA, Grobe N, Morris M, Chen A, Nieman MT, Adams GN, LaRusch G, Zhou Y, Bilodeau ML. Angiotensin 1–7 and Mas decrease thrombosis in Bdkrb2−/− mice by increasing NO and prostacyclin to reduce platelet spreading and glycoprotein VI activation. Blood J Am Soc Hematol. 2013;121(15):3023–32.
33. Stavrou EX, Fang C, Merkulova A, Alhalabi O, Grobe N, Antoniak S, Mackman N, Schmaier AH. Reduced thrombosis in Klkb1−/− mice is mediated by increased Mas receptor, prostacyclin, Sirt1, and KLF4 and decreased tissue factor. Blood J Am Soc Hematol. 2015;125(4):710–9.
34. Irmscher S, Döring N, Halder LD, Jo EA, Kopka I, Dunker C, Jacobsen ID, Luo S, Slevogt H, Lorkowski S, Beyersdorf N. Kallikrein cleaves C3 and activates complement. J Innate Immun. 2018;10(2):94–105.

35. Varga Z, Flammer AJ, Steiger P, Haberecker M, Andermatt R, Zinkernagel AS, Mehra MR, Schuepbach RA, Ruschitzka F, Moch H. Endothelial cell infection and endotheliitis in COVID-19. Lancet. 2020. https://doi.org/10.1016/S0140-6736(20)30937-5.
36. Bradley BT, Maioli H, Johnson R, Chaudhry I, Fink SL, Xu H, Najafian B, Marshall D, Lacy JM, Williams T, Yarid N. Histopathology and ultrastructural findings of fatal COVID-19 infections. MedRxiv. https://doi.org/10.1101/2020.04.17.20058545v1.
37. Varga Z, Flammer AJ, Steiger P, et al. Endothelial cell infection and endotheliitis in COVID-19. Lancet. https://doi.org/10.1016/S0140-6736(20)30937-5.
38. Helms J. High risk of thrombosis in patients in severe SARS-CoV-2 infection: a multicenter prospective cohort study. J Intensiv Care Med. 2020. https://doi.org/10.1007/s00134-020-06062.
39. Escher R, Breakey N, Lammle B. Severe COVID-19 infection associated with endothelial activation. Thromb Res. 2020;190:62.
40. Kayal S, Jaïs JP, Aguini N, Chaudiere J, Labrousse J. Elevated circulating E-selectin, intercellular adhesion molecule 1, and von Willebrand factor in patients with severe infection. Am J Respir Crit Care Med. 1998;157(3):776–8.
41. Aird WC. The role of the endothelium in severe sepsis and multiple organ dysfunction syndrome. Blood J Am Soc Hematol. 2003;101(10):3765–77.
42. Lowenstein CJ, Solomon SD. Severe COVID-19 is a microvascular disease. Circulation. 2020;142(17):1609–11.
43. Kranzhöfer R, Clinton SK, Ishii K, Coughlin SR, Fenton JW, Libby P. Thrombin potently stimulates cytokine production in human vascular smooth muscle cells but not in mononuclear phagocytes. Circ Res. 1996;79(2):286–94.
44. Loppnow H, Libby P. Proliferating or interleukin 1-activated human vascular smooth muscle cells secrete copious interleukin 6. J Clin Investig. 1990;85(3):731–8.
45. Chen D, Carpenter A, Abrahams J, Chambers RC, Lechler RI, McVey JH, Dorling A. Protease-activated receptor 1 activation is necessary for monocyte chemoattractant protein 1–dependent leukocyte recruitment in vivo. J Exp Med. 2008;205(8):1739–46.
46. Sugama Y, Tiruppathi C, Andersen TT, Fenton JW, Malik AB. Thrombin-induced expression of endothelial P-selectin and intercellular adhesion molecule-1: a mechanism for stabilizing neutrophil adhesion. J Cell Biol. 1992;119(4):935–44.
47. Kaplanski G, Marin V, Fabrigoule M, Boulay V, Benoliel AM, Bongrand P, Kaplanski S, Farnarier C. Thrombin-activated human endothelial cells support monocyte adhesion in vitro following expression of intercellular adhesion molecule-1 (ICAM-1; CD54) and vascular cell adhesion molecule-1 (VCAM-1; CD106). Blood J Am Soc Hematol. 1998;92(4): 1259–67.
48. Hiraiwa K, van Eeden SF. Nature and consequences of the systemic inflammatory response induced by lung inflammation. Lung Inflamm. 2014; 79.
49. Corrales-Medina VF, Musher DM, Shachkina S, Chirinos JA. Acute pneumonia and the cardiovascular system. Lancet. 2013;381(9865):496–505. https://doi.org/10.1016/S0140-6736(12)61266-5.
50. Shi S, Qin M, Shen B, et al. Association of cardiac injury with mortality in hospitalized patients with COVID-19 in Wuhan, China. JAMA Cardiol. 2020. https://doi.org/10.1001/jamacardio.2020.0950.11.
51. Li B, Liu Y, Hu T, Zhang Y, Zhang C, Li T, Wang C, Dong Z, Novakovic VA, Hu T, Shi J. Neutrophil extracellular traps enhance procoagulant activity in patients with oral squamous cell carcinoma. J Cancer Res Clin Oncol. 2019;145:1695–707.
52. Zuo Y, Yalavarthi S, Shi H, Gockman K, Zuo M, Madison JA, Blair CN, Weber A, Barnes BJ, Egeblad M, Woods RJ, Kanthi Y, Knight JS. Neutrophil extracellular traps in COVID-19. JCI Insight. 2020. https://doi.org/10.1172/jci.insight.13899.9.
53. Zuo Y, Yalavarthi S, Shi H, Gockman K, Zuo M, Madison JA, Blair CN, Weber A, Barnes BJ, Egeblad M, Woods RJ. Neutrophil extracellular traps in COVID-19. JCI Insight. 2020.

54. Nakazawa F, Kannemeier C, Shibamiya A, Song Y, Tzima E, Schubert U, Koyama T, Niepmann M, Trusheim H, Engelmann B, Preissner KT. Extracellular RNA is a natural cofactor for the (auto-)activation of factor VII-activating protease (FSAP). Biochem J. 2005;385:831–8.
55. Massberg S, Grahl L, von Bruehl ML, Manukyan D, Pfeiler S, Goosmann C, Brinkmann V, Lorenz M, Bidzhekov K, Khandagale AB, Konrad I. Reciprocal coupling of coagulation and innate immunity via neutrophil serine proteases. Nat Med. 2010;16(8):887–96.
56. Semeraro F, Ammollo CT, Morrissey JH, Dale GL, Friese P, Esmon NL, Esmon CT. Extracellular histones promote thrombin generation through platelet-dependent mechanisms: involvement of platelet TLR2 and TLR4. Blood J Am Soc Hematol. 2011;118(7):1952–61.
57. ClinicalTrials.gov. Covid-19: possible role of neutrophil extracellular traps (NETSINCOVID) identifier: NCT04412382. 2020.
58. Dolhnikoff M, Duarte-Neto AN, de Almeida Monteiro RA, da Silva LFF, de Oliveira EP, Saldiva PHN, Mauad T, Negri EM. Pathological evidence of pulmonary thrombotic phenomena in severe COVID-19. J Thromb Haemost. 2020;18(6):1517–9.
59. Fox SE, Akmatbekov A, Harbert JL, Li G, Brown JQ, Vander Heide RS. Pulmonary and cardiac pathology in African American patients with COVID-19: an autopsy series from New Orleans. Lancet Respir Med. 2020;8(7):681–6.
60. Carsana L, Sonzogni A, Nasr A, Rossi R, Pellegrinelli A. Pulmonary post mortem findings in a large series of COVID-19 cases from Northern. medRxiv. 2020.
61. Ackermann M, Verleden SE, Kuehnel M, Haverich A, Welte T, Laenger F, Vanstapel A, Werlein C, Stark H, Tzankov A, Li WW. Pulmonary vascular endothelialitis, thrombosis, and angiogenesis in Covid-19. N Engl J Med. 2020;383(2):120–8.
62. Chen T, Wu D, Chen H, Yan W, Yang D, Chen G, Ma K, Xu D, Yu H, Wang H, Wang T, Guo W, Chen J, Ding C, Zhang X, Huang J, Han M, Li S, Luo X, Zhao J, Ning Q. Clinical characteristics of 113 deceased patients with coronavirus disease 2019: retrospective study. BMJ. 2020; 368:m1091. https://doi.org/10.1136/bmj.m1091. Erratum in: BMJ. 2020; 368: m1295.
63. Zhou X, Cheng Z, Luo L, Zhu Y, Lin W, Ming Z, Chen W, Hu Y. DIC in COVID-19. Thromb Res. 2021.
64. Wada H, Ohiwa M, Kaneko T, Tamaki S, Tanigawa M, Takagi M, Mori Y, Shirakawa S. Plasma level of tumor necrosis factor in disseminated intravascular coagulation. Am J Hematol. 1991;37(3):147–51.
65. Wada H, Tamaki S, Tanigawa M, Takagi M, Mori Y, Deguchi A, Katayama N, Yamamoto T, Deguchi K, Shirakawa S. Plasma Level of IL-1β in Disseminated Intravascular Goagulation. Thromb Haemost. 1991;65(04):364–8.
66. Gao T, Hu M, Zhang X, Li H, Zhu L, Liu H, Dong Q, Zhang Z, Wang Z, Hu Y, Fu Y. Highly pathogenic coronavirus N protein aggravates lung injury by MASP-2-mediated complement over-activation. MedRxiv. 2020.
67. Sinkovits G, Mező B, Réti M, Müller V, Iványi Z, Gál J, Gopcsa L, Reményi P, Szathmáry B, Lakatos B, Szlávik J. Complement overactivation and consumption predicts in-hospital mortality in SARS-CoV-2 infection. Front Immunol. 2021;12:866.
68. Magro C, Mulvey JJ, Berlin D, Nuovo G, Salvatore S, Harp J, Baxter-Stoltzfus A, Laurence J. Complement associated microvascular injury and thrombosis in the pathogenesis of severe COVID-19 infection: a report of five cases. Transl Res. 2020;220:1–13.
69. Bajzar L, Morser J, Nesheim M. TAFI, or plasma procarboxypeptidase B, couples the coagulation and fibrinolytic cascades through the thrombin-thrombomodulin complex. J Biol Chem. 1996;271(28):16603–8.
70. Van de Wouwer M, Plaisance S, De Vriese A, Waelkens E, Collen D, Persson J, Daha MR, Conway EM. The lectin-like domain of thrombomodulin interferes with complement activation and protects against arthritis. J Thromb Haemost. 2006;4(8):1813–24.
71. Mold C, Gewurz H, Du Clos TW. Regulation of complement activation by C-reactive protein. Immunopharmacology. 1999;42(1–3):23–30.

72. Guan W, Ni Z, Hu Y. Clinical characteristics of coronavirus disease 2019 in China. N Engl J Med. 2020. https://doi.org/10.1056/NEJMoa2002032.
73. Tang N, Bai H, Chen X, Gong J, Li D, Sun Z. Anticoagulant treatment is associated with decreased mortality in severe coronavirus disease 2019 patients with coagulopathy. J Thromb Haemost. 2020;18:1094–9. https://doi.org/10.1111/jth.14817.
74. Lippi G, Plebani M, Henry BM. Thrombocytopenia is associated with severe coronavirus disease 2019 (COVID-19) infections: a meta-analysis. Clin Chim Acta. 2020;506:145–8.
75. Yang X, Yang Q, Wang Y, Wu Y, Xu J, Yu Y, Shang Y. Thrombocytopenia and its association with mortality in patients with COVID-19. J Thromb Haemost. 2020;18 (6):1469–72.
76. Weyrich AS, Zimmerman GA. Platelets in lung biology. Annu Rev Physiol. 2013; 75: 569–591.
77. Koupenova M, Clancy L, Corkrey HA, Freedman JE. Circulating platelets as mediators of immunity, inflammation, and thrombosis. Circ Res. 2018;122(2):337–51.
78. Assinger A. Platelets and infection—an emerging role of platelets in viral infection. Front Immunol. 2014;5:649.
79. Koupenova M, Vitseva O, MacKay CR, Beaulieu LM, Benjamin EJ, Mick E, Kurt-Jones EA, Ravid K, Freedman JE. Platelet-TLR7 mediates host survival and platelet count during viral infection in the absence of platelet-dependent thrombosis. Blood J Am Soc Hematol. 2014;124(5):791–802.
80. Zaid Y, Puhm F, Allaeys I, Naya A, Oudghiri M, Khalki L, Limami Y, Zaid N, Sadki K, Ben El Haj R, Mahir W. Platelets can associate with SARS-Cov-2 RNA and are hyperactivated in COVID-19. Circ Res. 2020;127(11):1404–18.
81. Wang D, Hu B, Hu C, Zhu F, Liu X, Zhang J, Wang B, Xiang H, Cheng Z, Xiong Y, Zhao Y, Li Y, Wang X, Peng Z. Clinical characteristics of 138 hospitalized patients with 2019 novel coronavirus-infected pneumonia in Wuhan, China. JAMA. 2020. https://doi.org/10.1001/jama.2020.1585.
82. Zhou F, Yu T, Du R. Clinical course and risk factors for mortality of adult inpatients with COVID-19 in Wuhan, China: a retrospective cohort study. Lancet. 2020.
83. Guo T, Fan Y, Chen M, et al. Cardiovascular implications of fatal out comes of patients with coronavirus disease 2019 (COVID-19). JAMA Cardiol. 2020. https://doi.org/10.1001/jamacardio.2020.1017.
84. Eltzschig HK, Carmeliet P. Hypoxia and inflammation. N Engl J Med. 2011;364(7):656–65. https://doi.org/10.1056/NEJMra0910283.
85. Hosogai N, Fukuhara A, Oshima K, et al. Adipose tissue hypoxia in obesity and its impact on adipocytokine dysregulation. Diabetes. 2007;56(4):901–11.
86. Trayhurn P, Wood IS. Adipokines: inflammation and the pleiotropic role of white adipose tissue. Br J Nutr. 2004;92:347–55.
87. Grimmer B, Kuebler WM. The endothelium in hypoxic pulmonary vasoconstriction. J Appl Physiol. 2017;123:1635–46.
88. Gupta N, Zhao YY, Evans CE. The stimulation of thrombosis by hypoxia. Thromb Res. 2019;181:77–83.
89. Gupta N, Sahu A, Prabhakar A, Chatterjee T, Tyagi T, Kumari B, Khan N, Nair V, Bajaj N, Sharma M, Ashraf MZ. Activation of NLRP3 inflammasome complex potentiates venous thrombosis in response to hypoxia. Proc Natl Acad Sci. 2017;114(18):4763–8.
90. Gonzalez FJ, Xie C, Jiang C. The role of hypoxia-inducible factors in metabolic diseases. Nat Rev Endocrinol. 2019;15(1):21–32.
91. Yaya S, Yeboah H, Charles CH, Otu A, Labonte R. Ethnic and racial disparities in COVID-19-related deaths: counting the trees, hiding the forest. BMJ Glob Health. 2020; 5 (6):e002913.
92. Papageorgiou N, Providencia R, Saberwal B, Sohrabi C, Tyrlis A, Atieh AE, Lim WY, Creta A, Khanji M, Rusinova R, Chooneea B. Ethnicity and COVID-19 cardiovascular complications: a multi-center UK cohort. Am J Cardiovasc Dis. 2020;10(4):455.

93. Liao S, Woulfe T, Hyder S, Merriman E, Simpson D, Chunilal S. Incidence of venous thromboembolism in different ethnic groups: a regional direct comparison study. J Thromb Haemost. 2014;12(2):214–9.
94. White RH, Keenan CR. Effects of race and ethnicity on the incidence of venous thromboembolism. Thromb Res. 2009;123:S11–7.
95. Zakai NA, McClure LA. Racial differences in venous thromboembolism. J Thromb Haemost. 2011;9(10):1877–82.
96. Edelstein LC, Simon LM, Montoya RT, Holinstat M, Chen ES, Bergeron A, Kong X, Nagalla S, Mohandas N, Cohen DE, Dong JF. Racial differences in human platelet PAR4 reactivity reflect expression of PCTP and miR-376c. Nat Med. 2013;19(12):1609–16.
97. Esenwa C, Unda SR, Altschul DJ, Patel NK, Malaviya A, Seiden J, Lendaris A, Moncrieffe K, Labovitz DL. The effect of race on composite thrombotic events in patients with COVID-19. Thromb Res. 2021;199:10–3.
98. Rodriguez F, Solomon N, de Lemos JA, Das SR, Morrow DA, Bradley SM, Elkind MS, Williams IV JH, Holmes D, Matsouaka RA, Gupta D. Racial and ethnic differences in presentation and outcomes for patients hospitalized with COVID-19: findings from the American heart association's COVID-19 cardiovascular disease registry. Circulation. 2020.
99. Ji HL, Zhao R, Matalon S, Matthay MA. Elevated plasmin (ogen) as a common risk factor for COVID-19 susceptibility. Physiol Rev. 2020.
100. Bevilacqua MP, Pober JS, Majeau GR, Cotran RS, Gimbrone RA Jr. Interleukin-1 (IL-1) induces biosynthesis and cell surface expression of pro-coagulant activity in human vascular endothelial cells. J Exp Med. 1984;160:618–23.
101. Nawroth PP, Handley DA, Esmon CT, Stern DM. Interleukin-1 induces endothelial cell procoagulant while suppressing cell-surface anticoagulant activity. Proc Natl Acad Sci U S A. 1986;83:3460–4.
102. Nawroth PP, Stern DM. Modulation of endothelial cell hemostatic properties by tumor necrosis factor. J Exp Med. 1986;163:740–5.
103. Freedman JE, Larson MG, Tanriverdi K, O'Donnell CJ, Morin K, Hakanson AS, Vasan RS, Johnson AD, Iafrati MD, Benjamin EJ. Relation of platelet and leukocyte inflammatory transcripts to body mass index in the Framingham heart study. Circulation. 2010; 122: 119–29.
104. Lutsey PL, Cushman M, Steffen LM, Green D, Barr RG, Herrington D, Ouyang P, Folsom AR. Plasma hemostatic factors and endothelial markers in four racial/ethnic groups: the MESA study. J Thromb Haemost. 2006;4(12):2629–35.
105. Folsom AR, Basu S, Hong CP, Heckbert SR, Lutsey PL, Rosamond WD, Cushman M. Reasons for differences in the incidence of venous thromboembolism in black versus white Americans. Am J Med. 2019;132(8):970–6.
106. Zakai NA, McClure LA, Judd SE, Safford MM, Folsom AR, Lutsey PL, Cushman M. Racial and regional differences in venous thromboembolism in the United States in 3 cohorts. Circulation. 2014;129(14):1502–9.
107. Zakai N, Lutsey P, Folsom A, Cushman M. Black-white differences in venous thrombosis risk: the longitudinal investigation of thromboembolism etiology (LITE). Blood. 2010;116 (21):478.
108. Foley JH, Conway EM. Cross talk pathways between coagulation and inflammation. Circ Res. 2016;118(9):1392–408.
109. Foreman KE, Vaporciyan AA, Bonish BK, Jones ML, Johnson KJ, Glovsky MM, Eddy SM, Ward PA. C5a-induced expression of P-selectin in endothelial cells. J Clin Investig. 1994;94 (3):1147–55.
110. A Phase 2 Clinical Trial to Assess the Safety and Efficacy of Complement 3 Inhibitor, AMY-101, in Patients With Acute Respiratory Distress Syndrome Due to COVID-19 (SAVE). Available on: ClinicalTrials.gov. https://clinicaltrials.gov/ct2/show/NCT04395456 ?term=complement+inhibitor&cond=Covid19&draw=2&rank=2. ClinicalTrials.gov Identifier: NCT04395456. Last updated on: February 21, 2021. Last accessed on: December 27, 2021.

111. Ravulizumab and COVID-19. Available on: ClinicalTrials.gov. Link: https://clinicaltrials.gov/ct2/show/NCT04570397?term=complement+inhibitor&cond=Covid19&draw=2&rank=7. ClinicalTrials.gov Identifier: NCT04570397. Last updated on: January 14, 2021. Last accessed on: December 27, 2021.
112. Colman RW. Hemostasis and thrombosis: basic principles and clinical practice. Lippincott Williams & Wilkins. 2006.

Chapter 10
Pathogenesis of CoViD19—Miscellaneous Mechanisms

Key Questions

- What major regulatory and cellular pathogenetic mechanisms are involved in the pathogenesis of complicated CoViD19?
- What are the links between homeostatic regulatory dysfunction and CoViD19 complications?
- What are the dynamics of the neuropeptide system in CoViD19?
- What is the role of viral injury and associated viral cellular interactions in CoViD19?
- What cellular stress mechanisms and cell death modalities may be involved in CoViD19?

10.1 Introduction

The complex pathogenetic background of CoViD19 has presented a challenge to clinicians and researchers worldwide. Several distinct pathogenetic mechanisms and systems that are activated, may be dysregulated and may act in synergism or intersect with each other. Respiratory and circulatory failure induced by the SARS CoV2 invasion and consequent dysregulations remain central to the pathology (Fig. 10.3). In addition to the renin-angiotensin system (RAS), the hyper-immune-inflammatory mechanisms and exaggerated cytokinetic activity, prothrombotic mechanisms, and a range of other cellular pathogenetic processes are linked with the development of CoViD19 complications.

Cardiovascular complications constitute a significant portion of the CoViD19 associated complications. Cardiovascular risk factors and pre-existing cardiovascular disease are linked with an increased risk of mortality in CoViD19. Advanced

U. Mallick, *Cardiovascular Complications of COVID-19*,
https://doi.org/10.1007/978-3-030-90065-6_10

CoViD19 accompanies unstable homeostasis and hemostasis that disturb coagulation balance, produce local and systemic micro and macrovascular events, tissue injury ultimately resulting in multi-organ dysfunction and failure, including cardiovascular injury. Dysregulation of RAS, immune-inflammatory reactions, and endothelial dysfunction play a crucial role in promoting thrombotic and proinflammatory pathways. Furthermore, the inter relationship between the innate immune mechanisms, such as the complement system, cytokines, and other inflammatory culprits NETs and inflammasomes, and pro coagulation, encompasses the vascular endothelial structures [1–5].

Several regulatory systems are implicated in CoViD19 complications. The proinflammatory effects of the kallikrein-kinin system (KKS) and release of acute-phase proteins in the acute phase of CoViD19 may be linked with symptoms of pain and fatigue [6–8]. The KKS is also implicated in prothrombotic activities and may cross-talk with other regulatory systems such as RAS [9]. The association of the KKS and CoViD19 complications, especially cardiovascular diseases, needs to be better understood. An association of raised BNP has been observed in CoViD19 patients especially in association with cardiovascular disease [10] and critically ill patients [11]. The natriuretic peptides are important markers of cardiovascular decompensation, however may also be raised in sepsis without evidence of cardiovascular involvement [12]. Proinflammatory cytokines such as IL-6 that play a central role in CoViD19 pathogenesis, influence the secretion of BNP (brain natriuretic peptide) and ANP (atrial natriuretic peptide) [13]. Another important hemodynamic regulator endothelin-1 (ET 1) appears to be associated with the severity of CoViD19 [14]. The endothelin 1 (ET 1) is a potent vasoconstrictor involved in the regulation of vascular hemodynamics, reflects the severity of cardiovascular diseases such as hypertension and heart failure [15]. The direct viral damage appears to contribute towards the organic pathogenesis including lungs and heart in severe CoViD19. Several reports and studies demonstrate the presence of SARS CoV2 viral particles in multiple organs and tissues in CoViD19 [16–19]. However, direct viral attacks by SARS CoV2 appear to be focal rather than broad dissemination. The direct viral injury has drawn a significant interest of researchers worldwide, however remains inconclusive and is subject to further exploration.

Although involvement or association of several important regulators and mechanisms is observed in CoViD19, exact mechanisms that lead to the development of complications in CoViD19 are not fully understood. It remains unclear how these mechanisms are regulated in CoViD19. Several intracellular processes mark the severity of CoViD19, such as mitochondrial dysfunction, ER stress (endoplasmic reticular stress), (Fig. 10.1) and various modalities of cell death that appear to be connected to the host and viral mechanisms. A multitude of mediators and signaling pathways play a vital role in these processes that lead to CoViD19 complications and may serve as a potential therapeutic target. Identification and mapping, of these pathogenetic mechanisms and their complex interactions, is strongly needed in association with the clinical, biochemical, and prognostic aspects of CoViD19. The cross-talk mechanisms between various homeostatic

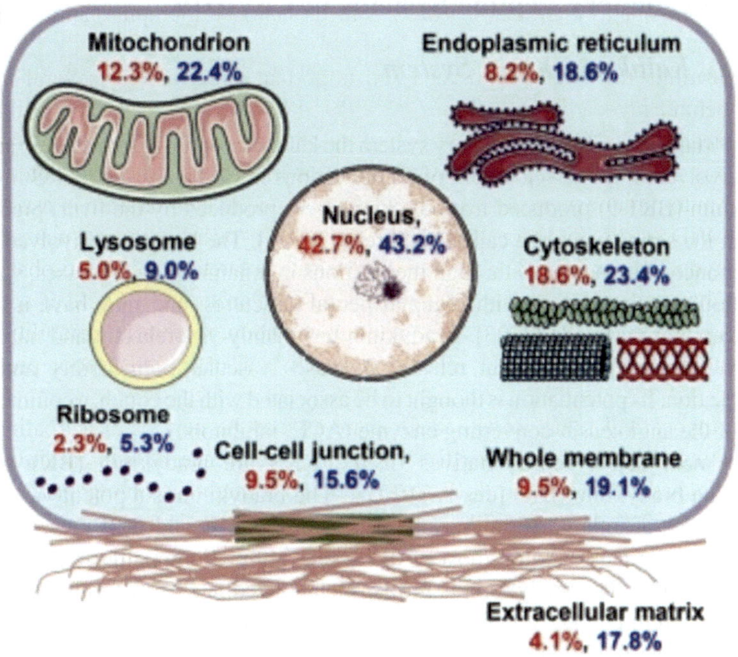

Fig. 10.1 Pulmonary cell structures and CoViD19. Schematic of changes in cell components within lung tissue from patients diagnosed with COVID-19. Red and blue fonts represent up- and downregulated proteins detected in lungs from patients diagnosed with COVID-19 compared to control lung tissue. *Source* Figure 1d. Leng, L., Cao, R., Ma, J., Mou, D., Zhu, Y., Li, W., Lv, L., Gao, D., Zhang, S., Gong, F. and Zhao, L., 2020. Pathological features of COVID-19-associated lung injury: a preliminary proteomics report based on clinical samples. Signal transduction and targeted therapy, 5(1), pp.1–9. https://www.nature.com/articles/s41392-020-00355-9

regulators must be further explored to differentiate between the beneficial and harmful effects in CoViD19 patients.

This chapter is aimed to enhance the understanding of the pathogenesis of CoViD19 complications. In this chapter, we identify and describe a variety of pathogenetic mechanisms and regulatory factors from the emerging literature that may be associated with CoViD19. We provide an introduction into the association of regulatory systems and associated mechanisms and their dynamics in relation to the cardiovascular and other complications observed in CoViD19. We also review the salient features of the SARS CoV2 related viral injury and several cellular mechanisms including intracellular stress and organellar dysfunction that ultimately lead to the tissue damage and dysfunction in CoViD19. We illustrate the pathogenetic structure of these mechanisms in association with the molecular processes and discuss their implications. Several mechanisms described here, may serve as potential therapeutic targets in CoViD19 and are currently being explored.

10.2 Regulatory Peptide Systems in CoViD19

10.2.1 Kallikrein-Kinin System

An important homeostasis regulatory system the kallikrein-kinin system (KKS) appears to be involved in the development of complications in CoViD19. The KKS involves bradykinin (BK1-9) produced from the kininogen (produced by the liver) precursors through the serine peptidase called kallikrein [20, 21]. The kinins are involved in the maintenance of homeostasis through their actions in inflammatory processes, vascular relaxation, and interaction with regional neural structures, and may have a role in cardiovascular diseases [22, 23]. Bradykinin has mainly vasorelaxant and natriuretic activity, induces prostaglandin release, increases vascular permeability and fluid extravasation. Its potentiation is thought to be associated with the cough, a common side effect of the angiotensin-converting enzyme (ACE) inhibitors.

The main active representatives of the KKS are bradykinin (BK) and its metabolite bradykinin (BK) [des-Arg9]-BK. The bradykinin is a potent vasodilator and mediator of inflammation that interacts with the B1R and B2R receptors [24]. These receptors are found on most of the tissues but predominantly in the vascular endothelial cells. The bradykinin is further metabolized into other forms such as BK 1-7 and 1-5 through ACE, which is most commonly known of the several peptides involved in the bradykinin-metabolizing mechanism [27]. Other peptides are also involved in this process, and include ACE 2, aminopeptidase P (APP), NEP, endothelin-converting enzyme (ECE)-1, carboxypeptidase N (CPN), and dipeptidylpeptidaseIV (DPPIV) [25–28].

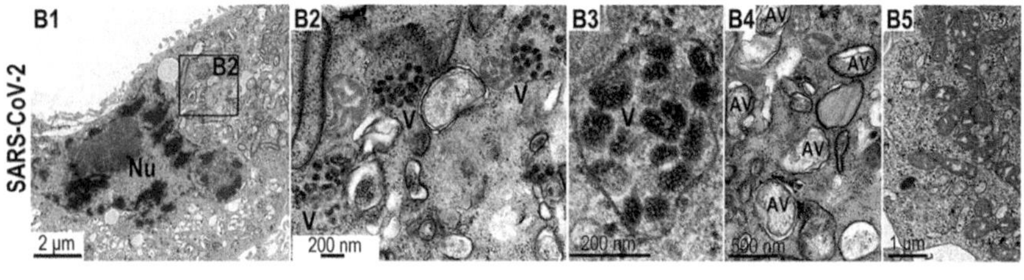

Fig. 10.2 TEM micrographs of HPAEpiC cells of SARS-CoV-2-infected group. TEM micrographs of HPAEpiC cells of SARS-CoV-2-infected group in a study conducting ultrastructural analysis of host cells i.e., alveolar epithelium (Human pulmonary alveolar epithelial cells-primary human alveolar type 2: HPAEpiC - human AT2 cell-derived cell line) and its adjacent microvascular endothelium and pulmonary microvascular endothelial cells (HULEC-5a - human pulmonary microvascular endothelial cell line), following SARS-CoV-2 infection. b1 The overall image of the infected cell. The area indicated by the black box is enlarged in. b2.The micrograph of clusters of virus particles (V) within cell body. b3 Enlarged image of virus indicated in b2. b4 A large amount of autophagic vacuoles (AV) in the infected HPAEpiC cells. b5 The micrograph of fragmented mitochondria (M) in the infected HPAEpiC cells. *Source* Figure 7c. Wang, P., Luo, R., Zhang, M., Wang, Y., Song, T., Tao, T., Li, Z., Jin, L., Zheng, H., Chen, W. and Zhao, M., 2020. A cross-talk between epithelium and endothelium mediates human alveolar–capillary injury during SARS-CoV-2 infection. Cell death & disease, 11(12), pp.1–17. https://www.nature.com/articles/s41419-020-03252-9. Published by Springer Nature Group

The RAS and KKS may cross-talk at several levels [29, 30]. The KKS and RAS may be upregulated or an increase in RAS may be associated with a decrease in KKS in a stimulus-dependent manner [31]. ACE2 downregulates Kallikrein Kinin System (KKS). The ACE2 hydrolyzes [des-Arg9]-BK into inactive breakdown products [32]. A decrease in the ACE2 in CoViD19 may be associated with hyperactivation of KKS and increase local and systemic clotting mechanisms [33]. Through regulation of the vessel wall tissue factor, the B2R, AT2R, and Mas work in concert to counterbalance the prothrombotic impact of the AT1R [34, 35].

An increase in the bradykinin is also associated with an increase in systemic inflammatory response [36] and may activate complement C3 system [37]. The ACE2 hydrolyzes bradykinin active metabolite DABK(desArg-9-bradykinin) [32]. Downregulation of the ACE2 increases DABK levels leading to increased signaling of the B1R, causing an increase in inflammation [38]. The activation of B2R induces the enhancement of the regional blood flow, may confer tissue protection and reflect the cardioprotective role [22]. The pro-inflammatory cytokines may induce the expression of B1R [23, 39], also found in the cardiac fibroblasts. The TLR4 that bind SARS CoV2, are also found on cardiac fibroblasts, once activated may increase the B1R mRNA and protein levels [39]. A loss of homeostatic balance associated with CoViD19 related to the ACE2 downregulation or via the pro-inflammatory cytokines may result in lung injury and cardiovascular damage in the complicated disease. Further investigations are required to evaluate the potential role of this kallikrein-kinin system in CoViD19 therapy.

10.2.2 Endothelin System

Endothelin-1, a potent vasoconstrictor, has been described as a marker of severity of CoViD19 [14]. The endothelin system is mainly composed of three endogenous 21 amino acid peptides ET 1, ET 2, and ET 3, known to interact with two types of receptors ET/A and ET/B, (that may antagonize each other), and possible other subtypes [40]. Various enzymes such as endothelin converting enzymes, metalloproteinases (MMPs), and mast cell enzymes (Chymase) are involved in the formation of ET 1, whereas enzymes such as carboxypeptidase cathepsin A are involved in the lysosomal degradation of ET1.

The endothelin receptors are found in a variety of vascular cells (endothelial cells, vascular smooth muscle cells), myocardium (endocardial endothelial cells, myocytes, fibroblasts). It plays a pro-inflammatory role through inducing pro-inflammatory mechanisms, secretion of cytokines such as Interleukin-6 (IL-6), monocyte chemoattractant protein-1 (MCP-1), tumor necrosis factor-α (TNF-α)], various enzymes, and production of cell adhesion molecules such as I-CAM 1 and endoplasmic reticulum stress [41] (Cytokine) [42–44].

The endothelin is a well-recognized marker of cardiovascular risk [45, 46]. The endothelin and RAS play an important role in the pathogenesis of cardiovascular diseases and may cross-talk at several levels [47]. The interaction between ET-1 and the RAS, an important pathogenetic mechanism in hypertension, and related cardiovascular damage may play a role in the development of cardiovascular complications in CoViD19.

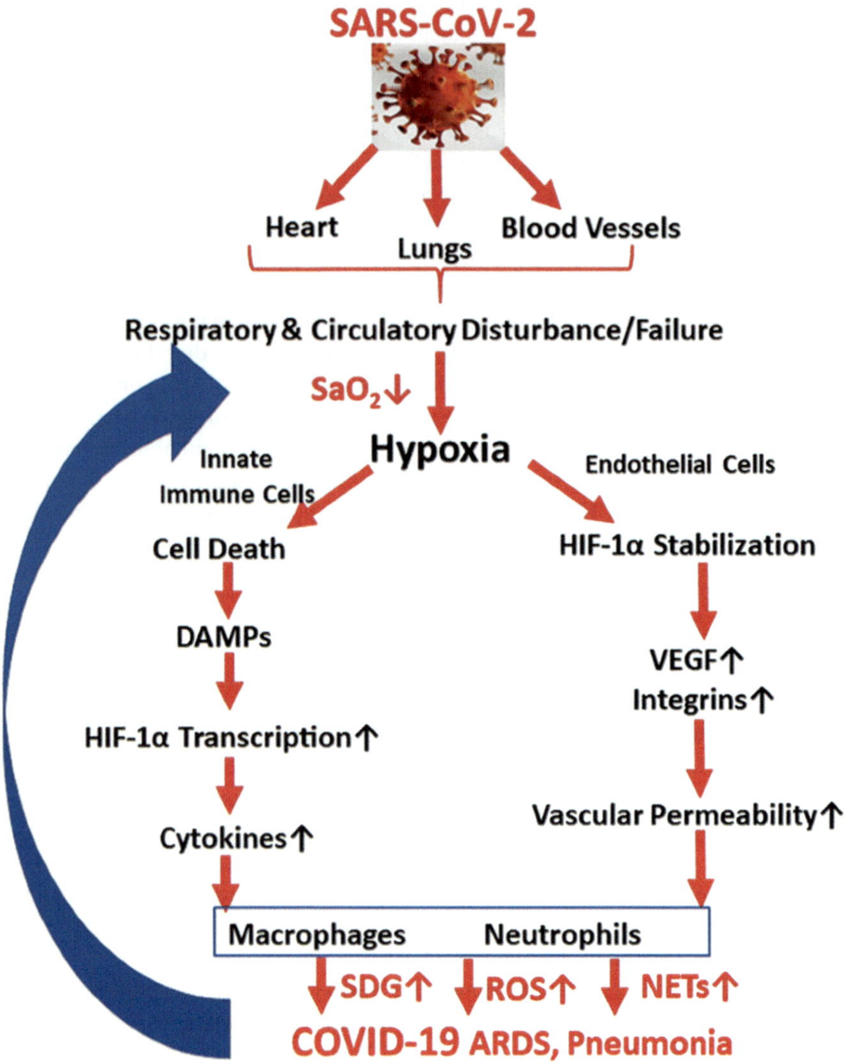

Fig. 10.3 Proposed pathological mechanisms and disease outcomes of COVID-19 involving hypoxia and HIF-1α-dependent detrimental cell signaling pathways. SARS-Cov-2—severe acute respiratory syndrome coronavirus 2, HIF-1α—hypoxia inducible factor 1α, ARDS—acute respiratory distress syndrome, DAMPs—damage associated molecular patterns, VEGF—vascular endothelial growth factor, NETs—neutrophil extracellular traps, ROS—reactive oxygen species, SDG—secretory degranulation. *Source* Figure 1. Serebrovska, Z.O., Chong, E.Y., Serebrovska, T. V., Tumanovska, L.V. and Xi, L., 2020. Hypoxia, HIF-1α, and COVID-19: from pathogenic factors to potential therapeutic targets. Acta Pharmacologica Sinica, 41(12), pp.1539–1546. https://www.nature.com/articles/s41401-020-00554-8. Published by Springer Nature Group

The CoViD19 is associated with a high immune-inflammatory burden. The inflammatory mediators including cytokines may play a part in the development of cardiovascular dysfunction through the interaction of neurohormones and the immune system [48]. Due to the possible role of NF-κB in the hyper-cytokinetic activity in CoViD19, pharmacological inactivation of the NF-κB signaling pathway may represent a potential therapeutic target [49]. The ET1 has been described as a biomarker of severity of risk associated with CoViD19, and NF-kB (nuclear factor-kappa B) mediation of endothelin expression may be an important mechanism [14, 50]. The NF-kB is a complex cellular protein system linked with the transcription of several genes involved in host immunity, inflammation, cellular proliferation, and apoptosis [51] and is associated with cytokine storm through various mechanisms.

Furthermore, racial and age-related differences in circulating ET-1 have been found, indicating an association between the high incidence of hypertension and heart failure in black individuals and older adults [15, 52, 53].

Further studies are required to establish the role of the endothelin, the genetic variations in ET-1 genes, NF-kB (nuclear factor-kappa B) mediation of endothelin expression, and the interaction of endothelin with other pathogenetic mechanisms involved in the development of CoViD19 complications.

10.2.3 Natriuretic Peptide System

Neurophysiological pathways are extremely important pathophysiological mechanisms in heart failure known for decades [54, 55]. Natriuretic Peptides (NPs) are cardiovascular protective and lower blood pressure, maintain fluid volume homeostasis and reduce cardiovascular fibrosis (reviewed in Pandey,2005). BNP are signaling molecules with natriuretic and vascular smooth muscle–relaxing activity that regulates cardiovascular, skeletal, and kidney function. These are of three types: ANP, B-type natriuretic peptide (BNP), and C-type natriuretic peptide (CNP). ANP is expressed and stored in the granules in atrial walls and released from atrial wall stretching and BNP is most predominantly expressed in ventricles and regulated by ventricular wall stretching. The biologically active, circulating form of BNP (BNP77–108) is a C-terminal fragment from prohormone BNP 1–108. The N-terminal fragment of BNP (NT-proBNP) coexists in blood with the C-terminal fragment. Circulating levels of both N-and C-terminal peptides have been used in clinical studies in association with cardiovascular diseases [56]. The neuropeptides are established markers of heart failure [57]. Serum BNP levels are also elevated in association with inflammatory conditions, sepsis, and septic shock [58, 59]. Data show that serum NT-proBNP may be used as markers of cardiac dysfunction in sepsis and may help to differentiate between survivors and non-survivors of severe sepsis. [60]. Studies show that inflammation may increase levels of NT pro BNP more than BNP, resulting in an increased NT pro BNP/BNP ratio [61]. The serum BNP activity reflects immunomodulatory activity in addition to vasodilatory, diuretic, and natriuretic properties in sepsis and septic shock, and plays an important role in the modulation of the production of inflammatory mediators in macrophages. Data show that BNP regulates the production of major inflammatory molecules, such as reactive oxygen- and nitrogen species (ROS and RNS), leukotriene B4 (LTB4), prostaglandin E2 (PGE2); modulates the cytokines (TNF-α, IL-12, and IL-10) profile, and affects cell motility [62]. An association between the pro-inflammatory cytokine IL6 and elevated serum BNP levels has been explored in heart failure. Elevated serum IL6 and BNP levels may independently predict morbidity and mortality in patients with congestive heart failure [63]. BNP levels are increased in conditions with raised levels of IL-1β and other cytokines including post-MI and progressive HF [64, 65]. High BNP levels may be seen in inflammatory conditions even in the absence of cardiovascular diseases (as previous).

Patients with severe CoViD 19 appear to have significantly raised plasma NT pro-BNP levels. In a retrospective cohort of 799 patients analysis data of 113 deceased and 161 recovered patients, the incidence of heart failure was recorded at 49% (41/83) and N-terminal pro-brain natriuretic peptide serum levels were markedly higher in the deceased patients (800.0 pg/mL) than in recovered patients (72.0 pg/mL) [66]. In another study, the highest BNP levels were observed in patients with elevation in Troponin likely to be linked with myocardial injury. The overall cohort of 187 patients admitted with CoViD 19 had serum NT-pro BNP levels of 268.4 pg/mL (75.3–689.1), normal Troponin group had 141.4 pg/mL (39.3–303.6) and elevated Troponin group had NT-pro BNP levels of 817.4 pg/mL (336.0–1944.0) $P < 0.001$ [67].

Patients with metabolic risk factors have worse outcomes in CoViD 19. Raised BNP levels have been found in severe CoViD 19 diabetics. In a single-center, retrospective, observational study of 193 patients with severe CoViD19 showed high levels of BNP in patients with diabetes mellitus 665 pg/mL versus non-diabetics 259 pg/ mL and in non-survivors 970 pg/mL (323 to 2535) versus survivors 46 pg/mL (31 to 267) < 0.001 (Normal NT-proBNP < 285 pg/mL) [68].

Increased serum BNP activity is also an important marker of myocardial involvement in CoViD 19. As seen in heart failure of other etiologies, increased serum BNP levels are also associated with poor outcomes in CoViD 19. Association of heart failure with proinflammatory cytokines increased levels of protease (ADAM 17) activity in HF, and upregulation of serum ACE2 activity in HF are likely important underlying mechanisms in cardiovascular complications in CoViD 19. Raised BNP serum levels with hyperinflammatory stress associated with complicated CoViD 19 further add to the possibility of association of these mechanisms with these complications.

Imaging evaluation of cardiac function provides an objective assessment of the cardiac structural and functional status. Due to the elevation of serum levels of biomarkers of heart failure in both myocardial injury and sepsis, it may be difficult to distinguish between these possible etiological mechanisms of the development of heart failure. Lack of cardiac imaging data may limit accurate assessment of the exact cause of heart failure in CoViD 19. Furthermore, detailed classification of

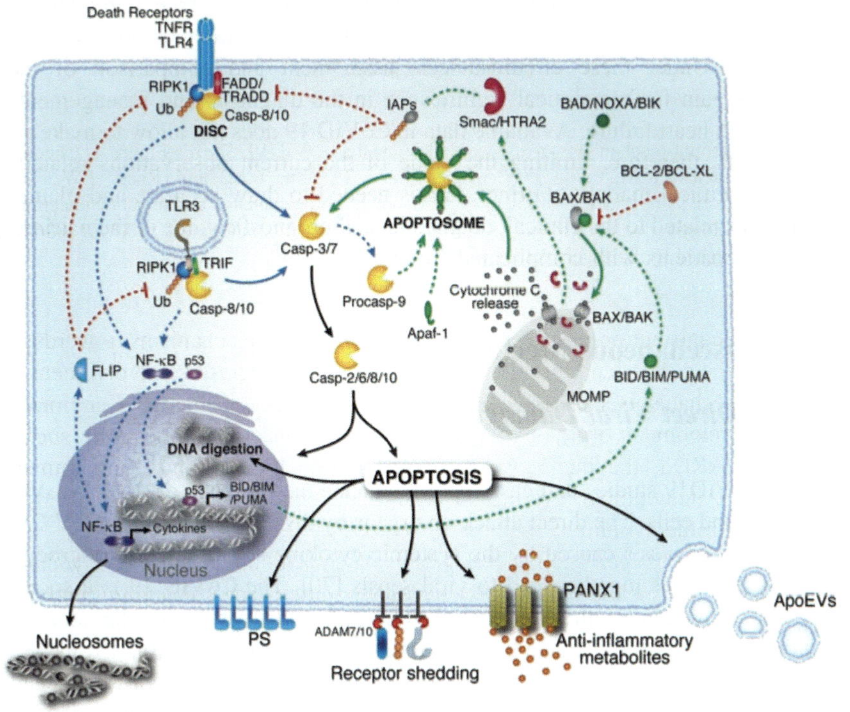

Fig. 10.4 Pathways to apoptosis. Apoptosis is triggered through two major pathways referred to as the intrinsic and extrinsic pathways. The intrinsic pathway is activated by oligomerization of the B-cell lymphoma-2 (BCL-2) family proteins BAK and BAX. BAK/BAX oligomers form pores in the mitochondrial outer membrane, leading to the release of cytochrome c into the cytosol. Activation of BAK/BAX is regulated by proapoptotic (e.g., BAD and BID) or antiapoptotic (e.g., BCL-2) BCL-2 family proteins. Cytochrome c binds to Apaf-1, which recruits procaspase-9, forming the apoptosome. In the apoptosome, caspase-9 is activated by autoproteolytic cleavage, initiating the caspase-processing cascade. The extrinsic pathway is activated by engagement of membrane receptors such as Tumor necrosis factor (TNF) receptor 1 (TNFR1), death receptors, or Toll-Like Receptors (TLRs). These proteins induce the formation of signaling complexes involving TNFR1-associated death domain protein (TRADD) or Fas-associated death domain protein (FADD), receptor-interacting serine/threonine protein kinase 1 (RIPK1) and procaspase-8. Ubiquitylation of RIPK1 by cellular inhibitors of apoptosis (cIAPs) stabilizes the complex and induces the activation of the transcription factor NFκB. FLIP, also present in the DISC, limits caspase-8 activity while promoting cell survival, cell proliferation, and the production of proinflammatory cytokines. Imbalances in this pathway, such as those imposed by cellular stress, allow the activation of caspase-8 and caspase-10, which in turn triggers the caspase activation cascade. Once active, executioner caspases (i.e., caspase-2, -6, -8 and -10) bring about programmed apoptotic death. Apoptotic cells release messengers in the form of nucleosomal structures, shed receptors, anti-inflammatory metabolites or molecules packaged in apoptotic extracellular vesicles (ApoEVs). Phosphatidylserine (PS) molecules exposed on the outer surface of the plasma membrane function as “eat me” signals for phagocytes. *Source* Figure 3. Bertheloot, D., Latz, E. and Franklin, B.S., 2021. Necroptosis, pyroptosis and apoptosis: an intricate game of cell death. Cellular & Molecular Immunology, 18(5), pp.1106–1121. https://www.nature.com/articles/s41423-020-00630-3. Published by Springer Nature Group

heart failure subtypes ie HFrEF and HFpEF according to recent guidelines is important for evaluation of risk and targeted treatment strategies and prognostic value [69]. Under these circumstances, assessment and comparison of these parameters gain further clinical significance in the diagnosis and management of patients with heart failure. Available data in CoViD 19 does not allow to make such comparisons, therefore, limiting the value of the current observations related to these biochemical markers. Further data is needed to draw accurate and plausible conclusions related to the clinical, diagnostic, and prognostic value of the natriuretic peptides in patients with complicated CoViD 19.

10.3 Miscellaneous Mechanisms

10.3.1 Direct Viral Damage

Several CoViD19 studies and case reports indicate the presence of SARS CoV2 in the tissues and cells. The direct attack on organs by disseminated SARS-CoV-2, the immune pathogenesis caused by the systemic cytokine storm, and the microcirculation dysfunctions together lead to viral sepsis [70]. The CoViD 19 is associated with viral infection of the endothelial cells and other cardiovascular structures resulting in direct viral damage to the vasculature and heart (Fig. 10.2). It has been suggested that pericytes may be infected by the SARS-CoV-2 virus and cause capillary endothelial cell/microvascular dysfunction, which may cause individual cell necrosis [71]. The endotheliopathy has been suggested to affect multiple organs in complicated CoViD19, suggesting a possible role in multi-organ failure. The endothelial cell infection and the endotheliitis may serve as underlying mechanisms linked to the vascular dysfunction and thrombotic events in the lung, kidney, and possibly the heart and other organs [72, 73].

Viral association with myocarditis is well known. Possible pathogenetic mechanisms of direct viral cardiac invasion in CoViD 19 include ACE 2 mediated viral cell entry in cardiomyocytes, pericytes or fibroblasts infection and dissemination of the virus [71]. The SARS CoV 2 may directly reside within the heart and cause myocardial injury. In a case reporting myocarditis in CoViD 19, the patient underwent an endomyocardial biopsy, which demonstrated low-grade myocardial inflammation and the absence of myocyte necrosis, with localization of SARS-CoV-2 within the macrophages, but not cardiomyocytes. [74].

Viral targeting of the host protein translational machinery results in direct cytotoxicity in the heart [75–77]. The mechanisms involved in the development of viral cell injury are complex. As a result of the viral infection, several cellular signaling pathways are activated. These pathways and mechanisms regulate viral entry, replication, release, and evasion from the host immune reactions [78]. Virus-induced cardiac dysfunction is also facilitated by viral proteinases that act on host proteins involved in the regulation of protein translation, transcription, cardiac contraction, signaling transduction, and host structural proteins [79, 80], for instance viral proteinase 2 A action on serum response factors (a muscle-enriched transcriptional factor controlling the expression of many cardiac contractile and regulatory genes) [81] or through modulation of host and viral gene expression and differential expression of miRNAs as seen in CVB3 myocarditis. Dysfunctional mechanisms such as loss of cellular homeostasis, translation/transcription shutoff, contractile dysfunction, and apoptosis, as a result of viral proteinase activity, play an important role in the direct damage of the infected cells as seen in viral myocarditis.

Several receptors are involved in the process of viral recognition and mediation of the immune response. Once the viral genome is recognized, these receptors trigger an intracellular signaling cascade of type I interferons and proinflammatory cytokines [79]. Besides receptors, the involvement of co-receptors has also been demonstrated in the viral cell injury mechanisms. The co-receptors, such as the decay-accelerating factor (CD55), facilitate viral receptors such as coxsackievirus-adenovirus receptor (CAR) located in the intercalated disc and the cell–cell junctions of the AV node in the adult heart, in the pathogenesis of myocardial injury in CVB3 infection [82–84].

The Toll-like receptors (TLRs) play an important role in viral recognition as well as activation of the inflammatory mechanisms, and viral clearance. The TLRs (TLR3, TLR9, and MDA5) are important in viral recognition and antiviral responses and mediate immune response to the viral infection. Viral infections typically activate the innate immune system through toll-like receptors (TLRs) that recognize molecular patterns (pathogen-associated molecular patterns or PAMPs) [85]. The SARS-CoV-2 and related coronaviruses activate TLRs such as TLR3, TLR7, RIG1 and NLRP3 [86]. The SARS CoV2 spike protein binds with the extracellular domain of various TLRs including TLR1, TLR4, and TLR6, with the strongest binding with TLR4 [87]. The TLRs may be an important pathogenetic link in CoViD19 related cardiovascular injury in an ACE2 depleted environment [88, 89]. The interconnection of the TLRs and major shedases (ADAM17, CTSL) and NLRP3 inflammasome may contribute to the pro-inflammatory pool and subsequent cytokine burst leading to aggravated CoViD19-CVD comorbidity [90]. A negative feedback mechanism in TLRs suppresses the inflammatory response. Continued activation of the TLRs down-regulates proinflammatory cytokine production and resulting inflammatory responses, via a negative feedback loop involving ILs and TGF- β [91]. Evidence shows that in the acute setting, loss of TLR4 leads to better viral clearance and reduced cardiac injury [92], whereas loss of other TLRs (TLR 3 or 9 and MAD5 (melanoma differentiation-associated protein 5)) results in death during viral myocarditis [93, 94].

The TLR4 activation, is associated with thrombo-inflammation [95] through signaling platelets and subsequent increase in the TF protein, which is procoagulant [96, 97].

The Toll-like receptors (TLRs) are expressed on the cell surface of cardiomyocytes and myeloid cells [98, 99], that recognize damage-associated molecular patterns (DAMPs) such a Heat Shock Proteins 60 (HSP 60) and pathogen-associated molecular patterns (PAMPs) derived from the damaged host cells and pathogens, and activate the transcription factor nuclear factor-κB (NF-κB)

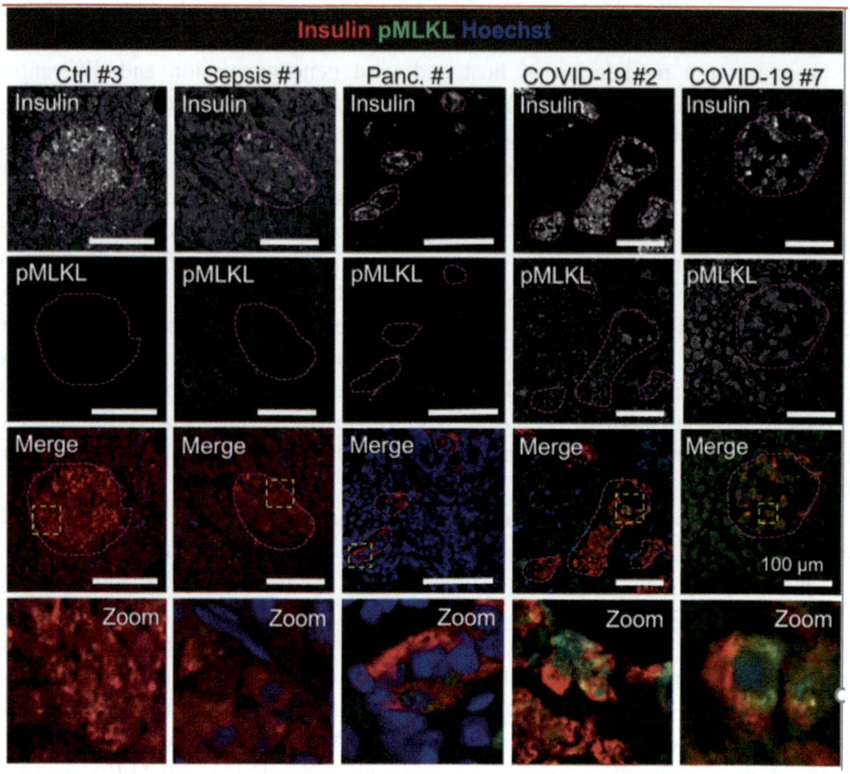

Fig. 10.5 SARS-CoV-2 infection leads to necroptosis in the pancreas. a Immunostainings of pancreas sections from non-COVID-19 patients (control, septic, and with pancreatitis) and from COVID-19 patients using antibodies against insulin and pMLKL marking necroptotic cells. Representative images from three independent experiments (n = 3) are shown. Scale bars, 100 μm. *Source* Copied and edited from Figure 4 Steenblock, C., Richter, S., Berger, I., Barovic, M., Schmid, J., Schubert, U., Jarzebska, N., von Mässenhausen, A., Linkermann, A., Schürmann, A. and Pablik, J., 2021. Viral infiltration of pancreatic islets in patients with COVID-19. Nature Communications, 12(1), pp.1–12. https://www.nature.com/articles/s41467-021-23886-3. Published by Springer Nature Group

leading to the expression of a wide range of inflammatory genes 89 [100]. Subjects with cardiovascular risk factors and obesity have altered levels of transcripts for some NF-κB pathway members and TLR2 in platelets [101]. Viral induction of the immune, proinflammatory, and prothrombotic mechanisms through TLRs showcases the mechanisms related to the cardiovascular injury induced by the viruses. The viral platelet interactions and related pathways involved in the thrombo-inflammation may play a role in the association of cardiovascular diseases and cardiometabolic risk factors with complicated CoViD19 and need further exploration. These mechanisms and pathways may be target of therapeutic interventions to help prevent cardiac injury in CoViD19 patients.

10.3.2 Endoplasmic Reticulum Stress

The endoplasmic reticulum (ER) homeostasis is crucial for cell functioning. The physiological stress or pathological conditions influence ER homeostasis. Several conditions such as hypoxia, ischemia, oxidative stress, viral diseases, and others are involved in the induction of mechanisms promoting the accumulation of misfolded or unfolded proteins in the ER, which further activate signal pathways to restore the ER homeostasis. Viruses may complete their lifecycle (host cell entry, production of viral proteins) through influencing the unfolded protein response (UPR), autophagy, signaling networks, and interconnection of these pathways is essential for the viral infection [102–105]. The "unfolded protein response" (UPR) and autophagy pathways, play important role in the regulation of protein homeostasis, apoptosis, and control of innate immunity, including viral particle clearance [106, 107]. Stressful conditions cause sequestration of the ER chaperone proteins in ER and result in activation of ER stress sensors (attached with the ER Chaperon proteins: glucose-regulated protein 78 (GRP78)). These sensors cause the release of ER transmembrane proteins (protein kinase-like ER-resident kinase (PERK), the activating transcription factor 6 (ATF6), and the inositol-requiring enzyme 1 (IRE1)) that lead to induction of the enzymes that cause degradation of unfolded protein to restore the homeostasis [108–110].

The coronavirus disease is associated with ER stress and the unfolded protein response (UPR) [111]. The SARS CoV2 may exploit the cell machinery, endoplasmic reticulum for multiplication. The viral glycoproteins may activate cellular transmembrane proteins, thereby generating the ER stress response to meet the need for folding and secretory capacity. In viral infections, mechanisms related to the viral and host immunity may lead to the development of the ER stress response. Interferon-induced antiviral response of the host is mediated by the ER transmembrane proteins, which helps to eliminate viral proteins and pathogenesis. The stress mechanisms including viral infections induce dysregulated ER stress response may ultimately lead to cell injury and death. Prolonged ER stress response leads to activation of the apoptotic pathways such as induction of C/EBP homologous protein (CHOP), activation of Jun N-terminal kinase (JNK), and cleavage of caspase-12 [112–114].

The ER stress and mediators play an important role in the development of cardiovascular diseases. Misfolded protein aggregates that are toxic to cardiomyocytes, found in various heart diseases [115, 116]. Several cardiovascular risk factors including hyperglycemia, hyperlipidemia, hyper-homocysteinemia, and hemodynamic shear stress, may trigger ER stress and endothelial cell dysfunction [117]. Angiotensin II receptor 1 (AT1R), an important component of RAS with a role in the pathogenesis of COVID19, may mediate ER stress in the endothelial cells [118]. Coxsackie B virus, adeno- and parvo-, viruses are known to cause myocarditis [119]. Several studies reveal the involvement of ER stress response in the development of cardiovascular complications, as a result of Coxsackievirus B3 [120–123], inflammatory conditions, and metabolic derangements [124, 125]. The pathogenetic mechanisms that determine the development of cardiovascular complications in CoViD 19 may share similarities with the mechanisms involved in the viral diseases resulting in similar complications. The exact mechanisms associated with ER stress in CoViD 19 are unclear and need further exploration.

10.3.3 Cell Death Modalities

Complicated CoViD19 is associated with obstructive and non-obstructive cardiovascular complications, acute respiratory distress syndrome (ARDS), and multi-organ failure. Cell death plays a major role in the pathogenesis of these complications and is linked with inflammation. (See Fig. 10.6). Multiple cell death modalities and mediators and signaling mechanisms may be involved in the development of complications in CoViD19. A direct viral injury or indirect mechanisms related to the illness in CoViD19 patients, induce cell death mechanisms and may harm the myocardial and vascular cells. The dysregulation of inflammation, immunomodulation, and regulatory mechanisms play a critical pathogenetic role in CoViD19. The stress conditions such as inflammation, and hyperimmune reactions may activate the major signaling processes autophagy, apoptosis, and necrosis. However, the complex interplay of the signaling mechanisms and pathways in patients with CoViD19 is not fully understood.

A variety of death cell pathways can be identified in the novel coronavirus disease including apoptosis, necroptosis, pyroptosis, and autophagy that may be associated with the severity of the disease and development of complications. The extrinsic death receptor pathway and an intrinsic mitochondrial-regulated pathway are highly integrated with apoptosis, necrosis, and autophagy 67 [126]. The activation/cleavage of caspase-8 reflects the extrinsic apoptotic pathway, whereas Bcl-2 plays an important role in the activation of the intrinsic pathway [127].

Data from pathology reports of complicated CoViD19 patients reveal cell death modalities in a variety of cardiovascular structures possibly indicating the underlying pathogenetic mechanisms that cause cardiovascular injury. The presence of cardiomyocyte necrosis and apoptosis [128–130] is associated with the development of myocarditis, heart failure, and various forms of myocardial injury associated with CoViD 19. The endothelial cell injury and associated dysfunction that leads to the vascular and thrombotic complications in CoViD 19, may be the result of induction of apoptosis and pyroptosis in these cells [73].

Pyroptosis is a form of lytic cell death mediated by the inflammasomes [131] marked by a rise in IL1 beta, may underlie lymphocytic depletion observed in CoViD19 known as a sign of CoVID19 severity. The different forms of cell death pyroptosis, apoptosis, and necroptosis are autonomous but may overlap and cross talk, and through collective interaction may circumvent pathogen mediated inhibition of different cell pathways giving rise to PANoptosis [132]. The combination of TNF-α and IFN-γ induced inflammatory cell death characterized by pyroptosis, apoptosis, and necroptosis (PANoptosis), which appears to be based on

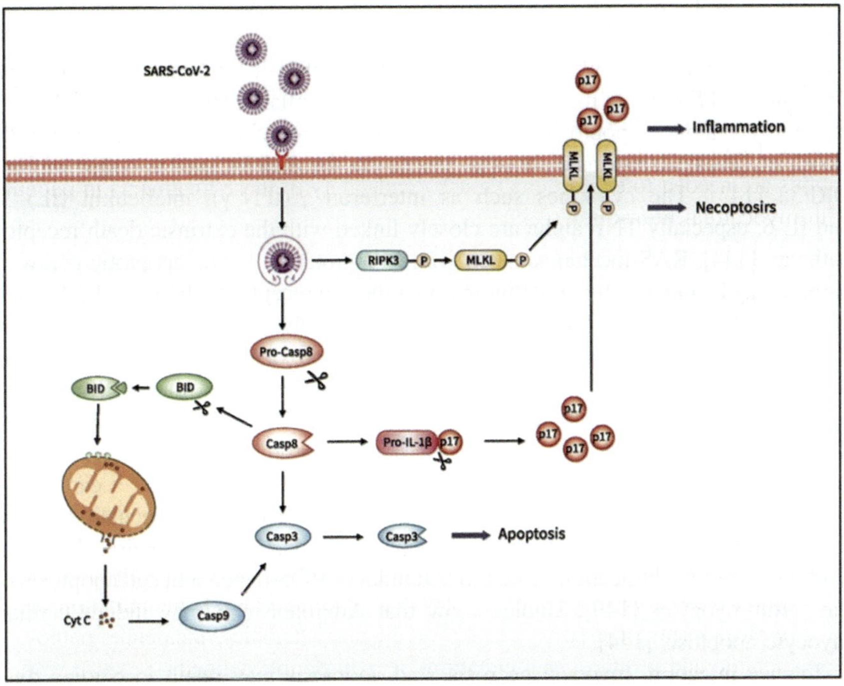

Fig. 10.6 Inflammatory response and cell death in CoViD19. A proposed model of SARS-CoV-2 infection induces inflammatory responses and cell death. SARS-CoV-2 infection induces the cell death through the activation of caspase-8. The activation of caspase-8 promotes pro-IL-1β cleavage, leading to the secretion of mature IL-1β (P17) through necroptosis pathway. *Source* Figure 6. Li, S., Zhang, Y., Guan, Z., Li, H., Ye, M., Chen, X., Shen, J., Zhou, Y., Shi, Z.L., Zhou, P. and Peng, K., 2020. SARS-CoV-2 triggers inflammatory responses and cell death through caspase-8 activation. Signal transduction and targeted therapy, 5(1), pp.1–10. https://www.nature.com/articles/s41392-020-00334-0. Published by Springer Nature Group

the cross-talk between the inflammasome/pyroptosis and apoptosis and necroptosis [133, 134]. The pyroptotic, apoptotic, and necroptotic cell death pathways interact to form a single molecular complex PANoptosome [132], that regulates PANoptosis. The PANoptosome complex provides a molecular scaffold allowing for the interactions and activation of the machinery required for inflammasome/ pyroptosis (such as NLRP3, ASC, caspase-1), apoptosis (caspase-8), and necroptosis [134]. The inflammatory cell death, PANoptosis, is induced by the coronavirus infection and impaired NLRP3 inflammasome function or pyroptosis can lead to negative consequences for the host [134]. Blocking cytokine-mediated leading to inflammatory death signaling pathways may benefit CoViD19 patients [135].

Apoptosis is programmed cell death characterized by nuclear and cellular fragmentations without inflammation, is found in CoViD19 and may be associated with the severity of the disease [136]. Apoptosis is also regarded as an innate antiviral defense mechanism, may inhibit viral expansion [137] and regulates inflammation [138, 139]. Both extrinsic death receptor pathways or intrinsic mitochondrial-regulated pathways may induce apoptosis [140–142]. (See Fig. 10.4). Terminal apoptotic pathway is common for both intrinsic and extrinsic pathways. The abnormal ER stress, mitochondrial dysfunction, inflammation, and several other factors may induce apoptosis in CoViD19. Induction of the apoptosis by SARS CoV2 involves the extrinsic pathway [143], via the SARS CoV2 encoded protein ORF3a [143]. The cytokines such as interferon γ (IFN γ), interleukin (IL) 1, and IL-6, especially TNF alpha are closely linked with the extrinsic death receptor pathway [144]. RAS mechanisms CoViD19 Angiotensin I. The apoptotic pathway signals may be induced by viral binding with the cell receptor without viral cell entry [145]. The intrinsic mitochondrial death pathway involves morphological damage to the cell as a result of apoptotic death signals. The peroxisome proliferator-activated receptors (PPARs) family are regulators of inflammation and metabolism, when activated reduce proinflammatory cytokines (IL-6 and INF γ) [146], are involved in the intrinsic apoptosis pathway. The PPARs are expressed in endothelial cells, vascular smooth muscle cells, and monocytes/macrophages and play a cardiovascular protective role [147]. Hypoxia amd other dysregulated RAS mechanisms may induce apoptosis in complicated CoViD19 and cause cardiac dysfunction. Hypoxia leads to excessive intracellular calcium and induces ROS-dependent cell apoptosis in the cardiomyocytes [149]. Studies show that Angiotensin II may induce cardiac myocyte apoptosis [144].

Intense infection, myocyte necrosis, and apoptosis may result in cardiac dysfunction. Cell death is a major component of ischemia–reperfusion injury and is posited as the central underlying cause of ventricular remodeling and cardiac dysfunction following myocardial infarction. Myocardial damage may be a consequence of apoptosis of the cardiomyocytes [150–155]. Various cardiovascular conditions heart failure, myocardial infarction, ischemia–reperfusion injury, dilated cardiomyopathy, myocarditis, and others exhibit apoptosis [156].

The Fas/Apolipoprotein 1 are membrane proteins /cell surface receptors (from tumor necrosis factor nerve growth factor receptor family), expressed in the activated mature T cells, play an important role in the immune response, also act as mediators of the apoptosis in association with a specific antibody or Fas Ligand [157, 158]. The Fas/Fas ligand pathway mediated endoplasmic reticulum stress (ER stress) induces apoptosis of the cardiomyocytes in acute myocarditis [159]. Elevated serum soluble Fas (sFas) and soluble Fas ligand (sFasL) levels are found in patients with myocarditis and dilated cardiomyopathy [150, 160–164]. Evidence shows that relatively high serum levels of Fas ligand and interleukin-10 cardiomyopathy and myocarditis may predict an increased risk of death [165, 166]. Persistent activation of the T cells precipitates apoptosis mediated by Fas/FasL interaction [167]. An association of apoptosis pathway with reduced lymphocyte and platelet counts has been previously explored in coronavirus patients who were found to have elevated soluble Fas ligand (sFasL) levels as compared to the healthy subjects [168].

Necrotic cell death is characterized by cytoplasmic swelling with eventual rupture of the plasma membrane, as well as swelling of organelles including the mitochondria. Neurohormonal activation leads to necrotic myocyte cell death. These mechanisms collectively trigger inflammation at the site of the injury [169]. In cardiomyocytes, necrosis is accompanied by an increase in cytosolic Ca^{2+} levels. Intracellular molecules "damage-associated molecular patterns" (DAMPs) detected by the innate immune system, cause inflammatory reaction provoking tissue damage and additional myocyte death". Evidence shows that necrotic myocardial cells release DAMPs that provoke fibroblast activation in vitro and trigger myocardial inflammation and fibrosis in vivo [170, 171]. Necroptosis is a programmed form of necrosis rupture of the plasma membrane and release of damage-associated molecular patterns [172] that is highly regulated by immune signaling pathways unlike necrosis [173]. Necroptosis may be involved in the CoViD19 associated lung injury and other organ injuries. (See Fig. 10.5). The higher levels of receptor-interacting kinase 3 (RIPK-3) that promotes signaling, leading to necroptosis, in CoViD19, may be linked with the development of ARDS in CoViD19 patients [174]. Similarly, the RIPK3 activity has been linked with cardiovascular diseases, and thrombotic complications [175]. The presence of necroptosis in CoViD19 may be a marker of cardiovascular complications in CoViD19. Further studies are needed to validate these mechanisms.

Autophagy is an adaptive cell response to physiological and stress mechanisms such as inflammation seen in acute settings as in sepsis or chronic settings as in cardiovascular or metabolic conditions. It is a highly conserved evolutionary process that regulates protein degradation, organelle turnover, and recycling of cellular components during cellular stress, and maintains cellular homeostasis. Excessive stress and dysregulated autophagy may eventually cause cell death [176, 177]. Autophagy is cell death occurring with massive autophagic vacuolization of the cytoplasm, a cell survival pathway activated by a variety of stresses that catalyzes the breakdown of intracellular organelles and proteins [178]. Autophagy is involved in viral clearance at multiple levels, hence also termed as "virophagy" may counter coronavirus infection, and may be inhibited by the coronaviruses [179]. The SARS CoV2 may exploit host cell machinery for survival and may induce autophagy via UPR induction in cells. Autophagy has been proposed as a potential therapeutic target in CoViD19 [179]. The NSP6, a protein that has an inducing effect on autophagosome formation, has been found to have mutations in an analysis, may impact intracellular survival of the virus, therefore, impacting pathogenicity [181]. Furthermore, autophagy and apoptosis may cross-talk. It has been speculated that over-accumulation of autophagosomes activates an apoptotic pathway that results in apoptotic death of the infected cells and disrupts the virus replication cycle [180].

Several factors including starvation, infection of host cells, excessive ER and oxidative stress, viral genome release, lysosomal damage may activate autophagy. In the cardiovascular system, autophagy ensures the maintenance of cardiovascular homeostasis and function. However, dysregulated autophagy associated with excessive or insufficient autophagy beyond a given threshold gives rise to cardiac disorders [182]. The autophagy/virophagy may serve as a potential therapeutic target in CoViD19 [183]. Furthermore, the dysregulated activity of NLRP3 inflammasome is linked with cytokine storms [184] involved in severe forms of CoViD19 [185], is associated with tissue damage [186]. The NLRP3 sense disturbance of cellular homeostasis may have a role in cell death-related inflammation [187], and antimicrobial defense, and induce pyroptotic and apoptotic cell death [188, 189]. The SARS CoV2 triggers activation of the Nod-like receptor family, pyrin domain-containing 3 (NLRP3) inflammasome pathway, and release of its products including the proinflammatory cytokines IL-6 and IL-1β [190]. The NLRP3 inflammasome signaling pathway and the pro-apoptotic mitochondrial signaling pathway associated with UPR/Autophagy pathways are important for the viral cycle of SARS-CoV-2, may be new targets for developing drugs for CoViD 19 [191].

Another cell death modality NETosis differs from other forms of cell death, such as necrosis and apoptosis. Viruses can stimulate neutrophils to produce Neutrophil Extracellular Traps (NETs), a network structure formed by freely circulating DNA expelled by neutrophils, and a variety of proteins. This process leads to cell death that is characterized by the destruction of the nuclear membrane before the plasmatic membrane. In dysregulated forms, this process generates an extreme systemic response with the production of cytokines, interferon I, and immune complexes, and may result in local and systemic damage. Neutrophil Extracellular Traps (NETs) consisting of circulating free DNA and histones are linked with inflammation, coagulation and thrombosis both locally and systemically in a variety of conditions [192]. Patients with CoViD19 have high levels of circulating free (cf-DNA) and DNA-myeloperoxidase complexes [193]. Elevated levels of these freely circulating complexes are correlated with the acuity of illness, inflammatory response, and severe disease. The circulating free RNA from SARS CoV 2 may trigger a coagulation cascade. Evidence shows that cf-RNA serves as a cofactor for auto-activation of factor VII-activating protease, thereby initiating coagulation [194]. Furthermore, an association of NETosis with the resurgence of non-infectious inflammatory illness in the CoViD19 patients recovering from the disease that might be referred to as “Post CoViD19 syndrome”, has been suggested [195]. The potential role of NETosis in CoViD19 i.e., the association between NETs activity and CoViD19 mortality/survival, between markers of NETosis and serum markers of inflammation and thrombosis, is currently being explored [196]. Further research is needed to define the interplay of cell death mechanisms, and their regulation in CoViD19. This will help to validate the potential role of these mechanisms as therapeutic targets in CoViD19 patients.

10.3.4 Mitochondrial Dysfunction

Mitochondria play a central role in ATP production via oxidative phosphorylation and act as the powerhouse of the cell [197, 198]. During the enzymatic activity of the electron transport chain reactive oxygen species (ROS) are produced in

Mitochondria [199]. Various stress factors trigger altered expression of mitochondrial and nuclear proteins resulting in oxidative stress. These include infections, inflammatory conditions, hypoxic and ischemic conditions, metabolic factors, and others. Cardiovascular and metabolic conditions such as atherosclerosis, hypertension, heart failure, and complications related to diabetes mellitus and obesity are precipitated by oxidative stress and associated inflammatory mechanisms.

Viral infections alter mitochondrial dynamics at various levels and impact mitochondrial functioning. The viruses may induce mtDNA degradation, alter mitochondrial metabolic pathways, impact mitochondrial membrane potential and modify the mitochondrial intracellular number and distribution, thereby influencing apoptosis, mitochondrial homeostasis, or evade mitochondrial antiviral signals [200–202].

Data show an association of CoViD19 with redox imbalance or oxidative stress [203, 204]. SARS CoV2 proteins may interact with the host cell mitochondrial proteins, and induce mitochondrial dysfunction exacerbating reactive oxygen species (ROS) production [205].

The ROS are generated by the Nox family NADPH is an abbreviation from nicotinamide adenine dinucleotide phosphate oxidases containing p22phox and NOX2. Increased NoX2 activation in CoViD19 is linked with CoViD19 complications including cardiovascular and thrombotic injury [203, 206]. Several mechanisms including dysregulated RAS may induce increased oxidative stress in CoViD19. The RAS plays an important role in cardiovascular physiology and pathological state.

The harmful impact of the Ang II/AT1 receptor pathway of RAS involves mechanisms resulting in oxidative stress, pro-inflammatory and prothrombotic effects. Ang II appears to cause the mitochondrial dysfunction that is observed in the development of cardiac and vascular dysfunction, through the protein kinase C–dependent pathway by activation of the endothelial cell NADPH oxidase and formation of peroxynitrite [207]. These mechanisms induce apoptosis and necrosis [208]. Sepsis triggers structural and functional abnormalities in the mitochondria, resulting in reduced energy supply and enhanced production of mitochondria-derived danger-associated molecular patterns (DAMPs), such as reactive oxygen species (ROS) [209] cardiolipin [210], cytochrome c [211] and others, ultimately resulting in complications of sepsis such as myocardial injury and multi-organ failure. Mitochondrial fragmentation and accumulation may result in the release of cytochrome c in the cytoplasm which triggers cellular apoptosis and cell death [212]. The association of mitochondrial dysfunction with increased oxidative stress and CoViD19 complications including cardiovascular injury warrants further exploration. Counterbalancing of the oxidative stress in CoViD19 or blocking ROS production may prevent exacerbation of CoViD19 [203, 204, 213].

10.4 Summary

The mechanisms underlying CoViD19 complications appear to be diverse, distinct, and powerful with local and systemic presence. However, certain mechanisms may overlap and act in a synergistic mode. The mechanisms implicated in the maintenance of homeostatic state may be dysregulated in CoViD19 and create a pathological imbalance, and if persistent and intense, may fail to restore the homeostasis and result in the development of complications implicating various structures, tissues, and organs. Among the most powerful mechanisms include the hyperinflammatory immune reaction and the renin-angiotensin system. Others including Kallikrein Kinin System (KKS), Endothelin (ET), and natriuretic peptides (NPs) also appear to be prominent in this interplay, leading to prothrombotic state and microvascular damage hallmark of the multi-organ failure. Besides, the proinflammatory cytokine release, the interaction of several inflammatory mechanisms including the NETosis, NLRP3 inflammasome mediated reactions, and processes related to the inflammatory cell death, indicate the potency and variety of inflammatory mechanisms activated in CoViD19 that generate excessive inflammation.

Direct viral injury an important mechanism has been sporadically described in the literature highlighting the pathogenetic processes in CoViD19 confirming the presence of viral particles in various tissues. The cardiac and vascular toxicity of the virus and the role of TLRs in the pro-inflammatory reactions may facilitate the development of the cardiovascular injury observed in CoViD19. The SARS CoV2 interacts with mitochondria at multiple levels, may disable the host defense mechanisms or through the exploitation of the cellular resources to survive and multiply. Several cellular mechanisms including mitochondrial dysfunction, excessive endoplasmic reticulum stress, unfolded protein response and involvement of various forms of cell death through direct and indirect viral mechanisms in CoViD19 indicate the pathogenetic nature of the CoViD19 complications including cardiovascular injury. Mechanisms regulating cell death in CoViD19 are poorly known. Apoptosis and severity of CoViD19 appear to be interlinked. Necroptosis and PANoptosis are associated with negative reactions in CoViD19 patients. Apoptosis and other forms of cell death leading to cardiomyocyte necrosis and apoptosis induced by SARS CoV 2 may reflect cardiovascular injury. Autophagy and apoptosis may cross-talk. It has been speculated that over-accumulation of autophagosomes activates an apoptotic pathway that results in apoptotic death of the infected cells and disrupts the virus replication cycle [180]. The inflammatory, immune, and thrombotic processes linked with various modalities of cell death associated with the development of CoViD19 complications must be further confirmed, along with their clinical and therapeutic implications.

Several regulatory mechanisms involved in the maintenance of homeostasis are impacted in severe CoViD19. The activation of the natriuretic peptide system appears to reflect the immune-inflammatory and cardiac instability known to be associated with the severity of CoViD19. The dysregulated KKS in CoViD19 may facilitate the viral impact of the SARS CoV2, through proinflammatory and prothrombotic processes, leading to cardiovascular injury. Similarly, the endothelin expression a well-known marker of cardiovascular risk appears to be associated with the severity of CoViD19 and needs further exploration.

A range of cross talk mechanisms between various reglatory systems, and between different organs may determine the clinical outcomes. Various interactions between lungs and kidneys or heart and kidneys may be recognized in CoViD19 patients reflecting the underlying pathogenetic interlinks that may further define clinical severity of the disease. Mechanisms related to the viral myocarditis and cytokine cardiomyopathy may reduce the glomerular filtration through hypotension, hypoperfusion, renal vein congestion [214]. Data also show that in patients with ARDS, the severity of the disease, diabetes, heart failure, and age, are associated with an increased risk of kidney damage [215] The high thrombo-inflammatory burden and cross-talk between various regulatory mechanisms in patients with CoViD19 may reflect these interlinks.

Furthermore, interaction between various pathogenetic mechanisms involved in CoViD19 that may contribute to the clinical features, severity, or risks associated with CoViD19 through the cross-talk mechanisms may be explained by the interactions between various regulatory peptide systems. For instance, the interaction through the cross talk mechanisms between ET-1 and the RAS in the pathogenesis of hypertension and related cardiovascular damage may have a role in the development of cardiovascular complications of CoViD19 [47]. The bradykinin and angiotensin precursors are generated in the liver and predominantly present in plasma. The Kallikrein Kinin System (KKS) may activate the complement system and generate pro-inflammatory and prothrombotic activity. The clinical features associated with the CoViD19 may be determined by the reciprocal interaction between the RAS, KKS, chymase in CoViD19 [216]. However, these interactions may also have a protective role. It is recognized that the endothelin system (ES) and natriuretic peptide system (NPs) may interact through several signaling mechanisms and multiple complex interactions, to maintain the blood pressure and vascular tone. The natriuretic peptides may offer support against inflammation through the cross-talk mechanisms or interaction with other peptides. It has been suggested that the atrial natriuretic peptide (ANP) may protect the heart from Ang II-induced remodeling by attenuating inflammation, at least partly through the endothelin 1/endothelin receptor A cascade [217]. The pathogenetic mechanisms in CoViD19 patients with complications may be tissue-specific, local, or systemic. Further exploration is needed to differentiate and define the cross talk mechanisms and further clarify the pathogenetic or protective implications of these interactions in CoViD19.The interaction of several potent inflammatory mediators, pathways, and mechanisms with various regulatory systems at multiple levels appear to be central to the CoViD19 pathology and need to be mapped. A thorough mapping of these pathogenetic mechanisms, viral mechanisms, viral signaling pathways, and the cellular and tissue damage in association with the biochemical, hematological, and clinical markers of CoViD19, and associated complications, is required. These associations must be explored using robust research modalities.

Summary Box

- Dysregulated endothelin and Kallikrein Kinin systems may induce pro-inflammatory and prothrombotic mechanisms in CoViD19.
- Serum BNP elevation in CoViD19 reflects inflammatory and cardiac instability.
- SARS CoV2 related direct viral injury may affect multiple organs including the heart, kidneys, gastrointestinal tract, liver, and brain.
- SARS CoV2 interaction with toll-like receptors (TLRs), may induce thrombo-inflammatory processes.
- Excessive endoplasmic reticular stress and unfolded protein response may be observed in severe CoViD19.
- Viruses interact with mitochondria at multiple levels, and SARS CoV2 may induce mitochondrial dysfunction.
- Cell death mechanisms involved in CoViD19 are associated with the severity of CoViD19.
- The synergistic effect of cytokines, such as TNF-α and IFN-γ, induces PANoptosis, inflammatory cell death, and contributes towards cytokine storm.
- Pathogenetic mechanisms involving the RAS and KKS, endothelin and NPs, KKS, and the complement system, may cross-talk and may induce a synergistic pathological impact.
- The intensity of the viral defense mechanisms, dysregulated inflammatory response, and loss of homeostasis indicate the severity of CoViD19.
- Matrix of pathogenetic mechanisms at local and systemic levels may cross-talk, and maybe tissue-specific, are dysregulated and cause homeostatic imbalance, thus facilitating CoViD19 complications.

References

1. Iba T, Levy JH. Inflammation and thrombosis: roles of neutrophils, platelets and endothelial cells and their interactions in thrombus formation during sepsis. J Thromb Haemost. 2018;16(2):231–41.
2. Noubouossie DF, Reeves BN, Strahl BD, Key NS. Neutrophils: back in the thrombosis spotlight. Blood. 2019;133(20):2186–97.
3. Subramaniam S, Jurk K, Hobohm L, Jäckel S, Saffarzadeh M, Schwierczek K, Wenzel P, Langer F, Reinhardt C, Ruf W. Distinct contributions of complement factors to platelet activation and fibrin formation in venous thrombus development. Blood. 2017;129(16):2291–302.
4. Wu C, Lu W, Zhang Y, Zhang G, Shi X, Hisada Y, Grover SP, Zhang X, Li L, Xiang B, Shi J. Inflammasome activation triggers blood clotting and host death through pyroptosis. Immunity. 2019;50(6):1401–11.

5. Bai B, Yang Y, Wang Q, Li M, Tian C, Liu Y, Aung LHH, Li PF, Yu T, Chu XM. NLRP3 inflammasome in endothelial dysfunction. Cell Death Dis. 2020;11(9):1–18.
6. Hall JM. Bradykinin receptors. Gen Pharmacol. 1997;28(1):1–6.
7. Marceau F, Hess JF, Bachvarov DR. The B1 receptors for kinins. Pharmacol Rev. 1998;50 (3):357–86.
8. Calixto JB, Cabrini DA, Ferreira J, Campos MM. Kinins in pain and inflammation. Pain. 2000;87(1):1–5.
9. Schmaier AH. The contact activation and kallikrein/kinin systems: pathophysiologic and physiologic activities. J Thromb Haemost. 2016;14(1):28–39.
10. Stefanini GG, Chiarito M, Ferrante G, Cannata F, Azzolini E, Viggiani G, De Marco A, Briani M, Bocciolone M, Bragato R, Corrada E. Early detection of elevated cardiac biomarkers to optimise risk stratification in patients with COVID-19. Heart. 2020;106 (19):1512–8.
11. Arentz M, Yim E, Klaff L, Lokhandwala S, Riedo FX, Chong M, Lee M. Characteristics and outcomes of 21 critically ill patients with COVID-19 in Washington State. JAMA. 2020;323 (16):1612–4.
12. Zakynthinos E, Kiropoulos T, Gourgoulianis K, Filippatos G. Diagnostic and prognostic impact of brain natriuretic peptide in cardiac and noncardiac diseases. Heart Lung. 2008;37 (4):275–85.
13. Witthaut R, Busch C, Fraunberger P, Walli A, Seidel D, Pilz G, Stuttmann R, Speichermann N, Verner L, Werdan K. Plasma atrial natriuretic peptide and brain natriuretic peptide are increased in septic shock: impact of interleukin-6 and sepsis-associated left ventricular dysfunction. Intensive Care Med. 2003;29(10):1696–702.
14. Farhangrazi ZS, Moghimi SM. Elevated circulating endothelin-1 as a potential biomarker for high-risk COVID-19 severity. Precis Nanomed. 2020;3:622–8.
15. Jankowich MD, Wu WC, Choudhary G. Association of elevated plasma endothelin-1 levels with pulmonary hypertension, mortality, and heart failure in African American individuals: the Jackson Heart Study. JAMA cardiology. 2016;1(4):461–9.
16. Varga Z, Flammer AJ, Steiger P, Haberecker M, Andermatt R, Zinkernagel AS, Mehra MR, Schuepbach RA, Ruschitzka F, Moch H. Endothelial cell infection and endotheliitis in COVID-19. The Lancet. 2020;395(10234):1417–8.
17. Wenzel P, Kopp S, Göbel S, Jansen T, Geyer M, Hahn F, Kreitner KF, Escher F, Schultheiss HP, Münzel T. Evidence of SARS-CoV-2 mRNA in endomyocardial biopsies of patients with clinically suspected myocarditis tested negative for COVID-19 in nasopharyngeal swab. Cardiovasc Res. 2020;116(10):1661–3.
18. Soleimani M. Acute kidney injury in SARS-CoV-2 infection: direct effect of virus on kidney proximal tubule cells. Int J Mol Sci. 2020;21(9):3275.
19. Morgan K, Samuel K, Vandeputte M, Hayes PC, Plevris JN. SARS-CoV-2 infection and the liver. Pathogens. 2020;9(6):430.
20. Regoli D, Barabé J. Pharmacology of bradykinin and related kinins. Pharmacol Rev. 1980;32:1–46.
21. Kakoki M, Smithies O. The kallikrein kinin system in health and in diseases of the kidney. Kidney Int. 2009;75:1019–30.
22. Manolis AJ, Marketou ME, Gavras I, Gavras H. Cardioprotective properties of bradykinin: role of the B 2 receptor. Hypertens Res. 2010;33(8):772–77.
23. Liesmaa I, Kuoppala A, Shiota N, Kokkonen JO, Kostner K, Mäyränpää M, Kovanen PT, Lindstedt KA. Increased expression of bradykinin type-1 receptors in endothelium of intramyocardial coronary vessels in human failing hearts. Am J Physiol-Heart Circ Physiol. 2005;288(5):H2317–22.
24. Leeb-Lundberg LM, Marceau F, Müller-Esterl W, Pettibone DJ, Zuraw BL. International Union of Pharmacology. XLV. Classification of the kinin receptor family: from molecular mechanisms to pathophysiological consequences. Pharmacol Rev. 2005;57:27–77.
25. Skidgel RA, Engelbrecht S, Johnson AR, and Erdös EG. Hydrolysis of substance P and neurotensin by converting enzyme and neutral endopeptidase. Peptides. 1984;5:769–76.

26. Hoang MV, Turner AJ. Novel activity of endothelin-converting enzyme: hydrolysis of bradykinin. Biochem J. 1997;327:23–26.
27. Kuoppala A, Lindstedt KA, Saarinen J, Kovanen PT, Kokkonen JO. Inactivation of bradykinin by angiotensin-converting enzyme and by carboxypeptidase N in human plasma. Am J Physiol Heart Circ Physiol. 2000;278:H1069–74.
28. Fryer RM, Segreti J, Banfor PN, Widomski DL, Backes BJ, Lin CW, Ballaron SJ, Cox BF, Trevillyan JM, Reinhart GA, et al. Effect of bradykinin metabolism inhibitors on evoked hypotension in rats: rank efficacy of enzymes associated with bradykinin-mediated angioedema. Br J Pharmacol. 2008;153:947–55.
29. Schmaier AH. The kallikrein-kinin and the renin-angiotensin systems have a multilayered interaction. Am J Physiol-Regul Integr Comp Physiol. 2003;285(1):R1–13.
30. Stoka V, Turk V. A structural network associated with the kallikrein-kinin and renin-angiotensin systems. Biol Chem. 2010;391(4):443–54. https://doi.org/10.1515/BC.2010.046 PMID: 20180650.
31. Su JB. Different cross-talk sites between the renin–angiotensin and the kallikrein–kinin systems. J Renin-Angiotensin-Aldosterone Syst. 2014;15(4):319–28.
32. Vickers C, Hales P, Kaushik V, Dick L, Gavin J, Tang J, Godbout K, Parsons T, Baronas E, Hsieh F, Acton S. Hydrolysis of biological peptides by human angiotensin-converting enzyme-related carboxypeptidase. J Biol Chem. 2002;277(17):14838–43.
33. Tolouian R, Vahed SZ, Ghiyasvand S, Tolouian A, Ardalan M. COVID-19 interactions with angiotensin-converting enzyme 2 (ACE2) and the kinin system; looking at a potential treatment. J Renal Inj Prev. 2020;9(2):e19–e19.
34. Fang C, Stavrou E, Schmaier AA, Grobe N, Morris M, Chen A, Nieman MT, Adams GN, LaRusch G, Zhou Y, Bilodeau ML. Angiotensin 1–7 and Mas decrease thrombosis in Bdkrb2−/− mice by increasing NO and prostacyclin to reduce platelet spreading and glycoprotein VI activation. Blood J Am Soc Hematol. 2013;121(15):3023–32.
35. Stavrou EX, Fang C, Merkulova A, Alhalabi O, Grobe N, Antoniak S, Mackman N, Schmaier AH. Reduced thrombosis in Klkb1−/− mice is mediated by increased Mas receptor, prostacyclin, Sirt1, and KLF4 and decreased tissue factor. Blood J Am Soc Hematol. 2015;125(4):710–9.
36. Jia H. Pulmonary angiotensin-converting enzyme 2 (ACE2) and inflammatory lung disease. Shock. 2016;46(3):239–48.
37. Irmscher S, Döring N, Halder LD, Jo EA, Kopka I, Dunker C, Jacobsen ID, Luo S, Slevogt H, Lorkowski S, Beyersdorf N. Kallikrein cleaves C3 and activates complement. J Innate Immun. 2018;10(2):94–105.
38. Sodhi CP, Wohlford-Lenane C, Yamaguchi Y, Prindle T, Fulton WB, Wang S, McCray PB Jr, Chappell M, Hackam DJ, Jia H. Attenuation of pulmonary ACE2 activity impairs inactivation of des-Arg9 bradykinin/BKB1R axis and facilitates LPS-induced neutrophil infiltration. Am J Physiol-Lung Cell Mol Physiol. 2018;314(1):L17–31.
39. Muñoz-Rodríguez C, Fernández S, Osorio JM, Olivares F, Anfossi R, Bolivar S, Humeres C, Boza P, Vivar R, Pardo-Jimenez V, Hemmings KE. Expression and function of TLR4-induced B1R bradykinin receptor on cardiac fibroblasts. Toxicol Appl Pharmacol. 2018;351:46–56.
40. Miyauchi T, Masaki T. Pathophysiology of endothelin in the cardiovascular system. Annu Rev Physiol. 1999;61:391.
41. Rautureau Y, Schiffrin EL. Endothelin in hypertension: an update. Curr Opin Nephrol Hypertens. 2012;21(2):128–36 [PubMed: 22257795].
42. Kowalczyk A, et al. The role of endothelin-1 and endothelin receptor antagonists in inflammatory response and sepsis. Arch Immunol Ther Exp (Warsz). 2015;63(1):41–52 [PubMed: 25288367].
43. Saleh MA, Pollock DM. Endothelin in renal inflammation and hypertension. Contrib Nephrol. 2011;172:160–70 [PubMed: 21893997].

44. De Miguel C, Pollock JS. Does endoplasmic reticulum stress mediate endothelin-1-induced renal inflammation? Am J Physiol Regul Integr Comp Physiol. 2013;305(2):R107–9 [PubMed: 23678028].
45. Rodeheffer RJ, Lerman A, Heublein DM, Burnett Jr JC. Increased plasma concentrations of endothelin in congestive heart failure in humans. Mayo Clini Proc. 1992;67(8):719–724. Elsevier.
46. Kiowski W, Kim J, Oechslin E, Sütsch G, Hunziker P, Müller P, Bertel O, Schmitt R, Jones R. Evidence for endothelin-1-mediated vasoconstriction in severe chronic heart failure. The Lancet. 1995;346(8977):732–6.
47. Rossi GP, Sacchetto A, Cesari M, Pessina AC. Interactions between endothelin-1 and the renin–angiotensin–aldosterone system. Cardiovasc Res. 1999;43(2):300–7.
48. Sharma R, Coats AJ, Anker SD. The role of inflammatory mediators in chronic heart failure: cytokines, nitric oxide, and endothelin-1. Int J Cardiol. 2000;72(2):175–86.
49. Kandasamy M. NF-κB signalling as a pharmacological target in COVID-19: potential roles for IKKβ inhibitors. Naunyn Schmiedebergs Arch Pharmacol. 2021;394(3):561–7.
50. Stow LR, Jacobs ME, Wingo CS, Cain BD. Endothelin-1 gene regulation. FASEB J. 2011;25(1):16–28.
51. Oeckinghaus A, Ghosh S. The NF-κB family of transcription factors and its regulation. Cold Spring Harbor Perspect Biol. 2009;1(4):a000034.
52. Dhaun N, Webb DJ. Endothelins in cardiovascular biology and therapeutics. Nat Rev Cardiol. 2019;16(8):491–502.
53. Ergul S, Parish DC, Puett D, Ergul A. Racial differences in plasma endothelin-1 concentrations in individuals with essential hypertension. Hypertension. 1996;28(4):652–5.
54. Packer M. The neurohormonal hypothesis: a theory to explain the mechanism of disease progression in heart failure. J Am Coll Cardiol. 1992;20:248–254. [PubMed] [Google Scholar.
55. Swedberg K. Importance of neuroendocrine activation in chronic heart failure. Impact on treatment strategies. Eur J Heart Fail. 2000;2:229–33. [PubMed] [Google Scholar].
56. Ramosand H, deBold AJ. Geneexpression, processing, and secretion of natriuretic peptides: physiologic and diagnostic implications. Heart Fail Clin. 2006;2(3):255–68.
57. Pfister R, Diedrichs H, Schiedermair A, Rosenkranz S, Hellmich M, Erdmann E, Schneider CA. Prognostic impact of NT-proBNP and renal function in comparison to contemporary multi-marker risk scores in heart failure patients. Eur J Heart Fail. 2008;10:315–20.
58. Ogawa T, de Bold AJ. Brain natriuretic Peptide production and secretion in inflammation. J Transplant. 2012;2012:962347. [PubMed].
59. Rudiger A, Gasser S, Fischler M, Hornemann T, von Eckardstein A, Maggiorini M. Comparable increase of B-type natriuretic peptide and amino-terminal pro-B-type natriuretic peptide levels in patients with severe sepsis, septic shock, and acute heart failure. Crit Care Med. 2006;34(8):2140–44.
60. Hoffmann U, Brueckmann M, Bertsch T, Wiessner M, Liebetrau C, Lang S, Haase KK, Borggrefe M, Huhle G. Increased plasma levels of NT-proANP and NT-proBNP as markers of cardiac dysfunction in septic patients. Clin Lab. 2005;51:373–9.
61. Jensen J, Ma L, Fu MLX, et al. Inflammation increases NT-proBNP and the NT-proBNP/BNP ratio. Clin Res Cardiol. 2010;99:445–52. https://doi.org/10.1007/s00392-010-0140-z.
62. Carotenuto F, Di Nardo P, Baldini PM. Brain Natriuretic Peptide (BNP) regulates the production of inflammatory mediators in human THP-1 macrophages. Regul Pept. 2008;148 (1–3):26–32. https://doi.org/10.1016/j.regpep.2008.02.009.
63. Maeda K, Tsutamoto T, Wada A, Mabuchi N, Hayashi M, Tsutsui T, Ohnishi M, Sawaki M, Fujii M, Matsumoto T, Kinoshita M. High levels of plasma brain natriuretic peptide and interleukin-6 after optimized treatment for heart failure are independent risk factors for morbidity and mortality in patients with congestive heart failure. J Am Coll Cardiol. 2000;36:1587–93. [PubMed] [Google Scholar].

64. Testa M, Yeh M, Lee P, Fanelli R, Loperfido F, Berman JW, LeJemtel TH. Circulating levels of cytokines and their endogenous modulators in patients with mild to severe congestive heart failure due to coronary artery disease or hypertension. J Am Coll Cardiol. 1996;28(4):964–71. [PubMed].
65. Omland T, Aakvaag A, Bonarjee VV, Caidahl K, Lie RT, Nilsen DW, Sundsfjord JA, Dickstein K. Plasma brain natriuretic peptide as an indicator of left ventricular systolic function and long-term survival after acute myocardial infarction. Comparison with plasma atrial natriuretic peptide and N-terminal proatrial natriuretic peptide. Circulation. 1996;93 (11):1963–9. [PubMed].
66. Chen T, Wu D, Chen H, Yan W, Yang D, Chen G, Ma K, Xu D, Yu H, Wang H, Wang T, Guo W, Chen J, Ding C, Zhang X, Huang J, Han M, Li S, Luo X, Zhao J, Ning Q. Clinical characteristics of 113 deceased patients with coronavirus disease 2019: retrospective study. BMJ. 2020;368:m1091. https://doi.org/10.1136/bmj.m1091. Erratum in: BMJ. 2020;368: m1295. PubMed PMID: 32217556.
67. Guo T, Fan Y, Chen M, et al. Cardiovascular implications of fatal out comes of patients with coronavirus disease 2019 (COVID-19). JAMA Cardiol. Published online March 27, 2020. https://doi.org/10.1001/jamacardio.2020.1017.
68. Yan Y, Yang Y, Wang F, et al. Clinical characteristics and outcomes of patients with severe covid-19 with diabetes. BMJ Open Diab Res Care. 2020;8:e001343. https://doi.org/10.1136/bmjdrc-2020-001343.
69. McDonagh TA, Metra M, Adamo M, Gardner RS, Baumbach A, Böhm M, Burri H, Butler J, Čelutkienė J, Chioncel O, Cleland JG. 2021 ESC Guidelines for the diagnosis and treatment of acute and chronic heart failure: Developed by the Task Force for the diagnosis and treatment of acute and chronic heart failure of the European Society of Cardiology (ESC) With the special contribution of the Heart Failure Association (HFA) of the ESC. European Heart Journal. 2021;42(36):3599–3726.
70. Li H, Liu L, Zhang D, Xu J, Dai H, Tang N, Su X, Cao B. SARS-CoV-2 and viral sepsis: observations and hypotheses. The Lancet. 2020;395(10235):1517–20.
71. Chen L, Li X, Chen M, Feng Y, Xiong C. The ACE2 expression in human heart indicates new potential mechanism of heart injury among patients infected with SARS-CoV-2. Cardiovasc Res. 2020;116(6):1097–100. https://doi.org/10.1093/cvr/cvaa078.
72. Bradley BT, Maioli H, Johnson R, Chaudhry I, Fink SL, Xu H, Najafian B, Marshall D, Lacy JM, Williams T, Yarid N. Histopathology and ultrastructural findings of fatal COVID-19 infections. MedRxiv. https://www.medrxiv.org/content/10.1101/2020.04.17.20058545v1.
73. Varga Z, Flammer AJ, Steiger P, et al. Endothelial cell infection and endotheliitis in COVID-19. Lancet. https://doi.org/10.1016/S0140-6736(20)30937-5.
74. Tavazzi G, Pellegrini C, Maurelli M, Belliato M, Sciutti F, Bottazzi A, Sepe PA, Resasco T, Camporotondo R, Bruno R, Baldanti F, Paolucci S, Pelenghi S, Iotti GA, Mojoli F, Arbustini E. Myocardial localization of coronavirus in COVID-19 cardiogenic shock. Eur J Heart Fail. 2020. https://doi.org/10.1002/ejhf.1828. epub ahead of print.
75. Lamphear BJ, Yan R, Yang F, Waters D, Liebig HD, Klump H, Kuechler E, Skern T, Rhoads RE. Mapping the cleavage site in protein synthesis initiation factor eIF-4 gamma of the 2A proteases from human coxsackievirus and rhinovirus. J Biol Chem. 1993;268:19200–3.
76. Liebig HD, Ziegler E, Yan R, Hartmuth K, Klump H, Kowalski H, Blaas D, Sommergruber W, Frasel L, Lamphear B. Purification of two picornaviral 2A proteinases: interaction with eIF-4 gamma and influence on in vitro translation. Biochemistry. 1993;32:7581–8.
77. Joachims M, Van Breugel PC, Lloyd RE. Cleavage of poly(A)-binding protein by enterovirus proteases concurrent with inhibition of translation in vitro. J Virol. 1999;73:718–27.
78. Garmaroudi FS, Marchant D, Hendry R, Luo H, Yang D, Ye X, Shi J, McManus BM. Coxsackievirus B3 replication and pathogenesis. Future Microbiol. 2015;10:629–53. https://doi.org/10.2217/fmb.15.5.

79. Esfandiarei M, McManus BM. Molecular biology and pathogenesis of viral myocarditis. Annu Rev Pathol. 2008;3:127–55. https://doi.org/10.1146/annurev.pathmechdis.3.121806.151534.
80. Luo H, Wong J, Wong B. Protein degradation systems in viral myocarditis leading to dilated cardiomyopathy. Cardiovasc Res. 2010;85:347–56. https://doi.org/10.1093/cvr/cvp225.
81. Wong J, Zhang J, Yanagawa B, Luo Z, Yang X, Chang J, McManus B, Luo H. Cleavage of serum response factor mediated by enteroviral protease 2A contributes to impaired cardiac function. Cell Res. 2012;22:360–71. https://doi.org/10.1038/cr.2011.114.
82. Knowlton KU. Coxsackievirus and adenovirus receptor (CAR) mediates atrioventricular-node function and connexin 45 localization in the murine heart. J Clin Invest. 2008;118:2758–70. https://doi.org/10.1172/JCI34777.
83. Lisewski U, Shi Y, Wrackmeyer U, Fischer R, Chen C, Schirdewan A, Jüttner R, Rathjen F, Poller W, Radke MH, Gotthardt M. The tight junction protein CAR regulates cardiac conduction and cell-cell communication. J Exp Med. 2008;205:2369–79. https://doi.org/10.1084/jem.20080897.
84. Coyne CB, Bergelson JM. Virus-induced Abl and Fyn kinase signals permit coxsackievirus entry through epithelial tight junctions. Cell. 2006;124:119–31. https://doi.org/10.1016/j.cell.2005.10.035.
85. Wang JP, Kurt-Jones EA, Finberg RW. Innate immunity to respiratory viruses. Cell Microbiol. 2007;9:1641–6.
86. Root-Bernstein R. Innate receptor activation patterns involving TLR and NLR synergisms in COVID-19, ALI/ARDS and sepsis cytokine storms: a review and model making novel predictions and therapeutic suggestions. Int J Mol Sci. 2021;22(4):2108.
87. Choudhury A, Mukherjee S. In silico studies on the comparative characterization of the interactions of SARS-CoV-2 spike glycoprotein with ACE-2 receptor homologs and human TLRs. J Med Virol. 2020;92(10):2105–13.
88. Qi YF, Zhang J, Wang L, Shenoy V, Krause E, Oh SP, Pepine CJ, Katovich MJ, Raizada MK. Angiotensin-converting enzyme 2 inhibits high-mobility group box 1 and attenuates cardiac dysfunction post-myocardial ischemia. J Mol Med. 2016;94(1):37–49.
89. Thankam FG, Dilisio MF, Dietz NE, Agrawal DK. TREM-1, HMGB1 and RAGE in the shoulder tendon: dual mechanisms for inflammation based on the coincidence of glenohumeral arthritis. PloS One. 2016;11(10):e0165492.
90. Thankam FG, Agrawal DK. Molecular chronicles of cytokine burst in COVID-19 patients with cardiovascular diseases; 2020.
91. Pittet JF, Griffiths MJ, Geiser T, Kaminski N, Dalton SL, Huang X, Brown LA, Gotwals PJ, Koteliansky VE, Matthay MA, Sheppard D. TGF-beta is a critical mediator of acute lung injury. J Clin Investig. 2001,107.1537 41.
92. Fairweather D, Yusung S, Frisancho S, Barrett M, Gatewood S, Steele R, Rose NR. IL-12 receptor beta 1 and Toll-like receptor 4 increase IL-1 beta- and IL-18-associated myocarditis and coxsackievirus replication. J Immunol. 2003;170:4731–7.
93. McCartney SA, Vermi W, Lonardi S, Rossini C, Otero K, Calderon B, Gilfillan S, Diamond MS, Unanue ER, Colonna M. RNA sensor-induced type I IFN prevents diabetes caused by a β cell-tropic virus in mice. J Clin Invest. 2011;121:1497–507. https://doi.org/10.1172/JCI44005.
94. Riad A, Westermann D, Escher F, Becher PM, Savvatis K, Lettau O, Heimesaat MM, Bereswill S, Volk HD, Schultheiss HP, Tschöpe C. Myeloid differentiation factor-88 contributes to TLR9-mediated modulation of acute coxsackievirus B3-induced myocarditis in vivo. Am J Physiol Heart Circ Physiol. 2010;298:H2024–31. https://doi.org/10.1152/ajpheart.01188.2009.
95. Rondina MT, Weyrich AS, Zimmerman GA. Platelets as cellular effectors of inflammation in vascular diseases. Circ Res. 2013;112:1506–19. https://doi.org/10.1161/CIRCRESAHA.113.300512PubMedAbstract|CrossRefFullText|GoogleScholar.

96. Rondina MT, Schwertz H, Harris ES, Kraemer BF, Campbell RA, Mackman N, et al. The septic milieu triggers expression of spliced tissue factor mRNA in human platelets. J Thromb Haemost. 2011;9:748–58. https://doi.org/10.1111/j.1538-7836.2011.04208.xPubMedAbstract|CrossRefFullText|GoogleScholar.
97. Matus V, Valenzuela JG, Hidalgo P, Pozo LM, Panes O, Wozniak A, et al. Human platelet interaction with E. coli O111 promotes tissue-factor-dependent procoagulant activity, involving Toll like receptor 4. PLoS One. 2017;12:e0185431. https://doi.org/10.1371/journal.pone.0185431. PubMed Abstract | CrossRef Full Text | Google Scholar.
98. Frantz S, Kobzik L, Kim YD, Fukazawa R, Medzhitov R, Lee RT, Kelly RA. Toll4 (TLR4) expression in cardiac myocytes in normal and failing myocardium. J Clin Invest. 1999;104:271–80. https://doi.org/10.1172/JCI6709.
99. Tavener SA, Long EM, Robbins SM, McRae KM, Van Remmen H, Kubes P. Immune cell Toll-like receptor 4 is required for cardiac myocyte impairment during endotoxemia. Circ Res. 2004;95:700–7. https://doi.org/10.1161/01.RES.0000144175.70140.8c.
100. Kawai T, Akira S. The role of pattern-recognition receptors in innate immunity: update on Toll-like receptors. Nat Immunol. 2010;11:373–84. https://doi.org/10.1038/ni.1863.
101. Freedman JE, Larson MG, Tanriverdi K, O'Donnell CJ, Morin K, Hakanson AS, Vasan RS, Johnson AD, Iafrati MD, Benjamin EJ. Relation of platelet and leukocyte inflammatory transcripts to body mass index in the Framingham heart study. Circulation. 2010;122:119–29. LinkGoogle Scholar.
102. Fung TS, Liu DX. Coronavirus infection, ER stress, apoptosis and innate immunity. Front Microbiol. 2014;5.
103. Fung TS, Liu DX. Human coronavirus: host-pathogen interaction. Annu Rev Microbiol. 2019;73:529–57.
104. Lim Y, Ng Y, Tam J, Liu D. Human coronaviruses: a review of virus-host interactions. Diseases. 2016;4:26.
105. Abdoli A, Alirezaei M, Mehrbod P, Forouzanfar F. Autophagy: the multi-purpose bridge in viral infections and host cells. Rev Med Virol. 2018;28:1–15.
106. Senft D, Ronai ZA. UPR, autophagy, and mitochondria crosstalk underlies the ER stress response. Trends Biochem Sci. 2015;40:141–8.
107. Grootjans J, Kaser A, Kaufman RJ, Blumberg RS. The unfolded protein response in immunity and inflammation. Nat Rev Immunol. 2016;16:469–84.
108. Lin JH, Walter P, Yen TS. Endoplasmic reticulum stress in disease pathogenesis. Annu Rev Pathol. 2008;3:399–425.
109. Yoshida H. ER stress and diseases. The FEBS Journal. 2007;274(3):630–658.
110. Szegezdi E, Logue SE, Gorman AM, Samali A. Mediators of endoplasmic reticulum stress-induced apoptosis. EMBO Rep. 2006;7(9):880–5.
111. Fung TS, Huang M, Liu DX. Coronavirus-induced ER stress response and its involvement in regulation of coronavirus–host interactions. Virus Res. 2014;194:110–23.
112. Marciniak SJ, Yun CY, Oyadomari S, Novoa I, Zhang Y, Jungreis R, Nagata K, Harding HP, Ron D. CHOP induces death by promoting protein synthesis and oxidation in the stressed endoplasmic reticulum. Genes Dev. 2004;18:3066–77.
113. Urano F, Wang X, Bertolotti A, Zhang Y, Chung P, Harding HP, Ron D. Coupling of stress in the ER to activation of JNK protein kinases by transmembrane protein kinase IRE1. Science. 2000;287:664–6.
114. Szegezdi E, Fitzgerald U, Samali A. Caspase-12 and ER-stress-mediated apoptosis: the story so far. Ann N Y Acad Sci. 2003;1010:186–94.
115. Sanbe A, Osinska H, Saffitz JE, Glabe CG, Kayed R, Maloyan A, Robbins J. Desmin-related cardiomyopathy in transgenic mice: a cardiac amyloidosis. Proc Natl Acad Sci U S A. 2004;101:10132–6. https://doi.org/10.1073/pnas.0401900101.131.
116. Weekes J, Morrison K, Mullen A, Wait R, Barton P, Dunn MJ. Hyperubiquitination of proteins in dilated cardiomyopathy. Proteomics. 2003;3:208–16. https://doi.org/10.1002/pmic.200390029.

117. Lenna S, Han R, Trojanowska M. Endoplasmic reticulum stress and endothelial dysfunction. IUBMB Life. 2014;66(8):530–7.
118. Haas MJ, Onstead-Haas L, Lee T, Torfah M, Mooradian AD. Angiotensin II receptor one (AT1) mediates dextrose induced endoplasmic reticulum stress and superoxide production in human coronary artery endothelial cells. Int J Cardiol. 2016;220:842–50.
119. Dennert R, Crijns HJ, Heymans S. Acute viral myocarditis. Eur Heart J. 2008;29(17):2073–82.
120. Knowlton KU. CVB infection and mechanisms of viral cardiomyopathy. Curr Top Microbiol Immunol. 2008;323:315–35.
121. Tam PE. Coxsackievirus myocarditis: interplay between virus and host in the pathogenesis of heart disease. Viral Immunol. 2006;19(2):133–46.
122. He B. Viruses, endoplasmic reticulum stress, and interferon responses. Cell Death Differ. 2006; 3(3):393–403.
123. Braakman I, van Anken E. Folding of viral envelope glycoproteins in the endoplasmic reticulum. Traffic. 2000;1(7):533–9.
124. Zhang K, Kaufman RJ. From endoplasmic-reticulum stress to the inflammatory response. Nature. 2008;454(7203):455–62.
125. Ozcan L, Tabas I. Role of endoplasmic reticulum stress in metabolic disease and other disorders. Annu Rev Med. 2012;63:317–28.
126. Biala AK, Kirshenbaum LA. The interplay between cell death signaling pathways in the heart. Trends Cardiovasc Med. 2014;24:325–31. https://doi.org/10.1016/j.tcm.2014.08.002.
127. Chen M, Wang J. Initiator caspases in apoptosis signaling pathways. Apoptosis. 2002;7 (4):313–9.
128. Fernández-Ruiz I. Microthrombi cause cardiac injury in COVID-19. Nat Rev Cardiol. 2021:1–1.
129. Jacobs W, Lammens M, Kerckhofs A, Voets E, Van San E, Van Coillie S, Peleman C, Mergeay M, Sirimsi S, Matheeussen V, Jansens H. Fatal lymphocytic cardiac damage in coronavirus disease 2019 (COVID-19): autopsy reveals a ferroptosis signature. ESC Heart Fail. 2020;7(6):3772–81.
130. Scarl RT, Balada-LIasat JM, Nowacki N, Solaro RJ, Williams J, Li J. Myocardial injury, inflammation and prothrombotic response are associated with outcomes of COVID-19 patients; 2021.
131. Kovacs SB, Miao EA. Gasdermins: effectors of pyroptosis. Trends Cell Biol. 2017;27 (9):673–84.
132. Christgen S, Zheng M, Kesavardhana S, Karki R, Malireddi RS, Banoth B, Place DE, Briard B, Sharma BR, Tuladhar S, Samir P. Identification of the PANoptosome: a molecular platform triggering pyroptosis, apoptosis, and necroptosis (PANoptosis). Front Cell Infect Microbiol. 2020;10.
133. Fornasari PM. SARS-CoV-2 protease-dependent human cell infection induces immunological response imbalance and neutrophils “Proteolytic Storm”. Proteolysis inhibitors can prevent and treat Covid-19. J Cardiol Res Rev Rep. 2021;SRC/JCRRR-139(2):135.https://doi.org/10.47363/JCRRR/2021.
134. Zheng M, Williams EP, Malireddi RS, Karki R, Banoth B, Burton A, Webby R, Channappanavar R, Jonsson CB, Kanneganti TD. Impaired NLRP3 inflammasome activation/pyroptosis leads to robust inflammatory cell death via caspase-8/RIPK3 during coronavirus infection. J Biol Chem. 2020;295(41):14040–52.
135. Karki R, Sharma BR, Tuladhar S, Williams EP, Zalduondo L, Samir P, Zheng M, Sundaram B, Banoth B, Malireddi RS, Schreiner P. Synergism of TNF-α and IFN-γ triggers inflammatory cell death, tissue damage, and mortality in SARS-CoV-2 infection and cytokine shock syndromes. Cell. 2021;184(1):149–68.
136. Taghiloo S, Aliyali M, Abedi S, Mehravaran H, Sharifpour A, Zaboli E, Eslami-Jouybari M, Ghasemian R, Vahedi-Larijani L, Hossein-Nattaj H, Amjadi O. Apoptosis and immunophenotyping of peripheral blood lymphocytes in Iranian COVID-19 patients: clinical and laboratory characteristics. J Med Virol. 2021;93(3):1589–98.

137. Kaminskyy V, Zhivotovsky B. To kill or be killed: how viruses interact with the cell death machinery. J Intern Med. 2010;267(5):473–82.
138. Roulston A, Marcellus RC, Branton PE. Viruses and apoptosis. Ann Rev Microbiol. 1999;53 (1):577–628.
139. Freundt EC, Yu L, Goldsmith CS, Welsh S, Cheng A, Yount B, Liu W, Frieman MB, Buchholz UJ, Screaton GR, Lippincott-Schwartz J. The open reading frame 3a protein of severe acute respiratory syndrome-associated coronavirus promotes membrane rearrangement and cell death. J Virol. 2010;84(2):1097–109.
140. Tajiri S, Oyadomari S, Yano S, Morioka M, Gotoh T, Hamada JI, Ushio Y, Mori M. Ischemia-induced neuronal cell death is mediated by the endoplasmic reticulum stress pathway involving CHOP. Cell Death Differ. 2004;11(4):403–15.
141. Nakagawa T, Zhu H, Morishima N, Li E, Xu J, Yankner BA, Yuan J. Caspase-12 mediates endoplasmic-reticulum-specific apoptosis and cytotoxicity by amyloid-beta. Nature. 2000;403(6765):98–103.
142. Rasheva VI, Domingos PM. Cellular responses to endoplasmic reticulum stress and apoptosis. Apoptosis. 2009;14(8):996–1007.
143. Ren Y, Shu T, Wu D, Mu J, Wang C, Huang M, Han Y, Zhang XY, Zhou W, Qiu Y, Zhou X. The ORF3a protein of SARS-CoV-2 induces apoptosis in cells. Cell Mol Immunol. 2020;17(8):881–3.
144. Haudek SB, Taffet GE, Schneider MD, Mann DL. TNF provokes cardiomyocyte apoptosis and cardiac remodeling through activation of multiple cell death pathways. J Clin Investig. 2007;117(9):2692–701.
145. Sharma A, Garcia G, Arumugaswami V, Svendsen CN (2020) Human iPSC-derived cardiomyocytes are susceptible to SARS CoV-2 infection. bioRxiv. 2020:2020.04.21.051912.
146. Darwish I, Mubareka S, Liles WC. Immunomodulatory therapy for severe influenza. Expert Rev Anti Infect Ther. 2011;9(7):807–22.
147. Ren Y, Sun C, Sun Y, Tan H, Wu Y, Cui B, Wu Z. PPAR gamma protects cardiomyocytes against oxidative stress and apoptosis via Bcl-2 upregulation.Vascul Pharmacol. 2009;51:169–174. https://doi.org/10.1016/j.vph.2009.06.004.
148. Kajstura J, Cigola E, Malhotra A, Li P, Cheng W, Meggs LG, Anversa P. Angiotensin II induces apoptosis of adult ventricular myocytes in vitro. J Mol Cell Cardiol. 1997;29 (3):859–70.
149. Kuo CY, Chiu YC, Lee AY, Hwang TL. Mitochondrial Lon protease controls ROS-dependent apoptosis in cardiomyocyte under hypoxia. Mitochondrion. 2015;23:7–16. https://doi.org/10.1016/j.mito.2015.04.004.
150. Toyozaki T, Hiroe M, Saito T, et al. Levels of soluble Fas in patients with myocarditis, heart failure of unknown origin, and in healthy volunteers. Am J Cardiol. 1998;81:798–800.
151. Toyozaki T, Hiroe M, Tanaka M, et al. Levels of soluble Fas ligand in myocarditis. Am J Cardiol. 1998;82:246–248.30313233.
152. Kagi D, Vignaux F, Ledermann B, et al. Fas and perforin pathways as major mechanisms of T cell-mediated cytotoxicity. Science. 1994;265:528–30.
153. Nagata S. Apoptosis by death factor. Cell. 1997;88:355–65.
154. Haunstetter A, Izumo S. Apoptosis: basic mechanisms and implications for cardiovascular disease. Circ Res. 1998;82:1111–29.
155. Ishiyama S, Hiroe M, Nishikawa T, et al. The Fas/Fas ligand system is involved in the pathogenesis of autoimmune myocarditis in rats. J Immunol. 1998;161:4695–701.
156. Fliss H, Gattinger D. Apoptosis in ischemic and reperfused rat myocardium. Circ Res. 1996;79:949–56.
157. Trauth BC, Klas C, Peters AM, Matzku S, Möller P, Falk W, Debatin KM, Krammer PH. Monoclonal antibody-mediated tumor regression by induction of apoptosis. Science. 1989;245(4915):301–5 PubMed PMID: 2787530.

158. Suda T, Takahashi T, Golstein P, Nagata S. Molecular cloning and expression of the Fas ligand, a novel member of the tumor necrosis factor family. Cell. 1993;75(6):1169–78 PubMed PMID: 7505205.
159. Woodruff JF. Viral myocarditis. A review. Am J Pathol. 1980;101:425–84.
160. Toyozaki T, Hiroe M, Tanaka M, et al. Levels of soluble Fas ligand in myocarditis. Am J Cardiol. 1998;82:246–8.
161. Nishigaki K, Minatoguchi S, Seishima M, et al. Plasma Fas ligand, an inducer of apoptosis, and plasma soluble Fas, an inhibitor of apoptosis, in patients with chronic congestive heart failure. J Am Coll Cardiol. 1997;29:1214–20.
162. Okuyama M, Yamaguchi S, Nozaki N, et al. Serum levels of soluble form of Fas molecule in patients with congestive heart failure. Am J Cardiol. 1997;79:1698–701.
163. Kawakami H, Shigematsu Y, Ohtsuka T, et al. Increased circulating soluble form of Fas in patients with dilated cardiomyopathy. Jpn Circ J. 1998;62:873–6.
164. Yamaguchi S, Yamada M, Okuyama M, et al. Elevated circulating levels and cardiac secretion of soluble Fas ligand in patients with congestive heart failure. Am J Cardiol. 1999;83:1500–3.
165. Sheppard R, Bedi M, Kubota T, Semigran MJ, Dec W, Holubkov R, Feldman AM, Rosenblum WD, McTiernan CF, McNamara DM, IMAC Investigators. Myocardial expression of Fas and recovery of left ventricular function in patients with recent onset cardiomyopathy. J Am Coll Cardiol. 2005;46(6):1036–42.
166. Nishii M, Inomata T, Takehana H, Takeuchi I, Nakano H, Koitabashi T, Nakahata J, Aoyama N, Izumi TJ. Serum levels of interleukin-10 on admission as a prognostic predictor of human fulminant myocarditis. Am Coll Cardiol. 2004;44(6):1292–7.
167. Dhein J, Walczak H, Bäumler C, Debatin KM, Krammer PH. Autocrine T-cell suicide mediated by APO-1/(Fas/CD95). Nature. 1995;373(6513):438–41. PubMed PMID: 7530335.
168. Chen RF, Chang JC, Yeh WT, Lee CH, Liu JW, Eng HL, Yang KD. Role of vascular cell adhesion molecules and leukocyte apoptosis in the lymphopenia and thrombocytopenia of patients with severe acute respiratory syndrome (SARS). Microbes Infect. 2006;8(1):122–7.
169. Cho YS, Park SY, Shin HS, Chan FK. Physiological consequences of programmed necrosis, an alternative form of cell demise. Mol Cells. 2010;29:327–32. https://doi.org/10.1007/s10059-010-0066.
170. Zhang W, Lavine KJ, Epelman S, Evans SA, Weinheimer CJ, Barger PM, Mann DL. J Am Heart Assoc. 2015;4(6):e001993.
171. Epelman S, Liu PP, Mann DL. Role of innate and adaptive immune mechanisms in cardiac injury and repair. Nat Rev Immunol. 2015;15(2):117–29. [PubMed] [Ref list].
172. Linkermann A, Green DR. Necroptosis. N Engl J Med. 2014;370(5):455–65.
173. Hanson B. Necroptosis: a new way of dying? Cancer Biol Ther. 2016;17(9):899–910.
174. Nakamura H, Kinjo T, Arakaki W, Miyagi K, Tateyama M, Fujita J. Serum levels of receptor-interacting protein kinase-3 in patients with COVID-19. Crit Care. 2020;24(1):1–3.
175. DeRoo E, Zhou T, Liu B. The Role of RIPK1 and RIPK3 in Cardiovascular Disease. Int J Mol Sci. 2020;21(21):8174.
176. Ferdous A, Battiprolu PK, Ni YG, Rothermel BA, Hill JA. FoxO, autophagy, and cardiac remodeling. J Cardiovasc Transl Res. 2010;3:355–64. [CrossRef] [PubMed].
177. Xie M, Morales CR, Lavandero S, Hill JA. Tuning flux: autophagy as a target of heart disease therapy. Curr Opin Cardiol. 2011;26:216–22. [CrossRef] [PubMed].
178. Ma X, Liu H, Foyil SR, Godar RJ, Weinheimer CJ, Hill JA, Diwan A. Impaired autophagosome clearance contributes to cardiomyocyte death in ischemia/reperfusion injury. Circulation. 2012;125(25):3170–81. [PubMed] [Ref list].
179. Carmona-Gutierrez D, Bauer MA, Zimmermann A, Kainz K, Hofer SJ, Kroemer G, Madeo F. Digesting the crisis: autophagy and coronaviruses. Microbial Cell. 2020;7(5):119.
180. Shojaei S, Suresh M, Klionsky DJ, Labouta HI, Ghavami S. Autophagy and SARS-CoV-2 infection: a possible smart targeting of the autophagy pathway; 2020.

181. Benvenuto D, Angeletti S, Giovanetti M, Bianchi M, Pascarella S, Cauda R, Ciccozzi M, Cassone A. Evolutionary analysis of SARS-CoV-2: how mutation of Non-Structural Protein 6 (NSP6) could affect viral autophagy. J Infect. 2020;81(1):e24–7.
182. Rothermel BA, Hill JA. Myocyte autophagy in heart disease: friend or foe? Autophagy. 2007;3:632–4.
183. Mijaljica D, Klionsky DJ. Autophagy/virophagy: a "disposal strategy" to combat COVID-19; 2020.
184. Lin L. et al. An NLRP3 inflammasome-triggered cytokine storm contributes to streptococcal toxic shock-like syndrome (STSLS). PLoS Pathog. 2019; 15.
185. Chen C. et al. Thalidomide combined with low-dose glucocorticoid in the treatment of COVID-19 pneumonia. 1–6; 2020. Preprints.
186. van den Berg DF, Te Velde AA. Severe COVID-19: NLRP3 inflammasome dysregulated. Front Immunol. 2020;11:1580.
187. Gaidt MM, Hornung V. The NLRP3 inflammasome renders cell death pro-inflammatory. J Mol Biol. 2018;430(2):133–41.
188. Aachoui Y, Sagulenko V, Miao EA, Stacey KJ. Inflammasome-mediated pyroptotic and apoptotic cell death, and defense against infection. Curr Opin Microbiol. 2013;16(3): 319–26.
189. He Y, Hara H, Núñez G. Mechanism and regulation of NLRP3 inflammasome activation. Trends Biochem Sci. 2016;41(12):1012–21.
190. Freeman TL, Swartz TH. Targeting the NLRP3 inflammasome in severe COVID-19. Front Immunol. 2020;11:1518.
191. Nabirotchkin S, Peluffo AE, Bouaziz J, Cohen D. Focusing on the unfolded protein response and autophagy related pathways to reposition common approved drugs against COVID-19; 2020. Preprints 2020, 2020030302. https://doi.org/10.20944/preprints202003.0302.v1.
192. Li B, Liu Y, Hu T, Zhang Y, Zhang C, Li T, Wang C, Dong Z, Novakovic VA, Hu T, Shi J. Neutrophil extracellular traps enhance procoagulant activity in patients with oral squamous cell carcinoma. J Cancer Res Clin Oncol. 2019;145:1695–707.
193. Zuo Y, Yalavarthi S, Shi H, Gockman K, Zuo M, Madison JA, Blair CN, Weber A, Barnes BJ, Egeblad M, Woods RJ, Kanthi Y, Knight JS. Neutrophil extracellular traps in COVID-19. JCI Insight. 2020. https://doi.org/10.1172/jci.insight.138999.
194. Nakazawa F, Kannemeier C, Shibamiya A, Song Y, Tzima E, Schubert U, Koyama T, Niepmann M, Trusheim H, Engelmann B, Preissner KT. Extracellular RNA is a natural cofactor for the (auto-)activation of factor VII-activating protease (FSAP). Biochem J. 2005;385:831–8.
195. Sawadogo SA, Dighero-Kemp B, Ouédraogo DD, Hensley L, Sakandé J. How NETosis could drive "Post-COVID-19 syndrome" among survivors. Immunol Lett. 2020.
196. ClinicalTrials.gov. Covid-19: Possible Role of Neutrophil Extracellular Traps (NETSINCOVID) Identifier: NCT04412382. Last updated June 02, 2020.
197. Jia G, Aroor AR, Sowers JR. Estrogen and mitochondria function in cardiorenal metabolic syndrome. Prog Mol Biol Transl Sci. 2014;127:229–49.
198. Kayar SR, Banchero N. Volume density and distribution of mitochondria in myocardial growth and hypertrophy. Respir Physiol. 1987;70:275–86. [CrossRef].
199. Galluzzi L, Kepp O, Trojel-Hansen C, et al. Mitochondrial control of cellular life, stress, and death. Circ Res. 2012;111:1198–207.
200. Anand SK, Tikoo SK. Viruses as modulators of mitochondrial functions. Adv Virol. 2013;2013.
201. Claus C, Liebert UG. A renewed focus on the interplay between viruses and mitochondrial metabolism. Arch Virol. 2014;159(6):1267–77.
202. Glingston RS, Deb R, Kumar S, Nagotu S. Organelle dynamics and viral infections: at cross roads. Microbes infect. 2019;21(1):20–32.
203. Loffredo L, Violi F. COVID-19 and cardiovascular injury: a role for oxidative stress and antioxidant treatment? Int J Cardiol. 2020;312:136.

204. Delgado-Roche L, Mesta F. Oxidative stress as key player in severe acute respiratory syndrome coronavirus (SARS-CoV) infection. Arch Med Res. 2020.
205. Shenoy S. Coronavirus (Covid-19) sepsis: revisiting mitochondrial dysfunction in pathogenesis, aging, inflammation, and mortality. Inflamm Res. 2020:1–9.
206. Violi F, Oliva A, Cangemi R, Ceccarelli G, Pignatelli P, Carnevale R, Cammisotto V, Lichtner M, Alessandri F, De Angelis M, Miele MC. Nox2 activation in Covid-19. Redox Biol 2020;36:101655.
207. Doughan AK, Harrison DG, Dikalov SI. Molecular mechanisms of angiotensin II-mediated mitochondrial dysfunction: linking mitochondrial oxidative damage and vascular endothelial dysfunction. Circ Res. 2008;102:488–96.
208. Indo HP, Yen HC, Nakanishi I, Matsumoto KI, Tamura M, Nagano Y, Matsui H, Gusev O, Cornette R, Okuda T, Minamiyama Y. A mitochondrial superoxide theory for oxidative stress diseases and aging. J Clin Biochem Nutr. 2015;56(1):1–7.
209. Yao X, Carlson D, Sun Y, Ma L, Wolf SE, Minei JP, Zang QS. Mitochondrial ROS induces cardiac inflammation via a pathway through mtDNA damage in a pneumonia-related sepsis model. PLoS One. 2015;10:e0139416. [CrossRef] [PubMed].
210. Chakraborty K, Raundhal M, Chen BB, Morse C, Tyurina YY, Khare A, Oriss TB, Huff R, Lee JS, St Croix CM, et al. The mito-DAMP cardiolipin blocks IL-10 production causing persistent inflammation during bacterial pneumonia. Nat Commun. 2017;8:13944. [CrossRef].
211. Eleftheriadis T, Pissas G, Liakopoulos V, Stefanidis I. Cytochrome c as a potentially clinical useful marker of mitochondrial and cellular damage. Front Immunol. 2016;7:279. [CrossRef] [PubMed].
212. Jiang HK, Wang YH, Sun L, et al. Aerobic interval training attenuates mitochondrial dysfunction in rats postmyocardial infarction: roles of mitochondrial network dynamics. Int J Mol Sci. 2014;15:5304–22.
213. Schönrich G, Raftery MJ, Samstag Y. Devilishly radical NETwork in COVID-19: oxidative stress, neutrophil extracellular traps (NETs), and T cell suppression. Adv Biol Regul. 2020;77:100741.
214. Ronco C, Reis T. Kidney involvement in COVID-19 and rationale for extracorporeal therapies. Nat Rev Nephrol. 2020;16(6):308–10.
215. Panitchote A, Mehkri O, Hastings A, Hanane T, Demirjian S, Torbic H, Mireles-Cabodevila E, Krishnan S, Duggal A. Factors associated with acute kidney injury in acute respiratory distress syndrome. Ann Intensiv Care 2019;9(1):1–10.
216. Abassi Z, Skorecki K, Hamo-Giladi DB, Kruzel-Davila E, Heyman SN. Kinins and chymase: the forgotten components of the renin-angiotensin system and their implications in COVID-19 disease. Am J Physiol-Lung Cell Mol Physiol. 2021;320(3):L422–9.
217. Fujita S, Shimojo N, Terasaki F, Otsuka K, Hosotani N, Kohda Y, Tanaka T, Nishioka T, Yoshida T, Hiroe M, Kitaura Y. Atrial natriuretic peptide exerts protective action against angiotensin II-induced cardiac remodeling by attenuating inflammation via endothelin-1/ endothelin receptor A cascade. Heart Vessel. 2013;28(5):646–57.

Chapter 11
Myocardial Injury in CoViD19

Key Questions

- What is a myocardial injury in CoViD19?
- What is the occurrence of myocardial injury in CoViD19?
- What are the variabilities in the presentation of myocardial injury in CoViD19?
- What are the key challenges in the recognition of myocardial injury in CoViD19?
- Which biomarker may help recognize myocardial injury in CoViD19?
- What are the prognostic implications of myocardial injury in CoViD19?
- Which crucial pathogenetic mechanisms lead to myocardial injury in CoViD19?

11.1 Introduction

Cardiovascular diseases are common worldwide and pose a significant risk of death and morbidity burden [1]. The CoViD19 patients especially those with severe disease may exhibit multi-systemic complications, among which the obstructive and non-obstructive cardiovascular diseases constitute a significant proportion of the morbidity and mortality associated with CoViD19 [2–4]. Myocardial injury is defined by at least one cardiac troponin concentration above the 99th percentile upper reference limit [5]. Data indicate that the development of the myocardial injury in CoViD19 is associated with poor prognosis [6].

The cardiovascular manifestations of the CoViD19 exhibit significant variabilities and complexities (Fig. 11.1). The complications such as uncontrolled blood

U. Mallick, *Cardiovascular Complications of COVID-19*,
https://doi.org/10.1007/978-3-030-90065-6_11

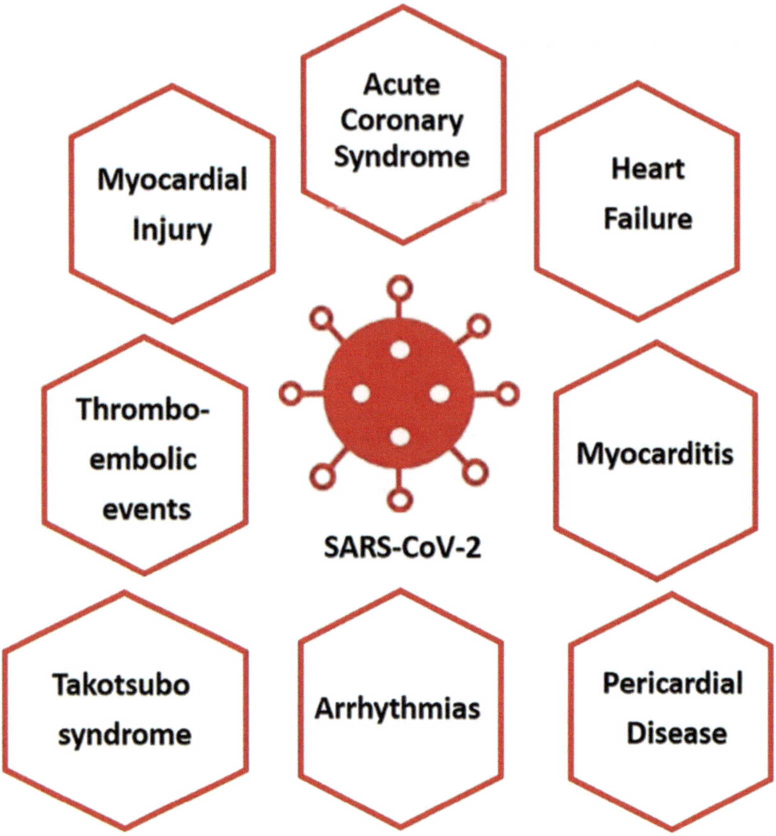

Fig. 11.1 Cardiovascular involvement in CoViD19. *Source* Figure 1. Polito, M.V., Silverio, A., Bellino, M. et al. Cardiovascular Involvement in COVID-19: What Sequelae Should We Expect? Cardiol Ther (2021). https://doi.org/10.1007/s40119-021-00232-8. https://link.springer.com/article/10.1007/s40119-021-00232-8. Published by Springer Nature

pressure, myocarditis, acute coronary events, acute cardiac failure, and arrhythmias or cardiogenic shock, are among several acute forms of cardiovascular complications that are found in association with severe CoViD19 [7, 8]. Nonspecific forms of myocardial injury, and non-ischemic cardiomyopathy, and sporadic cases of stress cardiomyopathy or Tako-Tsubo and coronary spasm have also been reported [9–11].

Uncertainties exist about the actual frequency of cardiovascular disease in CoViD19 patients. It is estimated that about 13–41% of patients with severe CoViD19 develop cardiovascular injury [12]. According to a meta-analysis of 53 studies involving 7,679 CoViD19 patients, about 21% of patients had the myocardial injury, and the severity of the disease was associated with a 4.74-fold increase in the risk of myocardial injury [13]. Several factors such as heterogeneity amongst the studies, confounding, lack of troponin standardized assays, or insufficient troponin evaluations are among several factors that may have led to an underestimation of the incidence of myocardial injury in CoViD19.

A significant amount of data reveal epidemiology and complex pathogenicity of the cardiovascular complications in CoViD19. Several obscurities revolve around defining the myocardial injury, the pathogenesis as well as its implications, which have presented as a challenge to the clinicians and the researchers. The CoViD19 patients on invasive therapies are more prone to cardiac injury due to increased stress factors such as hypoxemia, acid–base imbalance, metabolic stress, and mechanical and invasive procedures. Data from pathology and advanced cardiac imaging reports in the CoViD19 patients reveal various patterns of myocardial inflammation and indicate the presence of myocardial damage, supporting the occurrence of the myocardial injury in CoViD19 patients during the disease and post convalescence [8, 14]. However, several gaps exist in the knowledge, hence the term of non-specific myocardial injury has been used to describe the myocardial injury in CoViD19. The short-term and long-term outcomes of the myocardial injury in CoViD19 remain unclear. Further efforts are needed to draw plausible and concrete information.

Patients with acute coronary syndromes with CoViD19 have poor outcomes [15]. The acute coronary syndromes include the ST elevation and non-ST elevation myocardial infarction and unstable angina, are recognized as part of the classical spectrum of acute coronary pathology [16], although showed a considerable decline in the incidence during the CoViD19 pandemic [17], constitute a significant position among the CoViD19 complications, warranting further exploration.

This chapter is aimed to improve the current understanding of myocardial injury a frequent and potentially life-threatening complication of CoViD19. We present an overview of this potentially life-threatening complication of CoViD19, highlighting important epidemiological features, prognostic aspects, variabilities in the presentation, and explore the associated clinical impact. We describe several challenges faced by the healthcare community in recognition of the myocardial injury, including those related to the behavior of the associated biomarkers, as well as important mechanisms involved in the pathogenesis.

11.2 Epidemiology of Myocardial Injury

Myocardial injury is a common complication in patients with exacerbation of CoViD19 with higher rates of comorbidity and mortality [18]. Although several reports indicate a high incidence of myocardial injury in CoViD19 patients, controversies have been reported. Reports indicate that the incidence of myocardial injury may not be accurately estimated in CoViD19 studies [19] due to non-systematic use of cardiac-specific biomarkers such as hs-troponin (high-sensitivity cardiac troponin) and specific diagnostic tools in CoViD19 studies. Among the initial reports of the emerging pandemic, a much higher incidence of myocardial injury was reported. Analysis of a retrospective cohort of 54 patients admitted with CoViD19, shows myocardial injury developed in 24 (44.4%) of the patients, and 26 (48.1%) patients died in hospital. The death rate was higher in patients with myocardial injury as compared to those without 14 (60.9%) versus 8 (25.8%) respectively [20]. Another retrospective case series study of a cohort of 187 patients admitted with CoViD19 show a higher incidence of myocardial injury 27.8% (52/187), and a higher in-hospital mortality rate 59.6% (31/52) in those with elevated TnT levels compared with 8.9% (12 of 135) in those with normal TnT levels [21].

However, data from several pooled analyses reports indicate the incidence of myocardial injury in CoViD19 is around 20% [13, 22]. In a review of 26 CoViD19 studies including 11,685 patients, the weighted pooled prevalence of acute myocardial injury was 20% (ranged from 5 to 38% depending on the criteria used) [22] Another meta-analysis of 26 studies consisting of 8761 CoViD19 patients indicated an incidence of myocardial injury at 16.1–23.8% [23]. In a Chinese cohort of 416 patients admitted with CoViD19 about 19.7% (82) were reported to have a myocardial injury, had a significantly higher in-hospital mortality rate 51.2% (42 of 82) compared with those without myocardial injury 4.5% (15 of 335) [24]. Most of these studies indicate an association of increased mortality in CoViD19 patients with myocardial injury.

The pre-existing cardiovascular conditions increase the risk of death in hospitalized CoViD19 patients [25]. Several studies show an increased incidence of pre-existing cardiovascular metabolic risk factors in patients who develop a myocardial injury in CoViD19 [26, 27]. The risk has been reported to be higher in patients with previous cardiovascular disease or with older age, hypertension, diabetes mellitus or raised BMI [28, 29].

The myocardial injury is an important prognostic factor of CoViD19. According to a retrospective analysis of a cohort of 202 CoViD19 patients, the myocardial injury may increase the risk of death about five times ($HR = 5.382$, 95%CI 2.404–12.050, $P < 0.001$) [30]. However, the extent of the CV injury, along with associated short and long-term sequelae remains unclear. Studies indicate the persistence of post CoViD19 myocardial sequelae in a significant proportion of recovered patients. A prospective observational cohort study of 100 patients recently recovered from CoViD19 illness indicated cardiac involvement in 78 of 100 patients (78%) and ongoing myocardial inflammation in 60 of 100 patients (60%), independent of preexisting conditions, severity, and overall course of the acute illness, and time from the original diagnosis [14]. Studies show that patients with CoViD19 and myocardial injury may have a worse prognosis compared to the patients with non-CoViD19 ARDS pneumonia with myocardial injury indicating implication of other mechanisms or role of baseline comorbidities [31].

Significant variabilities exist in the forms of presentation of myocardial injury in CoViD19. The exact incidence of these forms is not well known. Among these include myocarditis and myopericarditis [32] or several forms of myocarditis such as acute, fulminant, or autoimmune myocarditis [33–35], or other forms of myocardial injury such as stress cardiomyopathy or Tako-Tsubo, and myocardial infarction with non-obstructive arteries [36].

Although the incidence of a severe and rapidly progressive form of myocarditis known as "fulminant myocarditis" is not well documented in CoViD19, sporadic cases and case reports describe the occurrence of this complication [37, 38] According to a study, the incidence of fulminant myocarditis was suspected in 7% of patients with a lethal outcome [39]. The intense immune- inflammatory turbulence in severe CoViD19 may drive the development of these complications through the infiltration of the myocardial tissue accompanied by myocardial structural and functional damage and hemodynamic compromise [40].

Several studies explore, the epidemiological relationship between the incidence of myocardial injury in CoViD19 patients with ARDS or other organic complications and prognostic implications. In a retrospective cohort study of 386 hospitalized CoViD19 patients investigating cardiac injury and mortality, about 70/386 (19.7%) patients with ARDS, 46/115 (40.0%) had a cardiac injury as compared to 30/271 (11.1%) patients without cardiac injury (<0.001) [41]. Other analyses further highlight the implications of CoViD19 related complications such as acute respiratory distress syndrome (ARDS) in relation to myocardial injury and mortality. The ARDS may pose a considerable risk towards mortality in patients with CoViD19 with cardiac injury [26, 41]. Although the reports clearly describe an increase in mortality risk in CoViD19 patients when a myocardial injury is present in these reports, others suggest a lack of association of the cardiac injury with an increased risk of ARDS or acute kidney injury (AKI) [42, 43]. According to a meta-analysis of 2389 CoViD19 patients from 13 studies exploring the association between cardiac injury and mortality, the cardiac injury was not significant for increased risk of ARDS (RR 2.57 [0.96, 6.85], $p = 0.06$; I^2: 84%) [43]. However, the report was further debated and controversies raised [44]. A retrospective analysis of 243 CoViD19 intubated patients and a subset of 506 patients with ARDS related to primary pneumonia was reported. In this report, the comparison of the incidence of the myocardial injury in CoViD19 patients with non CoViD19 ARDS pneumonia patients revealed similar rates between the two groups, however, after adjusting for the confounders such as age, renal impairment, and severity of illness, a lower incidence of the myocardial injury was noted in COVID19, indicating that mortality in CoViD19 myocardial injury may be related to the criticality of the illness [31]. The study further confirmed that elevation of serum troponin levels is associated with higher mortality in the CoViD19 group and among the non-survivors.

11.3 Definition, Presentation, and Challenges of Myocardial Injury

The actual definition of the myocardial injury, pathogenesis, and implications in CoViD19 patients, remain obscure due to several associated challenges in recognition and diagnostics and other factors. The variations in the manifestations of CoViD19 related cardiovascular disease particularly present an important challenge in the clinical settings. The multi-factorial nature of the cardiac harm, lack of robust data from dedicated clinical trials, non-systematic use of cardiac biomarkers in CoViD19 studies, lack of angiographic data, confounding, and several other factors including variabilities in the presentation, add to the perplexity in defining the myocardial injury in CoViD19 patients.

Multiple diagnostic complexities may be found in association with myocardial injury in CoViD19. The patients with CoViD19 may present with a variety of forms of myocardial injury, such as acute myocarditis, cardiogenic shock, with or without a hyperinflammatory picture or a previous history of CVD, or with mild or no respiratory symptoms [45]. Distinguishing between the clinical forms of myocardial injury, such as acute myocarditis or peri myocarditis and acute coronary syndromes may prove difficult for clinicians treating patients with CoViD19. Such challenges have been reported in the critical care settings in CoViD19 management. Data analysis of 22 CoViD19 patients admitted in the ICU showed 33% (7/22) patients had cardiomyopathy (defined based on clinical, echocardiographic, and biochemical parameters) of uncertain etiology [46].

Myocarditis has been proposed as an important entity among several mechanisms behind myocardial injury in CoViD19. The occurrence of myocarditis and myopericarditis as forms of presentation of the myocardial injury in CoViD19 patients is much debated [32]. Several forms of myocarditis such as acute, fulminant, or autoimmune myocarditis have been presented in the literature in association with CoViD19 [33–35]. Moreover, other forms of myocardial injury such as stress cardiomyopathy or Tako-Tsubo, and myocardial infarction with non-obstructive arteries have also been described among CoViD19 patients [36]. In a series of patients with CoViD19, who had ST-segment elevation, there was variability in the presentation, a high prevalence of non-obstructive disease, and a poor prognosis [47].

The myocardial injury in CoViD19 patients may be new or exacerbation of a pre-existing disease. Several studies report the occurrence of neo-cardiovascular disease in patients with CoViD19. According to a study involving patients who recovered from CoViD19, about a quarter of the patients had ischemic heart disease, the majority had no previous history of cardiovascular illness [48]. About 11.8% of patients, without underlying CVD among people who died from CoViD19, had substantial heart damage, (with elevated levels of cTnI or cardiac arrest during hospitalization) [15, 27].

11.4 Timing and Assessment of Myocardial Injury

The cardiovascular symptoms may be predominantly present at the time of initial patient presentation or may develop during the disease. According to a review, two patterns of myocardial injury have been described in CoViD19 indicating significant differences in the troponin levels between the survivors and non-survivors, and continuous tracking of troponin by the markers of inflammation among the non-survivors [49]. The involvement of different pathogenetic mechanisms in various stages of CoViD19 may reflect the temporal association of these mechanisms with the development of myocardial injury. An initial presentation of CoViD19 patients with predominantly cardiac symptomatology or development of the myocardial injury in a hospitalized patient at a later stage may reflect different pathogenetic routes.

Assessment of the myocardial injury and defining it in patients with CoViD19 may be a challenge. The myocardial injury may be associated with biochemical, electrical, structural, and functional modifications, recognized and assessed by different diagnostic techniques. A comprehensive analysis of the electrocardiographic, serum immunopathology, cardiac and coronary imaging indexes in addition to the neurohormonal and biochemical markers of myocardial injury is vital to accurately define the myocardial injury. Advanced imaging modalities such as cardiac magnetic resonance (CMR) imaging further provide a detailed assessment of the CoViD19 associated damage to the myocardium [50]. Studies have shown identifiable mechanisms in CoViD19 patients with elevated hsTnT, non-specific myocardial injury (with no cause of myocardial scarring in past) on CMR, classified as nonischemic heart disease-related, ischemic heart disease-related, or dual ischemic and non-ischemic pathology [51], and patterns of myocarditis [52].

Misclassification of myocardial injury as myocardial infarction has been previously reported [53]. The myocardial injury is defined by at least 1 cardiac troponin concentration above the 99th percentile upper reference limit [5]. Troponin elevation are most commonly caused by nonischemic myocardial injury, and type 2 myocardial infarction and myocardial injury, have poor short-term outcomes, with mortality rates >20% at 2 years [54]. Absence of ischemia determines the distinction between myocardial infarction and myocardial injury, with and without, respectively. Due to the intricacies in the definition of myocardial injury, interpretation of the term "myocardial injury" requires a cautious approach, in CoViD19 studies describing cardiac injury.

11.5 Biomarkers of Myocardial Injury

Serum troponin measurements provide means for important biochemical assessment of the myocardial damage. Data show that about 20% of CoViD19 hospitalized patients manifest a rise in troponin values [26]. The CoViD19 studies reporting cardiac injury utilize troponin as a marker of myocardial injury, however, controversies have been reported. The standardized parameter of troponin measurements used in diagnosing the myocardial injury, represented by a rise above the 99th percentile upper reference limit (URL), of serum high-sensitive cardiac troponin using standard assays, is utilized in most CoViD19 studies [55, 56]. However, reports suggest that troponin values exceeding the 99th percentile in the upper reference limit (URL) can only be observed in 8–12% of positive cases [57]. The controversies related to the use of troponin in studies reporting a myocardial injury in CoViD19 patients also appear to be related to timing or sequential use of troponins, non-systematic and selective use of troponin in CoViD19 studies, and other confounding factors [26, 58].

Elevated serum troponin levels are associated with higher mortality in CoViD19 and the presence of a cardiac injury detected by a rise in troponin is associated with a high risk of death in CoViD19 patients [26]. In a retrospective case series study of a cohort of 187 patients admitted with CoViD19, about 28% had elevated troponin levels and it was associated with higher mortality as compared to those with normal levels 9.6% versus 8.9%, respectively ($P < 0.001$) [59]. Patients with advanced CoViD19 with more critical illness more often have higher troponin levels [4]. Previous analyses report a higher frequency of elevated troponins in critically ill patients and prognostic significance and show that troponin is an independent predictor of mortality [60]. The rates of death may be much higher in CoViD19 patients with elevated troponin with a previous history of cardiovascular diseases [61].

The troponin elevations are common in many disease states such as acute peri-myocarditis, Tako-Tsubo, acute heart failure, and tachycardia. The troponin levels may also be elevated due to several non-cardiac conditions such as stroke, pulmonary embolism, sepsis, and renal failure. Since complicated CoViD19 accompanies a significant thromboembolic strain in the pulmonary vasculature, in the presence of associated right heart strain [62], the elevation of biochemical markers of myocardial injury might reflect cardiac injury related to these conditions.

Reports suggest that concomitant use of the markers of thrombosis and inflammation may be valuable in diagnosing the myocardial injury, staging of CoViD19, and risk stratification in CoViD19 patients [63]. The elevations of troponin may reflect a systemic illness in the advanced COVID-19 [64]. In critically ill patients, concomitant use of multiple biomarkers and diagnostic tools may facilitate improved recognition of the cardiac injury.

Although elevated serum troponin values are useful in detecting the myocardial injury in CoViD19, serum NT pro-BNP, markers of inflammation such as C reactive protein (CRP) or pro-inflammatory cytokines, and markers of thrombosis, and others may be utilized (Fig. 11.4). Several classical biomarkers of myocardial injury and inflammation have shown a powerful association with myocardial injury in patients with CoViD19 [21, 65]. According to a study, the extent of troponin elevation in CoViD19 patients modestly corresponded to the degree of elevation of high-sensitivity CRP (hsCRP) [66]. Elevated serum levels of Troponin T/I as a biomarker of myocardial injury, raised CRP and NT Pro BNP as markers of inflammation and myocardial dysfunction respectively, have been shown to have a positive association with the severity of CoViD19, also reflect a strong interlink between the inflammation, myocardial injury and ventricular dysfunction [66]. An elevation in the D-dimer, CK-MB, Troponin I, and CRP may reflect short-term mortality risk in patients with COVID-19 pneumonia [67]. A meta-analysis of 14 studies involving 3175 CoViD19 patients explored the association of CoViD19 related cardiac injury and outcome, confirmed the association of the elevated serum troponins, myoglobin, CK-MB, and NT-pro BNP levels in CoViD19 non-survivors as compared to the survivors. The levels of hs-cTnI (MD:34.54 pg/ml; 95% CI: 24.67 to 44.40 pg/ml; $I^2 = 88\%$), myoglobin (MD:186.81 ng/ml; 95% CI: 121.52 to 252.10 ng/ml; $I^2 = 88\%$), NT-pro BNP (MD:1183.55 pg/ml; 95% CI: 520.19 to 1846.91 pg/ml: $I^2 = 96\%$) and CK-MB (MD:2.49 ng/ml; 95% CI: 1.86 to 3.12 ng/ml; $I^2 = 90\%$) were significantly elevated among with non-survivors versus survivors with CoViD19 [42]. According to another meta-analysis of 29 CoViD19 studies exploring relationships between several cardiac markers and CoViD19 severity and mortality, the biomarkers CK-MB, cardiac troponin, procalcitonin (PCT), BNP, NT-pro BNP, and d-dimer levels were associated with the severity of CoViD19 and mortality [68]. Several other markers of myocardial injury such as creatinine kinase and myoglobin, and systemic inflammation including procalcitonin have also been evaluated in patients with CoViD19 and reports have suggested an association with CoViD19 severity and mortality [42, 68]. The role of serum pro-inflammatory cytokines such as TNF-α, IL-2R, IL-6, and IL-8, has also been explored in critical CoViD19 patients and a positive correlation with the serum troponin levels was observed [69–71], however, their clinical utility must be further validated. Efficient use of the prognostic markers may help identify patients at risk of developing cardiac injury and the systemic implications of CoViD19. Further evaluations are needed to determine the role of these biomarkers in CoViD19 patients with various degrees of disease severity in relationship with the myocardial injury, with and without previous cardiovascular disease, individually and in combination, as well as their dynamics in response to the therapeutic interventions.

11.6 Pathogenesis of the Myocardial Injury

The CoViD19 may adversely impact multiple cardiac and vascular structures including the electrical conduction system, the pericardium, the myocardium, and the endothelial system [72]. The acute cardiovascular complications in CoViD19 appear to be the consequence of new myocardial injury, underlying cardiometabolic risk factors, preexisting cardiovascular diseases, or several treatments administered to the CoViD19 patients [4, 73]. Other factors such as the strength of the intensity of viral infection [74], host natural immune defense systems, underlying cardiometabolic risk factors, age [75] and several genetic factors play a significant role in this process. Notable among these pathogenetic mechanisms include proinflammatory, hypercatecholaminic, hypoxic, hypercoagulability, hemodynamic compromise and direct viral damage that ultimately lead to myocardial injury.

The CoViD19 is a multi-systemic disease of intense thrombo-inflammatory nature that may affect lungs, kidneys, brain, gastrointestinal tract, and other organs and tissues that also appear to impact the heart. Intense immune and inflammatory mechanisms are highly pronounced in critically ill patients. The underlying biochemical, clinical, demographic, and genetic factors, as well as the comorbidities, may strengthen and maintain these mechanisms and may lead to the critical state in CoViD19. The processes that lead to the multi-organ injury in CoViD19 also facilitate the development of myocardial injury.

The lungs serve as the gateway for viral entry and act as the principal reservoir of the immune defense system and inflammation. In CoViD19, the lungs are the central pathogenetic core to the disease and appear to be a source of the dissemination of harmful reactions to the other organs, which may induce inflammation in the cardiovascular structures. Patients with ARDS in CoViD19 may exhibit cardiac inflammation, however, the extent of the myocardial damage may vary. A pathology report with cardiac biopsy from a patient with CoViD19 related ARDS showed a few interstitial mononuclear inflammatory infiltrates without substantial damage in the heart tissue [76]. Similarly, the thrombotic phenomena in the lungs adversely impact the heart. Data suggest that in CoViD19 patients, the thrombotic pulmonary complications such as pulmonary embolism (PE) or pulmonary microthrombi formation may exert negative cardiac impact [77, 78]. Whether the development of the myocardial injury is an independent process, or a result of the underlying multi-organ pathology is subject to further exploration.

The exploration of the pathogenetic factors behind the development of CoViD19 complications in research studies reveals several intricate direct and indirect reactions and mechanisms related to the virus that also appear to be linked with cardiac injury. A complex environment involving a range of viral processes, mediators, and signaling pathways that trigger and mediate cellular stress reactions, and dysfunctional mechanisms such as loss of cellular homeostasis, translation/transcription shutoff, contractile dysfunction, and apoptosis may promote myocardial injury. The major culprits that precipitate myocardial injury in CoViD19 include an increase in myocardial oxygen demand, high inflammatory burden with immunological turbulence with hyper-cytokinesis, dysregulated renin-angiotensin system, microvascular damage, hypercoagulability with disseminated intravascular coagulation [79], and overactivation of the complement system [80], hemodynamic and metabolic derangement, mechanisms related to the stress cardiomyopathy (Tako-Tsubo), or direct viral mechanisms (Figs. 11.2 and 11.3). Expression of a variety of elevated biomarkers indicating hyper-immune inflammatory, thrombotic, cardiac protein damage and dysfunction, such as D Dimers, CRP, troponins, cytokines, troponin, BNP, and several others, reflects these pathogenetic mechanisms in myocardial injury in CoViD19.

The myocardial injury in CoViD19 may be a new (neo myocardial injury in CoViD19 nMiCoV) or exacerbation of underlying risk (myocardial injury in CoViD19 due to pre-existing risk factors pMiCoV). Data show that infections and

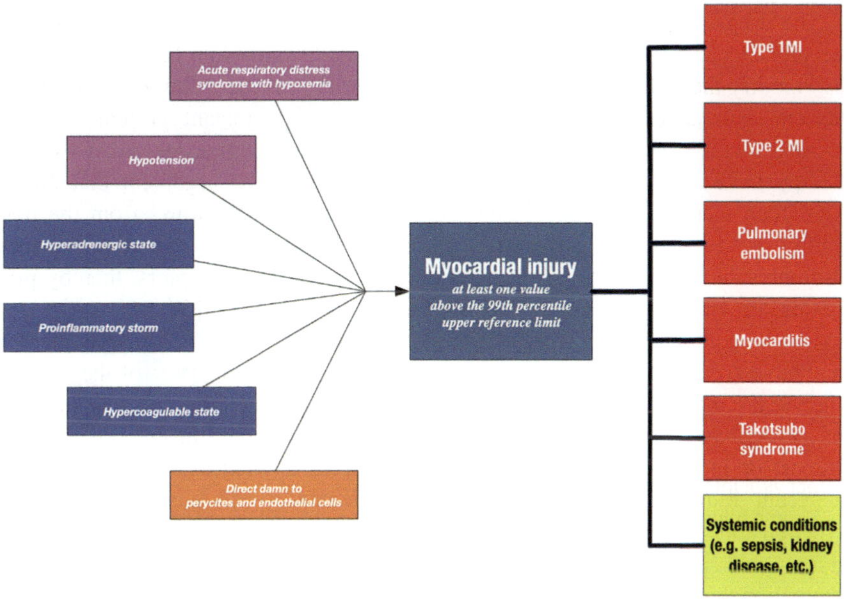

Fig. 11.2 Pathogenesis of myocardial injury in CoViD19. Pathophysiology of myocardial injury during acute SARS-CoV-2 infection and potential long-term sequelae following the recovery. MI myocardial infarction. *Source* Figure 2. Polito, M.V., Silverio, A., Bellino, M. et al. Cardiovascular Involvement in COVID-19: What Sequelae Should We Expect? Cardiol Ther (2021). https://doi.org/10.1007/s40119-021-00232-8. https://link.springer.com/article/10.1007/s40119-021-00232-8. Published by Springer Nature

inflammatory conditions increase the risk of acute coronary events in patients with pre-existing coronary artery disease or those with high-risk factor burden [81]. The pathogenesis of the development of a new myocardial injury in CoViD19 patients is unclear and may be the result of the interaction of the multifactorial pathogenetic nature of the disease and specific intricate mechanisms associated with the viral disease. Further clarification is needed to determine whether an acute myocardial injury and cardiac dysfunction exist at the time of presentation or myocardial injury develops with the intensification of the CoViD19 [82].

The infectious or inflammatory conditions are known to promote myocardial injury, decompensation of heart failure, and arrhythmias such as atrial fibrillation and other forms of cardiovascular diseases. The dynamics of immune pathogenetic responses in CoViD19 may mark variations in the severity of the disease at different stages [83, 84]. The role of hyper-immune-inflammatory mechanisms in new myocardial injury in CoViD19 appears crucial. Patients with complicated CoViD19 exhibit a high inflammatory burden recognized as cytokine storm release multiple cytokines and chemokines [85, 86] that may lead to vascular harm, prothrombotic reactions [87], atherosclerotic plaque instability, or myocardial inflammation and damage. The elevated biomarkers of the myocardial injury in CoViD19, strongly

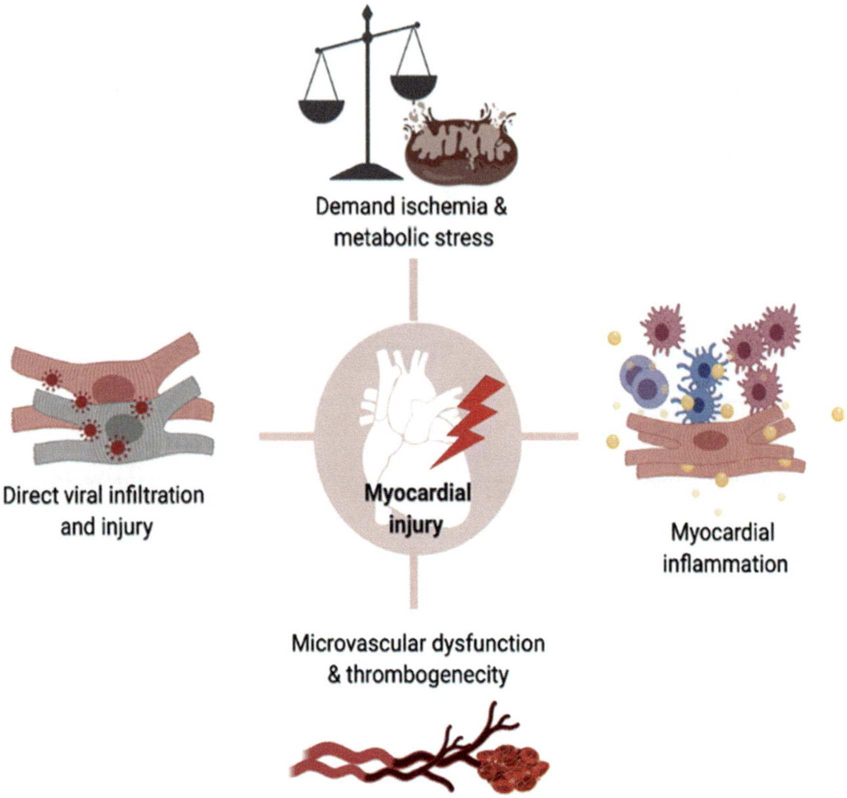

Fig. 11.3 Potential mechanisms of myocardial injury in COVID19. *Source* Figure 2. Cheng, P., Zhu, H., Witteles, R.M., Wu, J.C., Quertermous, T., Wu, S.M. and Rhee, J.W., 2020. Cardiovascular risks in patients with COVID-19: potential mechanisms and areas of uncertainty. Current cardiology reports, 22(5), pp. 1–6. https://link.springer.com/article/10.1007/s11886-020-01293-2. Published by Springer Nature

reflect the contribution of the immune-inflammatory mechanisms towards the severity of the disease and mortality. Furthermore, the progressive involvement and spread of mechanisms such as viral-induced dysregulation of the renin-angiotensin system, development of hypoxia due to the pulmonary complications such as pneumonia/ARDS, the intensity and spread of the hyper-immune-inflammatory mechanisms, induction of prothrombotic mechanisms, and microvascular injury, correlate with the evolutionary stage of CoViD19.

A myocardial oxygen supply/demand mismatch is a known cause of myocardial damage in CoViD19 and may be observed in conditions accompanying hypoxia or intense stressful mechanisms as observed in systemic sepsis. In the absence of an acute atherothrombotic event, in a clinical setting with overt myocardial ischemia, a significant inequity between the myocardial oxygen supply and/or demand results in type 2 Myocardial Infarction. Hopxia is associated with severe CoViD19 may

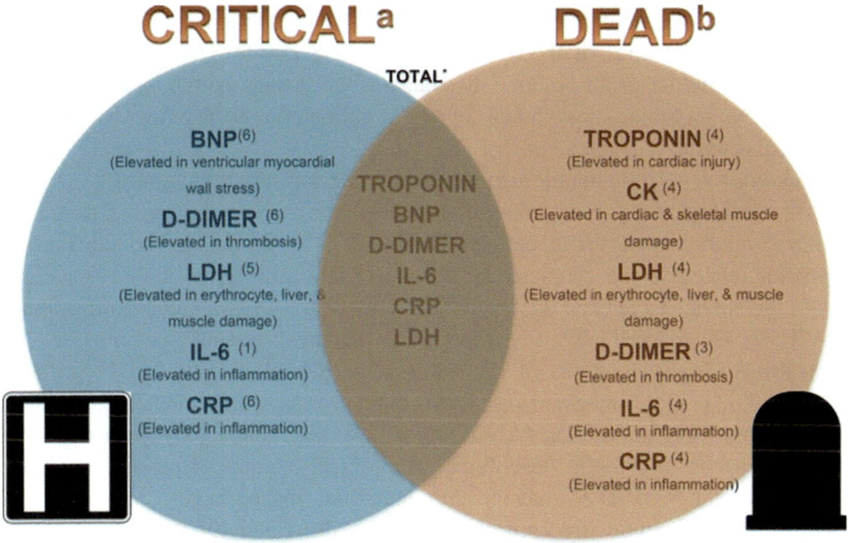

Fig. 11.4 Cardiac biomarkers in CoViD19. Analysis of association of cardiac biomarkers in COVID-19 patients. According to a metanalysis investigating prognostic significance of cardiac biomarkers in CoViD19 involving 2667 patients from 16 studies. (a) Significant difference seen in biomarkers in COVID-19 patients who were critically ill. (b) Significant difference seen in biomarkers in COVID-19 patients who died. *Significant difference seen in biomarkers in COVID-19 patients who died and/or were critically ill. Superscripts: total number of articles in each group. Biomarkers studied: Troponin, BNP, CK, CRP, LDH, D-dimer, IL-6. *Source* Figure 4. Sheth, A., Modi, M. and Dominic, P., 2021. Prognostic value of cardiac biomarkers in COVID-19 infection. Scientific reports, 11(1), pp. 1–9. https://www.nature.com/articles/s41598-021-84643-6. Published by Springer Nature Group

accompany intense pathogenetic mechanisms that mimic cardiac abnormalities. A case series of 2 patients with CoViD19 presented electrocardiographic abnormalities ie temporary SIQIIITIII morphology followed by reversible nearly complete atrioventricular block, and the second patient demonstrated ST-segment elevation accompanied by multifocal ventricular tachycardia. Hypoxia and inflammatory damage incurred by the virus were considered as the most likely underlying mechanisms of these ECG abnormalities in the severe stage of CoViD19 [88]. Hypoxia may induce inflammation and thrombosis.

The inflammatory and thrombotic processes may be induced via multiple pathways in CoViD19 involving the immune defense mechanisms, viral signaling processes, local and systemic regulatory mechanisms including dysregulated RAAS. The downregulation of ACE2 expression by SARS CoV2 infection was reported previously [89], is also observed in the heart [90, 91] may leave myocardial tissue susceptible to injury. Mechanisms involving pro-inflammatory cytokines and ACE2 depletion in the epicardial adipose tissue (EAT) that may induce cardiac inflammation have been proposed [92]. The immune defense processes may be dysregulated in CoViD19 and compounded with the loss of cardioprotective actions of the dysregulated RAAS due to SARS CoV2 induced mechanisms, induce prothrombotic mechanisms via several mediators and signaling mechanisms including endothelial damage ultimately leading to vascular and myocardial tissue damage.

The impact of inflammation in the heart is showcased in several pathology reports revealing the spread of the inflammatory infiltrates in the cardiac tissue and myocyte injury and death in patients with CoViD19, however, variations in the approach related to the characterization of the myocarditis in CoViD19 patients across the studies have been observed [93]. The cardiac inflammatory infiltration in CoViD19 is marked by a variety of features related or not to the myocarditis. Several patterns of myocarditis are described in CoViD19 patients. Distinguishing these mechanisms from other forms of cardiac inflammation, stress-induced or sepsis-related cardiomyopathy, and others may be a challenge [94]. According to a report describing pathological features of myocardial injury associated with CoViD19, mostly the interstitial macrophages, or features of multifocal lymphocytic myocarditis have been described [95]. Other CoViD19 reports suggest that features not typically associated with myocarditis such as focal cardiomyocyte necrosis, macro- or microvascular thrombi, inflammation, and intraluminal megakaryocytes, maybe more frequent than myocarditis [96]. Furthermore, a link between the cardiac inflammation and the duration of symptoms of CoViD19 has been suggested [91]. A cohort of sequential autopsies of 41 patients with CoViD19 revealed a positive correlation between cardiac inflammation with the duration of CoViD19 symptoms and hospitalization, and a positive trend in association with elevated cytokines [91]. Attempts have been made to explore links between the myocardial injury, inflammation, and cardiac dysfunction using advanced imaging techniques related to echocardiography and CMR, and myocardial sampling [52] with evidence of ongoing inflammation observed, post convalescence, in CoViD19 patients [48].

Studies show that about 60–70% of patients with fatal CoViD19 may have viremia [74, 97]. In another study, about 73% of patients with fatal CoViD19 had detectable SARS CoV2 in the myocardium at autopsy [91]. Mechanisms involving direct viral cardiac and vascular injury in CoViD19 have presented tremendous interest of the researchers with the publication of sporadic cases and pathology reports in the literature. In a case of a patient with CoViD19, low-grade myocardial inflammation and SARS CoV2 particles in the myocardial interstitial cells (absent from in the cardiomyocytes) with loss of cytoplasmic membrane integrity, indicated the implication of direct viral myocardial injury [98]. According to a case series of post mortem analysis of 12 patients with CoViD19, elevated troponins were associated with lymphocytic myocarditis (foci of lymphocytic inflammation associated with acute myocyte necrosis) with detectable SARS CoV2 RNA in one case [99]. Several other reports implicate direct viral damage of myocardial structure and endothelial cells, and features of endotheliitis [100, 101], although studies indicate the likelihood of misinterpretation of these findings [102]. Myocarditis especially in patients with no prior cardiovascular disease possibly a result of the direct viral myocardial and vascular injury caused by the SARS CoV2 implicates interaction with ACE2 found at the surface of the cardiomyocytes and vascular endothelium, remains vastly unknown [103].

The contribution of the mechanisms related to the immune-inflammation and thrombosis in CoViD19 related myocardial injury appears strong. The depletion of the cardioprotective shield due to the SARS COV2 induced downregulation of the protective arm of RAAS may make cardiac and vascular structures more vulnerable. The intensity and duration of the viral disease may further facilitate these mechanisms. The multisystemic propagation of CoViD19 appears to be a consequence of a cascade of intense dysregulated mechanisms and perturbed homeostasis and hemostasis, which may induce myocardial injury. Such associations may explain the temporal association of these mechanisms with the evolutionary stage of the disease. An early presentation of the myocardial injury may reflect exacerbation of a pre-existing overt disease and the associated inflammation, possibly triggered as a result of viral mechanisms. Whereas, the late development of the myocardial injury may be the result of intense immune-inflammatory mechanisms in synchrony with these factors. The cardiac inflammation may have long-term implications. Studies show a persistent myocardial inflammation in post convalescent CoViD19 patients indicating long term sequelae of the myocardial injury [14]. A role of CoViD19 related autoimmunity [104–106] in the development of long-term implications of the myocardial injury remains to be further explored.

Individual cases of acute myocarditis have emerged indicating myocardial involvement in the absence of angiographic evidence of coronary artery lesions in patients with CoViD19 with no signs or symptoms of interstitial pneumonia, supporting these mechanisms however no histopathological evidence has been provided [107]. Furthermore, several cases of fulminant myocarditis have been reported in china in patients with no previous history of CAD with the high inflammatory burden [108, 109].

The invasion of SARS CoV2 may be asymptomatic in individuals or minimally symptomatic for pulmonary complications, however, these patients may present with cardiovascular complications. According to a report similar viral load was detected in the asymptomatic and symptomatic patients, suggesting the transmission potential of asymptomatic or minimally symptomatic patients [110]. The development of cardiovascular complications in patients with mild or no respiratory symptoms may reflect a pathogenetic link between underlying clinically overt viral load and cardiovascular disease, due to an interplay between the SARS CoV2 and host viral defense mechanisms [111].

11.7 Summary

In summary, myocardial injury is a critical and frequent complication of the advanced CoViD19, with a higher incidence and fatality rate among patients with a critical illness or previous history of cardiovascular diseases or risk factor burden. Timely recognition of a specific type of myocardial injury in CoViD19 is important. Early and better-targeted management and treatment strategies must be applied in the management of myocardial injury in CoViD19 patients. Myocardial injury in CoViD19 presents in multiple forms. The exact prevalence of these variabilities and their implications remain unclear. The variabilities in the forms of myocardial injury in CoViD19 patients, and poor definition of myocardial injury, may adversely impact an accurate assessment of the individual risk and therefore, the clinical decision-making process.

In CoViD19 patients, identification, defining, and characterization of the myocardial injury may present a challenge. A cautious approach is warranted for an unbiased interpretation of the laboratory data in CoViD19 patients with a suspicion of myocardial injury. The variations in troponin elevation alone may be subject to misinterpretation for accurate detection of myocardial injury. An increased expression of other biomarkers such as BNP may be due to other systemic complications. Several mechanisms of cardiac injury such as myocarditis, stress cardiomyopathy or microvascular injury, or a high burden of infectious, hyper immunoinflammatory mechanisms, and the prothrombotic load may be identified in CoViD19 patients. Besides the cardiac disease, non-cardiac disease burden, such as associated renal complications may also complicate the interpretation of the biochemical markers of myocardial injury. A lack of careful interpretation of these data may have significant practical implications and may lead to poor patient management and application of poorly targeted therapies in CoViD19.

Recognition of myocardial injury or its forms requires a complex approach in CoViD19 patients. Distinguishing between the myocardial injury as a result of classic mechanisms involved in the ACS and those associated with SARS CoV2 such as hyperinflammatory stress is important. Patients with CoViD19 with a classical picture of an acute coronary event in absence of these inflammatory or immune markers may have a higher underlying native coronary risk. Tracking of the troponin by the hyperinflammatory or cytokine storm in patients with CoViD19 may suggest an acute myocardial injury related to the inflammatory and prothrombotic stress, which may be transitory, and may or may not be associated with an underlying cardiovascular disease. Utilizing a battery of biomarkers may be more effective in aiding the diagnosis of myocardial injury in CoViD19. The immune-inflammatory biomarkers together with markers of myocardial dysfunction in combination may be used to help to define the severity of disease or guide the evolution of the disease in CoViD19.

The CoViD19 patients at risk of myocardial injury must be identified early. Appropriate risk models must be developed for an early risk-stratification in patients with CoViD19. Risk assessment, however, may be a challenge. Advanced

CoViD19 significantly increased the risk of the development of myocardial injury, especially in patients with a high-risk factor burden or pre-existing cardiovascular and metabolic diseases. Several factors including clinical, demographic, multiple CoViD19 related viral-immune-inflammatory-thrombotic factors, conventional cardiometabolic risk factors, and comorbidities may reflect the individual risk profile in CoViD19 for a myocardial injury. Robust risk assessment modalities and novel approaches may be needed to determine the risk of myocardial injury in CoViD19 patients without underlying risk factors. Further studies are needed to better characterize the risk factors and determine risk estimation models.

The myocardial injury in patients with CoViD19 appears to have prognostic implications, although data on the long-term outcomes are not available. Regular evaluations and a follow-up may be needed for assessment of the cardiac damage and dysfunction, using appropriate diagnostic techniques. Among advanced imaging techniques, cardiac MRI is an effective tool for characterization of tissue with an acute myocardial injury [50]. The CMR may identify the myocardial injury patterns in CoViD19 patients with raised troponin and no previous history of the myocardial disease [51].

The management of myocardial injury in CoViD19 patients needs a multi-faceted approach, involving the electrocardiographic, echocardiographic, invasive, or non-invasive coronary imaging, and myocardial sampling techniques, especially in high-risk patients, guided by the clinical judgment and available expert guidelines to determine the appropriateness of these procedures. Multimodal identification of the myocardial injury involving multiple local and systemic viral-immune-inflammatory- thrombotic and specific markers that reflect the myocardial damage and dysfunction, together with the use of advanced cardiac imaging and other diagnostic modalities, is likely to be superior, however, such strategies need to be further evaluated. The healthcare professionals must be encouraged to adopt an aggressive approach in patients with CoViD19 related myocardial injury and use appropriate cardiac imaging modalities and other diagnostic tools. An early multidisciplinary assessment of the high-risk patients with myocardial injury may be considered involving critical care specialists, or virologists, and infectious diseases experts.

Pathogenesis of the myocardial injury in complicated CoViD19 involves multiple intricated immune-inflammatory stress and dysregulated mechanisms and dysfunctional homeostasis that also reflect variabilities in the clinical presentation, organ injury, and features of disease severity. Various culprits associated with the advanced CoViD19 may weaken the myocardial tissue and the cellular structures. The inflammatory thrombotic mechanisms dominate the pathogenetic profile of complicated CoviD19. Potent immune-inflammatory and prothrombotic processes interact and cause vascular damage and leak, reduce the oxygen supply, and may cause tissue destruction. The myocardial and vascular instability in CoViD19 is associated with a variety of clinical features of the complicated CoViD19. The development of arrhythmias (tachyarrhythmias, bradyarrhythmias), hypotension, and hypertension (with or without left ventricular hypertrophy), respiratory failure, anemia, and coronary artery spasm or embolism, may adversely impact the myocardial oxygen demand/supply. These mechanisms are known to promote type 2 myocardial infarction in the absence of a coronary atherothrombotic plaque.

The role of dysregulated cytokines appears to be crucial in the pathogenesis of myocardial injury in CoViD19. Similarly, other mechanisms related to the involvement of RAS mechanisms, especially in connection with the exposure to the activated AngII/AT1R pathway and downregulated ACE2, have also been identified. These mechanisms act as the pathogenetic substrate for CoViD19 associated promoters of myocardial injury. Other mechanisms, such as oxidative stress, endoplasmic reticular stress, mitochondrial dysfunction, range of cell death mechanisms, endothelial and myocardial cell damage, lead to dysfunctional homeostasis, and tissue damage, also facilitate the development of myocardial injury. The viral toxicity involves numerous direct and indirect mechanisms that may precipitate the myocardial injury via various mediators including the TLRs, or viral proteinases, signaling pathways, immune mechanisms, and induction of a variety of forms of cell death, through interaction with myocardial cells at multiple levels. These factors are also linked with the severity of CoViD19.

The gaps and weaknesses, in the understanding of epidemiological aspects of the myocardial injury in CoViD19, such as reporting of the prevalence, interlinks between myocardial injury and the underlying risk factors or with the CoViD19 related comorbidities, the utility of multiple biomarkers, and prognostication must be addressed using robust clinical research methodology and design. Specific disease management algorithms must be developed for the assessment and follow-up of patients with myocardial injury. The multifactorial pathogenetic nature of the myocardial injury may imply the use of unconventional therapeutic strategies in treating patients with CoViD19 related myocardial injury. These may include the use of anti-inflammatory and immune-modulatory agents in addition to the conventional anti-ischemic and cardioprotective treatments. However, further investigations are needed to explore the efficacy and safety of these treatments in patients with myocardial injury in CoViD19.

Summary Box

- Although, inconsistencies may surround in estimating the incidence of myocardial injury or defining the entity in CoViD19 studies and the long-term implications, the myocardial injury appears common in CoViD19 and significantly impacts prognosis.
- Myocardial injury in CoViD19 is associated with an increased risk of death and severity of the disease and in CoViD19 patients sequelae of the myocardial injury may last for longer periods post convalescence.
- CoViD19 related myocardial injury may present in several forms such as non-specific myocardial injury with variable patterns of inflammation or typical forms of myocarditis, however, characteristics, incidence, pathogenetic and prognostic implications remain poorly defined.

- The criticality of the underlying disease, duration of the symptoms, the intensity of the viral disease, development of organ injury appear to be associated with the development of myocardial injury in CoViD19.
- Measurement of troponin and associated dynamics must be complemented by CK MB, BNP, D Dimers, CRP, or perhaps pro-inflammatory cytokines, myoglobin, procalcitonin, in diagnosing the CoViD19 related myocardial injury.
- The myocardial injury should be better characterized in CoViD19 patients, judiciously using biochemical, histopathological, electrocardiographic, non-invasive, and invasive structural and functional assessments, guided by the clinical judgment in keeping with the level of risk.
- Critically ill patients and patients with a previous history of cardiovascular disease more often have much higher levels of serum biomarkers of myocardial injury.
- Cardiac extension of the immune-inflammatory infiltrates is led by intensity and duration of the viral disease, dysregulated homeostatic mechanisms involving RAS, immune regulation, thrombo-inflammation, cellular stress reactions, or viral toxicity.
- Variations in forms of myocardial injury reflects diversity of the pathogenetic mechanisms and intensity triggered by SARS CoV2, vulnerability of cardiac and vascular structures and immune defense mechanisms, and underlying individual risk factors.
- Long term immune-inflammatory impact of the CoViD19 and related biomarkers linked with the multifactorial pathogenetic process must be explored and evidence-based protocols must be developed to effectively manage myocardial injury in CoViD19 patients.

References

1. Roth GA, Mensah GA, Johnson CO, Addolorato G, Ammirati E, Baddour LM, Barengo NC, Beaton AZ, Benjamin, EJ, Benziger CP, Bonny A. Global burden of cardiovascular diseases and risk factors, 1990–2019: update from the GBD 2019 study. J Am Coll Cardiol. 2020;76 (25):2982–3021.
2. Yang J, Zheng Y, Gou X, Pu K, Chen Z, Guo Q, Ji R, Wang H, Wang Y, Zhou Y. Prevalence of comorbidities in the novel Wuhan coronavirus (COVID-19) infection: a systematic review and meta-analysis. Int J Infect Dis. 2020;10.
3. Onder G, Rezza G, Brusaferro S. Case-fatality rate and characteristics of patients dying in relation to COVID-19 in Italy. JAMA. 2020;323(18):1775–6.
4. Lala A, Johnson KW, Januzzi JL, Russak AJ, Paranjpe I, Richter F, Zhao S, Somani S, Van Vleck T, Vaid A, Chaudhry F. Prevalence and impact of myocardial injury in patients hospitalized with COVID-19 infection. J Am Coll Cardiol. 2020;76(5):533–46.
5. Thygesen K, Alpert JS, Jaffe AS, Chaitman BR, Bax JJ, Morrow DA, White HD, Executive Group on behalf of the Joint European Society of Cardiology (ESC)/American College of

Cardiology (ACC)/American Heart Association (AHA)/World Heart Federation (WHF) Task Force for the Universal Definition of Myocardial Infarction. Fourth universal definition of myocardial infarction (2018). J Am Coll Cardiol. 2018;72(18):2231–64.

6. Wei JF, Huang FY, Xiong TY, Liu Q, Chen H, Wang H, Huang H, Luo YC, Zhou X, Liu ZY, Peng Y. Acute myocardial injury is common in patients with COVID-19 and impairs their prognosis. Heart. 2020;106(15):1154–9.
7. Driggin E, Madhavan MV, Bikdeli B, Chuich T, Laracy J, Biondi-Zoccai G, Brown TS, Der Nigoghossian C, Zidar DA, Haythe J, Brodie D. Cardiovascular considerations for patients, health care workers, and health systems during the COVID-19 pandemic. J Am Coll Cardiol. 2020;75(18):2352–71.
8. Nishiga M, Wang DW, Han Y, Lewis DB, Wu JC. COVID-19 and cardiovascular disease: from basic mechanisms to clinical perspectives. Nat Rev Cardiol. 2020;17(9):543–58.
9. Rivero F, Antuña P, Cuesta J, Alfonso F. Severe coronary spasm in a COVID-19 patient. Catheter Cardiovasc Interv. 2020;97(5):E670-2.
10. Moretti F, Jeva F, Pedrinazzi C, Cacucci M, Marino M, Landolina M. Transient ST-segment elevation in coronavirus disease-2019. J Cardiovasc Med. 2021;22(5):417–9.
11. Almas T, Khedro T, Haadi A, Ahmed R, Alshaikh L, Al-Awaid AH, Panhwar MS, Virk HUH. COVID-19-induced takotsubo cardiomyopathy: venturing beyond the obvious. Ann Med Surg. 2021;65.
12. Aikawa T, Takagi H, Ishikawa K, Kuno T. Myocardial injury characterized by elevated cardiac troponin and in-hospital mortality of COVID-19: an insight from a meta-analysis. J Med Virol. 2021;93(1):51–5.
13. Gu ZC, Zhang C, Kong LC, Shen L, Li Z, Ge H, Lin HW, Pu J. Incidence of myocardial injury in coronavirus disease 2019 (COVID-19): a pooled analysis of 7,679 patients from 53 studies. Cardiovasc Diagn Therapy. 2020;10(4):667.
14. Puntmann VO, Carerj ML, Wieters I, Fahim M, Arendt C, Hoffmann J, Shchendrygina A, Escher F, Vasa-Nicotera M, Zeiher AM, Vehreschild M. Outcomes of cardiovascular magnetic resonance imaging in patients recently recovered from coronavirus disease 2019 (COVID-19). JAMA Cardiol. 2020;5(11):1265–73.
15. Zheng YY, Ma YT, Zhang JY, Xie X. COVID-19 and the cardiovascular system. Nat Rev Cardiol. 2020;17(5):259–60.
16. Thygesen K, Alpert JS, Jaffe AS, Chaitman BR, Bax JJ, Morrow DA, White HD, Mickley H, Crea F, Van de Werf F, Bucciarelli-Ducci C. Fourth universal definition of myocardial infarction (2018). Eur Heart J. 2019;40(3):237–69.
17. Araiza-Garaygordobil D, Montalto C, Martinez-Amezcua P, Cabello-Lopez A, Gopar-Nieto R, Alabrese R, Almaghraby A, Catoya-Villa S, Chacon-Diaz M, Kaufmann CC, Corbi-Pascual M. Impact of the COVID-19 pandemic on hospitalizations for acute coronary syndromes: a multinational study. QJM Int J Med. 2021.
18. Chen T, Wu D, Chen H, Yan W, Yang D, Chen G, Ma K, Xu D, Yu H, Wang H, Wang T, Guo W, Chen J, Ding C, Zhang X, Huang J, Han M, Li S, Luo X, Zhao J, Ning Q. Clinical characteristics of 113 deceased patients with coronavirus disease 2019: retrospective study. BMJ. 2020;26(368):m1091. https://doi.org/10.1136/bmj.m1091. Erratum. In: BMJ. 2020 Mar 31;368:m1295. PubMed PMID: 32217556.
19. Chapman AR, Bularga A, Mills NL. High-sensitivity cardiac troponin can be an ally in the fight against COVID-19. Circulation. 2020;141(22):1733–5.
20. He XW, Lai JS, Cheng J, Wang MW, Liu YJ, Xiao ZC, Xu C, Li SS, Zeng HS. Impact of complicated myocardial injury on the clinical outcome of severe or critically ill COVID-19 patients. Zhonghua Xin Xue Guan Bing Za Zhi. 2020;48(0):E011. https://doi.org/10.3760/cma.j.cn112148-20200228-00137. [Epub ahead of print] Chinese. PubMed PMID: 32171190.
21. Guo T, Fan Y, Chen M, et al. Cardiovascular implications of fatal out comes of patients with coronavirus disease 2019 (COVID-19). JAMA Cardiol. Published online March 27, 2020. https://doi.org/10.1001/jamacardio.2020.1017.

22. Bavishi C, Bonow RO, Trivedi V, Abbott JD, Messerli FH, Bhatt DL. Acute myocardial injury in patients hospitalized with COVID-19 infection: a review. Progr Cardiovasc Dis. 2020.
23. Prasitlumkum N, Chokesuwattanaskul R, Thongprayoon C, Bathini T, Vallabhajosyula S, Cheungpasitporn W. Incidence of myocardial injury in COVID-19-infected patients: a systematic review and meta-analysis. Diseases. 2020;8(4):40.
24. Shi S, Qin M, Shen B, et al. Association of cardiac injurywith mortality in hospitalized patients with COVID-19 in Wuhan, China. JAMA Cardiol. Published online March 25, 2020. https://doi.org/10.1001/jamacardio.2020.095011.
25. Ssentongo P, Ssentongo AE, Heilbrunn ES, Ba DM, Chinchilli VM. Association of cardiovascular disease and 10 other pre-existing comorbidities with COVID-19 mortality: a systematic review and meta-analysis. PloS One. 2020;15(8):e0238215.
26. Shi S, Qin M, Shen B, Cai Y, Liu T, Yang F, Gong W, Liu X, Liang J, Zhao Q, Huang H. Association of cardiac injury with mortality in hospitalized patients with COVID-19 in Wuhan, China. JAMA Cardiol. 2020;5(7):802–81.
27. Huang C, Wang Y, Li X, Ren L, Zhao J, Hu Y, Zhang L, Fan G, Xu J, Gu X, Cheng Z. Clinical features of patients infected with 2019 novel coronavirus in Wuhan, China. The Lancet. 2020;395(10223):497–506.
28. Chen T, Wu D, Chen H, Yan W, Yang D, Chen G, Ma K, Xu D, Yu H, Wang H, Wang T, Guo W, Chen J, Ding C, Zhang X, Huang J, Han M, Li S, Luo X, Zhao J, Ning Q. Clinical characteristics of 113 deceased patients with coronavirus disease 2019: retrospective study. BMJ. 2020;368:m1091. https://doi.org/10.1136/bmj.m1091. Erratum in: BMJ. 2020;368; m1295. PubMed PMID: 32217556; and other ref from myocardial injury.
29. Peng YD, Meng K, Guan HQ, Leng L, Zhu RR, Wang BY, He MA, Cheng LX, Huang K, Zeng QT. Clinical characteristics and outcomes of 112 cardiovascular disease patients infected by 2019-nCoV. Zhonghua Xin Xue Guan Bing Za Zhi. 2020;48:E004. https://doi.org/10.3760/cma.j.cn112148-20200220-00105.
30. Wang L, He WB, Yu XM, Liu HF, Zhou WJ, Jiang H. Prognostic value of myocardial injury in patients with COVID-19. Zhonghua Xin Xue Guan Bing Za Zhi. 2020;48(6):461–6.
31. Metkus TS, Sokoll LJ, Barth AS, Czarny MJ, Hays AG, Lowenstein CJ, Michos ED, Nolley EP, Post WS, Resar JR, Thiemann DR. Myocardial injury in severe COVID-19 compared with non–COVID-19 acute respiratory distress syndrome. Circulation. 2021;143 (6):553–65.
32. Fried JA, Ramasubbu K, Bhatt R, Topkara VK, Clerkin KJ, Horn E, Rabbani L, Brodie D, Jain SS, Kirtane AJ, Masoumi A. The variety of cardiovascular presentations of COVID-19. Circulation. 2020;141(23):1930–6.
33. Hu H, Ma F, Wei X, Fang Y. Coronavirus fulminant myocarditis treated with glucocorticoid and human immunoglobulin. Eur Heart J. 2020.
34. Sala S, Peretto G, Gramegna M, Palmisano A, Villatore A, Vignale D, De Cobelli F, Tresoldi M, Cappelletti AM, Basso C, Godino C. Acute myocarditis presenting as a reverse Tako-Tsubo syndrome in a patient with SARS-CoV-2 respiratory infection. Eur Heart J. 2020;41(19):1861–2.
35. Caraffa R, Marcolongo R, Bottio T, Rizzo S, Bifulco O, Bagozzi L, D'Onofrio A, Caforio AL, Jorgji V, Basso C, Gerosa G. Recurrent autoimmune myocarditis in a young woman during the coronavirus disease 2019 pandemic. ESC Heart Fail. 2021;8(1):756–60.
36. Meyer P, Degrauwe S, Van Delden C, Ghadri JR, Templin C. Typical takotsubo syndrome triggered by SARS-CoV-2 infection. Eur Heart J. 2020;41(19):1860–1860.
37. Richard I, Robinson B, Dawson A, Aya A, Ali R. An atypical presentation of fulminant myocarditis secondary to COVID-19 infection. Cureus. 2020;12(7).
38. Salamanca J, Díez-Villanueva P, Martínez P, Cecconi A, González de Marcos B, Reyes G, Salas C, Segovia J, Jiménez-Borreguero LJ, Alfonso F. COVID-19 "Fulminant Myocarditis" successfully treated with temporary mechanical circulatory support. Cardiovasc Imaging. 2020;13(11):2457–9.

39. Ruan Q, Yang K, Wang W, Jiang L, Song J. Clinical predictors of mortality due to COVID-19 based on an analysis of data of 150 patients from Wuhan, China. Intensive Care Med. 2020;46(5):846–8.
40. Tavazzi G, Pellegrini C, Maurelli M, Belliato M, Sciutti F, Bottazzi A, Sepe PA, Resasco T, Camporotondo R, Bruno R, Baldanti F. Myocardial localization of coronavirus in COVID-19 cardiogenic shock. Eur J Heart Fail. 2020;22(5):911–5.
41. Saleh SK, Oraii A, Soleimani A, Hadadi A, Shajari Z, Montazeri M, Moradi H, Talebpour M, Naseri AS, Balali P, Akhbari M. The association between cardiac injury and outcomes in hospitalized patients with COVID-19. Intern Emerg Med. 2020;15(8):1415–24.
42. Bansal A, Kumar A, Patel D, Puri R, Kalra A, Kapadia SR, Reed GW. Meta-analysis comparing outcomes in patients with and without cardiac injury and coronavirus disease 2019 (COVID19). Am J Cardiol. 2021;141:140–6.
43. Santoso A, Pranata R, Wibowo A, Al-Farabi MJ, Huang I, Antariksa B. Cardiac injury is associated with mortality and critically ill pneumonia in COVID-19: a meta-analysis. Am J Emerg Med. 2020.
44. Carver C, Jones N. Cardiac injury, ARDS and COVID-19 meta-analysis validity–correspondence in response to Santoso et al. Am J Emerg Med. 2020.
45. Fried JA, Ramasubbu K, Bhatt R, et al. The variety of cardiovascular presentations of COVID-19. Circulation. 2020.
46. Arentz M, Yim E, Klaff L, Lokhandwala S, Riedo FX, Chong M, et al. Characteristics and Outcomes of 21 Critically Ill Patients With COVID-19 in Washington State. JAMA [Internet]. 2020 Mar 19 [cited 2020 Mar 29]. https://jamanetwork.com/journals/jama/fullarticle/2763485.
47. Bangalore S, Sharma A, Slotwiner A, Yatskar L, Harari R, Shah B, Ibrahim H, Friedman GH, Thompson C, Alviar CL, Chadow HL. ST-segment elevation in patients with Covid-19—a case series. N Engl J Med. 2020;382(25):2478–80.
48. Kotecha T, Knight DS, Razvi Y, Kumar K, Vimalesvaran K, Thornton G, Patel R, Chacko L, Brown JT, Coyle C, Leith D. Patterns of myocardial injury in recovered troponin-positive COVID-19 patients assessed by cardiovascular magnetic resonance. Eur Heart J. 2021.
49. Clerkin KJ, Fried JA, Raikhelkar J, Sayer G, Griffin JM, Masoumi A, Jain SS, Burkhoff D, Kumaraiah D, Rabbani L, Schwartz A. COVID-19 and cardiovascular disease. Circulation. 2020;141(20):1648–55.
50. Demirkiran A, Everaars H, Amier RP, Beijnink C, Bom MJ, Götte MJ, van Loon RB, Selder JL, van Rossum AC, Nijveldt R. Cardiovascular magnetic resonance techniques for tissue characterization after acute myocardial injury. Eur Heart J Cardiovasc Imaging. 2019;20(7):723–34.
51. Knight DS, Kotecha T, Razvi Y, Chacko L, Brown JT, Jeetley PS, Goldring J, Jacobs M, Lamb LE, Negus R, Wolff A. COVID-19: myocardial injury in survivors. Circulation. 2020;142(11):1120–2.
52. Weckbach LT, Curta A, Bieber S, Kraechan A, Brado J, Hellmuth JC, Muenchhoff M, Scherer C, Schroeder I, Irlbeck M, Maurus S. Myocardial inflammation and dysfunction in COVID-19–associated myocardial injury. Circ Cardiovasc Imaging. 2021;14(1):e012220.
53. McCarthy C, Murphy S, Cohen JA, Rehman S, Jones-O'Connor M, Olshan DS, Singh A, Vaduganathan M, Januzzi JL, Wasfy JH. Misclassification of myocardial injury as myocardial infarction: implications for assessing outcomes in value-based programs. JAMA Cardiol. 2019;4(5):460–4.
54. Sandoval Y, Smith SW, Sexter A, Thordsen SE, Bruen CA, Carlson MD, Dodd KW, Driver BE, Hu Y, Jacoby K, Johnson BK. Type 1 and 2 myocardial infarction and myocardial injury: clinical transition to high-sensitivity cardiac troponin I. Am J Med. 2017;130(12):1431–2143.
55. Han H, Xie L, Liu R, Yang J, Liu F, Wu K, Chen L, Hou W, Feng Y, Zhu C. Analysis of heart injury laboratory parameters in 273 COVID-19 patients in one hospital in Wuhan, China. J Med Virol. 2020;92(7):819–23.

56. Wu Z, McGoogan JM. Characteristics of and important lessons from the coronavirus disease 2019 (COVID-19) outbreak in China: summary of a report of 72 314 cases from the Chinese center for disease control and prevention. JAMA. 2020;323(13):1239–42.
57. Lippi G, Plebani M. Laboratory abnormalities in patients with COVID-2019 infection. Clin Chem Lab Med (CCLM). 2020;58(7):1131–4.
58. Zhou F, Yu T, Du R, Fan G, Liu Y, Liu Z, Xiang J, Wang Y, Song B, Gu X, Guan L. Clinical course and risk factors for mortality of adult inpatients with COVID-19 in Wuhan, China: a retrospective cohort study. The Lancet. 2020;395(10229):1054–62.
59. Guo T, Fan Y, Chen M, et al. Association of cardiovascular disease and myocardial injury with outcomes of patients hospitalized with 2019-coronavirus disease (COVID-19). JAMA Cardiol. Published online March 27, 2020. https://doi.org/10.1001/jamacardio.2020.1017.
60. Lim W, Qushmaq I, Devereaux PJ, Heels-Ansdell D, Lauzier F, Ismaila AS, Crowther MA, Cook DJ. Elevated cardiac troponin measurements in critically ill patients. Arch Intern Med. 2006;166(22):2446–54.
61. Guo T, Fan Y, Chen M, Wu X, Zhang L, He T, Wang H, Wan J, Wang X, Lu Z. Cardiovascular implications of fatal outcomes of patients with coronavirus disease 2019 (COVID-19). JAMA Cardiol. 2020;5(7):811–8.
62. Li Y, Li H, Zhu S, Xie Y, Wang B, He L, Zhang D, Zhang Y, Yuan H, Wu C, Sun W. Prognostic value of right ventricular longitudinal strain in patients with COVID-19. Cardiovasc Imaging. 2020;13(11):2287–99.
63. Sandoval Y, Januzzi Jr JL, Jaffe AS. Cardiac troponin for the diagnosis and risk-stratification of myocardial injury in COVID-19: JACC review topic of the week. J Am Coll Cardiol. 2020.
64. Huber K, Goldstein P. Covid-19: implications for prehospital, emergency and hospital care in patients with acute coronary syndromes. Eur Heart J Acute Cardiovasc Care. 2020;9(3):222–8.
65. Shi S, Qin M, Shen B, et al. Association of cardiac injury with mortality in hospitalized patients with COVID-19 in Wuhan, China. JAMA Cardiol. (2020 Mar 27) [E-pub ahead of print)].
66. Guo T, Fan Y, Chen M, et al. Cardiovascular implications of fatal out comes of patients with coronavirus disease 2019 (COVID-19). JAMA Cardiol (2020 Mar 27) [E-pub ahead of print)].
67. Yang C, Liu F, Liu W, Cao G, Liu J, Huang S, Zhu M, Tu C, Wang J, Xiong B. Myocardial injury and risk factors for mortality in patients with COVID-19 pneumonia. Int J Cardiol. 2021;326:230–6.
68. Wungu CDK, Khaerunnisa S, Putri EAC, Hidayati HB, Qurnianingsih E, Lukitasari L, Humairah I. Meta-analysis of cardiac markers for predictive factors on severity and mortality of COVID-19. Int J Infect Dis. 2021;105:551–9.
69. Xia G, Fan D, Ma C, He Y, Wang M, Zhu Y, Zheng Q. Hyper-inflammatory response involves in cardiac injury among patients with coronavirus disease 2019. Am J Med Sci. 2021.
70. Zhou W, Song L, Wang X, Xu Z, Wang S, Wang J, Xu H, Zheng Y, Wang Y. Cardiac injury prediction and lymphocyte immunity and inflammation analysis in hospitalized patients with coronavirus disease 2019 (COVID-19). Int J Cardiol. 2021;326:237–42.
71. Alzahrani SH, Al-Rabia MW. Cardiac injury biomarkers and the risk of death in patients with COVID-19: a systematic review and meta-analysis. Cardiol Res Pract. 2021.
72. Sattar Y, Ullah W, Rauf H. COVID-19 cardiovascular epidemiology, cellular pathogenesis, clinical manifestations and management. Int J Cardiol Heart Vasc. 2020;29.
73. Agarwal MA, Ziaeian B, Lavie CJ, Fonarow GC. Cardiovascular disease in hospitalized patients with a diagnosis of coronavirus from the pre–COVID-19 era in United States: national analysis from 2016–2017. Mayo Clin Proc (Elsevier). 2020;95(12):2674–83.
74. Fajnzylber J, Regan J, Coxen K, Corry H, Wong C, Rosenthal A, Worrall D, Giguel F, Piechocka-Trocha A, Atyeo C, Fischinger S. SARS-CoV-2 viral load is associated with increased disease severity and mortality. Nat Commun. 2020;11(1):1–9.

75. Bae S, Kim SR, Kim MN, Shim WJ, Park SM. Impact of cardiovascular disease and risk factors on fatal outcomes in patients with COVID-19 according to age: a systematic review and meta-analysis. Heart. 2021;107(5):373–80.
76. Xu Z, Shi L, Wang Y, Zhang J, Huang L, Zhang C, Liu S, Zhao P, Liu H, Zhu L, Tai Y, Bai C, Gao T, Song J, Xia P, Dong J, Zhao J, Wang FS. Pathological findings of COVID-19 associated with acute respiratory distress syndrome. Lancet Respir Med. 2020;8(4):420–2. https://doi.org/10.1016/S2213-2600(20)30076-X. Epub 2020 Feb 18. Erratum in: Lancet Respir Med. 2020 Feb 25. PubMed PMID: 32085846.
77. Buja LM, Wolf DA, Zhao B, Akkanti B, McDonald M, Lelenwa L, Reilly N, Ottaviani G, Elghetany MT, Trujillo DO, Aisenberg GM. The emerging spectrum of cardiopulmonary pathology of the coronavirus disease 2019 (COVID-19): report of 3 autopsies from Houston, Texas, and review of autopsy findings from other United States cities. Cardiovasc Pathol. 2020;48:107233.
78. Ciceri F, Beretta L, Scandroglio AM, Colombo S, Landoni G, Ruggeri A, Peccatori J, D'Angelo A, De Cobelli F, Rovere-Querini P, Tresoldi M. Microvascular COVID-19 lung vessels obstructive thromboinflammatory syndrome (MicroCLOTS): an atypical acute respiratory distress syndrome working hypothesis. Crit Care Resusc. 2020;22(2):95.
79. Tang N, Li D, Wang X, Sun Z. Abnormal coagulation parameters are associated with poor prognosis in patients with novel coronavirus pneumonia. J Thromb Haemost. 2020;18 (4):844–7.
80. de Nooijer AH, Grondman I, Janssen NA, Netea MG, Willems L, van de Veerdonk FL, Giamarellos-Bourboulis EJ, Toonen EJ, Joosten LA. Complement activation in the disease course of coronavirus disease 2019 and its effects on clinical outcomes. J Infect Dis. 2021;223(2):214–24.
81. CowanLT, Lutsey PL, Pankow JS, Matsushita K, Ishigami J, Lakshminarayan K. In patient and out patient infection as a trigger of cardiovascular disease: the ARIC study. J Am Heart Assoc. 2018;7(22):e009683–e009683. https://doi.org/10.1161/JAHA.118.009683. Ref infection CAD?
82. Clerkin KJ, Fried JA, Raikhelkar J, Sayer G, Griffin JM, Masoumi A, Jain SS, Burkhoff D, Kumaraiah D, Rabbani L, Schwartz A, Uriel N. Coronavirus disease 2019 (COVID-19) and cardiovascular disease. Circulation. 2020 Mar 21. https://doi.org/10.1161/CIRCULATIONAHA.120.046941. [Epub ahead of print] PubMed PMID: 32200663.
83. Cao W, Li T. COVID-19: towards understanding of pathogenesis. Cell Res. 2020;30 (5):367–9.
84. Yang L, Liu S, Liu J, Zhang Z, Wan X, Huang B, Chen Y, Zhang Y. COVID-19: immunopathogenesis and immunotherapeutics. Signal Transduct Target Ther. 2020;5(1): 1–8.
85. Huang C, Wang Y, Li X, et al. Clinical features of patients infected with 2019 novel coronavirus in Wuhan, China. Lancet. 2020;395(10223):497–506. https://doi.org/10.1016/S0140-6736(20)30183-5.
86. Yang C, Jin Z. An acute respiratory infection runs into the most common noncommunicable epidemic—COVID-19 and cardiovascular diseases. JAMA Cardiol. Published online March 25, 2020. https://doi.org/10.1001/jamacardio.2020.0934.
87. Bester J, Pretorius E. Effects of IL-1β, IL-6 and IL-8 on erythrocytes, platelets and clot viscoelasticity. Sci Rep. 2016;6(1):1–10.
88. He J, Wu B, Chen Y, et al. Characteristic electrocardiographic manifestations in patients with COVID-19 [published online ahead of print, 2020 Mar 29]. Can J Cardiol. 2020; S0828–282X(20)30301–9. https://doi.org/10.1016/j.cjca.2020.03.028.
89. Silhol F, Sarlon G, Deharo JC, Vaïsse B. Downregulation of ACE2 induces overstimulation of the renin–angiotensin system in COVID-19: should we block the renin–angiotensin system? Hypertens Res. 2020:1–3.
90. Sharma A, Garcia Jr G, Wang Y, Plummer JT, Morizono K, Arumugaswami V, Svendsen CN. Human iPSC-derived cardiomyocytes are susceptible to SARS-CoV-2 infection. Cell Rep Med. 2020;1(4):100052.

91. Bearse M, Hung YP, Krauson AJ, Bonanno L, Boyraz B, Harris CK, Helland TL, Hilburn CF, Hutchison B, Jobbagy S, Marshall MS. Factors associated with myocardial SARS-CoV-2 infection, myocarditis, and cardiac inflammation in patients with COVID-19. Modern Pathol. 2021:1–13.
92. Malavazos AE, Goldberger JJ, Iacobellis G. Does epicardial fat contribute to COVID-19 myocardial inflammation? Eur Heart J. 2020;41(24):2333–2333.
93. Mele D, Flamigni F, Rapezzi C, Ferrari R. Myocarditis in COVID-19 patients: current problems. Int Emerg Med. 2021:1–7.
94. Siripanthong B, Nazarian S, Muser D, Deo R, Santangeli P, Khanji MY, Cooper LT Jr, Chahal CAA. Recognizing COVID-19–related myocarditis: the possible pathophysiology and proposed guideline for diagnosis and management. Heart Rhythm. 2020;17(9):1463–71.
95. Basso C, Leone O, Rizzo S, De Gaspari M, van der Wal AC, Aubry MC, Bois MC, Lin PT, Maleszewski JJ, Stone JR. Pathological features of COVID-19-associated myocardial injury: a multicentre cardiovascular pathology study. Eur Heart J. 2020;41(39):3827–35.
96. Buja L, Stone J. A novel coronavirus meets the cardiovascular system: society for cardiovascular pathology symposium 2021. Cardiovasc Pathol Off J Soc Cardiovasc Pathol. 2021.
97. Eberhardt KA, Meyer-Schwickerath C, Heger E, Knops E, Lehmann C, Rybniker J, Schommers P, Eichenauer DA, Kurth F, Ramharter M, Kaiser R. RNAemia corresponds to disease severity and antibody response in hospitalized COVID-19 patients. Viruses. 2020;12 (9):1045.
98. Tavazzi G, Pellegrini C, Maurelli M, Belliato M, Sciutti F, Bottazzi A, Sepe PA, Resasco T, Camporotondo R, Bruno R, Baldanti F, Paolucci S, Pelenghi S, Iotti GA, Mojoli F, Arbustini E. Myocardial localization of coronavirus in COVID-19 cardiogenic shock. Eur J Heart Fail. 2020. https://doi.org/10.1002/ejhf.1828. [Epub ahead of print] PubMed PMID: 32275347.
99. Bradley BT, Maioli H, Johnson R, Chaudhry I, Fink SL, Xu H, Najafian B, Marshall D, Lacy JM, Williams T, Yarid N. Histopathology and ultrastructural findings of fatal COVID-19 infections. MedRxiv. https://www.medrxiv.org/content/10.1101/2020.04.17.20058545v1.
100. Fox SE, Li G, Akmatbekov A, Harbert JL, Lameira FS, Brown JQ, Vander Heide RS. Unexpected features of cardiac pathology in COVID-19 infection. Circulation. 2020;142 (11):1123–5.
101. Fox SE, Lameira FS, Rinker EB, Vander Heide RS. Cardiac Endotheliitis and multisystem inflammatory syndrome after COVID-19. Ann Intern Med. 2020;173(12):1025–7.
102. Bullock HA, Goldsmith CS, Zaki SR, Martines RB, Miller SE. Difficulties in differentiating coronaviruses from subcellular structures in human tissues by electron microscopy. Emerg Infect Dis. 2021;27(4):1023.
103. Zheng YY, Ma YT, Zhang JY, Xie X. COVID-19 and the cardiovascular system. Nat Rev Cardiol. Published online March 5, 2020. https://doi.org/10.1038/s41569-0200360-5.
104. McMillan P, Uhal BD. COVID-19–A theory of autoimmunity to ACE-2. MOJ Immunol. 2020;7(1):17.
105. Townsend A. Autoimmunity to ACE2 as a possible cause of tissue inflammation in Covid-19. Med Hypotheses. 2020;144:110043.
106. McMillan P, Dexhiemer T, Neubig RR, Uhal BD. COVID-19—a theory of autoimmunity against ACE-2 explained. Front Immunol. 2021;12:499.
107. Inciardi RM, Lupi L, Zaccone G, et al. Cardiac involvement in a patient with coronavirus disease 2019 (COVID-19). JAMA Cardiol. Published online March 27, 2020. https://doi.org/10.1001/jamacardio.2020.1096.
108. Zeng JH, Liu YX, Yuan J, Wang FX, Wu WB, Li JX, Wang LF, Gao H, Wang Y, Dong CF, Li YJ, Xie XJ, Feng C, Liu L. First case of COVID-19 complicated with fulminant myocarditis: a case report and insights. Infection. 2020 Apr 10. https://doi.org/10.1007/s15010-020-01424-5. [Epub ahead of print] PubMed PMID: 32277408.

109. Hu H, Ma F, Wei X, Fang Y. Coronavirus fulminant myocarditis saved with glucocorticoid and human immunoglobulin. Eur Heart J (2020 Mar 16) [E-pub ahead of print].
110. Zou L, Ruan F, Huang M, Liang L, Huang H, Hong Z, Yu J, Kang M, Song Y, Xia J, Guo Q, Song T, He J, Yen HL, Peiris M, Wu J. SARS-CoV-2 viral load in upper respiratory specimens of infected patients. N Engl J Med. 2020;382(12):1177–9. https://doi.org/10.1056/NEJMc2001737. Epub 2020 Feb 19. PubMed PMID: 32074444; PubMed Central PMCID: PMC7121626.
111. Fung SY, Yuen KS, Ye ZW, Chan CP, Jin DY. A tug-of-war between severe acute respiratory syndrome coronavirus 2 and host antiviral defence: lessons from other pathogenic viruses. Emerg Microbes Infect. 2020;9(1):558–70. https://doi.org/10.1080/22221751.2020.1736644. eCollection 2020. Review. PubMed PMID: 32172672; PubMed Central PMCID:PMC7103735.

Chapter 12
Heart Failure in CoViD19

Key Questions

- What is the epidemiological association of heart failure in CoViD19
- Does heart failure contribute to the CoViD19 associated risk?
- What are the prognostic implications of heart failure in CoViD19?
- What peculiarities exist in the behavior of biomarkers in cardiac failure in CoViD19?
- What are the main determinants of heart failure in CoViD19?

12.1 Epidemiology

The CoViD19 pandemic, among other cardiovascular complications, has drawn a special focus on the potentially lethal cardiac complication "heart failure" at multiple levels and has even led to the restructuring of care of heart failure patients [1, 2]. Several important features related to heart failure, such as an increased susceptibility of patients with chronic cardiac failure towards developing CoViD19, an elevated risk of developing CoViD19 complications in patients heart failure, and development of de novo heart failure in CoViD19 patients, have come under debate and remain poorly understood. Besides, heart failure in CoViD19 may present in multiple forms of severity and a pose significant therapeutic challenge. The forms of clinical presentation may range from fluid imbalance to cardiogenic shock or even death.

Data show that heart failure is a common and serious complication in severe CoViD19. Heart failure may present in de novo form (without a history of prior cardiovascular disease) in CoViD19 patients or as an exacerbation of the pre-existing heart failure. The previous history of heart failure and the background

U. Mallick, *Cardiovascular Complications of COVID-19*,
https://doi.org/10.1007/978-3-030-90065-6_12

cardiovascular risk factors, appear to be associated with increased mortality in CoViD19 patients. In a retrospective study of 799 patients admitted with CoViD19, data of 274 patients (113 deceased and 161 recovered) were analyzed. The study showed that heart failure was among the most common critical complications during the exacerbation of CoViD19. About 49% (41/83) of patients had heart failure and patients with preexisting cardiovascular disease had worse outcomes. The incidence of de novo heart failure in CoViD19 patients was reported at 19% (21/109) in patients with no previous history of cardiovascular diseases or hypertension and was higher in the deceased 20/41 (49%) than recovered patients 1/68 (1%) [3]. In a retrospective, multicenter study of 191 patients admitted with CoViD19 about 52% (28 of 54) of the deceased patients had a diagnosis of heart failure as compared to 12% (16 of 137) of the survivors. According to the demographic data, the burden of risk factors such as hypertension, coronary heart disease, and diabetes mellitus, was much higher in the non-survivors (54) as compared to survivors (137) about 48% versus 23%, 31% versus 14%, and 24% versus 1% respectively [4]. Several other studies have reported an increased risk of mortality due to heart failure in CoViD19. In a multi-center observational study of 8910 CoViD19 patients from Asia, America, and North America, the risk of in-hospital death due to heart failure was 15.3%, versus 5.6% among those without heart failure [5]. Although data on specific forms of heart failure in CoViD19 is scarce, studies report the association of poor outcomes in CoViD19 patients with right heart failure. A retrospective study of 110 consecutive hospitalized patients with CoViD19, demonstrated an association of right ventricular dilatation in about 31% (32/110) of patients with CoViD19 and a significant association with increased mortality [6]. Studies further confirm the increased risk of mortality when right ventricular dysfunction is present in CoViD19 patients [7].

12.2 Role of Comorbidities in Heart Failure with CoViD19

The pathogenesis of heart failure in CoViD19 appears to be multi-factorial (Fig. 12.2), likely to be the consequence of several underlying comorbidities associated with CoViD19 criticality, including the development of multi-organ dysfunction, ARDS, pulmonary thromboembolic conditions, and various forms of myocardial ischemic and inflammatory complications. Analyses have explored predictors of adverse outcomes of heart failure among hospitalized CoViD19 patients (Fig. 12.4). A retrospective study involving 803 hypertensive patients with CoViD19 showed average systolic blood pressure as an independent predictor for the development of heart failure (hazard ratio (HR) per 10 mmHg 1.89, 95% confidence interval (CI): 1.15, 3.13) [8].

Patients with chronic lung conditions and a history of smoking have increased susceptibility towards CoViD19 [9, 10], manifest more severe disease [9] and

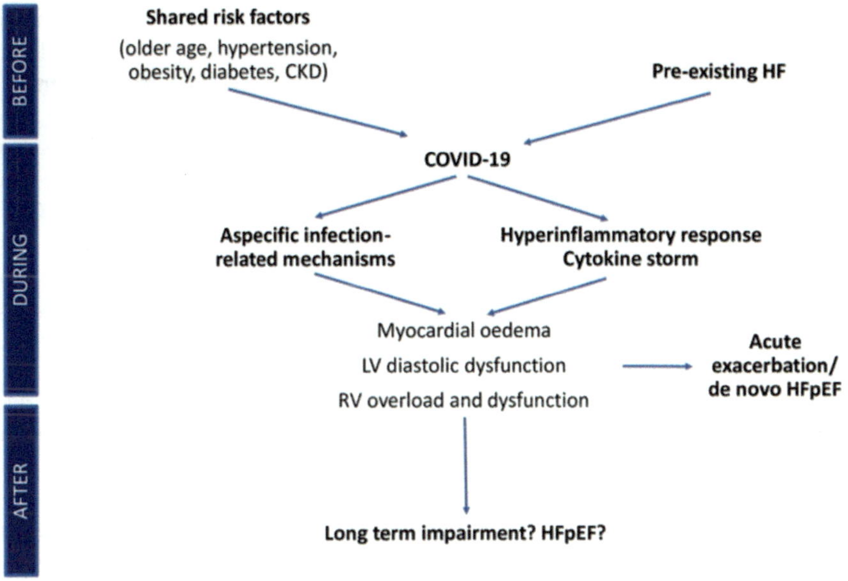

Fig. 12.1 The short- and long-term relationship between COVID-19 and HFpEF. CKD, chronic kidney disease; COVID-19, Coronavirus Disease 2019; HF, heart failure; HFpEF, heart failure with preserved ejection fraction; LV, left ventricular; RV, right ventricular. *Source* Figure 1. Zaccone, G., Tomasoni, D., Italia, L., Lombardi, C.M. and Metra, M., 2021. Myocardial Involvement in COVID-19: an Interaction Between Comorbidities and Heart Failure with Preserved Ejection Fraction. A Further Indication of the Role of Inflammation. Current heart failure reports, pp.1–8. https://link.springer.com/article/10.1007/s11897-021-00509-y. By Springer Nature

an increase in mortality in CoViD19 [11, 12]. Studies show that sepsis and respiratory diseases contribute to the decompensation of heart failure [13, 14]. The ARDS is a major complication in CoViD19 patients. The association of ARDS in CoViD19 may increase the risk for developing heart failure [15]. Other lung conditions associated with advanced CoViD19 such as thrombotic pulmonary disease, or pulmonary hypertension, may induce right heart injury and determine the development of heart failure or decompensation of pre existing cardiac failure in patients with CoViD19 (Fig. 12.3). Similarly, the association of the multi-organ injury, especially various forms of renal parenchymal or vascular complications promote heart failure pathogenesis in CoViD19 patients with advanced disease.

Heart Failure and myocardial injury may share common grounds in patients with CoViD19 with a significant overlap in the diagnostic and etiopathogenetic mechanisms. The development of myocardial injury may increase susceptibility towards developing heart failure and a pre-existing heart failure makes may increase susceptibility towards myocardial injury. The heart failure in CoViD19 may be a consequence of a newly developed cardiac injury or decompensation of a previously existing cardiovascular disease or severely dysregulated blood pressure

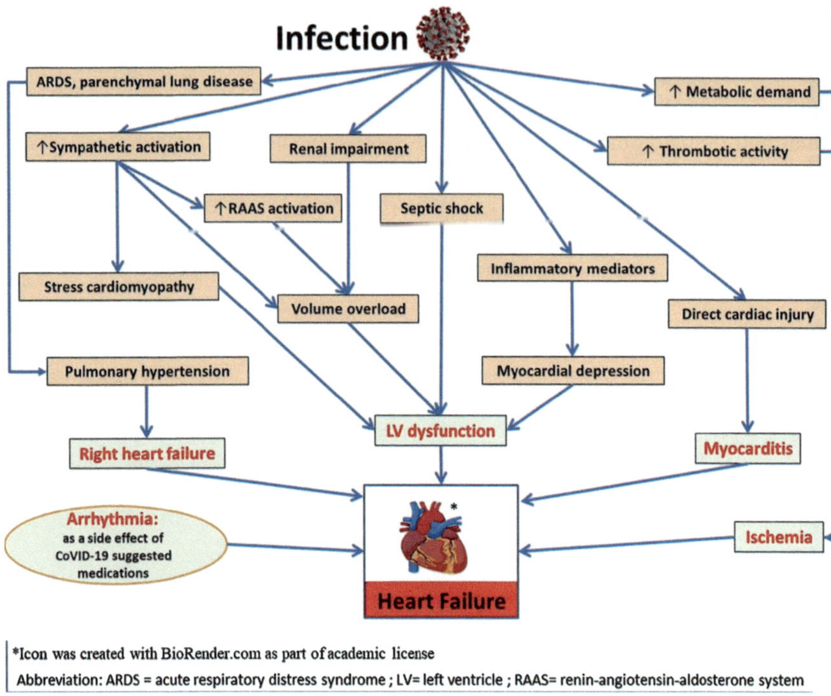

Fig. 12.2 Mechanisms heart failure in CoViD19. *Source* Figure 1. Bader, F., Manla, Y., Atallah, B. and Starling, R.C., 2021. Heart failure and COVID-19. Heart failure reviews, 26(1), pp.1–10. https://link.springer.com/article/10.1007/s10741-020-10008-2. By Springer Nature Group

secondary to the hyperinflammatory stress or underlying ischemic, metabolic, hemodynamic, or infectious turbulence. Occurrence of the cases of decompensated heart failure or cardiogenic shock in the absence of a previous history of cardiovascular disease has been reported in patients with CoViD 19 [16]. An acute CoViD19 related myocarditis, arrhythmia, or an acute ischemic event may present as acute heart failure warranting a careful work up in the exploration of heart failure in the CoViD19 patients.

12.3 Biomarkers of Heart Failure in CoViD19

The N-terminal pro-brain natriuretic peptide is used as a standard biomarker for biochemical detection of myocardial dysfunction in subjects with CoViD 19. Other biomarkers of myocardial injury and inflammatory stress including high-sensitivity C-reactive protein (hsCRP), interleukin-6 (IL-6), interleukin-10 (IL-10) are also used to further refine and define diagnostic and management strategies. In a retrospective study of 799 patients admitted with CoViD 19, data of 113 deceased and

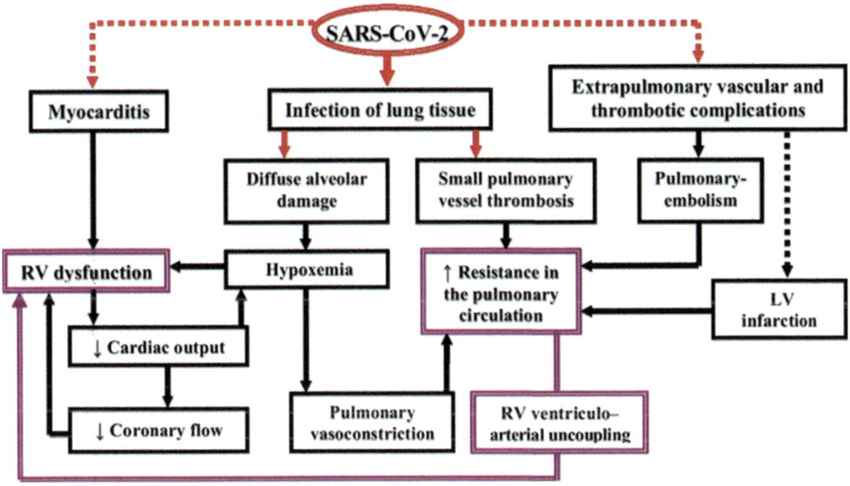

Fig. 12.3 Pathogenesis of right heart failure in CoViD19. Pathophysiologic role of heart–lung interactions for the development and progression of life-threatening RV dysfunction during SARS-COV-2 infection. The bold red arrows indicate the major direct impact of the virus on the lung tissue. The red dotted arrows indicate other possible direct cardiovascular damages of the virus with prognostic relevance. *Source* Figure 1. Dandel, M., 2021. Heart–lung interactions in COVID-19: prognostic impact and usefulness of bedside echocardiography for monitoring of the right ventricle involvement. Heart Failure Reviews, pp.1–15. https://link.springer.com/article/10.1007/s10741-021-10108-7. Published by Springer Nature Group

161 recovered patients were analyzed. The N-terminal pro-brain natriuretic peptide concentrations were markedly higher in deceased patients (800.0 pg/mL) than in recovered patients (72.0 pg/mL). About 49% (85/173) patients had significantly raised value of NT pro-BNP, median (IQR) $\geq$ 285 pg/mL, in this cohort, and the higher values were more often seen in the deceased patients 85% 68 of 80 as compared to the survivors 18% 17 of 93 [3]. The elevated pro-inflammatory cytokines in CoViD19 that mark multi-organ dysfunction may indicate imminent heart failure, may be used in the assessment of heart failure or a future risk [17, 18]. Hyper cytokinesis is an important feature of severe CoViD19 with overexpression of several cytokines and chemokines that reflect injury to multiple organs due to the viral disease [19]. Elevated IL-6, IL-10, TNF-alpha imply heart failure-related mechanisms [20].

The association of raised BNP with ARDS has been previously indicated [21] and reflects an unfavorable course among patients with ARDS. Troponin, a marker of myocardial injury in CoViD19 patients, may be used when cardiac dysfunction is suspected and other markers of myocardial injury CKMB, myoglobin may be considered. Endothelin-1 (ET 1) an important hemodynamic regulator associated with heart failure, appears to be elevated with the severity of CoViD19 [22]. Serum ACE2 and ADAM-17 activity have also been explored in patients with heart failure and may have a role in CoviD19 [23–25]. Multiple biomarkers may be used in

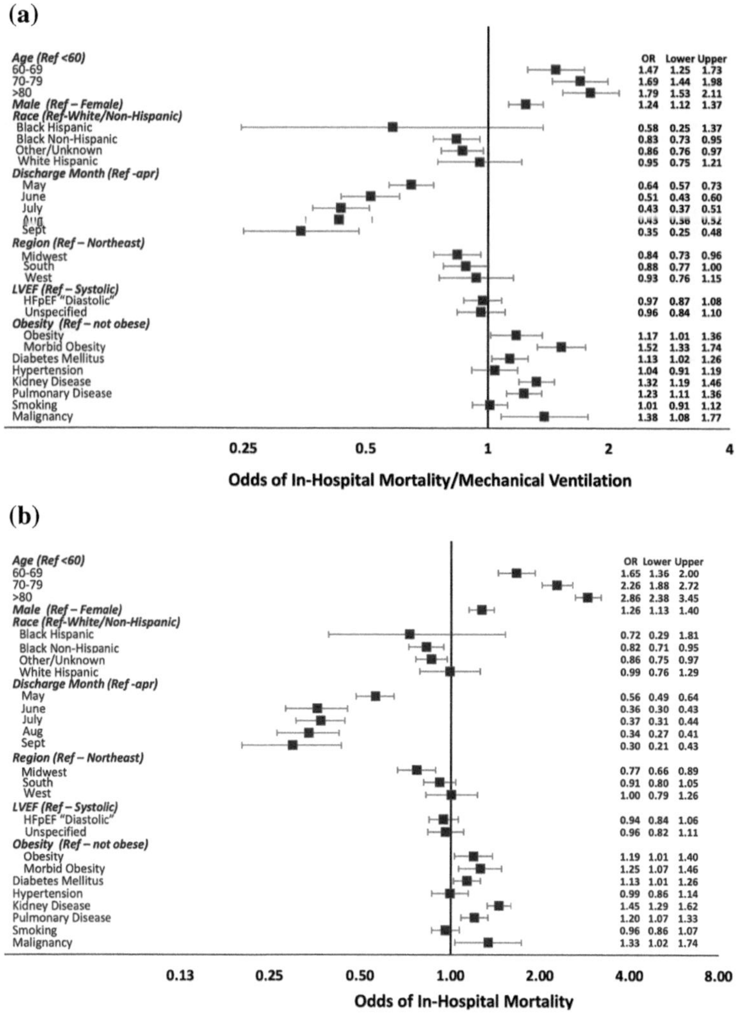

Fig. 12.4 Predictors of adverse in-hospital outcomes among HF patients hospitalized with COVID-19. **a** Predictors of in-hospital mortality or mechanical ventilatory need in HF patients hospitalized with COVID-19. This figure shows predictors of in-hospital mortality or mechanical ventilatory needs among patients with a history of HF hospitalized with COVID-19. Odds ratios are reported for clinical covariates of interest. Lower and upper bounds correspond to 95% confidence intervals [CI]. **b** Predictors of in-hospital mortality in HF patients hospitalized with COVID-19. This figure describes predictors of in-hospital mortality among patients with a history of HF hospitalized with COVID-19. COVID-19 = coronavirus disease-2019; HFpEF = heart failure with preserved ejection fraction; OR = odds ratio. *Source* Figure 2. Bhatt, A.S., Jering, K. S., Vaduganathan, M., Claggett, B.L., Cunningham, J.W., Rosenthal, N., Signorovitch, J., Thune, J.J., Vardeny, O. and Solomon, S.D., 2021. Clinical outcomes in patients with heart failure hospitalized with COVID-19. Heart Failure, 9(1), pp.65–73. https://www.jacc.org/doi/full/10.1016/j.jchf.2020.11.003. By Springer Nature Group

combination in the assessment of cardiac dysfunction of the CoViD19 patients. Elevation of the biomarkers may be secondary to systemic inflammation [26] and may be present with a normal cardiac function [27] warranting a cautious approach in the clinical settings. Several biomarkers, such as CRP, ferritin, D dimers, the markers of severity of CoViD19, also known to have an association with myocardial injury and inflammation may aid in risk assessment in CoViD19 patients in the assessment of heart failure and further risk. The detection of a variety of biomarkers in patients with CoViD19 related heart failure reflects the involvement of different pathogenetic mechanisms. An approach involving the use of multiple biomarkers in CoViD19 patients in combination, when heart failure is suspected, may be more effective as compared to the use of conventional heart failure serum markers. Immune, inflammatory, neurohormones, and markers of myocardial injury besides markers of severity of CoViD19 are particularly important.

A meticulous assessment and quantification of the myocardial dysfunction are essential for the confirmation of the diagnosis of heart failure. Besides the use of multiple biomarkers, several classical imaging techniques such as echocardiography, cardiac magnetic resonance imaging, and others may be used for detailed cardiac assessments. Precise measurements of the cardiac functional parameters through imaging techniques may help to understand the specific features and characteristics of the heart failure, and aid distinction between various forms, such as with HF with reduced ejection fraction (HFrEF) or with preserved ejection fraction (HFpEF), associated with the novel coronavirus disease CoViD19.

12.4 Pathogenetic Mechanisms of Heart Failure in CoViD19

The pathogenicity of heart failure in CoViD19 appears to involve RAS mechanisms, immune and inflammatory processes, hypoxia, dysregulated hemodynamic mechanisms, apoptosis, and several other processes triggered by the complex interaction between viral invasion, and the host defense and regulatory mechanisms. Expression and kinetics of a variety of blood proteins such as the Ang II, ACE 2, cytokines (TNF-α, IL-6, IL-10), hs C Reactive Protein high-sensitivity C-reactive protein (hs CRP), BNP, troponin, endothelin, showcase the association of heart failure and CoViD19. Elevated cytokine release is a prominent feature of the pathogenesis of severe CoViD19 [28]. The high inflammatory burden or cytokine storm appears to be linked with cardiac complications such as inflammatory or fulminant myocarditis, decompensation of heart failure, cardiogenic shock, and arrhythmias in CoViD19 patients. Hyper cytokine release is cardiotoxic [29–31], and interaction of the immune system and the neurohormones involving cytokines, cardiac structural changes, and dysfunction [32] are interlinked via several mechanisms including immune toxicity of the myocardium or vascular structures, impacting myocardial cell contractility [33], cellular stress mechanisms or extracellular matrix remodeling and fibrosis [34, 35], Data show that TNF-α levels are markedly elevated in advanced heart failure [29, 36], and the BNP and IL-6 independently predict mortality in heart failure [37]. The cardiac inflammatory load in association with cytokine storm and other hyperinflammatory mechanisms, also noticed with multi-organ dysfunction in CoViD19, are likely mechanisms underlying heart failure in this viral disease. In CoViD19, an elevated CRP, IL-6, IFN-γ, IL-1, and TNF-α adversely impact the cardiovascular system among other organs [19]. The prolonged cardiac inflammation may be determined by the enhanced signaling of the cytokine related mechanisms [38] that are also markers of future cardiovascular risk [17, 18]. Patients with preexisting CVD or heart failure have an increased underlying inflammatory activity and enhanced inflammatory stress due to CoViD19 is likely to increase the risk of heart failure and related complications.

SARS CoV2 uses ACE2 as a receptor for viral cell entry and RAS mechanisms are dysregulated in CoViD19 and represent a prominent pathognomonic feature of the severe disease. Elevated ACE2 activity, a known marker of the severity of heart failure [39], may increase the susceptibility of patients with cardiac diseases for CoViD19 and disease severity. Whether the upregulation of ACE2 activity in heart failure is a cause, or a consequence of the adaptive or maladaptive mechanism in heart failure, is subject to debate. The SARS CoV2 downregulates ACE2, and the associated dysregulation that results in Ang II elevation and the consequent deleterious pro-inflammatory, prothrombotic and vasoplegic impact may adversely impact the cardiac function for instance via interfering with cardiac vasculature or harming myocardium. The involvement of another co-player in this process, an important enzyme disintegrin ADAM 17 TACE protease, which is known to mediate ectodomain shedding of the ACE2 [40], further supports the role of these mechanisms in CoViD19 related heart failure. Evidence suggests that ADAM 17 protease activity is also upregulated in the heart failure [24, 25]. Mechanisms involved in the upregulation of ADAM 17 in heart failure and enhanced ACE 2 activity in HF, also involve increase cytokine production and may explain the role of RAS-Inflammatory pathways in the development of HF in patients with complicated CoViD 19 [41–43]. These markers further justify the risk of cardiac complications including heart failure, in patients with cardiometabolic risk factors including diabetes mellitus with CoViD19 [44, 45]. Role of several other vasoactive systems such as prostaglandins and catecholamines or cellular processes including, mitochondrial damage and oxidative stress [46], cell death, cellular immune-metabolic interactions [47] are likely to be important in the pathogenesis of heart failure in CoViD19 patients. The iatrogenicity of CoViD19 treatments such as immune agents (chloroquine/hydroxychloroquine, interferon-alpha 2B) or antiviral drugs (Lopinavir/ritonavir) needs further considerations.

12.5 Summary

In summary, heart failure HF is a common complication in CoViD19. It may be associated with worse outcomes especially in patients with preexisting cardiovascular disease or a high risk-factor burden. Evaluation of underlying myocardial, electrical, vascular, or associated inflammatory stress, related to sepsis and multi-organ injury must be performed to assess the risk and pathogenetic severity of heart failure in CoViD19 patients. A battery of biochemical markers may aid a better risk assessment. The BNP, and markers of myocardial injury such as troponin, or markers of immune-inflammatory stress such as CRP, cytokines, and others that indicate the severity of disease such as ferritin, D Dimers may be utilized. Likely mechanisms involved in the development of heart failure in CoViD 19, involve a spectrum of inflammatory, immunological, humoral, infectious, metabolic, ischemic, and other stress mechanisms that may result in heart failure due to a myocardial injury or hemodynamic decompensation. Among these mechanisms, the dysregulated RAS and hyperinflammatory mechanisms appear to be the most likely culprits that may act in synergism and ultimately result in heart failure. Further studies are required in a larger variety of cohorts to generate robust clinical, imaging, and biochemical data, especially the mechanisms related to the direct viral injury and associated inflammatory mechanisms. This will help to better characterize and determine the etiopathogenesis and clinical course of heart failure in CoViD19. The imaging investigations such as CMR hold a significant value for detection of myocardial sequelae that are associated with CoViD19 and underlying heart failure [48] and may help detecting the myocardial injury earlier [49]. Heart failure in CoViD19 needs to be better characterized and improved strategies are needed for disease staging and phenotyping in CoViD19 patients. Right heart failure with associated CoViD19 pulmonary disease and prognostic implications warrant a careful approach in patient management with timely recognition and treatment and require further exploration. Heart failure with preserved ejection fraction (HFpEF) appears to be closely linked with CoViD19 (Fig. 12.1) and its short and long term implications need to be better understood. The role of the conventional and unconventional biomarkers in CoViD19 needs to be further validated and mechanisms involved in CoViD19 related cardiac damage need to be determined. Adaptations are necessary to improve therapeutic options for CoViD19 related heart failure and the models of care of heart failure services.

Summary Box

- Heart failure increases the risk for severe CoViD19 disease and complications.
- Pre-existing cardiac failure and cardiometabolic risk factors are associated with worse outcomes.

- A new heart failure in CoViD19 patients may reflect a new myocardial injury, elevated ischemic or inflammatory stress, arrhythmia, or significant pulmonary disease burden.
- Further research is needed to define heart failure, phenotyping, stagging, and outcomes in CoViD19 patients.
- The beta natriuretic peptide and markers of myocardial injury like troponin aid in diagnosing heart failure, however, immune-inflammatory markers along with markers of severity of CoViD19 may improve the estimation.
- Among the variety of pathogenetic mechanisms, dysregulated inflammatory and vasoactive mechanisms are prominent.
- Delivery of heart failure care has been significantly restructured during the CoViD19 pandemic, vulnerable population groups must be prioritized.
- Robust studies should address the impact of the pandemic on the outcomes in patients with heart failure and CoViD19.

References

1. Shah PB, Welt FG, Mahmud E, Phillips A, Kleiman NS, Young MN, Sherwood M, Batchelor W, Wang DD, Davidson L, Wyman J. Triage considerations for patients referred for structural heart disease intervention during the COVID-19 pandemic: an ACC/SCAI position statement. Cardiovasc Interv. 2020;13(12):1484–8.
2. Virani SA, Clarke B, Ducharme A, Ezekowitz JA, Heckman GA, McDonald M, Mielniczuk LM, Swiggum E, Van Spall HG, Zieroth S, Society CHF. Optimizing access to heart failure care in Canada during the COVID-19 pandemic. Can J Cardiol. 2020;36 (7):1148–51.
3. Chen T, Wu D, Chen H, Yan W, Yang D, Chen G, Ma K, Xu D, Yu H, Wang H, Wang T, Guo W, Chen J, Ding C, Zhang X, Huang J, Han M, Li S, Luo X, Zhao J, Ning Q. Clinical characteristics of 113 deceased patients with coronavirus disease 2019: retrospective study. BMJ. 2020;368:m1091. https://doi.org/10.1136/bmj.m1091. Erratum in: BMJ. 2020;368: m1295. PubMed PMID: 32217556.
4. Zhou F, Yu T, Du R. Clinical course and risk factors for mortality of adult inpatients with COVID-19 in Wuhan, China: a retrospective cohort study. Lancet. 2020.
5. Mehra MR, Desai SS, Kuy S, Henry TD, Patel AN. Cardiovascular disease, drug therapy, and mortality in Covid-19. N Engl J Med. 2020;382(25):e102.
6. Argulian E, Sud K, Vogel B, Bohra C, Garg VP, Talebi S, Lerakis S, Narula J. Right ventricular dilation in hospitalized patients with COVID-19 infection. Cardiovasc Imaging. 2020;13(11):2459–61.
7. Li Y, Li H, Zhu S, Xie Y, Wang B, He L, Zhang D, Zhang Y, Yuan H, Wu C, Sun W. Prognostic value of right ventricular longitudinal strain in patients with COVID-19. Cardiovasc Imaging. 2020;13(11):2287–99.
8. Ran J, Song Y, Zhuang Z, Han L, Zhao S, Cao P, Geng Y, Xu L, Qin J, He D, Wu F. Blood pressure control and adverse outcomes of COVID-19 infection in patients with concomitant hypertension in Wuhan China. Hypertens Res. 2020;43(11):1267–76.

9. Reddy RK, Charles WN, Sklavounos A, Dutt A, Seed PT, Khajuria A. The effect of smoking on COVID-19 severity: a systematic review and meta-analysis. J Med Virol. 2021;93 (2):1045–56.
10. Olloquequi J. COVID-19 Susceptibility in chronic obstructive pulmonary disease. Eur J Clin Investig. 2020;50(10):e13382.
11. Docherty AB, Harrison EM, Green CA, Hardwick HE, Pius R, Norman L, Holden KA, Read JM, Dondelinger F, Carson G, Merson L. Features of 20 133 UK patients in hospital with covid-19 using the ISARIC WHO Clinical Characterisation Protocol: prospective observational cohort study. BMJ. 2020;369.
12. Pranata R, Soeroto AY, Huang I, Lim MA, Santoso P, Permana H, Lukito AA. Effect of chronic obstructive pulmonary disease and smoking on the outcome of COVID-19. Int J Tuberc Lung Dis. 2020;24(8):838–43.
13. Walker AM, Drozd M, Hall M, Patel PA, Paton M, Lowry J, Gierula J, Byrom R, Kearney L, Sapsford RJ, Witte KK. Prevalence and predictors of sepsis death in patients with chronic heart failure and reduced left ventricular ejection fraction. J Am Heart Assoc. 2018;7(20): e009684.
14. Alon D, Stein GY, Korenfeld R, Fuchs S. Predictors and outcomes of infection-related hospital admissions of heart failure patients. PloS One. 2013;8(8):e72476.
15. Metkus TS, Sokoll LJ, Barth AS, Czarny MJ, Hays AG, Lowenstein CJ, Michos ED, Nolley EP, Post WS, Resar JR, Thiemann DR. Myocardial injury in severe COVID-19 compared with non–COVID-19 acute respiratory distress syndrome. Circulation. 2021;143 (6):553–65.
16. Fried JA, Ramasubbu K, Bhatt R, et al. The variety of cardiovascular presentations of COVID-19. Circulation. 2020.
17. Ziegler L, Gajulapuri A, Frumento P, Bonomi A, Wallén H, de Faire U, Rose-John S, Gigante B. Interleukin 6 trans-signalling and risk of future cardiovascular events. Cardiovasc Res. 2019;115(1):213–21.
18. Ferrante G, Condorelli G. Interleukin-6 trans-signalling and risk of future cardiovascular events: a new avenue for atheroprotection? 2019.
19. Huang C, Wang Y, Li X, Ren L, Zhao J, Hu Y, Zhang L, Fan G, Xu J, Gu X, Cheng Z. Clinical features of patients infected with 2019 novel coronavirus in Wuhan China. The Lancet. 2020;395(10223):497–506.
20. Kumar A, Parrillo JE, Kumar A. Clinical review: myocardial depression in sepsis and septic shock. Crit Care. 2002;6(6):1–9.
21. Karmpaliotis D, Kirtane AJ, Ruisi CP, Polonsky T, Malhotra A, Talmor D, Kosmidou I, Jarolim P, de Lemos JA, Sabatine MS, Gibson CM. Diagnostic and prognostic utility of brain natriuretic Peptide in subjects admitted to the ICU with hypoxic respiratory failure due to noncardiogenic and cardiogenic pulmonary edema. Chest. 2007;131(4):964–71.
22. Farhangrazi ZS, Moghimi SM. Elevated circulating endothelin-1 as a potential biomarker for high-risk COVID-19 severity. Precis Nanomed. 2020;3:622–8.
23. Sama IE, Ravera A, Santema BT, van Goor H, ter Maaten JM, Cleland JGF, Rienstra M, Friedrich AW, Samani NJ, Ng LL, Dickstein K, Lang CC, Filippatos G, Anker SD, Ponikowski P, Metra M, van Veldhuisen DJ, Voors AA. Circulating plasma concentrations of angiotensin-converting enzyme 2 in men and women with heart failure and effects of renin–angiotensin–aldosterone inhibitors. Eur Heart J.2020;41(19):1810–17. https://doi.org/10.1093/eurheartj/ehaa373.
24. Lambert DW, Yarski M, Warner FJ, et al. Tumor necrosis factor{alpha} convertase (ADAM17) mediates regulated ectodomain shedding of the severe-acute respiratory syndrome-coronavirus (SARSCoV) receptor, angiotensin-converting enzyme-2 (ACE2). J Biol Chem. 2005;280:30113–9.
25. Fedak PW, Moravec CS, McCarthy PM, et al. Altered expression of disintegrin metalloproteinases and their inhibitor in human dilated cardiomyopathy. Circulation. 2006;113:238–45.

26. Zakynthinos E, Kiropoulos T, Gourgoulianis K, Filippatos G. Diagnostic and prognostic impact of brain natriuretic peptide in cardiac and noncardiac diseases. Heart Lung. 2008;37(4):275–85.
27. Knight DS, Kotecha T, Razvi Y, Chacko L, Brown JT, Jeetley PS, Goldring J, Jacobs M, Lamb LE, Negus R, Wolff A. COVID-19: Myocardial injury in survivors. Circulation. 2020;142(11):1120–2.
28. Mehta P, McAuley DF, Brown M, Sanchez E, Tattersall RS, Manson JJ. COVID-19: consider cytokine storm syndromes and immunosuppression. The Lancet. 2020;395(10229):1033–4.
29. Levine B, Kalman J, Mayer L, Fillit HM, Packer M. Elevated circulating levels of tumor necrosis factor in severe chronic heart failure. N Engl J Med. 1990;323(4):236–41.
30. Matsumori A, Yamada T, Suzuki H, et al. Increased circulating cytokines in patients with myocarditis and cardiomyopathy. Br Heart J. 1994;72:561–66.
31. Jamal FA, Khaled SK. The cardiovascular complications of chimeric antigen receptor T cell therapy. Curr Hematol Malig Rep. 2020;15(2):130–2.
32. Sharma R, Coats AJ, Anker SD. The role of inflammatory mediators in chronic heart failure: cytokines, nitric oxide, and endothelin-1. Int J Cardiol. 2000;72(2):175–86.
33. Keira N, Tatsumi T, Matoba S, Shiraishi J, Yamanaka S, Akashi K, Kobara M, Asayama J, Fushiki S, Fliss H, Nakagawa M. Lethal effect of cytokine-induced nitric oxide and peroxynitrite on cultured rat cardiac myocytes. J Mol Cell Cardiol. 2002;34(5):583–96.
34. Hedayat M, Mahmoudi MJ, Rose NR, Rezaei N. Proinflammatory cytokines in heart failure: double-edged swords. Heart Fail Rev. 2010;15(6):543–62.
35. Chou CH, Hung CS, Liao CW, Wei LH, Chen CW, Shun CT, Wen WF, Wan CH, Wu XM, Chang YY, Wu VC. IL-6 trans-signalling contributes to aldosterone-induced cardiac fibrosis. Cardiovasc Res. 2018;114(5):690–702.
36. McMurray J, Abdullah I, Dargie H, Shapiro D. Increased concentrations of tumour necrosis factor in "cachectic" patients with severe heart failure. Br Heart J. 1991;66:356–8.
37. Maeda K, Tsutamoto T, Wada A, Mabuchi N, Hayashi M, Tsutsui T, Ohnishi M, Sawaki M, Fujii M, Matsumoto T, Kinoshita M. High levels of plasma brain natriuretic peptide and interleukin-6 after optimized treatment for heart failure are independent risk factors for morbidity and mortality in patients with congestive heart failure. J Am Coll Cardiol. 2000;36:1587–93. [PubMed] [Google Scholar].
38. Guzik TJ, Mohiddin SA, Dimarco A, Patel V, Savvatis K, Marelli-Berg FM, Madhur MS, Tomaszewski M, Maffia P, D'Acquisto F, Nicklin SA. COVID-19 and the cardiovascular system: implications for risk assessment, diagnosis, and treatment options. Cardiovasc Res. 2020;116(10):1666–87.
39. Epelman S, Tang WH, Chen SY, Van Lente F, Francis GS, Sen S. Detection of soluble angiotensin-converting enzyme 2 in heart failure: insights into the endogenous counter-regulatory pathway of the renin-angiotensin-aldosterone system. J Am Coll Cardiol. 2008;52(9):750–4. https://doi.org/10.1016/j.jacc.2008.02.088.
40. Lambert DW, Yarski M, Warner FJ, et al. Tumor necrosis factor-alpha convertase (ADAM17) mediates regulated ectodomain shedding of the severe–acute respiratory syndrome-coronavirus (SARS-CoV) receptor, angiotensin-converting enzyme-2 (ACE2). J Biol Chem. 2005;280:30113.
41. de Queiroz TM, Lakkappa N, Lazartigues E. ADAM17-mediated shedding of inflammatory cytokines in hypertension. Front Pharmacol. 2020;11:1154.
42. Seals DF, Courtneidge SA. The ADAMs family of metalloproteases: multidomain proteins with multiple functions. Genes Dev. 2003;17(1):7–30.
43. Liu H, Wang H, Cheng D, Wang Q, Pei Z, Zhu N, Fang W, Yu Q. Potential role of a disintegrin and metalloproteinase-17 (ADAM17) in age-associated ventricular remodeling of rats. RSC Adv. 2019;9(25):14321–30.
44. Fagyas M, Uri K, Siket IM, Fulop GA, Csato V, Darago A, Boczan J, Banyai E, Szentkiralyi IE, Maros TM, Szerafin T, Edes I, Papp Z and Toth A. New perspectives in the renin-angiotensin-aldosterone system (RAAS) II: albumin suppresses angiotensin converting enzyme (ACE) activity in human. PLoS One. 2014;9:e87844.

45. Uri K, Fagyas M, Mányiné Siket I, Kertesz A, Csanadi Z, Sandorfi G, Clemens M, Fedor R, Papp Z, Edes I, Toth A. New perspectives in the renin-angiotensin-aldosterone system (RAAS) IV: circulating ACE2 as a biomarker of systolic dysfunction in human hypertension and heart failure. PLoS One. 2014;9(4):e87845.
46. Dai DF, Johnson SC, Villarin JJ, Chin MT, Nieves-Cintrón M, Chen T, Marcinek DJ, Dorn GW, Kang YJ, Prolla TA, Santana LF. Mitochondrial oxidative stress mediates angiotensin II–induced cardiac hypertrophy and Gαq overexpression–induced heart failure. Circ Res. 2011;108(7):837–46.
47. Ketelhuth DF, Lutgens E, Bäck M, Binder CJ, Van den Bossche J, Daniel C, Dumitriu IE, Hoefer I, Libby P, O'Neill L, Weber C. Immunometabolism and atherosclerosis: perspectives and clinical significance: a position paper from the Working Group on Atherosclerosis and Vascular Biology of the European Society of Cardiology. Cardiovasc Res. 2019;115(9):1385–92.
48. Ojha V, Verma M, Pandey NN, Mani A, Malhi AS, Kumar S, Jagia P, Roy A, Sharma S. Cardiac magnetic resonance imaging in coronavirus disease 2019 (COVID-19): a systematic review of cardiac magnetic resonance imaging findings in 199 patients. J Thorac Imaging. 2021;36(2):73–83.
49. Shchendrygina A, Nagel E, Puntmann VO, Valbuena-Lopez S. COVID-19 myocarditis and prospective heart failure burden. Expert Rev Cardiovasc Ther. 2021;19(1):5–14.

Chapter 13
Hypertension in CoViD19

Key Questions

- What are the implications of hypertension in CoViD19?
- What is the occurrence of hypertension in CoViD19?
- Does pre existing hypertension elevate risk in CoViD19?
- What complexities are associated with hypertension and CoViD19?
- What pathogenic mechanisms may determine the severity of CoViD19 in patients with hypertension?
- What mechanisms impact blood pressure control in CoViD19 patients?
- What is the prognostic significance of hypertension in CoViD19?

13.1 Epidemiology

Hypertension is highly prevalent in complicated CoViD19 and appears to be associated with poor outcomes [1]. The global trends of hypertension indicate a pandemic-like situation with about 30% of individuals affected by the disease in the low- and middle-income countries and only one in three are aware of the disease [2, 3]. Likely, data reporting CoViD19, describe the high prevalence of hypertension, with prevalence even higher in severe or critical patients [4]. However, several controversies have emerged related to the hypertension-related data in CoViD19 [5, 6] and CoViD19-hypertension interlinks. The global trends and recent CoViD19 analyses, nevertheless, point to a high prevalence of hypertension in CoViD19, which may have an incidence as high as 56% [7] and an elevated risk of morbidity

U. Mallick, *Cardiovascular Complications of COVID-19*,
https://doi.org/10.1007/978-3-030-90065-6_13

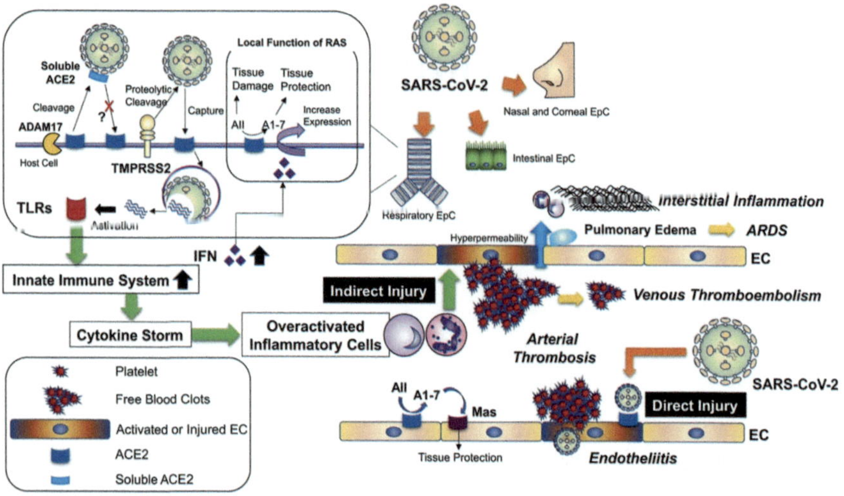

Fig. 13.1 Potential pathogenetic mechanisms and vascular complications in CoViD19. Possible mechanism of SARS-CoV-2-induced vascular complications. ACE2 angiotensin-converting enzyme 2, ADAM17 a disintegrin and metalloprotease 17, AII angiotensin II, A1-7 angiotensin 1–7, ARDS acute respiratory distress syndrome, EC endothelial cell, EpC epithelial cell, IFN interferon, SARS-CoV-2 severe acute respiratory syndrome coronavirus 2, TLRs Toll-like receptors, TMPRSS2 transmembrane serine protease 2, RAS renin-angiotensin system. *Source* Figure 1. Shibata, S., Arima, H., Asayama, K., Hoshide, S., Ichihara, A., Ishimitsu, T., Kario, K., Kishi, T., Mogi, M., Nishiyama, A. and Ohishi, M., 2020. Hypertension and related diseases in the era of COVID-19: a report from the Japanese Society of Hypertension Task Force on COVID-19. Hypertension Research, 43(10), pp. 1028–1046. https://www.nature.com/articles/s41440-020-0515-0. By Springer Nature Group

and mortality in patients with hypertension who contract CoViD19 despite the risk of confounding [8]. However, the significance of hypertension as an independent risk factor in CoViD19 needs to be further validated [9].

Data indicate that patients with chronic hypertension who contract CoViD19 may have severe disease and poor outcomes. In a cohort of 1,590 patients from 575 hospitals, preexisting hypertension was independently associated with severe COVID19 (hazard ratio 1.575, 95% CI: 1.07–2.32) after adjusting for age and smoking status [10]. The criticality of CoViD19 is associated with cardiovascular diseases [11, 12], also appears to be reflected in association with hypertension. Data suggest that patients with critical CoViD19 more often have co-existing hypertension than non-critical patients, among the comorbidities. In a retrospective single-center study of 138 hospitalized patients with CoViD19 reported prevalence of co-existing hypertension was 43/138 (31.2%), much higher in those admitted in the intensive care unit (ICU) 21/36 (58.3%), as compared to the non-ICU 22/102 (21.6%) patients [13]. In a retrospective case series, among a cohort of 799 patients admitted with CoViD19, analysis of data of 113 deceased and 161 recovered patients, showed a higher prevalence of chronic hypertension in the deceased

Study name	Odds ratio	Lower limit	Upper limit	p-Value	HT	N-HT	Total	Relative weight
Zhang G et al. 3	4,42	2,27	8,61	0,00	26 / 54	29 / 167	55 / 221	6,38
Zhang JJ et al. 3	1,89	0,91	3,94	0,09	22 / 42	36 / 98	58 / 140	5,75
Guan W et al. 3	2,01	1,35	2,99	0,00	41 / 165	132 / 934	173 / 1099	9,78
Huang C et al. 3	1,09	0,17	6,88	0,93	2 / 6	11 / 35	13 / 41	1,40
Liu W et al. 3	2,26	0,39	12,96	0,36	2 / 8	9 / 70	11 / 78	1,53
Wang D et al. 3	5,09	2,26	11,48	0,00	21 / 43	15 / 95	36 / 138	5,05
Wang Z et al. 3	7,08	1,59	31,54	0,01	5 / 9	9 / 60	14 / 69	2,02
Chen C et al. 3	3,64	1,48	8,96	0,00	14 / 49	10 / 101	24 / 150	4,42
Wu C et al. 3	2,38	1,17	4,85	0,02	23 / 39	61 / 162	84 / 201	5,93
Xiang T et al. 3	15,20	2,19	105,42	0,01	4 / 6	5 / 43	9 / 49	1,27
Wan S et al. 3	1,06	0,31	3,67	0,92	4 / 13	36 / 122	40 / 135	2,74
Deng Q et al 3	1,53	0,67	3,51	0,31	24 / 36	43 / 76	67 / 112	4,94
Guo T et al. 3	6,64	3,29	13,38	0,00	33 / 61	19 / 126	52 / 187	6,04
Li X et al. 3	2,21	1,52	3,21	0,00	104 / 166	165 / 382	269 / 548	10,13
Simone A et al 3	2,92	1,31	6,52	0,01	48 / 60	37 / 64	85 / 124	5,13
Mao L et al. 3	3,22	1,67	6,18	0,00	32 / 51	56 / 163	88 / 214	6,53
Feng Y et al 3	5,29	3,41	8,22	0,00	72 / 145	52 / 331	124 / 476	9,18
Li J et al. 3	2,59	2,00	3,36	0,00	173 / 362	213 / 816	386 / 1178	11,78
	2,98	2,37	3,75	0,00	650 / 1315	938 / 3845	1588 / 5160	

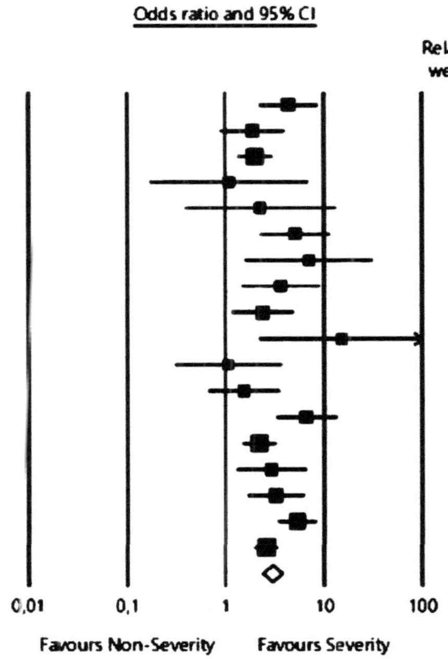

I^2: 49.89; p=0.009

Random Effects

Fig. 13.2 Hypertension and COVID19 severity. Meta-analysis with forest plot presenting the OR and 95% CI for severity or mortality of COVID-19 according to the presence of hypertension. *Source* Figure 2C. de Almeida-Pititto, B., Dualib, P.M., Zajdenverg, L., Dantas, J.R., De Souza, F.D., Rodacki, M. and Bertoluci, M.C., 2020. Severity and mortality of COVID 19 in patients with diabetes, hypertension and cardiovascular disease: a meta-analysis. Diabetology & metabolic syndrome, 12(1), pp. 1–12. https://link.springer.com/article/10.1186/s13098-020-00586-4. By Springer Nature Group

Study name	Odds ratio	Lower limit	Upper limit	p-Value	HT	N-HT	Total	Relative weight
	Statistics for each study				Severe / Total			
Giamarellos-Bourboulis et al	1,50	0,37	6,06	0,57	6 / 10	22 / 44	28 / 54	3,08
Zhang J et al 4	1,39	0,22	8,92	0,73	5 / 11	3 / 8	8 / 19	1,84
Guan W et al 4	3,53	2,08	5,99	0,00	24 / 165	43 / 934	67 / 1099	12,30
Chen et al. 4	2,86	1,71	4,80	0,00	54 / 93	59 / 181	113 / 274	12,63
Wu C et al. 4	2,69	0,97	7,48	0,06	16 / 23	28 / 61	44 / 84	5,20
Fan J et al. 4	1,13	0,13	9,94	0,92	2 / 10	2 / 11	4 / 21	1,36
Deng Y et al. 4	3,16	1,67	5,96	0,00	40 / 58	69 / 167	109 / 225	10,07
Yuan M et al. 4	35,00	1,66	738,65	0,02	5 / 5	5 / 22	10 / 27	0,72
Zhou F et al. 4	3,05	1,57	5,92	0,00	26 / 58	28 / 133	54 / 191	9,55
Zheng KI et al. 4	8,07	3,04	21,37	0,00	12 / 22	18 / 139	30 / 161	5,59
Ruan Q et al. 4	1,91	0,97	3,77	0,06	29 / 52	39 / 98	68 / 150	9,27
Li J et al. 4	3,89	2,67	5,66	0,00	77 / 362	53 / 816	130 / 1178	16,43
Wang L et al 4	1,54	0,89	2,65	0,12	32 / 138	33 / 201	65 / 339	11,98
	2,88	2,22	3,74	0,00	328 / 1007	402 / 2815	730 / 3822	

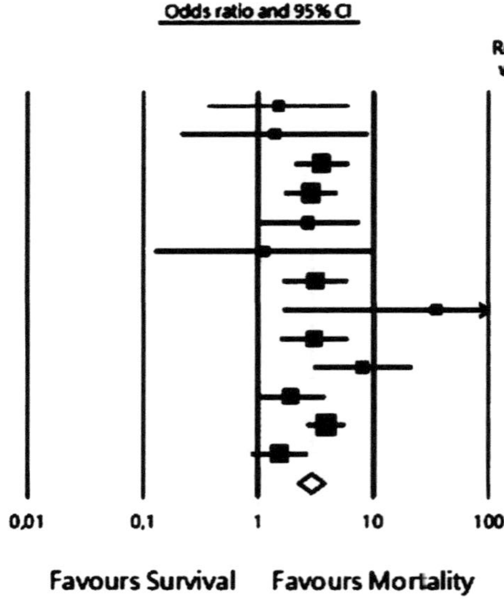

$I^2=35.57; p=0.098$

Random Effects

Fig. 13.3 Hypertension and COVID19 mortality. Meta-analysis with forest plot presenting the OR and 95% CI for severity or mortality of COVID-19 according to the presence of hypertension. *Source* Figure 2D. de Almeida-Pititto, B., Dualib, P.M., Zajdenverg, L., Dantas, J.R., De Souza, F.D., Rodacki, M. and Bertoluci, M.C., 2020. Severity and mortality of COVID 19 in patients with diabetes, hypertension and cardiovascular disease: a meta-analysis. Diabetology & metabolic syndrome, 12(1), pp. 1–12. https://link.springer.com/article/10.1186/s13098-020-00586-4. By Springer Nature Group

patients as compared to those who recovered 48% (54) versus 24% (39). The blood pressure measurements were performed on admission, and patients with a critical disease on admission were older and had hypertension. The analysis was, however, unadjusted for age [14].

Several risk factors accompanying hypertension are also common comorbidities in CoViD19 and key risk determinants, may interfere with the risk assessment process. Results of a pooled analysis of 2893 CoViD19 patients suggest that hypertension may have up to 2.5-fold higher risk of severe and fatal COVID19, especially among the older subjects [15, 16]. Studies further suggest poor outcomes and significantly higher risk of mortality in CoViD19 patients with hypertension, who are untreated as compared to those on hypertensive treatments [45]. However, whether hypertension is an independent risk factor for poor outcomes remains to be further explored.

Data highlighting the in-hospital blood pressure trends and associations in CoViD19 are scarce, however, indicate a high risk. A retrospective analysis of 803 hypertensive patients (diagnosed on admission) with CoViD19, showed a poor BP control was independently associated with higher risks of adverse outcomes of CoViD19 [17]. Another retrospective cohort study including 2864 CoViD19 patients, of which 1628 were hypertensive, aimed to investigate the association between in-hospital blood pressure (BP) control and CoViD19–related outcomes and to compare the effects of different antihypertension treatments. The study showed that poor BP control during the hospitalization had worse clinical outcomes (blood pressure $\geq$ grade 2 (OR 3.03, 95% CI: 1.83-5.03, $P < 0.001$). The length of time from the symptoms-onset to normothermia, inflammatory resorption, and viral shedding increased with the elevated blood pressure grade [18].

13.2 Complexities in Hypertension and CoViD19

Several factors, such as type of hypertension (whether primary or secondary), the severity stage or form of hypertension (whether it is multidrug-resistant or controlled on a single drug), or the duration of hypertension, or presence of underlying target organ damage, may strongly impact the prognosis in subjects with hypertension. These factors are likely to have an impact on the dynamics of blood pressure control and outcomes in CoViD19 patients. Due to the paucity of data, the behavior and trends of hypertension in CoViD19 are not well understood.

Chronic hypertension and CoViD19 adversely impact each other. The duration of the chronic hypertension, advanced age, frailty, and associated organ damage may render a significant vulnerability to the key vascular structures and the heart. Chronic hypertension may induce myocardial structural and functional changes, and microvascular and macrovascular dysfunction involving multiple vascular territories (central and peripheral including cerebrovascular, and renal territories). These factors often lead to a greater predisposition towards, heart failure, coronary artery disease, or arrhythmias such as atrial fibrillation, and stroke. Patients with chronic hypertension with CoViD19 are particularly at high risk due to the underlying risk burden for hypertension, and more often exhibit complications.

There is a significant overlap in the comorbidities between associated with CoViD19 and hypertension [19]. Data from the initial CoViD19 studies suggested factors such as advanced age, male sex, and various cardiovascular and metabolic risk factors such as obesity and diabetes, are associated with disease severity and poor outcomes in CoViD19 [20, 21] (Figs. 13.2 and 13.3). A large observational cohort study of 20,133 CoViD19 in-patients confirmed the age, male sex, and obesity as independent predictors of mortality [22]. These factors are already recognized as important risk factors for hypertension across the world populations among several others [23]. Analyses confirm a significant association of the three risk factors, hypertension, obesity and diabetes, with increased risk of severe COVID19 on admission [24]. Later data from several large analyses further validated the association of these factors in CoViD19 patients as well as their contribution towards the risk and poor outcomes. Larger studies assessing joint associations of multiple risk factors in CoViD19 patients, confirmed advanced age and male sex, as predictors of 30-day mortality in the nursing home residents with CoViD19, with hypertension a very frequent occurrence (4116/5256 (78%)), however not a predictor [25] as well as independent association of diabetes mellitus with in-hospital mortality in CoViD19 [26] (a condition commonly associated with hypertension).

Furthermore, data investigating the association of comorbidities in CoViD19 reveal hypertension is important comorbidity, also show age as an important risk factor for the severe disease [27]. According to an analysis of Italian CoViD19 related deaths, hypertension affected 73.8% of patients, the average age of patients was 78.5 years (median 80 years, range 31–103 years) [28]. However, interconnection of hypertension and CoViD19 severity, appear to have been confounded by age and multimorbidity in several reports describing hypertension in connection with CoViD19 severity [21, 29, 30]. Advanced age is an important cardiovascular risk factor, with strong implications in the analytical process of the data related to hypertension concerning CoViD19. Patients with advanced age usually have an increased prevalence of hypertension and have worse outcomes [21]. Furthermore, the older adults frequently manifest uncontrolled hypertension, often have isolated, mild systolic hypertension [32]. The intricacies related to the frailty in advanced age, burden of risk factors, including diagnosed and undiagnosed cardiovascular and organ dysfunction, and poor outcomes, are likely to impact the associations between hypertension and CoViD19 and outcomes.

Adjustments of the variables including age and comorbidities as predictors of poor outcome in CoViD19 may suppress the predictability of hypertension-related mortality [33], and failure to adjust for age in the larger datasets [34], may have led to an overestimation of the association of hypertension with increased risk of CoViD19 mortality, as predicted in the earlier studies [20, 35]. Several controversies exist in the hypertension-related data in CoViD19 [6, 36]. Although reports reaffirm that in the COVID19 outbreak, mortality is predicted by age, and the presence of comorbidities, however also suggest, lack of significant interference of hypertension in the mortality [37]. Other analyses have also shown the significant contribution of the cardiovascular, metabolic risk factors and hypertension, towards fatal CoViD19 outcomes, however a higher impact on mortality in the younger subjects [5]. The presence of important comorbidities like obesity, diabetes may interfere in the evidence linking the outcome of hypertension and CoViD19 [38].

Several weaknesses may be observed in the earlier reports describing hypertension-related severity in CoViD19. These reports may not have included relevant studies, have heterogeneity, or have failed to adjust for confounding factors [39], or may be subject to interpretation bias [21, 40]. Furthermore, in the earlier CoViD19 studies, important data may have been lacking, and confounding may exist concerning the data collection methods, diagnostic methodology, variations in the study design, and sample size [41, 42]. A lack of adjustment of the confounding factors [24] or criteria for defining hypertension in the studies, or inadequate follow up, may have resulted in errors in an accurate estimation of the true incidence and outcomes of hypertension in subjects with CoViD19 [7, 21, 43, 44]. Moreover, the hypertension may co-exist historically, or diagnosed at or during the admission, and the dynamics of blood pressure during the admission may not be available or lack clarity in the CoViD19 study reports The relevant conclusions may be based on the descriptive associations, more often, than upon the actual causal relationship between the variable and the outcome.

Other important clinical aspects of association of hypertension with CoViD19 such as characteristics of uncontrolled hypertension, treated versus untreated and others also require further clarity. Presence of uncontrolled hypertension may influence the outcome of CoViD19 subjects. Uncontrolled hypertension in CoViD19 patients may contribute to decompensation of the heart disease, critical disease, and increase mortality [17]. An elevated pulse pressure is an important marker of these poor outcomes. However, analyses may suggest a possible lack of adverse consequences of uncontrolled BP in hypertensive patients with CoViD19 [45, 46]. Further studies with robust designs are needed to validate these associations.

In acute settings of infections, hyperinflammatory conditions, hypertension may acquire an accelerated or even malignant form that may complicate with an acute myocardial injury, acute cardiac decompensation, arrhythmias, or acute coronary event or stroke. Rapid onset of heart failure with systolic blood pressure > 140 mmHg, may induce hypertensive acute decompensation of heart failure. The potential deleterious impact of hypertension especially in association with CoViD19 may have significant implications on the management. The intensity of the viral infection, duration of symptoms, presence of other comorbidities including kidney disease, underlying cardiometabolic risk factors, as well as hospital environment, may lead to poor BP control during the hospital stay and impact the clinical outcomes.

Other complexities associated with hypertension may be related to the multi-factorial interaction of key risk factors, such as hypercholesterolemia, diabetes mellitus, renovascular disease, adrenal, and other vascular or endocrinological factors, that lead to hypertension. Endocrinological or renovascular hypertension is often difficult to control. Although, CoViD19 and endocrinological correlation have been shown in small studies and case reports [47, 48], and worsening of the endocrinological disease has been reported with CoViD19 [49], data regarding behavior of secondary forms of hypertension in CoViD19 are not available.

Hypertension and renal disease are interconnected and hold a two-way relationship [50]. The renal implications in hypertension further add to the complexities in the management of hypertension, and often precipitate complications. Data show that renal diseases are among the important complications in severe CoViD19 [51], may further exacerbate the viral disease and contribute towards poor outcomes [52, 53]. Association of hypertension and trends towards severe morbidity and mortality in CoViD19 patients, have been seen in patients with kidney disease [54]. The peculiarities of hypertension in association with renal disease in CoViD19, and the impact of hypertension in the decompensation of renal and heart conditions during CoViD19, need to be further investigated. Further exploration of the behavior and trends of hypertension, and the interplay of various types and forms of the severity of hypertension in CoViD19, is required.

13.3 CoViD19 Susceptibility and Hypertension

The controversy around the use of treatment with ACEi /ARBs in CoViD19 hypertensive patients [55] was addressed by the expert group statements recommending continuation of the use of these therapies in CoViD19 patients [56–58].

The drugs angiotensin-converting enzyme inhibitors (ACEi) and angiotensin II receptor blockers (ARBs) act by blocking the ACE/Angiotensin II/AT1R pathway, also modify the inflammatory molecules such as intercellular adhesion molecule-1, vascular cell adhesion molecule-1, monocyte chemoattractant protein-1, tumor necrosis factor-α, and C-reactive protein. Patients with hypertension on ACEi/ARB therapy have an increased expression of ACE2 [59]. The argument that ACEi/ARBs can increase the susceptibility towards SARS CoV2, draws from the possibility of an increase in expression of the ACE2 due to these therapies that may also enhance the SARS CoV2 interaction with the ACE 2 receptors, thereby promoting the viral invasion of cells in the lungs to invade cells [60, 61].

On the contrary, it has been argued and demonstrated that ACEi/ARB therapy may have a protective role in CoViD19 through the overexpression of the ACE 2. The ACE2 may induce anti-inflammatory, and cardioprotective mechanisms and may even have a role in repairing the lung injury as shown in the experimental studies, or in repairing organs harboring the ACE 2, such as kidneys [61, 62]. A recent retrospective multi-center study, included 1128 adult patients with hypertension diagnosed with COVID19 demonstrated a lower risk of all-cause mortality in patients taking ACEi/ARBs compared to the non-users [63]. An international, open science, cohort analysis, aimed to determine whether the use of ACEIs or ARBs is associated with increased susceptibility to COVID19 in patients with hypertension. The analysis of 1 355 349 antihypertensive users, (363 785 ACEI or ARB monotherapy users, 248 915 CCB (Calcium Channel Blockers) or THZ (Thiazide) monotherapy users, 711 799 ACEI or ARB combination users, and 473 076 CCB or THZ combination users) indicated that ACEI or ARB use was not associated with a clinically significant increase in the risk of COVID19 diagnosis or hospital admission-related outcomes [64].

13.4 Pathogenesis

Several pathogenetic processes reflecting etiological interactions and host mechanisms reveal the complexities related to the severity of CoViD19 in patients with hypertension. Such processes may determine possible increased predisposition of the hypertensive patients towards CoViD19, may act as prognostic determinants in CoViD19 patients with hypertension, and may be associated with poor BP control in CoViD19 patients. In patients with hypertension, infections, hyperinflammatory stress, multi-organ failure may exacerbate the underlying etiopathogenetic risk factors, such as renal disease, humoral and catecholaminergic turbulence, vascular non-compliance, increased cardiac afterload, augmenting damage to the already affected environment. Worsening and intensification of these conditions promote the development of cardiovascular complications in CoViD19 when hypertension is present. Patients with CoViD19 with complications may also have low blood pressure in association with the septic, cardiac complications that accompany vasoplegia, factors leading to low cardiac output, or mechanisms impacting hemodynamic and fluid balance.

Several stress mechanisms are associated with infectious illnesses that may make BP control a challenge. Poor BP control in CoViD19 patients is likely to be secondary to the impact of multiple factors such as hypoxia, dysregulated immune, inflammatory process, and vasoactive control systems, and iatrogenic factors lead to a poor fluid balance and inappropriate hemodynamic control, especially when underlying risk factors and organ or tissue vulnerability are present in CoViD19 patients.

Data suggest that during the infective conditions, concomitant comorbidities such as hypertension carry significant prognostic value [65]. An exact estimation of the direct risk of developing the complications may not be possible, however, these are likely to be more common due to the mechanisms involving vascular viral injury, cytokine storm, and associated inflammatory stress [66] (Fig. 13.1). Hypertension is associated with chronic low inflammatory stress among other cardiovascular diseases [67]. Innate and adaptive immune mechanisms participate in blood pressure elevation and end organ damage [68]. The association of immune-inflammation and hypertension with endothelial dysfunction and hyperinflammatory state with elevated levels of Ang II, chemokines, and cytokines, including interleukin-6 (IL-6) and tumor necrosis factor-α (TNF-α) [69], also observed in severe CoViD19 [70], may determine a poor BP control or unfavorable disease outcome.

Inflammation is a key mechanism in the initiation, progression, and complications of the interactions of several pathogenetic factors involved in hypertension. Several inflammatory molecules such as intercellular adhesion molecule-1 (ICAM-1), vascular cell adhesion molecule-1 (VCAM-1), monocyte chemoattractant protein-1 (MCP-1), tumor necrosis factor-α (TNF-α), and C-reactive protein (CRP) are involved in cardiovascular diseases. Increases in the levels of plasma pro-inflammatory cytokines (PICs) and other markers of inflammation are associated with the progression of hypertension, whereas immune suppression produces beneficial outcomes [71, 72].

Vascular injury as a result of the viral invasion in already vulnerable vasculature may have a deleterious impact. Specific pathophysiological mechanisms related to the SARS CoV2 involving an interplay of the virus with vascular endothelial bed ACE 2 receptors, increased Angiotensin II activity, an imbalance between RAS components /axes, appear to have a direct role in the development of cardiovascular complications in CoViD19, that also include hypertension. Angiotensin II adversely influences vascular integrity via a variety of mechanisms, such as endothelial dysfunction [73], oxidative stress [74] and others, thereby facilitating the development of hypertension, may be excessively available in CoViD19 [75]. The endothelial cell dysfunction promotes proinflammatory excess and vascular dysfunction. Similarly, overexpression of endothelin in CoViD19 [76], an important pathogenetic determinant of hypertension [77] may contribute to elevated blood pressure in CoViD19 patients. Endothelin, a potent vasoconstrictor, and RAS interaction promotes elevation in blood pressure and related complications [78], are dysregulated in CoViD19.

Drug-induced hypertension is an important entity [79]. Several drug classes including non steroidal anti inflammatory drugs (NSAIDs), and corticosteroids, used in the management of CoViD19 may contribute towards poor blood pressure control in hypertensives, or exacerbation of borderline hypertension, warranting a precautious approach in CoViD19 management.

The cellular stress mechanisms and redox signaling lead to impaired cellular homeostasis in CoViD19 and pathogenesis of complications. The mechanisms involving a variety of oxidative redox proteomics, mitochondrial oxidative stress, endoplasmic reticular stress, are interlinked with immune-inflammatory processes and cell death mechanisms. Such mechanisms are known to promote hypertension [80] and require further exploration in CoViD19.

Several metabolic and immune-inflammatory processes, linked with metabolic conditions such as obesity or diabetes, are dysregulated in CoViD19 [81] and impact cardiovascular system, promote hypertension [82]. A mosaic of molecular, and tissue mechanisms inflammatory, vasoactive, endothelial dysfunction, increased insulin resistance, other local and systemic reactions, and vascular stiffness, adversely impact vascular tissue structure, function, and compliance leading to complications.

PPARγ (peroxisome proliferator-activated receptor-gamma) are among the family of orphan receptors. "PPARs", are an important regulator of blood pressure, when impaired promote hypertension. PPARγ influence blood pressure by modulating renal, vascular, and immune function [83]. The PPARγ complex, are involved in severe COVID19 lung disease and have a role in the major monocyte/macrophage-mediated inflammatory storm [84]. Furthermore, these receptors may be a potential target in CoViD19 treatment [85] due to their role in the suppression of anti inflammatory processes.

Overactivation of the sympathetic system is associated with hypertension [92]. Such mechanisms may play a role in CoViD19 related comorbidities [93, 94] including hypertension. Cases of Tako-tsubo cardiomyopathy and stroke have been reported in CoViD19 patients [95, 96] reflecting these mechanisms. Sympathetic overactivation may contribute to the development of hypertension in CoViD19 that is associated with hyperimmune reactions, dysregulated RAS, and other processes, and risk factors as aging and male gender. Several CoViD19 cardiac manifestations and adverse glycemic dysregulation may reflect autonomic dyshomeostasis in patients with diabetes mellitus during COVID19 [97]. Data suggest autonomic dysfunction interacts with the immune system via neuroinflammatory pathways and cholinergic pathways and also controls the respiratory system [98]. These mechanisms may contribute towards poor blood pressure control and have practical implications in the management of CoViD19 related blood pressure variations.

13.5 Summary

Hypertension appears to be a prevalent condition in patients with complicated CoViD19, and adversely impacts the disease and the outcome, although the prognostic implications in CoViD19 need to be further validated. Evidence suggests that patients hospitalized with CoViD19 have elevated blood pressure, and may have poor blood pressure control. Elevated blood pressure during the hospital stay appears to increase the risk of severe CoViD19 disease.

Chronic or co-existing hypertension is a more frequent association in CoViD19 patients, and hypertensive patients more often have severe CoViD9. The association of hypertension and the criticality of the CoViD19 may reflect bidirectional pathogenetic risks. Improved blood pressure control in the community and avoidance of viral infection in hypertensive individuals may help to minimize the risk associated with CoViD19. Effective preventive measures may be adopted in patients with hypertension and related risk factors to diminish the risk.

Chronic or background hypertension in patients with CoViD19 with target organ damage to the heart, and associated vasculature or involving other organs, may further aggravate the risk of cardiovascular complications. The links between the cardiometabolic risk factors, hypertension, and severity of CoViD19, imply the need for a comprehensive approach to addressing these risk factors. Older adults require additional precautions due to the elevated risk associated with CoViD19 and hypertension.

Studies indicate the development of new hypertension in CoViD19 patients without a previous history of elevated blood pressure. The newly diagnosed hypertension and poor blood pressure control in CoViD19 patients during the admission, mark poor outcomes. Although studies provide evidence of the development of new hypertension in CoViD19 patients, further data are needed to draw plausible conclusions. The existing data underscore the significance of monitoring CoViD19 patients at risk and recognizing and treating elevated blood pressure early. A better BP control in CoViD19 patients during hospitalization may help to improve the outcomes.

Secondary forms or multi-drug resistant hypertension need special considerations due to the associated complexities in management and elevated risk. Accelerated or uncontrolled hypertension carries a higher risk of critical complications, such as cardiac decompensation, arrhythmias, or cerebrovascular injury, or renal disease [99–101].

Infectious or inflammatory conditions may result in extreme fluctuations in hypertension, thereby further aggravating the risk. Blood pressure variations in the acute settings of complicated CoViD19 may be caused by several factors such as sepsis, dehydration, catecholamine stress, or other vasoplegic factors. Hyperinflammation and RAS appear to play a significant role in the initiation and perpetuation of these factors. The underlying pathogenic mechanisms linking hypertension and severity and prognosis of CoViD19 infection needs to be elucidated.

Ensuring optimum blood pressure control may be a challenge to the clinicians in the acute settings of CoViD19. Characteristics and behavior of hypertension remain vastly undefined in CoViD19. Traits related to the phenotypic and severity-related variations of hypertension in CoVID19 need to be further explored. Management of patients with hypertension in CoViD19 warrants a more cautious approach, also due to the associated renal pathology, and the risk of cardiovascular and metabolic factors. Iatrogenicity of the drugs used in CoViD19 management may induce elevated blood pressure, therefore need to be cautiously used. Patients may require frequent monitoring and adjustment of the medication.

The actual impact of the BP control in hypertensive CoViD19 patients, needs further exploration. Standard protocols and guidelines must be used to ensure effective management of hypertension in CoViD19 patients. Whether hypertension increases the susceptibility for CoViD19 remains unclear. Expert guidances on the use of ACEi or ARBs currently recommend the continuation of the use of these drugs in patients CoViD19. Several large studies describing hypertension during the COVID19 pandemic, although have generated stronger data, the observational or retrospective designs may reflect weaknesses of the evidence base. Well-conducted studies using sound designs, methodology, and robust outcomes, will allow better characterize hypertension, estimation of the risks and the outcomes in CoViD19 patients. This will help define variations and behavior of hypertension in this population, and evaluate effective and safe treatment choices.

Summary Box

- Hypertension is a common association with CoViD19 and negatively impacts the disease.
- Pre-existing hypertension is significantly linked with the severity of CoViD19.
- Comorbidities and older age are likely to aggravate the risk associated with hypertension in CoViD19.

- The infectious, hyperimmune, and pro-inflammatory nature of CoViD19 drives elevated blood pressure in CoViD19 with a major role of dysregulated RAS mechanisms.
- A cautious approach is needed in the use of drugs in CoViD19 management that may elevate blood pressure.
- Evidence suggests a lack of increased susceptibility to CoViD19 due to the antihypertensive drugs such as ACEi/ARBs.
- Effective blood pressure control must be ensured in hypertensive subjects and extra precautions must be taken to avoid CoViD19.
- Characteristics, severity, behavior, and phenotypic variations of hypertension in CoViD19 are not well understood.
- Further studies are needed to determine the impact of hypertension on CoViD19 fatality.
- Robust trials are needed to investigate the epidemiological, and causal associations of various forms and severities of hypertension and CoViD19, especially the long-term prognostic implications.

References

1. Guan WJ, Ni ZY, Hu Y, Liang WH, Ou CQ, He JX et al. China medical treatment expert group for CoViD19. Clinical characteristics of coronavirus disease 2019 in China. N Engl J Med 2020. Epub ahead of print.
2. Touyz RM, Schiffrin EL. A compendium on hypertension: new advances and future impact. Circ Res. 2021;128(7):803–7.
3. Schutte AE, Srinivasapura Venkateshmurthy N, Mohan S, Prabhakaran D. Hypertension in low-and middle-income countries. Circ Res. 2021;128(7):808–26.
4. Du Y, Zhou N, Zha W, Lv Y. Hypertension is a clinically important risk factor for critical illness and mortality in COVID19: A meta-analysis. Nutr Metab Cardiovasc Dis. 2021;31 (3):745–55.
5. Tadic M, Saeed S, Grassi G, Taddei S, Mancia G, Cuspidi C. Hypertension and COVID19: ongoing controversies. Front Cardiovas Med. 2021; 8.
6. Li G, Li H, Lu J. No adequate evidence indicating hypertension as an independent risk factor for COVID19 severity. Clin Res Cardiol. 2021;110(1):146–7.
7. Richardson S, Hirsch JS, Narasimhan M, Crawford JM, McGinn T, Davidson KW, Barnaby DP, Becker LB, Chelico JD, Cohen SL, Cookingham J. Presenting characteristics, comorbidities, and outcomes among 5700 patients hospitalized with COVID19 in the New York City area. JAMA. 2020;323(20):2052–9.
8. Kario K, Morisawa Y, Sukonthasarn A, Turana Y, Chia YC, Park S, Wang TD, Chen CH, Tay JC, Li Y, Wang JG. COVID-19 and hypertension—evidence and practical management: guidance from the HOPE Asia network. J Clin Hypert. 2020;22(7):1109–19.
9. Tadic M, Cuspidi C, Grassi G, Mancia G. COVID-19 and arterial hypertension: hypothesis or evidence? J Clin Hypert. 2020;22(7):1120–6.
10. Guan WJ, Liang WH, Zhao Y, Liang HR, Chen ZS, Li YM, Liu XQ, Chen RC, Tang CL, Wang T, Ou CQ. Comorbidity and its impact on 1590 patients with COVID19 in China: a nationwide analysis. Eur Resp J. 2020; 55(5).

11. Xie Y, You Q, Wu C, Cao S, Qu G, Yan X, Han X, Wang C, Zhang H. Impact of cardiovascular disease on clinical characteristics and outcomes of coronavirus disease 2019 (COVID19). Circul J. 2020; CJ-20.
12. Cummings MJ, Baldwin MR, Abrams D, Jacobson SD, Meyer BJ, Balough EM, Aaron JG, Claassen J, Rabbani LE, Hastie J, Hochman BR. Epidemiology, clinical course, and outcomes of critically ill adults with COVID19 in New York city: a prospective cohort study. The Lancet. 2020;395(10239):1763–70.
13. Wang D, Hu B, Hu C, Zhu F, Liu X, Zhang J, Wang B, Xiang H, Cheng Z, Xiong Y, Zhao Y. Clinical characteristics of 138 hospitalized patients with 2019 novel coronavirus–infected pneumonia in Wuhan, China. JAMA. 2020;323(11):1061–9.
14. Chen T, Wu D, Chen H, Yan W, Yang D, Chen G, Ma K, Xu D, Yu H, Wang H, Wang T, Guo W, Chen J, Ding C, Zhang X, Huang J, Han M, Li S, Luo X, Zhao J, Ning Q. Clinical characteristics of 113 deceased patients with coronavirus disease 2019: retrospective study. BMJ. 2020 Mar 26;368:m1091. doi: https://doi.org/10.1136/bmj.m1091. Erratum in: BMJ. 2020 Mar 31;368:m1295. PubMed PMID: 32217556.
15. Lippi G, Wong J, Henry BM. Hypertension and its severity or mortality in Coronavirus Disease 2019 (COVID19): a pooled analysis. Pol Arch Intern Med. 2020 Mar 31. doi: https://doi.org/10.20452/pamw.15272. [Epub ahead of print] PubMed PMID: 32231171.
16. Lippi G, Wong J, Henry BM. Hypertension and its severity or mortality in Coronavirus Disease 2019 (COVID19): a pooled analysis. Polish Arch Int Med. 2020.
17. Ran J, Song Y, Zhuang Z, Han L, Zhao S, Cao P, Geng Y, Xu L, Qin J, He D, Wu F. Blood pressure control and adverse outcomes of COVID19 infection in patients with concomitant hypertension in Wuhan, China. Hypert Res. 2020; 43(11):1267–1276.
18. Chen R, Yang J, Gao X, Ding X, Yang Y, Shen Y, He C, Xiang H, Ke J, Yuan F, Cheng R. Influence of blood pressure control and application of renin-angiotensin-aldosterone system inhibitors on the outcomes in COVID-19 patients with hypertension. J Clin Hypert. 2020;22 (11):1974–83.
19. Whelton PK, Carey RM, Aronow WS, Casey DE, Collins KJ, Dennison Himmelfarb C, DePalma SM, Gidding S, Jamerson KA, Jones DW, MacLaughlin EJ. 2017 ACC/AHA/ AAPA/ABC/ACPM/AGS/APhA/ASH/ASPC/NMA/PCNA guideline for the prevention, detection, evaluation, and management of high blood pressure in adults: a report of the American College of Cardiology/American Heart Association Task Force on Clinical Practice Guidelines. J Am Coll Cardiol. 2018;71(19):e127-248.
20. Shi Y, Yu X, Zhao H, Wang H, Zhao R, Sheng J. Host susceptibility to severe COVID19 and establishment of a host risk score: findings of 487 cases outside Wuhan. Crit Care. 2020;24(1):1–4.
21. Wu C, Chen X, Cai Y, Zhou X, Xu S, Huang H, Zhang L, Zhou X, Du C, Zhang Y, Song J. Risk factors associated with acute respiratory distress syndrome and death in patients with coronavirus disease 2019 pneumonia in Wuhan, China. JAMA Int Med. 2020;180 (7):934–43.
22. Docherty AB, Harrison EM, Green CA, Hardwick HE, Pius R, Norman L, Holden KA, Read JM, Dondelinger F, Carson G, Merson L. Features of 20 133 UK patients in hospital with CoViD19 using the ISARIC WHO Clinical Characterisation Protocol: prospective observational cohort study. Bmj. 2020; 369.
23. Hall JE, do Carmo JM, da Silva AA, Wang Z, Hall ME. Obesity-induced hypertension: interaction of neurohumoral and renal mechanisms. Circul Res. 2015; 116(6):991–1006.
24. Denova-Gutiérrez E, Lopez-Gatell H, Alomia-Zegarra JL, López-Ridaura R, Zaragoza-Jimenez CA, Dyer-Leal DD, Cortés-Alcala R, Villa-Reyes T, Gutiérrez-Vargas R, Rodríguez-González K, Escondrillas-Maya C. The association of obesity, type 2 Diabetes, and hypertension with severe coronavirus disease 2019 on admission among Mexican patients. Obesity. 2020;28(10):1826–32.
25. Panagiotou OA, Kosar CM, White EM, Bantis LE, Yang X, Santostefano CM, Feifer RA, Blackman C, Rudolph JL, Gravenstein S, Mor V. Risk factors associated with all-cause 30-day mortality in nursing home residents with COVID19. JAMA Int Med. 2021.

26. Barron E, Bakhai C, Kar P, Weaver A, Bradley D, Ismail H, Knighton P, Holman N, Khunti K, Sattar N, Wareham NJ. Associations of type 1 and type 2 diabetes with COVID19-related mortality in England: a whole-population study. Lancet Diab Endoc. 2020;8(10):813–22.
27. Fathi M, Vakili K, Sayehmiri F, Mohamadkhani A, Hajiesmaeili M, Rezaei-Tavirani M, Eilami O. The prognostic value of comorbidity for the severity of COVID19: a systematic review and meta-analysis study. PloS One. 2021; 16(2):e0246190.
28. COVID19 Surveillance Group. Characteristics of COVID19 patients dying in Italy: report based on available data on March 20th, 2020. Rome, Italy: Instituto Superiore Di Sanita. (2020). www. epice ntro. iss. it/coron aviru s/bolle ttino/Repor t-COVI D-2019_20_marzo _eng. pdf. Accessed, 20.
29. Clerkin KJ, Fried JA, Raikhelkar J, Sayer G, Griffin JM, Masoumi A, Jain SS, Burkhoff D, Kumaraiah D, Rabbani L, Schwartz A. COVID19 and cardiovascular disease. Circulation. 2020;141(20):1648–55.
30. Guo T, Fan Y, Chen M, Wu X, Zhang L, He T, Wang H, Wan J, Wang X, Lu Z. Cardiovascular implications of fatal outcomes of patients with coronavirus disease 2019 (COVID19). JAMA cardiology. 2020;5(7):811–8.
31. Vokonas PS, Kannel WB, Cupples LA. Epidemiology and risk of hypertension in the elderly: the Framingham study. J Hypert Suppl Off J Internat Soc Hypert. 1988; 6(1):S3–9.
32. Hyman DJ, Pavlik VN. Characteristics of patients with uncontrolled hypertension in the United States. N Engl J Med. 2001;345(7):479–86.
33. Iaccarino G, Grassi G, BForghi C, Ferri C, Salvetti M, Volpe M. Age and multimorbidity predict death among COVID19 patients: results of the SARS-RAS study of the Italian Society of Hypertension. Hypertension. 2020; 76(2):366–72.
34. Deng G, Yin M, Chen X, Zeng F. Clinical determinants for fatality of 44,672 patients with COVID19. Crit Care. 2020;24:1–3.
35. Shi Y, Yu X, Zhao H, Wang H, Zhao R, Sheng J. Host susceptibility to severe COVID19 and establishment of a host risk score: findings of 487 cases outside Wuhan. Crit Care. 2020: 24(1):1–4.
36. Li X, Xu S, Yu M, Wang K, Tao Y, Zhou Y, Shi J, Zhou M, Wu B, Yang Z, Zhang C. Risk factors for severity and mortality in adult COVID19 inpatients in Wuhan. J Allergy Clin Immun. 2020; 146(1):110–8.
37. Li G, Li H, Lu J. No adequate evidence indicating hypertension as an independent risk factor for COVID19 severity. Clin Res Cardiol. 2021; 110(1):146–7.
38. Iaccarino G, Grassi G, Borghi C, Ferri C, Salvetti M, Volpe M. Age and multimorbidity predict death among COVID19 patients: results of the SARS-RAS study of the Italian Society of Hypertension. Hypertension. 2020;76(2):366–72.
39. Bae S, Kim SR, Kim MN, Shim WJ, Park SM. Impact of cardiovascular disease and risk factors on fatal outcomes in patients with COVID19 according to age: a systematic review and meta-analysis. Heart. 2021;107(5):373–80.
40. Williamson EJ, Walker AJ, Bhaskaran K, Bacon S, Bates C, Morton CE, Curtis HJ, Mehrkar A, Evans D, Inglesby P, Cockburn J. Factors associated with COVID19-related death using Open SAFELY. Nature. 2020;584(7821):430–6.
41. Li B, Yang J, Zhao F, Zhi L, Wang X, Liu L, Bi Z, Zhao Y. Prevalence and impact of cardiovascular metabolic diseases on COVID19 in China. Clin Res Cardiol. 2020;109 (5):531–8.
42. Chen C, Yan JT, Zhou N, Zhao JP, Wang DW. Analysis of myocardial injury in patients with COVID19 and association between concomitant cardiovascular diseases and severity of COVID19. Zhonghua Xin Xue Guan Bing Za Zhi. 2020;48:E008–E008.
43. Wu C, Chen X, Cai Y, Zhou X, Xu S, Huang H, Zhang L, Zhou X, Du C, Zhang Y, Song J. Risk factors associated with acute respiratory distress syndrome and death in patients with coronavirus disease 2019 pneumonia in Wuhan, China. JAMA Int Med. 2020; 180 (7):934–43.

44. Yang J, Zheng Y, Gou X, Pu K, Chen Z, Guo Q, Ji R, Wang H, Wang Y, Zhou Y. Prevalence of comorbidities in the novel Wuhan coronavirus (COVID19) infection: a systematic review and meta-analysis. Int J Infect Dis. 2020; 10.
45. Emami A, Javanmardi F, Pirbonyeh N, Akbari A. Prevalence of underlying diseases in hospitalized patients with COVID19: a systematic review and meta-analysis. Arch Acad Emerg Med. 2020; 8(1).
46. Denova-Gutiérrez E, Lopez-Gatell H, Alomia-Zegarra JL, López-Ridaura R, Zaragoza-Jimenez, CA, Dyer-Leal, DD, Cortés-Alcala R, Villa-Reyes T, Gutiérrez-Vargas R, Rodríguez González, K, Escondrillas-Maya C. The association of obesity, type 2 Diabetes, and hypertension with severe coronavirus disease 2019 on admission among Mexican patients. Obesity. 2020; 28(10):1826–32.
47. Zhou F, Yu T, Du R, Fan G, Liu Y, Liu Z, Xiang J, Wang Y, Song B, Gu X, Guan L. Clinical course and risk factors for mortality of adult inpatients with COVID19 in Wuhan, China: a retrospective cohort study. The Lancet. 2020;395(10229):1054–62.
48. Grasselli G, Zangrillo A, Zanella A, Antonelli M, Cabrini L, Castelli A, Cereda D, Coluccello A, Foti G, Fumagalli R, Iotti G. Baseline characteristics and outcomes of 1591 patients infected with SARS CoV2 admitted to ICUs of the Lombardy Region, Italy. JAMA. 2020;323(16):1574–81.
49. Richardson S, Hirsch JS, Narasimhan M, Crawford JM, McGinn T, Davidson KW, Barnaby DP, Becker LB, Chelico JD, Cohen SL, Cookingham J. Presenting characteristics, comorbidities, and outcomes among 5700 patients hospitalized with COVID19 in the New York City area. Jama. 2020; 323(20):2052–9.
50. Ran J, Song Y, Zhuang Z, Han L, Zhao S, Cao P, Geng Y, Xu L, Qin J, He, D, Wu F. Blood pressure control and adverse outcomes of COVID19 infection in patients with concomitant hypertension in Wuhan, China. Hypert Res. 2020; 43(11):1267–76.
51. Sheppard JP, Nicholson BD, Lee J, McGagh D, Sherlock J, Koshiaris C, Oke J, Jones NR, Hinton W, Armitage L, Van Hecke O. Association between blood pressure control and coronavirus disease 2019 outcomes in 45 418 symptomatic patients with hypertension: an observational cohort study. Hypertension. 2021;77(3):846–55.
52. Gao C, Cai Y, Zhang K, Zhou L, Zhang Y, Zhang X, Li Q, Li W, Yang S, Zhao X, Zhao Y. Association of hypertension and antihypertensive treatment with COVID19 mortality: a retrospective observational study. Eur Heart J. 2020;41(22):2058–66.
53. Haider SS, Shaikh F, Rayasam V, Kumar, D, Helmstetter N. Bilateral Adrenal Gland Infarction in the Setting of COVID19 Infection. In *TP100. TP100 UNEXPECTED COVID19 CASE REPORTS* (pp. A4075-A4075). American Thoracic Society. 2021.
54. Martino M, Aboud N, Cola MF, Giancola G, Ciarloni A, Salvio G, Arnaldi G. Impact of COVID19 pandemic on psychophysical stress in patients with adrenal insufficiency: the CORTI-COVID study. J Endocrinol Invest. 2021;44(5):1075–84.
55. Durcan E, Turan S, Sahin S, Sulu C, Taze SS, Kavla Y, Ozkaya HM, Kadioglu P. Psychosocial effects and clinic reflections of the COVID19 outbreak in patients with acromegaly and Cushing's disease. Pituitary. 2021; 1–11.
56. Wadei HM, Textor SC. The role of the kidney in regulating arterial blood pressure. Nat Rev Nephrol. 2012;8(10):602–9.
57. Hirsch JS, Ng JH, Ross DW, Sharma P, Shah HH, Barnett RL, Hazzan AD, Fishbane S, Jhaveri KD, Abate M, Andrade HP. Acute kidney injury in patients hospitalized with COVID19. Kidney Int. 2020;98(1):209–18.
58. Chan L, Chaudhary K, Saha A, Chauhan K, Vaid A, Zhao S, Paranjpe I, Somani S, Richter F, Miotto R, Lala A. AKI in hospitalized patients with COVID19. J Am Soc Nephrol. 2021;32(1):151–60.
59. Cheng Y, Luo R, Wang K, Zhang M, Wang Z, Dong L, Li J, Yao Y, Ge S, Xu G. Kidney disease is associated with in-hospital death of patients with COVID19. Kidney Int. 2020;97 (5):829–38.
60. Uribarri A, Núñez-Gil IJ, Aparisi A, Becerra-Muñoz VM, Feltes G, Trabattoni D, Fernández-Rozas I, Viana-Llamas MC, Pepe M, Cerrato E, Capel-Astrua T. Impact of renal

function on admission in COVID19 patients: an analysis of the international HOPE COVID19 (Health Outcome Predictive Evaluation for COVID19) Registry. J Nephrol. 2020;33(4):737–45.

61. Are patients with hypertension and diabetes mellitus at increased risk for COVID19 infection? Fang L, Karakiulakis G, Roth M Lancet Respir Med. 2020 Apr; 8(4):e21.
62. Kuster GM, Pfister O, Burkard T, Zhou Q, Twerenbold R, Haaf P, Widmer AF, Osswald S. SARS-CoV2: should inhibitors of the renin-angiotensin system be withdrawn in patients with COVID19? Eur Heart J. 2020 Mar 20. pii: ehaa235. doi:https://doi.org/10.1093/eurheartj/ehaa235. [Epub ahead of print] PubMed PMID: 32196087.
63. American Heart Association (AHA), Heart Failure Society of America (HFSA) and American College of Cardiology (ACC). Patients taking ACE-i and ARBs who contract COVID19 should continue treatment, unless otherwise advised by their physician. 2020; 21.
64. International Society of Hypertension. A statement from the International Society of Hypertension on COVID19. 2020. Available on: https://ish-world.com/a-statement-from-the-international-society-of-hypertension-on-covid-19/. Accessed on 25 December 2021.
65. Li XC, Zhang J, Zhuo JL. The vasoprotective axes of the renin-angiotensin system: physiological relevance and therapeutic implications in cardiovascular, hypertensive and kidney diseases. Pharmacol Res. 2017;125:21–38.
66. Ferrario CM, Jessup J, Chappell MC, Averill DB, Brosnihan KB, Tallant EA, Diz DI, Gallagher PE. Effect of angiotensin-converting enzyme inhibition and angiotensin II receptor blockers on cardiac angiotensin-converting enzyme 2. Circulation. 2005;111(2605–2610):9.
67. Furuhashi M, Moniwa N, Mita T, Fuseya T, Ishimura S, Ohno K, Shibata S, Tanaka M, Watanabe Y, Akasaka H, Ohnishi H, Yoshida H, Takizawa H, Saitoh S, Ura N, Shimamoto K, Miura T. Urinary angiotensin-converting enzyme 2 in hypertensive patients may be increased by olmesartan, an angiotensin II receptor blocker. Am J Hypertens. 2015;28:15–21.
68. Imai Y, Kuba K, Rao S, Huan Y, Guo F, Guan B, Yang P, Sarao R, Wada T, Leong-Poi H, Crackower MA, Fukamizu A, Hui CC, Hein L, Uhlig S, Slutsky AS, Jiang C, Penninger JM. Angiotensin-converting enzyme 2 protects from severe acute lung failure. Nature. 2005;436:112–6.
69. Zhang P, Zhu L, Cai J, Lei F, Qin JJ, Xie J, Liu YM, Zhao YC, Huang X, Lin L, Xia M, Chen MM, Cheng X, Zhang X, Guo D, Peng Y, Ji YX, Chen J, She ZG, Wang Y, Xu Q, Tan R, Wang H, Lin J, Luo P, Fu S, Cai H, Ye P, Xiao B, Mao W, Liu L, Yan Y, Liu M, Chen M, Zhang XJ, Wang X, Touyz RM, Xia J, Zhang BH, Huang X, Yuan Y, Rohit L, Liu PP, Li H. Association of Inpatient Use of Angiotensin Converting Enzyme Inhibitors and Angiotensin II Receptor Blockers with Mortality Among Patients With Hypertension Hospitalized With COVID19. Circ Res. 2020 Apr 17.doi: https://doi.org/10.1161/CIRCRESAHA.120.317134. [Epub ahead of print] PubMed PMID: 32302265.
70. Morales DR, Conover MM, You SC, Pratt N, Kostka K, Duarte-Salles T, Fernández-Bertolín S, Aragón M, DuVall SL, Lynch K, Falconer T. Renin–angiotensin system blockers and susceptibility to COVID19: an international, open science, cohort analysis. Lanc Dig Health. 2021;3(2):e98-114.
71. Al-Baadani AM, Elzein FE, Alhemyadi SA, Khan OA, Albenmousa AH, Idrees MM. Characteristics and outcome of viral pneumonia caused by influenza and Middle East respiratory syndrome-coronavirus infections: a 4-year experience from a tertiary care center. Annals Thor Med. 2019;14(3):179.
72. Chalmers JD, Singanayagam A, Hill AT. Systolic blood pressure is superior to other haemodynamic predictors of outcome in community acquired pneumonia. Thorax. 2008;63(8):698–702. https://doi.org/10.1136/thx.2008.095562.
73. Ferrario CM, Strawn WB. Role of the renin-angiotensin-aldosterone system and proinflammatory mediators in cardiovascular disease. Am J Cardiol. 2006;98:121–8.
74. Caillon A, Paradis P, Schiffrin EL. Role of immune cells in hypertension. Br J Pharmacol. 2019;176(12):1818–28.

75. De Miguel C, Rudemiller NP, Abais JM, Mattson DL. Inflammation and hypertension: new understandings and potential therapeutic targets. Curr Hypertens Rep. 2015;17(1):507.
76. Shi Y, Wang Y, Shao C, Huang J, Gan J, Huang X, Bucci E, Piacentini M, Ippolito, G, Melino G. COVID19 infection: the perspectives on immune responses. 2020.
77. Schillaci G, Pirro M, Gemelli F, Pasqualini L, Vaudo G, Marchesi S, Siepi D, Bagaglia F, Mannarino E. Increased C-reactive protein concentrations in never-treated hypertension: the role of systolic and pulse pressures. J Hypertens. 2003;21:1841–6.
78. Stumpf C, John S, Jukic J, Yilmaz A, Raaz D, Schmieder RE, Daniel WG, Garlichs CD. Enhanced levels of platelet P selectin and circulating cytokines in young patients with mild arterial hypertension. J Hypertens. 2005;23:995–1000.
79. Sundar UM, Ugusman A, Chua HK, Latip J, Aminuddin A. Piper sarmentosum promotes endothelial nitric oxide production by reducing asymmetric dimethylarginine in tumor necrosis factor-α-induced human umbilical vein endothelial cells. Front Pharmacol. 2019;10:1033.
80. Brown DI, Griendling KK. Regulation of signal transduction by reactive oxygen species in the cardiovascular system. Circ Res. 2015;116(3):531–49.
81. Vieira C, Nery L, Martins L, Jabour L, Dias R, Simões e Silva AC. Downregulation of membrane-bound angiotensin converting enzyme 2 (ACE2) receptor has a pivotal role in COVID19 immunopathology. Curr Drug Targ. 2021; 22(3):254–81.
82. Farhangrazi ZS, Moghimi SM. Elevated circulating endothelin-1 as a potential biomarker for high-risk COVID19 severity. Precis Nanomed. 2020;3:622–8.
83. Lüscher TF, Seo BG, Bühler FR. Potential role of endothelin in hypertension. Controversy on endothelin in hypertension. Hypertension. 1993; 21(6_pt_1):752–7.
84. Rossi GP, Sacchetto A, Cesari M, Pessina AC. Interactions between endothelin-1 and the renin–angiotensin–aldosterone system. Cardiovasc Res. 1999;43(2):300–7.
85. Grossman A, Messerli FH, Grossman E. Drug-induced hypertension–An unappreciated cause of secondary hypertension. Eur J Pharmacol. 2015;763:15–22.
86. Griendling KK, Camargo LL, Rios FJ, Alves-Lopes R, Montezano AC, Touyz RM. Oxidative stress and hypertension. Circ Res. 2021;128(7):993–1020.
87. Batabyal R, Freishtat N, Hill E, Rehman M, Freishtat, R, Koutroulis I. Metabolic dysfunction and immunometabolism in COVID19 pathophysiology and therapeutics. Int J Obes. 2021; 1–7.
88. Koenen M, Hill MA, Cohen P, Sowers JR. Obesity, adipose tissue and vascular dysfunction. Circ Res. 2021;128(7):951–68.
89. Fang S, Livergood MC, Nakagawa P, Wu J, Sigmund CD. Role of the peroxisome proliferator activated receptors in hypertension. Circ Res. 2021;128(7):1021–39.
90. Desterke C, Turhan AG, Bennaceur-Griscelli A, Griscelli F. PPARγ cistrome repression during activation of lung monocyte-macrophages in severe COVID19. Iscience. *2020;* 23 (10):101611.
91. Qin X, Huang C, Wu K, Li Y, Liang X, Su M, Li R. Anti–coronavirus disease 2019 (COVID-19) targets and mechanisms of puerarin. J Cell Mol Med. 2021;25(2):677–85.
92. Julius S. Autonomic nervous dysfunction in essential hypertension. Diab Care. 1991;14 (3):249–59.
93. Porzionato A, Emmi A, Barbon S, Boscolo-Berto R, Stecco C, Stocco E, Macchi V, De Caro R. Sympathetic activation: a potential link between comorbidities and COVID-19. FEBS J. 2020;287(17):3681–8.
94. Goldstein DS. The extended autonomic system, dyshomeostasis, and COVID19. Clin Auton Res. 2020; 1–17.
95. Minhas AS, Scheel P, Garibaldi B, Liu G, Horton M, Jennings M, Jones SR, Michos ED, Hays AG. Takotsubo syndrome in the setting of COVID19. Case Reports. 2020;2(9):1321–5.
96. Sellner J, Taba P, Öztürk S, Helbok R. The need for neurologists in the care of COVID-19 patients. Eur J Neurol. 2020;27(9):e31–2.
97. Lim S, Bae JH, Kwon HS, Nauck MA. Reply to: autonomic dyshomeostasis in patients with diabetes mellitus during COVID19. Nat Rev Endocrinol. 2021; 1–1.

98. Kenney MJ, Ganta CK. Autonomic nervous system and immune system interactions. Compr Physiol. 2014;4:1177–200.
99. Parati G, Ochoa JE, Lombardi C, Bilo G. Assessment and management of blood-pressure variability. Nat Rev Cardiol. 2013;10(3):143.
100. Yang M, Pan X, Liang Z, Huang X, Duan M, Cai H, Jiang G, Wen, X, Chen L. Association between blood pressure variability and the short-term outcome in patients with acute spontaneous subarachnoid hemorrhage. Hypert Res. 2019; 42(11):1701–7.
101. Webster J, Petrie JC, Jeffers TA, Lovell HG. Accelerated hypertension—patterns of mortality and clinical factors affecting outcome in treated patients. QJM: An Int J Med. 1993; 86(8):485–99.

Chapter 14
Cardiac Arrhythmias in CoViD19

Key Questions

- How common are cardiac arrhythmias in CoViD19?
- What is the importance of cardiac arrhythmias in CoViD19?
- What types of arrhythmias may be observed in CoViD19?
- How may arrhythmias impact CoViD19 patients?
- Which factors may contribute to the development of arrhythmias in CoViD19?
- What complexities are associated with arrhythmias in CoViD19 patients?

14.1 Epidemiology of Arrhythmias in CoViD19

Severe CoViD19 accompanies a variety of pro arrhythmogenic factors and conditions related to the infectious and hyperinflammatory nature of the disease (Fig. 14.1). Patients with complicated CoViD19 may develop conduction system abnormalities in the heart leading to rhythm abnormalities of varying severities [1]. Particular factors that are likely to be important precipitants of the arrhythmic complications in CoViD19, such as hypoxic lung conditions, sepsis, hyperinflammatory stress, are well-recognized triggers of the coronary and myocardial complications i.e. cardiac and vascular injury that enhance the risk of arrhythmias.

Data indciate that cardiac arrhythimas are frequently associated with CoViD19 and the incidence of different types of cardiac arrhythmias may vary. Several studies investigating characteristics and features of the novel coronavirus disease CoViD19, report the occurrence, and association of cardiac arrhythmias. The frequency, severity, and duration of arrhythmias may vary in relation to the burden of the underlying stress factors and the cardiovascular fitness. The patients with

U. Mallick, *Cardiovascular Complications of COVID-19*,
https://doi.org/10.1007/978-3-030-90065-6_14

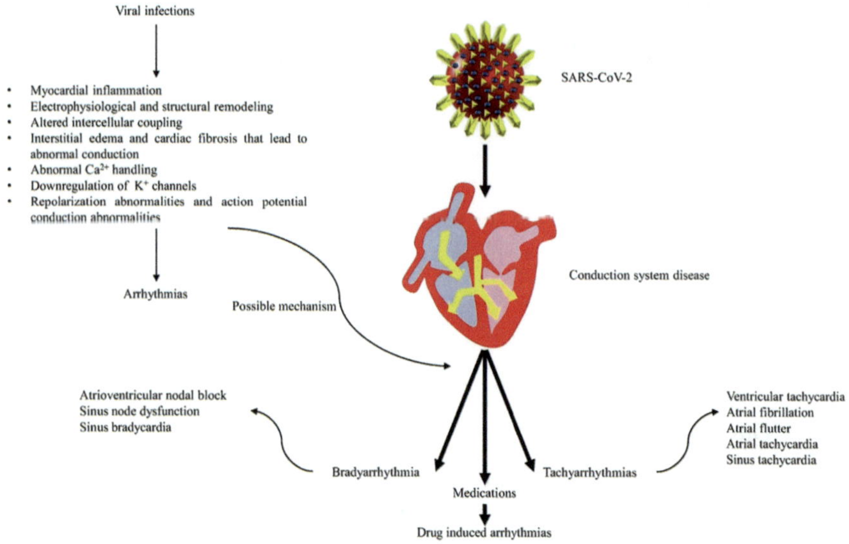

Fig. 14.1 Arrhythmia manifestations of COVID-19 and possible mechanisms. *Source* Figure 1. Babapoor-Farrokhran, S., Rasekhi, R.T., Gill, D., Babapoor, S. and Amanullah, A., 2020. Arrhythmia in COVID-19. SN Comprehensive Clinical Medicine, pp.1-6. https://link.springer.com/article/10.1007/s42399-020-00454-2. By Springer Nature Group

CoViD19 may have increased heart rates in sinus rhythm such as tachycardia or worsening of the pre-existing arrhythmias i.e. faster rates of atrial fibrillation known prior to contracting the viral disease or may develop new arrhythmias, often associated with severe disease. The arrhythmias may present early in the acute phase or during the recovery phase of the disease [47, 48]; however, are most likely to occur in the critical state of CoViD19. Studies further indicate that the development of cardiac injury in CoViD19 patients, frequently associated with severe disease, promotes arrhythmias.

Palpitations may present as the initial symptom in CoViD19. In a cohort study of 137 CoViD19 hospitalized patients, about 7.3% of patients presented with palpitations as the initial symptom [46]. In a retrospective analysis of data of 4526 hospitalized CoViD19 patients from four continents, about 18% (827/4526) of patients developed cardiac arrhythmia during the hospitalization [2]. Other analyses showed the incidence of arrhythmias in CoViD19 patients ranged from 17% to 30% [6, 38]. A study reporting cardiac arrhythmia as the most frequent cardiac complication, showed that the risk of developing arrhythmia appears to be higher among CoViD19 patients with elevated underlying cardiac risk due to pre-existing cardiac disease or a new cardiac injury. In a large survey investigating cardiovascular disease in 3011 CoViD19 hospitalized patients, about 349/3011 (11.6%, 95% confidence interval (CI)) patients were diagnosed with a cardiac complications during hospitalization. In this study, cardiac arrhythmia/conduction disorders were the most common cardiac complications, occurring in $n = 258/3011$ (8.6%) patients (7.6-9.6,

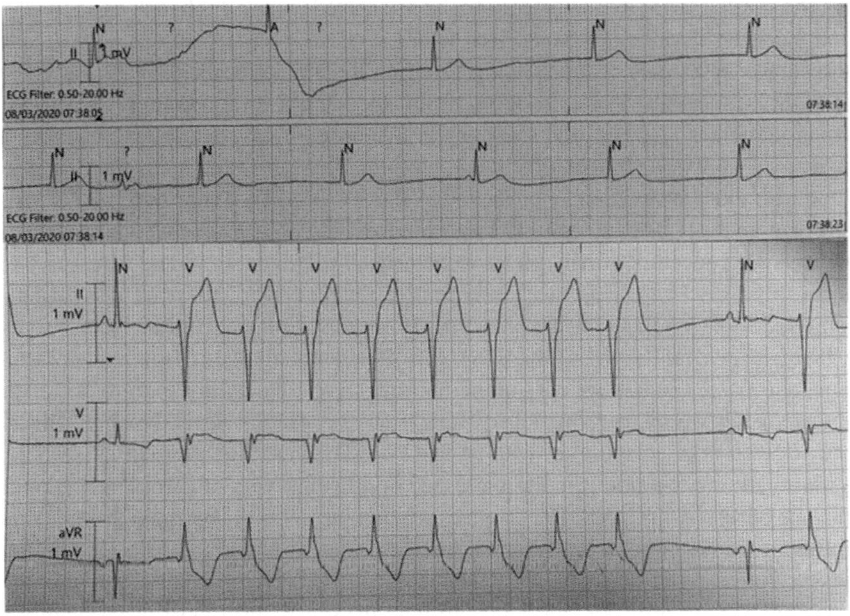

Fig. 14.2 Electrocardiography strips showing intermittent junctional bradycardia and non-sustained ventricular tachycardia in a confirmed COVID-19 patient. *Source* Figure 1 Chia, P.L., Tan, K., Tan, L.W., Chin, P.S. and Foo, D., 2020. Rhythm blues in the time of coronavirus disease 2019 (COVID-19): how the cardiac electrophysiologist adapts to a viral pandemic in Singapore. Journal of Interventional Cardiac Electrophysiology, 58, pp. 269–272. https://link.springer.com/article/10.1007/s10840-020-00782-2#Fig1. By Springer Nature Group

95% confidence interval (CI) [3]. Among these supraventricular tachycardia *n* = 189/3011, 6.3% (5.4–7.1, 95% CI) and atrial fibrillation *n* = 142/3011, 4.7% (4.0–5.5, 95% CI) were most common. In the overall cohort about 453/3011 (15.1%) had a prior history of cardiac arrhythmia/conduction disorder and about *n* = 463/3011 (15.4%) patients had pe-existing coronary artery disease. The burden of pre-existing cardiac disease was higher among CoViD19 patients who developed a cardiac injury. Among *n* = 349/3011 patients who developed cardiac complications, about 82 (23.5%) patients had pre-existing cardiac arrhythmia/conduction disorder as compared to 371/2662 (14%) of those without development of cardiac complications during the study. In this study, among patients with cardiac complications, about 258 patients developed cardiac arrhythmia/conduction disorder representing 73.9% (69.3–78.5, 95% CI) of patients with cardiac complications (n = 349) versus 8.6% (7.6–9.6, 95% CI) of the total cohort (*n* = 3011). In the overall cohort, nearly one-third of patients n = 937/3011 (31.0%) had a history of cardiac disease, whereas, n =147/349 (42.2%) patients with cardiac complications had a pre-existing history of a cardiac disease versus n = 790/2662 (29.8%) patients without the cardiac complications, *P*-value <0.001. The authors concluded that there was a low incidence of cardiac complications during hospital admission, despite a frequent history of cardiovascular disease [3].

The cardiac arrhythmias appear to be associated with a high risk of morbidity and mortality in patients hospitalized with CoViD19 and may significantly impact the clinical outcomes of the disease. The CoViD19 is associated with a variety of arrhythmic manifestations, ranging from the benign to potentially life-threatening outcomes [4]. The frequency of cardiac arrhythmias appears to be higher in severe CoViD19 as compared to the non-severe disease. Cardiac arrhythmias were found in about 60% (51/75) of fatal CoViD19 cases [5]. According to the retrospective analysis of data from 4526 hospitalized CoViD19 patients, about 43% of patients who developed arrhythmias were mechanically ventilated and 51% survived to hospital discharge [2]. In a retrospective single-center study, of 138 patients admitted with CoViD19 related pneumonia, arrhythmias were reported in 16.7% (23/138) of the general cohort and 44.4% (16/36) of patients admitted in the intensive care unit, and 6.9% (7/102) patients in the non-intensive care setting *P*-value <.001. In this study the overall mortality rate of 4.3% was observed [6]. Several reports indicate the association of arrhythmias with critical CoViD19 and high mortality [7–9].

Furthermore, variations in the incidence of different types of cardiac arrhythmias may be observed in CoViD19. Cardiac arrhythmias in CoViD19 range from benign forms of tachycardia or bradycardia, atrial fibrillation (AF), atrial flutter, to more severe forms, such as Torsade de Point due to QT prolongations, polymorphic ventricular tachycardia, or ventricular arrhythmias due to fever in Brugada syndrome [10, 11, 51] (Fig. 14.2). In a retrospective case series study of a cohort of 187 patients admitted with CoViD19, Ventricular Tachycardia (VT)/Ventricular Fibrillation (VF) was found in 5.9% (11) patients as a complication of the disease [12]. Larger multinational studies investigating cardiac arrhythmias in 4526 CoViD19 hospitalized patients have shown a high frequency of (81.8%) atrial arrhythmias, representing the majority, with bradyarrhythmia and ventricular arrhythmias in 22.6 and 20.7% of patients, respectively. Regional differences in types of arrhythmias have been confirmed in line with previous findings with Asian region with a higher burden of bradyarrhythmias and lower burden of tachyarrhythmias [2]. Analysis of the 12-lead ECGs and telemetry of 115 patients admitted with CoViD19 included 69 patients admitted to the medical intensive care unit (MICU) and 46 patients admitted to a general medicine ward, revealed that an atrial tachyarrhythmia that had not been present on admission, was recorded on a subsequent 12-lead ECG in 19 patients (16.5%), all admitted to the MICU (27.5% of MICU patients). In contrast, no patient admitted to the general inpatient service developed atrial arrhythmias ($p = 0.00002$). These arrhythmias included atrial fibrillation (AF) in 12 patients, atrial flutter in 6 patients, and atrial tachycardia in 1 patient. The authors observed that Atrial arrhythmias are common among patients with CoViD19 who require admission to an intensive care unit and are often followed by hemodynamic deterioration [51].

Studies further show that atrial fibrillation is frequently associated with CoViD19. A large survey investigating cardiovascular disease in 3011 CoViD19 hospitalized patients showed atrial fibrillation ($n = 142$, 4.7%) was the most common form of arrhythmia, and malignant ventricular rhythm disturbances were least common n = 14 patients (0.5%) [3]. Atrial fibrillation has been reported as the most common form of arrhythmia associated with CoViD19 with a history of atrial fibrillation, present in about 19% of hospitalized CoViD19 patients [13] and adversely impacted the outcome. Another report based on a survey of 1197 respondents involving 76 countries across 6 continents investigating CoViD19 associated arrhythmia, described AF as the most common occurrence (21%) [14]. The AF has been described as a risk associated with CoViD19 patients? [15]. Although, the incidence of new-onset AF in CoViD19 hospitalized patients is not well known,ccording to reports, the new onset AF incidence may vary between 3.6 to 6.7% as a new ECG abnormality [16, 17]. Small case series and sporadic cases reporting the occurrence of heart block in association with CoViD19 have been reported [18, 53], and the overall incidence appears to be low. An analysis reporting incidence of arrhythmia in CoViD19 patients describes the occurence of atrioventricular/ventricular block (11.8%) as the highest among arrhythmia, exceeding the ratio of sinus tachycardia (7.5%), sinus bradycardia (8%), atrial arrhythmias (7%), and ventricular arrhythmias (4%) [54, 55]. The evidence further suggests an occurrence of electrocardiographic QT-prolongation in CoViD19 patients, known to have potentially fatal pro-arrhythmic impact. The QT-prolongation is most commonly associated with the use of drugs used in the treatment of CoViD19, such as chloroquine (CQ), hydroxychloroquine (HCQ), azithromycin, ritonavir/lopinavir, etc. [55, 56]. (For further details about cardiac toxicity of drugs used in the treatment of CoViD19 please refer to Chap. 5 in this book).

14.2 Pathogenesis of Arrhythmias in CoViD19

A myriad of molecular, proteomic reactions, cellular stress mechanisms that promote homeostatic dysfunction are associated with viral invasion in CoViD19, may induce myocardial and conduction tissue instability, and may facilitate cardiac arrhythmias. The etiopathogenesis of arrhythmias is complex and heterogeneous. Several viral and hyperinflammatory conditions are known to promote arrhythmias [19] and may have long term cardiac implications [20]. Sepsis is known to carry a high risk of atrial and life-threatening arrhythmias [21]. According to a retrospective analysis of 136 CoViD19 hospitalized patients, investigating cardiac arrest, about 119/136 (87.5%) patients had respiratory compromise as a cause of the cardiac arrest. The data show that the initial rhythm at cardiac arrest was asystole in 89.7% patients, pulseless electrical activity (PEA) in 4.4%, and shockable rhythm in 5.9% patients [22]. Cardiac injury may promote fatal arrhythmias, and severe and prolonged arrhythmias may cause a cardiac injury. Elevation of troponin in CoViD19 patients was observed in malignant arrhythmia indicating the underlying myocardial damage [12]. For further details about mechanisms related to cardiac injury in CoViD19 please refer to Chap. 11 in this book.

Classical cardiovascular risk factors commonly observed in patients with CoViD19 such as advanced age, hypertension, diabetes mellitus, coronary heart disease, or other forms of background preexisting cardiovascular disease or newly developed cardiac injury may compromise cardiac fitness or decompensate myocardium and generate arrhythmias. Myocardial injury may be associated with scarring observed in CoViD19 patients [23] and may increase long term risk of developing arrhythmias [24]. A higher burden of cardiometabolic risk factors or presence of preexisting cardiovascular disease in patients with CoViD19 are likely to contribute to the development of arrhythmias. In the retrospective analysis of data of 4526 hospitalized CoViD19 patients from four continents, cardiac comorbidities were common among patients with cardiac arrhythmias: 69% had hypertension, 42% diabetes, 30% had heart failure, and 24% had coronary artery disease [2].

CoViD19 related acute lung injury and sepsis appear to play an important role in the development of arrhythmias. These complications are associated with a multitude of pro-arrhythmogenic complex pathogenetic mechanisms, such as pulmonary hypoxic and metabolic stress, cardiopulmonary micro, and macrovascular damage, hyperactivity of prothrombotic factors, catecholaminergic stress and unfavorable hemodynamics. The core pathogenetic culprit mechanisms linked with CoViD19 in particular cytokine storm with hyperinflammatory stress, dysregulated RAS, microvascular and prothrombotic burden, electrolyte imbalance (hypokalemia, hypomagnesemia), and other factors that promote myocardial injury and dysfunction may further lead to the development of arrhythmias. The uncontrolled inflammation and immune dysregulation related phenomena in particular, known as potential initators and mediators of cardiac arrhythmias, may play a key role in arrhythmogenicity [25, 26]. The pro-inflammatory cytokines may promote arrythmias via substrate-triggered cardiac electrical and structural remodeling. The activated macrophages and macrophage-secreted pro-inflammatory cytokines are known with a signficant pro-arrhythmogenic potential [57, 58]. Several pro-inflammatory cytokines including IL-6 and IL-1β, IL-2, IL-8, IL-17, G-CSF, GM-CSF, IP-10, MCP-1, CCL-3, and TNF-α are known in association with canonical immune-inflammatory stress in severe CoViD19 [59–61]. The IL-6 plays a critical role in the pathophysiology of several cardiac disorders including arrhythmias, may contribute to the modulation of ICa,L and IK currents precipitating cardiac instability, and may also regulate ICaL and density [62]. The elevated immune inflammatory biomarkers, such as C-reactive protein (CRP) and IL-6, may mark the inflammatory burden in CoViD19 [27], may thus assist in determining the cardiac risk. Similarly, interactions between cytokines and autoantibodies that may induce AF have been investigated [31]. Several RAS and immune mechanisms are linked with the development of atrial fibrillation. An important correlation between elevated ACE 2 levels, or Ang II and atrial fibrillation has been previously described [28, 29, 30, 31].

The viral invasion may induce cardiac myocyte damage directly leading to myocardial dysfunction and the development of arrhythmia. Arrhythmogenic mechanisms involving activated NF-κB that may affect mRNA expression of the pore-forming (Kv4,2 and Kv4.3) and regulatory/auxiliary beta subunit

(KChIP2) subunits of fast transient outward potassium current (Ito,f) may promote arrhythmia by affecting the action potential (AP) troponin CoViD19 [27]. The NF-κB is a key transcription factor critical for regulation of cardiac inflammatory signaling pathways, and coronaviruses are known to use various signalling pathways, including the NF-κB pathway of the host cell, by differentially activating its transcription factors and downstream target genes for their replication [63, 64].

Several mechanisms associated with CoViD19 may influence cardiac electrophysiology and promote arrhythmias. The altered metabolic activity in the cardiac tissue may generate arrhythmias. Reports suggest that sympathetic overactivation in CoViD19 with excessive catecholamine release [33, 34] may underlie arrhythmogenesis in CoViD19 patients [35]. Sympathetic stimulation is also known to contribute to metabolic dysfunction, an important feature associated with the CoViD19 that may precipitate arrhythmias [36]. Cardiac electrical stability relies on the effective maintenance of sodium and calcium homeostasis that may be adversely impacted under the hyper-inflammatory stresss environment reated to the viral disease. Metabolic activity impacts the expression and function of repolarizing potassium currents, and alterations in the metabolic activity may determine changes in calcium homeostasis impacting excitation-contraction coupling. Anomalies impacting the energy metabolism and ion homeostasis interlinks may alter cardiac electrophysiological stability and promote arrhythmias in CoViD19. The sympathetic activation has a proinflammatory role, may impact immune modulation, and promotes M1 polarization, and may contribute towards ventricular arrhythmogenesis [65].

Furthermore, patients with CoViD19 treated with certain drugs may develop iatrogenic forms of cardiac arrhythmias. These drugs include hydrochloroquine, chloroquine, or azithromycin, which may result in electrocardiographic QT prolongation. Cardiac toxicity, associated with antiviral therapy such as ribavirin and interferon, may cause arrhythmias and requires close monitoring [37]. Concomitant inflammatory stress with elevated C-reactive protein (CRP), IL-6 with potentially arrhythmogenic drugs in CoViD19 may increase the risk of QT prolongation [27].

The critical CoViD19 accompanies ventilatory and hemodynamic compromise leading to decompensation of multiple body systems ultimately causing multi-organ failure and death. The pulmonary pathology in CoViD19 is complex with a variety of pathological injuries in pulmonary parenchyma, vasculature, and hemodynamics, as well as micro and macro prothrombotic processes that exert adverse hemodynamic and structural stress on the right heart, thereby increasing the risk of arrhythmias including atrial fibrillation [39]. Other factors such as an increased atrial stretch, stiffness, elevated right ventricular pressures synchronised with the thrombo inflammatory burden of CoViD19 may lead to cardiac rhythmic turbulences and acute functional decline [40, 41]. Although underlying individual cardiometabolic risk factors and potential mechanisms related to the acute viral and immune-inflammatory stress and other hemodynamic regulatory mechanisms may help delineate the core pathognesis of the cardiac arrhythmias in CoViD19, the exact associations of viral induced mechanisms that adversely impact the cardiac structural and electrophysiological integrity and cellular homeostasis and precise signaling pathways yet remain to be further determined.

14.3 Summary

Cardiac arrhythmias frequently occur with CoViD19, although, their true incidence is not fully known. The arrhythmias appear to be associated with high morbidity and mortality among patients hospitalized with CoViD19 infection. The incidence of various types of arrhythmias associated with CoViD19 and their relevant clinical outcomes need further exploration. Palpitations may present as the initial symptom in CoViD19. Arrhythmias may present early in the acute phase or may develop during the recovery phase of the viral disease [27, 39, 42, 43], or may even occur post CoViD19 recovery, the evidence indicating the features and associated trends needs to be further strenghtened. Despite gaps in data, cardiac arrhythmias appear to be among the most common cardiac complications of CoViD19 and adversley impact patient outcomes. A higher frequency of tachyarrhythmias and atrial fibrillation appears to be common among various types of arrhythmias observed in association with CoViD19. Patients with critical CoViD19 and a high burden of comorbidities, including cardiovascular or metabolic risk factors, more often have arrhythmias, therefore require closer monitoring and enhanced measures to minimize the serious risk of developing complications. Special precautions with the use of effective prevention strategies are needed for risk mitigation, related to arrhythmias, in critical CoViD19 patients.

The arrhythmogenicity of CoViD19 appears to contribute to the poor outcomes observed in severe CoViD19 patients. Cardiac arrhythmias may result in serious comorbidities and fatality, including stroke, and sudden cardiac death. Acute cardiac decompensation, acute coronary syndromes, cardiogenic shock, cerebrovascular injury, or cardiac arrest are notable life threatening complications of cardiac arrhythmias. Persistent and severe forms of cardiac arrhythmias may cause myocardial injury, hemodynamic compromise, and generate a prothrombotic state resulting in complications that determine a high risk of morbidity and mortality.

Both acute infectious inflammatory stress as well as pre-existing risk burden contribute towards arrhythmogenic risk associatedwith CoViD19. The arrhythmogenicity may be due to the viral injury or sepsis or may be driven by the associated cardiacor metabolic co-morbidities or a range of risk factors. There may be ethnic or regional differences in the incidence of cardiacarrhythmias across the globe [2]. Patients with CoViD19 with elevated underlying cardiac risk appear to be particularly prone to arrhythmias indicating that the underlying burden of pre-existing cardiac risk may have a significant contribution towards the risk of developing arrhythmias. Although, the historical links between the viral conditions, sepsis, inflammatory conditions, and arrhythmias may help understand the association of arrhythmias in CoViD19 patients, several factors related to the viral infectivity, viral cardiac affinity, host immune reactivity, genetic and several other factors may distinctly impact the arrhythmogenic burden associated with CoViD19.

The heterogeneity in the pathogenesis of arrhythmias in CoViD19 and pathogenetic complexities may justify the use of non-conventional diagnostic and therapeutic methods in the management of CoViD19 patients. CoViD19 is a high thrombo-inflammatory state with significantly elevated thrombotic risk and vascular damage and arrhythmias may further potentiate the risk of prothrombotic complications in CoViD19. Dampening of the inflammatory stress using pharmacological interventions may help minimize arrhythmic risk in CoViD19 patients [23, 27, 40, 44] and associated complications. Prompt recognition and effective management of arrhythmias and associated cardiac damage in CoViD19 may help reduce the associated morbidity and mortality. A lower intervention threshold should be used in the high-risk patients who develop CoViD19.

Individual risk assessments are important for effective prevention, especially in patients with cardiac damage due to the viral disease and in subjects with high cardio-metabolic risk burden. The risk of myocardial injury and scarring in CoViD19 patients, and persistence of the sequelae post convalescence warrants a further careful long term approach. The development of such complications may dictate the need for prolonged cardiac surveillance in CoViD19 patients due to the long-term risk of arrhythmogenicity. An early implementation of aggressive preventive measures and close monitoring are key tools in combating such risks. Advanced cardiac investigations including imaging modalities such as CMR, and cardiac telemetry tools may be used to determine the risk and early prevention of arrhythmias and consequent complications in CoViD19 patients at high risk. Further data are needed to better describe the forms and characteristics of cardiac arrhythmias in CoViD19, identify markers of risk, and develop better strategies for optimal management and risk mitigation.

A multitude of factors related to the viral invasion, the intensity of the disease, hypoxic-immune-inflammatory-metabolic stress of CoViD19, sympathetic overstimulation, and several others that promote underlying myocardial injury and multi-organ damage, contribute towards the arrhythmogenicity of CoViD19. Serum electrolytes, and markers of myocardial injury and dysfunction such as troponin [12, 41–46], CKMB, LDH, and markers of CoViD19 severity including elevated CRP, D Dimers, ferritin, pro-inflammatory cytokines such as IL-6, may aid in risk estimation of the cardiac arrhythmias. Markers of inflammation such as CRP may help predict the risk of arrhythmias [22, 46]. The associations of these markers and the predictability of the risk in CoViD19 patients, however, need to be further assessed using robust research methodology. Furthermore, the cardiotoxicity of drugs used in CoViD19 poses an important risk. Awareness must be raised among healthcare professionals with regards to a judicious use of these drugs in the management of CoViD19. Expert recommendations are needed for an effective management of the cardiotoxicity of drugs with arrhythmogenic potential used in the management of CoViD19 patients, along with practical guidance regarding potential drug interactions and the dose adjustments. We recommend the use of expert clinical guidelines in the management of cardiac arrhythmias in CoViD19 patients. As observed with other cardiac interventions, reductions in the procedural volume of electrophysiology procedures were observed with CoViD19 internationally (2). Strict measures and protocols need to be adapted in th healthcare institutions for the effective delivery of cardiac interventions while minimizing the risk of contagion.

Summary Box

- Cardiac arrhythmias are among the top most common cardiovascular complications of CoViD19.
- Tachyarrhythmias appear to be most common among cardiac arrhythmias, and atrial fibrillation is the most common form of tachyarrhythmia in CoViD19.
- Ventricular arrhythmias that display a high potential of fatality occur with a more critical disease however appear to have a lower frequency in CoViD19.
- Arrhythmias may decompensate the cardiovascular disease or trigger a cardiovascular disease; risks may be higher in CoViD19 patients.
- Viral and inflammatory conditions including sepsis have known associations with cardiac arrhythmias.
- A pre-existing cardiac risk, a new cardiac injury, and the criticality of CoViD19 associated inflammatory and dysregulated mechanisms determine cardiac arrhythmogenicity in CoViD19 subjects.
- Serum immune-inflammatory markers may have a role in the assessment of the risk of cardiac arrhythmias in CoViD19 patients.
- Suppressing the inflammatory activity may diminish the arrhythmic burden in CoViD19 patients.
- Cardiotoxic drugs used in CoViD19 may cause arrhythmias and must be used cautiously.
- Further research is needed to determine the patterns of cardiac arrhythmias in CoViD19, to assess potential risk determinants and their connections with CoViD19 comorbidities.

References

1. Kochav SM, Coromilas E, Nalbandian A, Ranard LS, Gupta A, Chung MK, Gopinathannair R, Biviano AB, Garan H, Wan EY. Cardiac arrhythmias in COVID19 infection. Circul Arrhyth Electrophys. 2020;13(6):e008719.
2. Coromilas EJ, Kochav S, Goldenthal I, Biviano A, Garan H, Goldbarg S, Kim JH, Yeo I, Tracy C, Ayanian S, Akar J. Worldwide survey of COVID19–associated arrhythmias. Circul Arrhyth Electrophys. 2021;14(3):e009458.
3. Linschoten M, Peters S, van Smeden M, Jewbali LS, Schaap J, Siebelink HM, Smits PC, Tieleman RG, van der Harst P, van Gilst WH, Asselbergs FW. Cardiac complicationsXE "cardiac complications" in patients hospitalised with COVID19. Eur Heart J Acute Cardiovasc Care. 2020;9(8):817–23.

4. Gopinathannair R, Merchant FM, Lakkireddy DR, Etheridge SP, Feigofsky S, Han JK, Kabra R, Natale A, Poe S, Saha SA, Russo AM. COVID19 and cardiac arrhythmias: a global perspective on arrhythmia characteristics and management strategies. J Interv Card Electrophysiol. 2020;59:329–36.
5. Du Y, Tu L, Zhu P, Mu M, Wang R, Yang P, Wang X, Hu C, Ping R, Hu P, Li T. Clinical features of 85 fatal cases of COVID19 from Wuhan. A retrospective observational study. Am J Respir Crit Care Med. 2020; 201(11):1372–9.
6. Wang D, Hu B, Hu C, Zhu F, Liu X, Zhang J, Wang B, Xiang H, Cheng Z, Xiong Y, Zhao Y, Li Y, Wang X, Peng Z. Clinical Characteristics of 138 Hospitalized Patients With 2019 Novel Coronavirus-Infected Pneumonia in Wuhan, China. JAMA. 2020 Feb 7. doi: https://doi.org/10.1001/jama.2020.1585. [Epub ahead of print] PubMed PMID: 32031570; PubMed Central PMCID: PMC7042881.
7. Mehra MR, Desai SS, Kuy S, Henry, TD, Patel AN. Cardiovascular disease, drug therapy, and mortality in CoViD19. New England J Med. 2020; 382(25):e102.
8. Wetterslev M, Jacobsen PK, Hassager C, Jøns C, Risum N, Pehrson S, Bastiansen A, Andreasen AS, Tjelle Kristiansen K, Bestle MH, Mohr T. Cardiac arrhythmias in critically ill patients with coronavirus disease 2019: A retrospective population-based cohort study. Acta Anaesthesiologica Scandinavica. 2021.
9. Bhatla A, Mayer MM, Adusumalli S, Hyman MC, Oh E, Tierney A, Moss J, Chahal AA, Anesi G, Denduluri S, Domenico CM. COVID19 and cardiac arrhythmias. Heart Rhythm. 2020;17(9):1439–44.
10. Kochav SM, Coromilas E, Nalbandian A, Ranard LS, Gupta A, Chung MK, Gopinathannair R, Biviano AB, Garan H, Wan EY. Cardiac arrhythmias in COVID19 infection. Circul Arrhyth Electrophy. 2020; 13(6):e008719.
11. Sorgente A, Capulzini L, Brugada P. The known into the unknown: Brugada syndrome and COVID19. Jankelson L, Karam G, Becker ML, Chinitz LA, Tsai MC. QT prolongation, torsades de pointes, and sudden death with short courses of chloroquine or hydroxychloroquine as used in COVID19: a systematic review. Heart Rhythm. 2020; 17(9):1472–9.
12. Guo T, Fan Y, Chen M, et al. Cardiovascular implications of fatal outcomes of patients with coronavirus disease 2019 (COVID19). JAMA Cardiol. Published online March 27, 2020. doi:10.1001/ jamacardio. 2020.1017)
13. Inciardi RM, Adamo M, Lupi L, Cani DS, Di Pasquale M, Tomasoni D, Italia L, Zaccone G, Tedino C, Fabbricatore D, Curnis A. Characteristics and outcomes of patients hospitalized for COVID19 and cardiac disease in Northern Italy. Eur Heart J. 2020;41(19):1821–9.
14. Gopinathannair R, Merchant FM, Lakkireddy DR, Etheridge SP, Feigofsky S, Han JK, Kabra R, Natale A, Poe S, Saha SA, Russo AM. COVID19 and cardiac arrhythmias: a global perspective on arrhythmia characteristics and management strategies. J Intervent Card Electrophy. 2020; 59:329–36.
15. Sanchis-Gomar F, Perez-Quilis C, Lavie CJ. Should atrial fibrillation be considered a cardiovascular risk factor for a worse prognosis in COVID19 patients? Eur Heart J. 2020;41 (32):3092–3.
16. Angeli F, Spanevello A, De Ponti R, Visca D, Marazzato J, Palmiotto G, Feci D, Reboldi G, Fabbri LM, Verdecchia P. Electrocardiographic features of patients with COVID19XE "CoViD19" pneumonia. Eur J Intern Med. 2020;78:101–6.
17. Gawałko M, Kapłon-Cieślicka A, Hohl M, Dobrev D, Linz D. COVID19 associated atrial fibrillation: Incidence, putative mechanisms and potential clinical implications. 2020
18. Mahdawi TE, Wang H, Haddadin FI, Al-Qaysi D, Wylie JV. Heart block in patients with coronavirus disease 2019: A case series of 3 patients infected with SARS-CoV-2. HeartRhythm Case Reports. 2020;6(9):652–6.
19. Baksi AJ, Kanaganayagam GS, Prasad SK. Arrhythmias in viral myocarditis and pericarditis. Cardiac Electrophy Clin. 2015;7(2):269–81.
20. Pavlicek V, Kindermann I, Wintrich J, Mahfoud F, Klingel K, Böhm M, Ukena C. Ventricular arrhythmias and myocardial inflammation: Long-term follow-up of patients with suspected myocarditis. Int J Cardiol. 2019;274:132–7.

21. Shahreyar M, Fahhoum R, Akinseye O, Bhandari S, Dang G, Khouzam RN. Severe sepsis and cardiac arrhythmias. Annals Translat Med. 2018; 6(1).
22. Shao F, Xu S, Ma X, Xu Z, Lyu J, Ng M, Cui H, Yu C, Zhang Q, Sun P, Tang Z. In-hospital cardiac arrest outcomes among patients with COVID19 pneumonia in Wuhan, China. Resuscitation. 2020;151:18–23.
23. Ojha V, Verma M, Pandey NN, Mani A, Malhi AS, Kumar S, Jagia P, Roy A, Sharma S. Cardiac magnetic resonance imaging in coronavirus disease 2019 (COVID19): a systematic review of cardiac magnetic resonance imaging findings in 199 patients. J Thorac Imaging. 2021;36(2):73–83.
24. Puntmann VO, Carerj ML, Wieters I, Fahim M, Arendt C, Hoffmann J, Shchendrygina A, Escher F, Vasa-Nicotera M, Zeiher AM, Vehreschild M. Outcomes of cardiovascular magnetic resonance imaging in patients recently recovered from coronavirus disease 2019 (COVID19). JAMA cardiology. 2020;5(11):1265–73.
25. Aviles RJ, Martin DO, Apperson-Hansen C, Houghtaling PL, Rautaharju P, Kronmal RA, Tracy RP, Van Wagoner DR, Psaty BM, Lauer MS, Chung MK. Inflammation as a risk factor for atrial fibrillation. Circulation. 2003;108(24):3006–10.
26. Issac TT, Dokainish H, Lakkis NM. Role of inflammation in initiation and perpetuation of atrial fibrillation: a systematic review of the published data. J Am Coll Cardiol. 2007;50 (21):2021–8.
27. Lazzerini PE, Boutjdir M, Capecchi PL. COVID19, arrhythmic risk, and inflammation: mind the gap! Circulation. 2020;142(1):7–9.
28. Walters TE, Kalman JM, Patel SK, Mearns M, Velkoska E, Burrell LM. Angiotensin converting enzyme 2 activity and human atrial fibrillation: increased plasma angiotensin converting enzyme 2 activity is associated with atrial fibrillation and more advanced left atrial structural remodelling. Ep Europace. 2017;19(8):1280–7.
29. Wu YX, Han X, Chen C, Zou LX, Dong ZC, Zhang YL, Li HH. Time series gene expression profiling and temporal regulatory pathway analysis of angiotensin II induced atrial fibrillation in mice. Front Physiol. 2019;10:597.
30. Li J, Wang S, Bai J, Yang XL, Zhang YL, Che YL, Li HH, Yang YZ. Novel role for the Immunoproteasome subunit PSMB10 in angiotensin II–induced atrial fibrillation in mice. Hypertension. 2018;71(5):866–76.
31. Liu Y, Shi Q, Ma Y, Liu Q. The role of immune cells in atrial fibrillation. J Mol Cell Cardiol. 2018;123:198–220.
32. Coromilas EJ, Kochav S, Goldenthal I, Biviano A, Garan H, Goldbarg S, Kim JH, Yeo I, Tracy C, Ayanian S, Akar J. Worldwide survey of COVID19–associated arrhythmias. Circul Arrhyth Electrophy. 2021; 14(3):e009458.
33. Giannitsi S, Tsinivizov P, Poulimenos LE, Kallistratos MS, Varvarousis D, Manolis AJ, Tsamakis K, Rizos E, Spandidos DA, Tsiptsios D, Triantafyllis AS. [Case Report] Stress induced (Takotsubo) cardiomyopathy triggered by the COVID19 pandemic. Exp Ther Med. 2020;20(3):2812–4.
34. Wang H, Tang X, Fan H, Luo Y, Song Y, Xu Y, Chen Y. Potential mechanisms of hemorrhagic stroke in elderly COVID19 patients. Aging (Albany NY). 2020;12(11):10022.
35. Nazari MA, Rosenblum JS, Haigney MC, Rosing DR, Pacak K. Pathophysiology and acute management of tachyarrhythmias in pheochromocytoma: JACC REVIEW TOPIC OF THE WEEK. J Am Coll Cardiol. 2020;76(4):451–64.
36. Gubbi S, Nazari MA, Taieb D, Klubo-Gwiezdzinska J, Pacak K. Catecholamine physiology and its implications in patients with COVID19. The Lancet Diabetes & Endocrinology. 2020.
37. Sakabe M, Yoshioka R, Fujiki A. Sick sinus syndrome induced by interferon and ribavirin therapy in a patient with chronic hepatitis C. J Cardiol Cases. 2013;8(6):173–5.
38. Li Y, Liu T, Liu M, Li YJ, Yang Y, Zhao J. Electrocardiogram abnormalities in patients with COVID-19. Zhong Hua Xin Lv Shi Chang Xue Za Zhi. 2020;24(2):128–32.
39. Nowroozpoor A, Malekmohammad M, Seyyedi SR, Hashemian SM. Pulmonary hypertension in Intensive care units: an updated review. Tanaffos. 2019;18(3):180.

40. Tsapenko MV, Tsapenko AV, Comfere TB, Mour GK, Mankad SV, Gajic O. Arterial pulmonary hypertension in noncardiac intensive care unit. Vasc Health Risk Manag. 2008;4 (5):1043.
41. Pinsky MR. The right ventricle: interaction with the pulmonary circulation. Crit Care. 2016;20(1):1–9.
42. Seecheran R, Narayansingh R, Giddings S, Rampaul M, Furlonge K, Abdool K, Bhagwandass N, Seecheran NA. Atrial arrhythmias in a patient presenting with coronavirus disease-2019 (COVID19) infection. J Invest Med High Impact Case Reports. 2020;8:2324709620925571.
43. Guzik TJ, Mohiddin SA, Dimarco A, Patel V, Savvatis K, Marelli-Berg FM, Madhur MS, Tomaszewski M, Maffia P, D'Acquisto F, Nicklin SA. COVID19 and the cardiovascular system: implications for risk assessment, diagnosis, and treatment options. Cardiovasc Res. 2020;116(10):1666–87.
44. Fudim M, Qadri YJ, Ghadimi K, MacLeod DB, Molinger J, Piccini JP, Whittle J, Wischmeyer PE, Patel MR, Ulloa L. Implications for neuromodulation therapy to control inflammation and related organ dysfunction in COVID19. J Cardiovasc Transl Res. 2020:1–6.
45. Boothe SD, Myers JD, Pok S, Sun J, Xi Y, Nieto RM, Cheng J, Jacot JG. The effect of substrate stiffness on cardiomyocyte action potentials. Cell Biochem Biophys. 2016;74 (4):527–35.
46. Liu K, Fang YY, Deng Y, Liu W, Wang MF, Ma JP, Xiao W, Wang YN, Zhong MH, Li CH, Li GC. Clinical characteristics of novel coronavirus cases in tertiary hospitals in Hubei Province. Chin Med J. 2020.
47. Issac TT, Dokainish H, Lakkis NM. Role of inflammation in initiation and perpetuation of atrial fibrillation: a systematic review of the published data. J Am Coll Cardiol. 2007; 50 (21):2021–8.
48. Coromilas EJ, Kochav S, Goldenthal I, Biviano A, Garan H, Goldbarg S, Kim JH, Yeo I, Tracy C, Ayanian S, Akar J. Worldwide survey of COVID19–associated arrhythmias. Circul Arrhyth Electrophy. 2021; 14(3):e009458.
49. Linschoten M, Peters S, van Smeden M, Jewbali LS, Schaap J, Siebelink HM, Smits PC, Tieleman RG, van der Harst P, van Gilst WH, Asselbergs FW. Cardiac complications in patients hospitalised with COVID19. Eur Heart J Acute Cardiovas Care. 2020; 9(8):817–23.
50. Guo T, Fan Y, Chen M, Wu X, Zhang L, He T, Wang H, Wan J, Wang X, Lu Z. Cardiovascular implications of fatal outcomes of patients with coronavirus disease 2019 (COVID19). JAMA Cardiol. 2020;5(7):811–8.
51. Jankelson, L, Karam G, Becker ML, Chinitz LA, Tsai MC, QT prolongation, torsades de pointes, and sudden death with short courses of chloroquine or hydroxychloroquine as used in COVID19: A systematic review. Heart Rhythm. 2020;17(9):1472–1479.
52. Colon, CM, Barrios, JG, Chiles, JW, McElwee SK, Russell DW, Maddox WR, Kay, GN. Atrial arrhythmias in COVID-19 patients. Clinical Electrophysiology. 2020;6(9):1189–1190.
53. Wang Y, Wang, Z, Tse G, Zhang L, Wan EY, Guo Y, Lip GY, Li G, Lu Z, Liu T. Cardiac arrhythmias in patients with COVID-19. Journal of Arrhythmia. 2020;36(5):827–836.
54. Li Y, Liu T, Liu M, Li YJ, Yang Y, Zhao J. Electrocardiogram abnormalities in patients with COVID-19. Zhong Hua Xin Lv Shi Chang Xue Za Zhi. 2020;24(2):128–32.
55. Chorin E, Wadhwani L, Magnani S, Dai M, Shulman E, Nadeau-Routhier C, Knotts R, Bar-Cohen R, Kogan E, Barbhaiya C, Aizer A. QT interval prolongation and torsade de pointes in patients with COVID-19 treated with hydroxychloroquine/azithromycin. Heart Rhythm. 2020;17(9):1425–1433.
56. Borba, Mayla Gabriela Silva, Fernando Fonseca Almeida Val, Vanderson Souza Sampaio, Marcia Almeida Araújo Alexandre, Gisely Cardoso Melo, Marcelo Brito, Maria Paula Gomes Mourão et al. "Effect of high vs low doses of chloroquine diphosphate as adjunctive therapy for patients hospitalized with severe acute respiratory syndrome coronavirus 2 (SARS-CoV-2) infection: a randomized clinical trial.' JAMA network open. 2020;3(4):e208857–e208857.
57. Chen M, Li X, Wang S, Yu L, Tang J, Zhou S. The Role of Cardiac Macrophage and Cytokines on Ventricular Arrhythmias. Frontiers in Physiology. 2020;11:1113.

58. Lewek J, Kaczmarek K, Cygankiewicz I, Wranicz JK, Ptaszynski P. Inflammation and arrhythmias: potential mechanisms and clinical implications. Expert Review of Cardiovascular Therapy. 2014;12(9):1077–1085.
59. Huang C, Wang Y, Li X, Ren L, Zhao J, Hu Y, Zhang L, Fan G, Xu J, Gu X, Cheng Z. Clinical features of patients infected with 2019 novel coronavirus in Wuhan, China. The Lancet. 2020;395(10223):497–506.
60. Cao X. COVID-19: immunopathology and its implications for therapy. Nature Reviews Immunology. 2020:20(5);269–270.
61. Xu Z, Shi L, Wang Y, Zhang J, Huang L, Zhang C, Liu S, Zhao P, Liu H, Zhu L, Tai Y. Pathological findings of COVID-19 associated with acute respiratory distress syndrome. The Lancet Respiratory Medicine. 2020;8(4):420–422.
62. Hagiwara Y, Miyoshi S, Fukuda K, Nishiyama N, Ikegami Y, Tanimoto K, Murata M, Takahashi, E, Shimoda K, Hirano T, Mitamura H. SHP2-mediated signaling cascade through gp130 is essential for LIF-dependent ICaL,[Ca2+] i transient, and APD increase in cardiomyocytes. Journal of Molecular and Cellular Cardiology. 2007;43(6):710–716.
63. Uhler C, Shivashankar GV. Mechano-genomic regulation of coronaviruses and its interplay with ageing. Nature Reviews Molecular Cell Biology. 2020;21(5):247–248.
64. Poppe M, Wittig S, Jurida L, Bartkuhn M, Wilhelm J, Müller H, Beuerlein K, Karl N, Bhuju S, Ziebuhr J, Schmitz ML. The NF-κB-dependent and-independent transcriptome and chromatin landscapes of human coronavirus 229E-infected cells. PLoS Pathogens. 2071;13(3):e1006286.
65. Chen M, Li X, Wang S, Yu L, Tang J, Zhou S. The Role of Cardiac Macrophage and Cytokines on Ventricular Arrhythmias. Frontiers in Physiology. 2020;11:111.

Chapter 15
Acute Coronary Syndromes in CoViD19

Key Questions

- How common is the occurrence of acute coronary syndromes in CoViD19?
- What are the risk implications of the association of acute coronary syndromes with CoViD19?
- Which factors associated with CoViD19 may promote the risk of acute coronary syndromes?
- What are the dynamics of ACS during the initial phase of CoViD19 pandemic?
- What are the challenges and complexities associated with acute coronary syndromes in CoViD19 patients?

15.1 Epidemiology of Acute Coronary Syndromes in CoViD19

A spectrum of cardiovascular conditions is observed in the CoViD19 patients, especially in cases with severe disease, and may present in typical and atypical forms of cardiac injury resulting in dysfunction or even cardiac death. Myocardial injury extensively introduced in the previous chapter (Chap. 11) takes the main stage among CoViD19 associated cardiovascular complications and may dangerously mask an acute coronary event. Distinguishing between the mechanisms associated with coronary or non-coronary mechanisms that may lead to cardiac injury and or associated complications is vital in guiding the most appropriate therapeutic intervention (Fig. 15.4). The intricacies related to multiple biochemical factors, infectious complexities, and practical challenges may hinder the prompt diagnosis of the culprit event and the delivery of effective therapeutic interventions.

U. Mallick, *Cardiovascular Complications of COVID-19*,
https://doi.org/10.1007/978-3-030-90065-6_15

The acute coronary event or coronary atherothrombosis appears to be a distinct entity from a non-specific myocardial injury commonly described in the CoViD19 literature. Several CoViD19 studies report the occurrence of acute coronary syndromes (ACS) both STEMI and non- STEMI [1–3], however, the exact prevalence in CoViD19 is not well known. Studies report a fall in the overall incidence of acute coronary syndromes during the pandemic. According to the reports this fall is likely to be due to under-reporting, avoidance, lack of presentation, or other reasons. Nevertheless, the association of ACS with CoViD19 appears significant [4, 5] and may have a significant prognostic impact. According to studies, the prevalence of ACS may vary between 4.5 and 25% among the CoViD19 patients [6–10]. According to an observational cohort study of 12598 hospitalized patients with ACS, about 4% of patients hospitalized with an ACS had CoViD19 [11].

Several small studies report the occurrence of STEMI in association with CoViD19 and indicate STEMI at the time of presentation or during the course of hospitalization (Fig. 15.2). In a retrospective cohort study of 28 CoViD19 patients, the STEMI was the first presentation in about 85.7% (24) patients with a diagnosis of CoViD19 [12]. In a case series report of 18 CoViD19 patients with STEMI, a total of 10 patients (56%) had ST-segment elevation at the time of presentation, and the other 8 patients had development of ST-segment elevation during hospitalization (median, 6 days) [13].

Data indicate that patients with acute coronary syndromes and CoViD19 have poor outcomes [14]. In a case series of 18 patients with CoViD19 mostly males (83%), about 67% (6/9) of patients with ST elevations who underwent coronary angiography had an obstructive epicardial coronary lesion. About 44% (8/18) of patients diagnosed with myocardial infarction had higher median peak troponin and D-dimer levels than the 56% (10/18) patients with noncoronary myocardial injury. The in-hospital case-fatality rate was 72% (13/18) (MI 4/13 and noncoronary myocardial injury 9/13) [13]. Data from an observational cohort study of 12,598 hospitalized patients with ACS showed poor outcomes in ACS with CoViD19. These patients had an increased incidence of in-hospital cardiac arrest (6.3% vs 3.0%), higher troponin levels, and were more likely to have presented in pulmonary edema (9.0 vs. 3.4%) or cardiogenic shock (9.6 vs. 3.9%) [11].

Data reporting angiographic findings in CoViD19 patients are scarce. The contagiousness and risks in CoViD19 impacted the management of ACS with under-utilization of coronary angiography, however, this led to the adaptations and adjustments in ACS management [5]. According to a registry report describing demographic characteristics, management strategies, and outcomes in of 1185 CoViD19 patients with STEMI, these patients are less likely to receive invasive angiography (78%) [16]. Other studies also confirm under-utilization of the invasive treatments in CoViD19 patients with ACS [11]. The reports of angiographic findings in ACS patients with CoViD19 indicate that a culprit lesion may not be identifiable by coronary angiography in approximately 40% of patients with CoViD19 with STEMI [12]. In another case series of 18 STEMI patients with CoViD19, about 9 (50%) STEMI patients underwent coronary angiography, and obstructive disease was found in 6 (67%) of these patients [13]. (Fig. 15.3).

15.2 Defining Acute Coronary Syndromes, Challenges in Presentation and Assessment

The acute coronary syndromes (ST-Elevation Myocardial Infarction (STEMI), Non-ST Elevation Myocardial Infarction (NSTEMI), or Unstable Angina (UA)) form a spectrum of coronary artery disease. Myocardial infarction is a form of myocardial injury. Diagnosis of MI requires evidence of myocardial ischemia and has various subtypes. The presentation of ACS as type 1 MI is due to the atherosclerotic plaque rupture resulting in myocardial damage, is characterized by plaque rupture, ulceration, erosion, or dissection resulting in coronary thrombosis [17]. Whereas the type 2 MI is infarction from myocardial oxygen supply–demand mismatch in the absence of atherothrombosis [17]. In CoViD19 distinction between non-specific myocardial injury and an ACS may be difficult due to non-specific rise and fall of troponin values or patients may present with type 2 MI secondary to oxygen supply/demand mismatch. A clinical judgment based upon the historical and electrocardiographic evidence is important to recognize the ACS complemented with confirmation of coronary obstruction.

Biochemical confirmation of the ACS with a rise in serum cardiac troponin levels above at least the 99th percentile of the upper reference range is generally used in CoViD19. Patients with ACS and CoViD19 appear to have worse biochemistry [11, 13, 18]. Coronary imaging techniques provide a visual assessment of the coronary obstruction, and angiographic visualization of the coronary arteries and mechanical restoration of the blood flow are gold-standard in the management of CAD. As an alternative to the invasive coronary angiography, CT angiography has been shown to have an important diagnostic value in CoViD19 patients with a high suspicion of coronary artery disease [19].

Several complexities may exist in distinguishing the non-specific myocardial injury from an acute coronary syndrome in CoViD19 patients (Fig. 15.1). Troponin elevation is most commonly caused by non-ischemic myocardial injury rather than acute myocardial infarction (MI) [20] that require evidence of myocardial ischemia. Patients with myocardial injury may be misclassified as T2MI [21]. Studies further show that a substantial percentage of patients coded as having T2MI actually have myocardial injury [21]. Troponin elevation may be non-specific in patients with sepsis. Complexities related to the infectious nature of the disease, and lack of protocols may hinder the angiographic confirmation of the coronary obstruction, coronary assessments, and delivery of the appropriate intervention. A lack of angiographic evidence of coronary obstruction in the settings of CoViD19 may pose a challenge to the treating clinician. Expert guidance has been published to help guide the management of patients with ACS in CoVD19 patients [22].

The use of serum biomarkers is pivotal in the diagnosis of acute coronary events. The intensity of the disease burden associated with CoViD19 may be associated with the elevation of multiple biomarkers that may confound the diagnostics. Elevated troponins may be seen in the absence of ACS and may portend short- and long-term outcomes [23, 24]. Higher troponin elevations have been seen in the

STEMI patients with CoViD19 as compared to CoViD19 patients with non-coronary myocardial injury, and these patients also had elevated D Dimer levels [13]. Elevated CRP and D Dimers have also been reported in studies investigating STEMI patients with CoViD19 [25]. Several biomarkers associated with severe CoViD19 may indicate elevated coronary risk. Elevation of markers of cardiac injury troponins, CKMB, myoglobin that also indicates poor outcomes [26]; and markers of CoViD19 severity such as C-reactive protein (CRP), interleukin 6 (IL-6), D Dimers [27] may aid diagnosis. Risk models predicting poor outcomes in CoViD19 patients with cardiac injury, based on a combination of biomarkers such as troponin and AST, and advanced age, have been proposed [28].

15.3 Pathogenesis of Acute Coronary Syndromes in CoViD19

Acute coronary syndromes are a consequence of a reduced blood supply to the myocardium causing damage to the myocardial cells. An erosion or rupture of an unstable atherosclerotic plaque and thrombosis causes a partial or complete mechanical coronary obstruction. Cardiovascular diseases (CVD) may be precipitated by acute respiratory infections [29, 30[. Several harmful mechanisms observed in sepsis [31], may lead to cardiovascular complications, also observed in CoViD19 may contribute towards cardiac complications including the ACS. The process of coronary atherothrombotic plaque erosion, instability and dislodging, and thrombosis is led by several inflammatory, immune, coagulation, cellular, and molecular mechanisms. Among these mechanisms hyper immune-inflammation and thrombosis, key components of the thrombo-inflammatory phenomenon observed in severe CoVID19 play a major role in the development of acute coronary complications in CoViD19, and endotheloppathy acts as a bridge bewteen these mechanisms Moreover, in CoViD19 multiple dysregulated mechanisms involving these routes may ultimately lead to the instability of the atherosclerotic plaque and coronary vasoplegia. The hemodynamic disturbance, oxidative stress, and toll-like receptors (TLR) activation (mediated by hyaluronic acid), observed in CoViD19 [32–35], may induce superficial plaque erosion through damage to the endothelial cells [36, 37]. The pathogenetic features and mechanisms related to the acuity and severity of CoViD19 lead to increased biomechanical stress on coronary arteries, variations in the coronary arterial tone, disturbance in homeostasis and hemostasis, hemodynamic malfunction, and altered myocardial metabolic balance that contribute to coronary vascular instabililty. Injury to the cardiovascular endothelial bed and cardiomyocytes promotes cardiovascular injury in CoViD19. In addition, mechanisms related to a direct viral injury to the endothelial vascular bed or myocardial cells may facilitate the development of ACS in CoViD19 patients. The exact associations of these mechanisms however remain to be further determined.

Inflammation, an important pathogenetic hallmark of CoViD19, plays a major role in acute coronary syndromes [38, 39]. Inflammation promotes the formation of an occlusive thrombus over a ruptured coronary plaque through endothelial dysfunction and procoagulant activity of the blood [15]. Several immune-inflammatory pathways result in an increased coronary and systemic inflammatory activity and prothrombotic conditions that dominate severe CoViD19. The hyper-immune and proinflammatory mechanisms involving cytokines, endothelial, platelet and leukocyte activation, activation of the procoagulant pathways and prothrombotic activities promote acute cardiac events such as myocardial infarction [40, 41].

The CoViD19 has a significantly elevated vascular and thrombotic risk [42]. Persistent inflammatory stress may serve as a marker of severity and prognosis in patients with high vascular risk. Data show exaggerated and persistent pro-inflammatory cytokine release in CoViD19 patients [43, 44]. Differential intracoronary cytokine expression in ruptured fibrous cap and intact fibrous cap associated with coronary thrombosis have been demonstrated [45]. The proinflammatory cytokines such as interleukin-6 have predictive value in the setting of acute coronary ischemia [46]. Data show that plasma concentrations of TNF-α are persistently elevated among post-MI patients at increased risk for recurrent coronary events [47]. These hyperinflammatory stress mechanisms involving systemic inflammation, immune cells, and inflammatory factors, and a cascade of other dysregulated processes associated with CoViD19, may result in an enhanced atherosclerotic plaque instability [36] ultimately leading to coronary plaque rupture and dislodging.

The microvascular damage and endothelial cell dysfunction appear to have a major role in the development of vascular instability and involve important RAS related mechanisms such as dysregulation of the ACE2 [48]. The ACE2 is highly expressed in pericytes, and appears to have a role in the development of microvascular dysfunction observed in CoViD19 patients [49], and may reflect higher tendencies for the acute coronary syndromes (ACS) [50] in CoViD19 patients. The mechanisms related to the develoment of thrombosis in the microvascular bed and coronary vessels in CoViD19 are complex with an important role of pericytes [51], endothelial cells, and cross-talk mechanisms [52] that may facilitate vasoplegia, hypercoagulability and prothrombotic reactions. These mechanisms and SARS CoV2-pericyte interactions [53] may suggest an important pathogenetic route to the development of acute coronary events in CoViD19. Microthrombi as a potential cause of STEMI associated with CoViD19 have been reported in the absence of epicardial coronary lesions [54], indicating peculiarities associated with the coronary events in the novel coronavirus disease. Data reporting STEMI in CoViD19 patients also suggest that an elevated burden of thrombus in patients with CoViD19 may be associated with STEMI [25]. In CoViD19, enhanced release of procoagulant factors, platelet activation, increased hematopoiesis, or formation of Neutrophil Extracellular Traps (NETs), and dysregulation of complement activation, promote thrombosis. For further details related to endotheliopathy and thrombosis in CoViD19, please refer to Chap. 9.

15.4 Summary

The acute coronary syndromes carry a high risk of morbidity and mortality, which is estimated to be higher when associated with CoViD19. Prompt recognition and treatment of the ACS improve outcomes. The prevalence of ACS in CoViD19 may not be well described in the literature. The clinicians treating the ACS in patients with CoViD19 may face challenges due to the overlapping clinical, biochemical picture and other features that may cloud distinguishing between the ACS and non-specific myocardial injury associated with CoViD19.

The biomarkers of ACS such as troponin appear to be significantly elevated in the ACS patients with CoViD19 as compared to the patients with non-specific myocardial injury related to the CoViD19. Concomitant use of other biomarkers such as markers of inflammation and thrombosis such as CRP, D Dimers, may assist in estimating the risk of developing ACS. Specific algorithms involving multiple biomarkers must be defined for short and long-term risk stratification of patients with ACS in CoViD19, and to help develop strategies to mitigate the risk of a coronary event.

Although the exact pathogenetic process of ACS in CoViD19 is not well understood, a combination of infectious, multiple harmful intense dysregulated hemostatic and homeostatic mechanisms, and burden of underlying risk factors appear to facilitate a coronary event. Systemic immune-inflammatory stress dysregulated blood cellular structures, a cascade of activated mechanisms that result in hypercoagulation, lead to a vasoplegic insult, prothrombotic state, and dislodging of the atherosclerotic plaque, coronary thrombosis, and obstruction. The cytokine storm, mechanisms related to direct or indirect viral toxicity causing damage to the vascular endothelial bed dysfunction, or activation of the complement system, inflammasomes, neutrophil extracellular traps, or platelet activation are remarkable in the development of ACS in CoViD 19. The induction of the erosion of coronary atherosclerotic plaque and enhanced plaque instability may be precipitated by the hyper immune-inflammatory mechanisms or myocardial depression secondary to increased myocardial oxygen demand and severe hemodynamic instability. The exact mechanisms behind the development of ACS in CoViD19 need to be better characterized.

Dynamics in the intensity and evolution of the pathogenetic mechanisms may be associated with the chronological variations observed in the presentation of ACS in CoViD19 patients. The presentation of ACS in the early phase of CoViD 19 is likely to be due to underlying cardiovascular risk factors and at a later stage as the severity of the disease progresses is likely to be due to the compounding of the harmful mechanisms associated with the disease severity and associated triggering factors.

Data show that patients with STEMI presenting with COVID19 infection may have a longer in-patient admission and higher rates of intensive care admission [25]. A low threshold is recommended for using the invasive hemodynamic supportive measures in patients with CoViD19 due to a higher likelihood of worse outcomes.

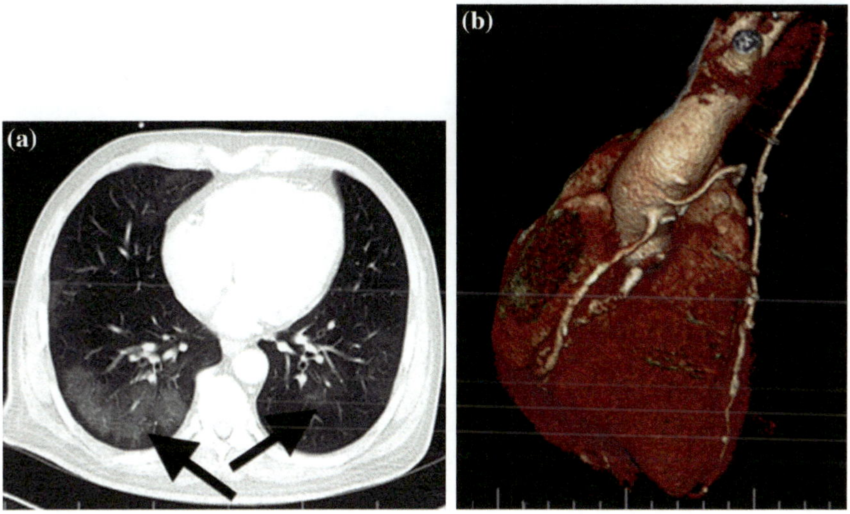

Fig. 15.1 The diagnosis of acute coronary syndrome should not be missed in a patient with COVID19. **a** CT angiogram demonstrates patchy peripheral predominant ground glass airspace opacity in the dependent lung segment. There was no evidence of pleural effusion, cavitation, or lymphadenopathy. Findings are typical of COVID-19 pneumonia, and should be included in the differential in geographic areas of disease outbreaks. **b** Coronary artery bypass grafts are patent without significant stenosis. *Source* Figure 1 Behzad, S., Velez, E., Najafi, M.H. and Gholamrezanezhad, A., 2020. Coronavirus disease 2019 (COVID-19) pneumonia incidentally detected on coronary CT angiogram: a do-not-miss diagnosis. Emergency radiology, 27, pp. 721–726. Coronavirus disease 2019 (COVID-19) pneumonia incidentally detected on coronary CT angiogram: a do-not-miss diagnosis | SpringerLink. By Springer Nature Group

A high risk of cardiac complications with severe CoVID19 related comorbidities and risk associated with contagiousness of the disease have prompted adaptations in the management of ACS in patients with CoViD19. Studies have explored the usefulness of other coronary imaging modalities such as CT coronary angiogram in these patients, which may be considered as an alternative coronary imaging modality in this population group.

The underutilization of the invasive therapeutic strategies in patients with ACS and CoViD19 is alarming. Visualization of the coronary lesions responsible for myocardial infarction and unstable angina is vital for diagnosing ACS, and for delivery of the effective therapeutic intervention, therefore improving the outcomes. CoViD19 may have negatively impacted time-dependent care of STEMI patients [55]. Special protocols have been developed to optimize treatment strategies and mitigate risk including the risk of spread of this contagion in patients with CoViD19 [56–58]. Further studies are needed to understand the ACS better in CoViD19, to detect early patients at risk, and adapt strategies to mitigate the risk. Several ongoing studies are investigating the role of risk factors, pre-existing cardiovascular disease, and associated outcomes in CoViD19 patients [59, 60, 61] the epidemiological [62] and therapeutic aspects.

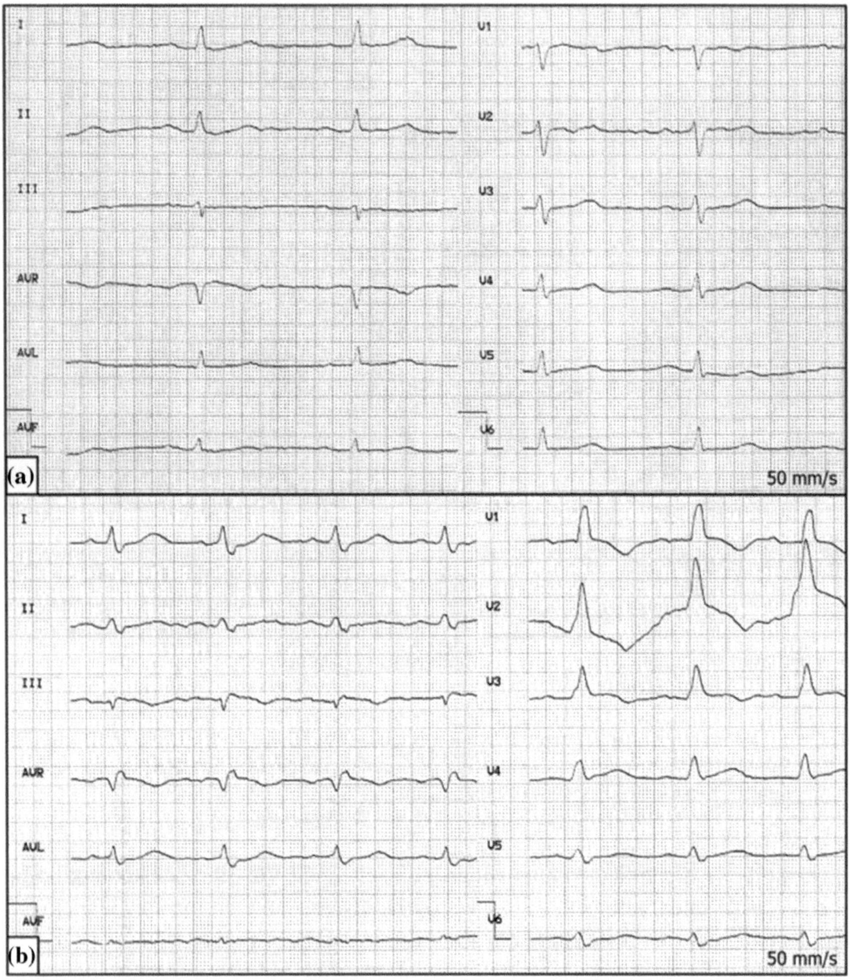

Fig. 15.2 Acute myocardial infarction due to coronary stent thrombosis in a symptomatic COVID-19 patient. **a** 12-lead ECG recording on admission with normal sinus rhythm. **b** Complete right bundle branch block and an ST-elevation in lead aVR. *Source* Figure 1 Hinterseer, M., Zens, M., Wimmer, R.J., Delladio, S., Lederle, S., Kupatt, C. and Hartmann, B., 2021. Acute myocardial infarction due to coronary stent thrombosis in a symptomatic COVID-19 patient. Clinical Research in Cardiology, 110, pp. 302–306. Acute myocardial infarction due to coronary stent thrombosis in a symptomatic COVID-19 patient | SpringerLink. By Springer Nature Group

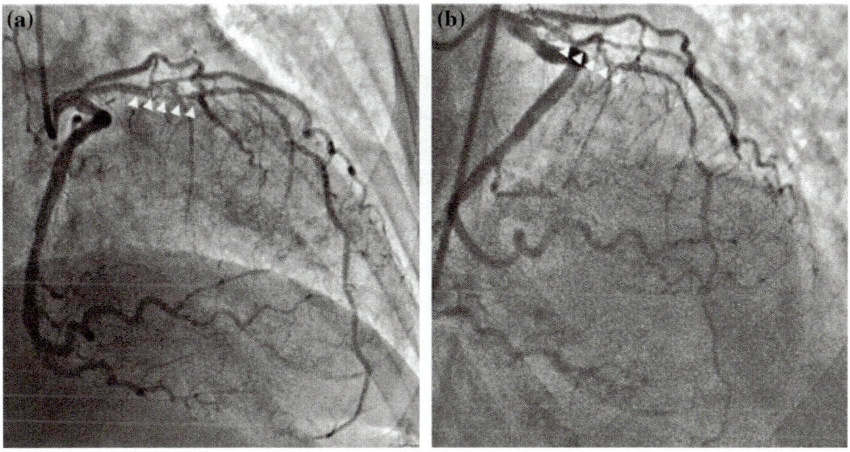

Fig. 15.3 Acute coronary syndrome precipitated by COVID19. Coronary angiography. Severe stenosis in the mid-segment of the left anterior descending artery (arrowheads) in bifurcation with a diagonal branch in the right anterior oblique and anterior–posterior cranial projections. *Source* Figure 3 Yousefi-Koma, A., Naghashzadeh, F., Figtree, G.A., Patel, S. and Galougahi, K.K., 2020. Multi-modality imaging of inflammation and ischemia for assessment of myocardial injury in Covid-19. Journal of Nuclear Cardiology, pp. 1–4. https://link.springer.com/article/10.1007/s12350-020-02233-x#Fig3. By Springer Nature Group

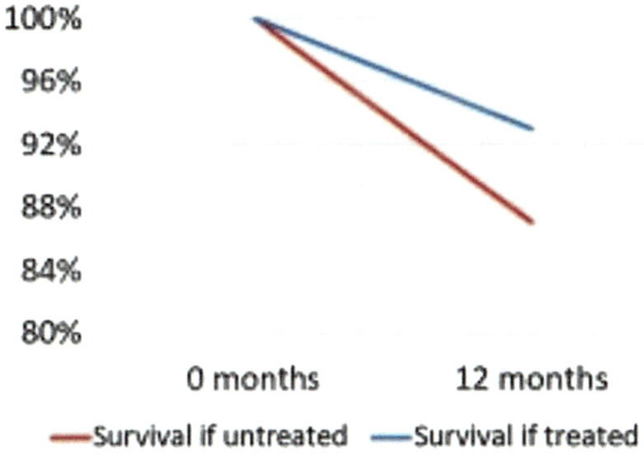

Fig. 15.4 Survival benefits of appropriate invasive management in patients with ST-elevation myocardial infarction (STEMI). *Source* Modified from Figure 1. Giordano, A., Biondi-Zoccai, G., Frati, G. and Bartorelli, A.L., 2020. Management of structural heart disease and acute coronary syndromes in the COVID-19 pandemic. Current atherosclerosis reports, 22(7), pp. 1–4. https://link.springer.com/article/10.1007/s11883-020-00849-5. By Springer Nature Group

Summary Box

- The ACS in CoViD19, are associated with poor outcomes.
- Diagnosing ACS in CoViD19 patients and distinction from other forms of myocardial injury may be a challenge.
- Troponin levels may reflect a systemic illness, may be higher in the ACS in CoViD19, versus non-specific myocardial injury, and should be used in conjunction with markers of thrombo-inflammation such as CRP, D Dimers and others for diagnosis and risk assessment
- Coronary angiography is the gold standard, is under-utilized in CoViD19, however, the role of CT coronary angiography must be considered.
- CoViD19 accompanies intense local and systemic immune-inflammatory mechanisms leading to the erosion of fibrous cap of coronary atherosclerotic plaque, or others enhancing plaque instability, together with prothrombotic processes, including hypercoagulation, platelet and complement activation, and vasoplegia associated with endothelial cell damage, ACE 2 depletion, and cytokine storm.
- Further studies are required to determine mechanisms that lead to the acute coronary syndromes in CoViD19, define risk assessment algorithms, and explore the potential unconventional therapeutic options.
- Strategies and protocols must be developed and implemented to optimize the management of ACS during the CoViD19 pandemic.

References

1. Metzler B, Siostrzonek P, Binder RK, Bauer A, Reinstadler SJ. Decline of acute coronary syndrome admissions in Austria since the outbreak of COVID-19: the pandemic response causes cardiac collateral damage. Eur Heart J. 2020;41(19):1852–3.
2. De Rosa S, Spaccarotella C, Basso C, Calabrò MP, Curcio A, Filardi PP, Mancone M, Mercuro G, Muscoli S, Nodari S, Pedrinelli R. Reduction of hospitalizations for myocardial infarction in Italy in the COVID-19 era. Eur Heart J. 2020;41(22):2083–8.
3. Solomon MD, McNulty EJ, Rana JS, Leong TK, Lee C, Sung SH, Ambrosy AP, Sidney S, Go AS. The Covid-19 pandemic and the incidence of acute myocardial infarction. N Engl J Med. 2020;383(7):691–3.
4. Tam CCF, Cheung KS, Lam S, Wong A, Yung A, Sze M, Lam YM, Chan C, Tsang TC, Tsui M, Tse HF. Impact of coronavirus disease 2019 (COVID-19) outbreak on ST-segment–elevation myocardial infarction care in Hong Kong, China. Circ: Cardiovasc Qual Outcomes. 2020;13(4):e006631.
5. Huber K, Goldstein P. Covid-19: implications for prehospital, emergency and hospital care in patients with acute coronary syndromes. Eur Heart J: Acute Cardiovasc Care. 2020;9(3):222–8.
6. Wang D, Hu B, Hu C, Zhu F, Liu X, Zhang J, Wang B, Xiang H, Cheng Z, Xiong Y, Zhao Y, Li Y, Wang X, Peng Z. Clinical characteristics of 138 hospitalized patients with 2019 novel coronavirus-infected Pneumonia in Wuhan, China. JAMA. 2020. https://doi.org/10.1001/

jama.2020.1585. [Epub ahead of print] PubMed PMID: 32031570; PubMed Central PMCID: PMC7042881.

7. Zouh Madjid M, Safavi-Naeini P, Solomon SD, Vardeny O. Potential effects of coronaviruses on the cardiovascular system: a review. JAMA Cardiol. 2020. https://doi.org/10.1001/jamacardio.2020.1286. [Epub ahead of print] PubMed PMID: 32219363.
8. Zhou F, Yu T, Du R, Fan G, Liu Y, Liu Z, Xiang J, Wang Y, Song B, Gu X, Guan L, Wei Y, Li H, Wu X, Xu J, Tu S, Zhang Y, Chen H, Cao B. Clinical course and risk factors for mortality of adult inpatients with COVID-19 in Wuhan, China: a retrospective cohort study. Lancet. 2020;395(10229):1054–1062. https://doi.org/10.1016/S0140-6736(20)30566-3. Epub 2020 Mar 11. Erratum in: Lancet. 2020;395(10229):1038; Lancet. 2020;395(10229):1038. PubMed PMID: 32171076.
9. Li B, Yang J, Zhao F, Zhi L, Wang X, Liu L, Bi Z, Zhao Y. Prevalence and impact of cardiovascular metabolic diseases on COVID-19 in China. Clin Res Cardiol. 2020. https://doi.org/10.1007/s00392-020-01626-9. [Epub ahead of print] Review. PubMed PMID: 32161990; PubMed Central PMCID: PMC7087935.
10. Chen T, Wu D, Chen H, Yan W, Yang D, Chen G, Ma K, Xu D, Yu H, Wang H, Wang T, Guo W, Chen J, Ding C, Zhang X, Huang J, Han M, Li S, Luo X, Zhao J, Ning Q. Clinical characteristics of 113 deceased patients with coronavirus disease 2019: retrospective study. BMJ. 2020;368:m1091.https://doi.org/10.1136/bmj.m1091.Erratum.In:BMJ.2020Mar31;368: m1295PubMed PMID: 32217556.
11. Rashid M, Wu J, Timmis A, Curzen N, Clarke S, Zaman A, Nolan J, Shoaib A, Mohamed MO, de Belder MA, Deanfield J. Outcomes of COVID-19 positive acute coronary syndrome patients: a multisource electronic healthcare records study from England. J Intern Med. 2021.
12. Stefanini GG, Montorfano M, Trabattoni D, Andreini D, Ferrante G, Ancona M, Metra M, Curello S, Maffeo D, Pero G, Cacucci M. ST-elevation myocardial infarction in patients with COVID-19: clinical and angiographic outcomes. Circulation. 2020;141(25):2113–6.
13. Bangalore S, Sharma A, Slotwiner A, Yatskar L, Harari R, Shah B, Ibrahim H, Friedman GH, Thompson C, Alviar CL, Chadow HL. ST-segment elevation in patients with Covid-19—a case series. N Engl J Med. 2020;382(25):2478–80.
14. Zheng YY, Ma YT, Zhang JY, Xie X. COVID-19 and the cardiovascular system. Nat Rev Cardiol. 2020;17(5):259–60.
15. Corrales-Medina VF, Musher DM, Shachkina S, Chirinos A. Acute pneumonia and the cardiovascular system. Lancet. 2013;381(9865):496–505. https://doi.org/10.1016/S0140-6736(12)61266-5.
16. Garcia S, Dehghani P, Grines C, Davidson L, Nayak KR, Saw J, Waksman R, Blair J, Akshay B, Garberich R, Schmidt C. Initial findings from the North American COVID-19 myocardial infarction registry. J Am Coll Cardiol. 2021;77(16):1994–2003.
17. Thygesen K, Alpert JS, Jaffe AS, Chaitman BR, Bax JJ, Morrow DA, White HD. Executive Group on behalf of the Joint European Society of Cardiology (ESC)/American College of Cardiology (ACC)/American Heart Association (AHA)/World Heart Federation (WHF) Task Force for the Universal Definition of Myocardial Infarction, 2018. Fourth universal definition of myocardial infarction. J Am Coll Cardiol. 2018;72(18), 2231–64.
18. Lala A, Johnson KW, Januzzi JL, Russak AJ, Paranjpe I, Richter F, Zhao S, Somani S, Van Vleck T, Vaid A, Chaudhry F. Prevalence and impact of myocardial injury in patients hospitalized with COVID-19 infection. J Am Coll Cardiol. 2020;76(5):533–46.
19. Cronin M, Wheen P, Armstrong R, Kumar R, McMahon A, White M, Sheehy N, McMahon G, Murphy RT, Daly C. CT coronary angiography and COVID-19: inpatient use in acute chest pain service. Open Heart. 2021;8(1), e001548.
20. Sandoval Y, Smith SW, Sexter A, Thordsen SE, Bruen CA, Carlson MD, Dodd KW, Driver BE, Hu Y, Jacoby K, Johnson BK. Type 1 and 2 myocardial infarction and myocardial injury: clinical transition to high-sensitivity cardiac troponin I. The Am J Med. 2017;130 (12):1431–9.

21. McCarthy C, Murphy S, Cohen JA, Rehman S, Jones-O'Connor M, Olshan DS, Singh A, Vaduganathan M, Januzzi JL, Wasfy JH. Misclassification of myocardial injury as myocardial infarction: implications for assessing outcomes in value-based programs. JAMA Cardiol. 2019;4(5):460–4.
22. Mahmud E, Dauerman HL, Welt FG, Messenger JC, Rao SV, Grines C, Mattu A, Kirtane AJ, Jauhar R, Meraj P, Rokos IC. Management of acute myocardial infarction during the COVID-19 pandemic. J Am Coll Cardiol. 2020.
23. Giannitsis E, Katus HA. Cardiac troponin level elevations not related to acute coronary syndromes. Nat Rev Cardiol. 2013;10(11):623.
24. Blich M, Sebbag A, Attias J, Aronson D, Markiewicz W. Cardiac troponin I elevation in hospitalized patients without acute coronary syndromes. The Am J Cardiol. 2008;101 (10):1384–8.
25. Choudry FA, Hamshere SM, Rathod KS, Akhtar MM, Archbold RA, Guttmann OP, Woldman S, Jain AK, Knight CJ, Baumbach A, Mathur A. High thrombus burden in patients with COVID-19 presenting with ST-segment elevation myocardial infarction. J Am Coll Cardiol. 2020;76(10):1168–76.
26. Qin JJ, Cheng X, Zhou F, Lei F, Akolkar G, Cai J, Zhang XJ, Blet A, Xie J, Zhang P, Liu YM. Redefining cardiac biomarkers in predicting mortality of inpatients with COVID-19. Hypertension. 2020;76(4):1104–12.
27. Tian W, Jiang W, Yao J, Nicholson CJ, Li RH, Sigurslid HH, Wooster L, Rotter JI, Guo X, Malhotra R. Predictors of mortality in hospitalized COVID-19 patients: a systematic review and meta-analysis. J Med Virol. 2020;92(10):1875–83.
28. Toraih EA, Elshazli RM, Hussein MH, Elgaml A, Amin M, El-Mowafy M, El-Mesery M, Ellythy A, Duchesne J, Killackey MT, Ferdinand KC. Association of cardiac biomarkers and comorbidities with increased mortality, severity, and cardiac injury in COVID-19 patients: a meta-regression and decision tree analysis. J Med Virol. 2020;92(11), 2473–88.
29. Cowan LT, Lutsey PL, Pankow JS, Matsushita K, Ishigami J, Lakshminarayan K. Inpatient and outpatient infection as a trigger of cardiovascular disease: the ARIC study. J Am Heart Assoc. 2018;7(22):e009683–e009683. https://doi.org/10.1161/JAHA.118.009683PubMed GoogleScholarCrossref.
30. Madjid M, Miller CC, Zarubaev VV, et al. Influenza epidemics and acute respiratory disease activity are associated with a surge in autopsy-confirmed coronary heart disease death: results from 8 years of autopsies in 34,892 subjects. Eur Heart J. 2007;28(10):1205–10.
31. Rittirsch D, Flierl MA, Ward PA. Harmful molecular mechanisms in sepsis. Nat Rev Immunol. 2008;8(10):776–87.
32. Khanmohammadi S, Rezaei N. Role of Toll-like receptors in the pathogenesis of COVID-19. J Med Virol. 2021;93(5):2735–9.
33. Root-Bernstein R. Innate receptor activation patterns involving TLR and NLR synergisms in COVID-19, ALI/ARDS and sepsis cytokine storms: a review and model making novel predictions and therapeutic suggestions. Int J Mol Sci. 2021;22(4):2108.
34. Laforge M, Elbim C, Frère C, Hémadi M, Massaad C, Nuss P, Benoliel JJ, Becker C. Tissue damage from neutrophil-induced oxidative stress in COVID-19. Nat Rev Immunol. 2020;20 (9):515–6.
35. Sattar Y, Ullah W, Rauf H. COVID-19 cardiovascular epidemiology, cellular pathogenesis, clinical manifestations and management. Int J Cardiol. Heart & Vasculature. 2020;29.
36. Crea F, Libby P. Acute coronary syndromes: the way forward from mechanisms to precision treatment. Circulation. 2017;136(12):1155–66.
37. Tomaniak M, Katagiri Y, Modolo R, de Silva R, Khamis RY, Bourantas CV, Torii R, Wentzel JJ, Gijsen FJ, van Soest G, Stone PH. Vulnerable plaques and patients: state-of-the-art. Eur Heart J. 2020;41(31):2997–3004.
38. Libby P. Molecular bases of the acute coronary syndromes. Circulation. 1995; 91:2844–50.
39. Ross R. Mechanisms of disease: atherosclerosis: an inflammatory disease. N Engl J Med. 1999;340:115–26.

40. Corrales-Medina VF, Madjid M, Musher DM. Role of acute infection in triggering acute coronary syndromes. Lancet Infect Dis. 2010;10(2):83–92.
41. Smeeth L, Thomas SL, Hall AJ, Hubbard R, Farrington P, Vallance P. Risk of myocardial infarction and stroke after acute infection or vaccination. N Engl J Med. 2004;351(25):2611–8.
42. McFadyen JD, Stevens H, Peter K. The emerging threat of (micro) thrombosis in COVID-19 and its therapeutic implications. Circ Res. 2020;127(4):571–87.
43. Hu B, Huang S, Yin L. The cytokine storm and COVID-19. J Med Virol. 2021;93(1):250–6.
44. Zhu H, Rhee JW, Cheng P, Waliany S, Chang A, Witteles RM, Maecker H, Davis MM, Nguyen PK, Wu SM. Cardiovascular complications in patients with COVID-19: consequences of viral toxicities and host immune response. Curr Cardiol Rep. 2020;22(5):1–9.
45. Chandran S, Watkins J, Abdul-Aziz A, Shafat M, Calvert PA, Bowles KM, Flather MD, Rushworth SA, Ryding AD. Inflammatory Differences in Plaque Erosion and Rupture in Patients With ST-Segment Elevation Myocardial Infarction. Journal of the American Heart Association. 2017;6(5):e005868.
46. Biasucci LM, Bitelli A, Liuzzo G, Altamura S, Caligiuri G, Monaco C, Rebuzzi AG, Ciliberto G, Maseri A. Elevated levels of interleukin-6 in unstable angina. Circulation. 1996;94:874–7.
47. Ridker PM, Rifai N, Pfeffer M, Sacks F, Lepage S, Braunwald E. Elevation of tumor necrosis factor-alpha and increased risk of recurrent coronary events after myocardial infarction. Circulation. 2000;101(18):2149–53. https://doi.org/10.1161/01.cir.101.18.2149.
48. Varga Z, Flammer AJ, Steiger P, Haberecker M, Andermatt R, Zinkernagel AS, Mehra MR, Schuepbach RA, Ruschitzka F, Moch H. Endothelial cell infection and endotheliitis in COVID-19. The Lancet. 2020;395(10234):1417–8.
49. Shi Y, Wang Y, Shao C, Huang J, Gan J, Huang X, Bucci E, Piacentini M, Ippolito G, Melino G. COVID-19 infection: the perspectives on immune responses. 2020.
50. Bairey Merz CN, Pepine CJ, Shimokawa H, Berry C. Treatment of coronary microvascular dysfunction. Cardiovasc Res. 2020;116(4), 856–70.
51. Avolio E, Madeddu P. Discovering cardiac pericyte biology: from physiopathological mechanisms to potential therapeutic applications in ischemic heart disease. Vascul Pharmacol. 2016;86:53–63.
52. Sweeney M, Foldes G. It takes two: endothelial-perivascular cell cross-talk in vascular development and disease. Front Cardiovasc Med. 2018;5:154.
53. Chen L, Li X, Chen M, Feng Y, Xiong C. The ACE2 expression in human heart indicates new potential mechanism of heart injury among patients infected with SARS-CoV-2. Cardiovasc Res. 2020;116(6):1097–100.
54. Guagliumi G, Sonzogni A, Pescetelli I, Pellegrini D, Finn AV. Microthrombi and ST-segment–elevation myocardial infarction in COVID-19. Circulation. 2020;142(8):804–9.
55. Roffi M, Guagliumi G, Ibanez B. The obstacle course of reperfusion for ST-segment–elevation myocardial in the COVID-19 pandemic. Circulation. 2020;141(24):1951–3.
56. Chieffo A, Stefanini GG, Price S, Barbato E, Tarantini G, Karam N, Moreno R, Buchanan GL, Gilard M, Halvorsen S, Huber K. EAPCI position statement on invasive management of acute coronary syndromes during the COVID-19 pandemic. Eur Heart J. 2020;41(19):1839–51.
57. Briedis K, Aldujeli A, Aldujeili M, Briede K, Zaliunas R, Hamadeh A, Stoler RC, McCullough PA. Considerations for management of acute coronary syndromes during the SARS-CoV-2 (COVID-19) pandemic. The Am J Cardiol. 2020.
58. Valente S, Anselmi F, Cameli M. Acute coronary syndromes during COVID-19: a simple short guide from Italy to assist in the management of ACS during the COVID-19 pandemic is presented. 2020.
59. Linschoten M, Asselbergs FW. CAPACITY-COVID: a European registry to determine the role of cardiovascular disease in the COVID-19 pandemic.

60. Assiut University Registry for ACS Patients During COVID-19 Pandemic—Full Text View —ClinicalTrials.gov. Assiut University Registry for ACS Patients During COVID-19 Pandemic. ClinicalTrials.gov Identifier: NCT04691609; Last updated: December 31, 2020.
61. Primary Angioplasty for STEMI During COVID-19 Pandemic (ISACS-STEMI COVID-19) Registry—Full Text View—ClinicalTrials.gov. Primary Angioplasty for STEMI During COVID-19 Pandemic (ISACS-STEMI COVID-19) Registry (ISACS-STEMI). ClinicalTrials.gov Identifier: NCT04412655; Last updated June 11, 2020.
62. Preventing Cardiac Complication of COVID-19 Disease With Early Acute Coronary Syndrome Therapy: A Randomised Controlled Trial—Full Text View—ClinicalTrials.gov. Preventing Cardiac Complication of COVID-19 Disease With Early Acute Coronary Syndrome Therapy: A Randomised Controlled Trial. (C-19-ACS)); ClinicalTrials.gov Identifier: NCT04333407; Last updated Apr 9, 2020.

Chapter 16
Diabetes Mellitus and COVID19

Key Questions

- What is the frequency of diabetes mellitus in CoViD19?
- Does diabetes mellitus add to the burden of CoViD19 morbidity and mortality?
- What are the prognostic implications of the association of diabetes and CoViD19?
- Does diabetes increase the risk of CoViD19 or vice-versa is true?
- What is the association of hyperglycemia and new-onset diabetes, with CoViD19?
- What are the major pathogenetic links between diabetes and CoViD19?
- What are the practical implications of the CoViD19 and diabetes interlinks that present the challenges in the management?
- What are the main concerns related to the antidiabetic treatments in CoViD19 patients?

16.1 Epidemiology

Diabetes mellitus is a highly prevalent condition worldwide, with an estimated 463 million people affected, and carries a significant morbidity and mortality burden [1, 2]. Several serious complications related to cardiovascular, renal diseases, and stroke are frequently found in association with diabetes mellitus. Multiple studies investigating CoViD19 confirm a significant association of the novel coronavirus disease at levels proportional to the spread of diabetes mellitus across the globe. Significant variabilities can be seen in the incidence reporting of diabetes mellitus in

U. Mallick, *Cardiovascular Complications of COVID-19*,
https://doi.org/10.1007/978-3-030-90065-6_16

CoViD19 studies, indicating a wide range and geographical variations in the incidence, 10.1% [3], 17% [4], 18.3% [5], 24,4% [6], 24% [7] and 34% [8]. According to a metanalysis of 7 studies conducted in China that included 1576 patients admitted with CoViD19, about 9.7% of patients had diabetes mellitus [9]. The data show that the burden of diabetes-associated CoViD19 is extremely high worldwide, and is particularly high in Europe and the Americas. Incidence may be even higher in South America [10, 11] and Africa where the majority of diabetes goes undiagnosed [12].

The association of diabetes with CoViD19 appears to be even higher with the severe or critical disease (Fig. 16.4). A retrospective study of 1099 CoViD19 hospitalized patients, showed an almost twice higher association of diabetes in the severe CoViD19 patients, 28/173 (16.2%), as compared to the non-severe subjects (53/926 (5.7%)). Among patients, who met the primary composite endpoint (admission to an intensive care unit (ICU), the use of mechanical ventilation, or death), the ratio of the diabetics was much higher 18/67 (26.9%), as compared to the group of patients who did not meet 63/1032 (6.1%) the primary composite endpoint [13]. A meta-analysis comparing the incidence of ICU/severe, and non-ICU/severe 1527 CoViD19 patients, showed about 9.27% patients had DM with a twice higher incidence in the ICU/severe group [14].

Furthermore, diabetic patients with severe CoViD19 appear to have a higher fatality as compared to non-diabetics (Fig. 16.5). A single-center retrospective observational study of 193 hospitalized CoViD19 patients, showed an increased mortality rate in patients with severe COViD19 with diabetes mellitus. In this study, 24.9% (48) patients had diabetes. Patients with severe CoViD19 and diabetes had a poor survival rate, as compared to those without, (HR 1.53 (95% CI 1.02 to 2.30; $p = 0.041$). The mortality rate was about 56% (108/193) in the overall cohort, and 81.3% (39/48) in the diabetics, as compared to 47.6% (69/145) in the non-diabetics $p < 0.001$ [15]. Analyses go a step further, marking diabetes mellitus as a risk factor for CoViD19. A retrospective study of a cohort of 174 hospitalized CoViD19 patients, investigating the impact of diabetes on the progression of CoViD19, suggested diabetes as a risk factor for the rapid progression and poor prognosis of CoViID19 [16].

Reports suggest that diabetes is a contributory factor towards mortality in CoViD19 patients in the older age group [16]. In a retrospective observational study of 1122 CoViD19 hospitalized patients in 88 U.S. hospitals, 451 patients had diabetes and/or uncontrolled hyperglycemia. CoViD19 patients with diabetes and uncontrolled hyperglycemia, were older than the counterparts (median age of 65 vs 61 years, $P = 0.005$) [17]. According to an analysis, among patients above age 65 years considered at higher risk of fatality, about 26.8% of patients appear to be diabetics [18]. According to a report among 46 fatal cases of SARS CoV2, 84% of patients were older than age 60, diabetes was a likely association with increased mortality [19]. Reports also suggest high fatality in the younger diabetic subjects with CoViD19 [20], especially younger adults with the critical disease [21].

Both type 1 and type 2 diabetics have increased risk of critical disease and mortality in CoViD19 [22]. Other studies confirm an increase in type 1 diabetes

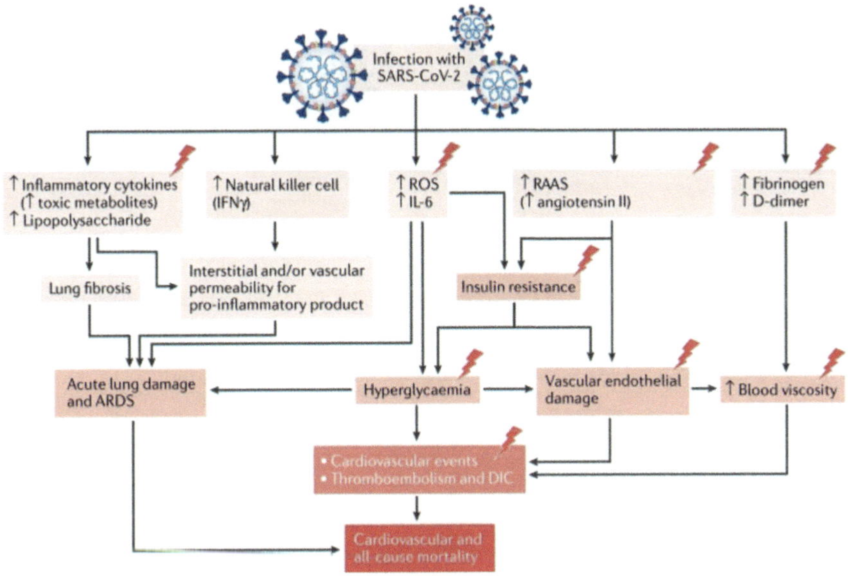

Fig. 16.1 Potential pathogenetic mechanisms in diabetes mellitus and CoViD19. Lightning bolts indicate mechanisms that are accentuated in patients with type 2 diabetes mellitus (T2DM). Text from the figure source. Infection with severe acute respiratory syndrome coronavirus 2 (SARS-CoV-2) (7,239) can lead to increased levels of inflammatory mediators in the blood, including lipopolysaccharide 240,241, inflammatory cytokines (9,43,242,243) and toxic metabolites. Modulation of natural killer cell activity (increased 9,39,50 or decreased 242,244) and IFNγ production can increase the interstitial and/or vascular permeability for pro-inflammatory products (243,245,246). In addition, infection with SARS-CoV-2 leads to increased reactive oxygen species (ROS) production (243,247,248). These effects lead to lung fibrosis 249, acute lung damage and acute respiratory distress syndrome (ARDS) 9,250. ROS production and viral activation of the renin–angiotensin–aldosterone system (RAAS) 249,251 (via increased angiotensin II expression) cause insulin resistance (39,252), hyperglycemia (253) and vascular endothelial damage (243,254,255), all of which contribute to cardiovascular events, thromboembolism and disseminated intravascular coagulation (DIC). Infection also causes increases in the clotting components fibrinogen 60,256 and D-dimer (43,242,257), leading to increases in blood viscosity (146,243) and vascular endothelial damage, and associated cardiovascular events, thromboembolism and DIC. COVID-19, coronavirus disease 2019. *Source* Figure 1. Lim, S., Bae, J.H., Kwon, H.S. and Nauck, M.A., 2021. COVID-19 and diabetes mellitus: from pathophysiology to clinical management. Nature Reviews Endocrinology, 17(1), pp. 11–30. https://www.nature.com/articles/s41574-020-00435-4. By Springer Nature Group

mellitus related mortality observed during the CoViD19 pandemic [23]. Association of diabetes with the severity of CoViD19 and risk of death is compounded by the concomitant presence of cardiovascular conditions and risk factors.

Studies have indicated that obesity and diabetes increase risk of SARS CoV2 infection, and suggest that obesity may potentiate the prognostic risk of diabetes in CoViD19 subjects [5]. The cardiometabolic conditions frequently compound in CoViD19. In a case series of 5700 CoViD19 patients admitted in hospitals in the

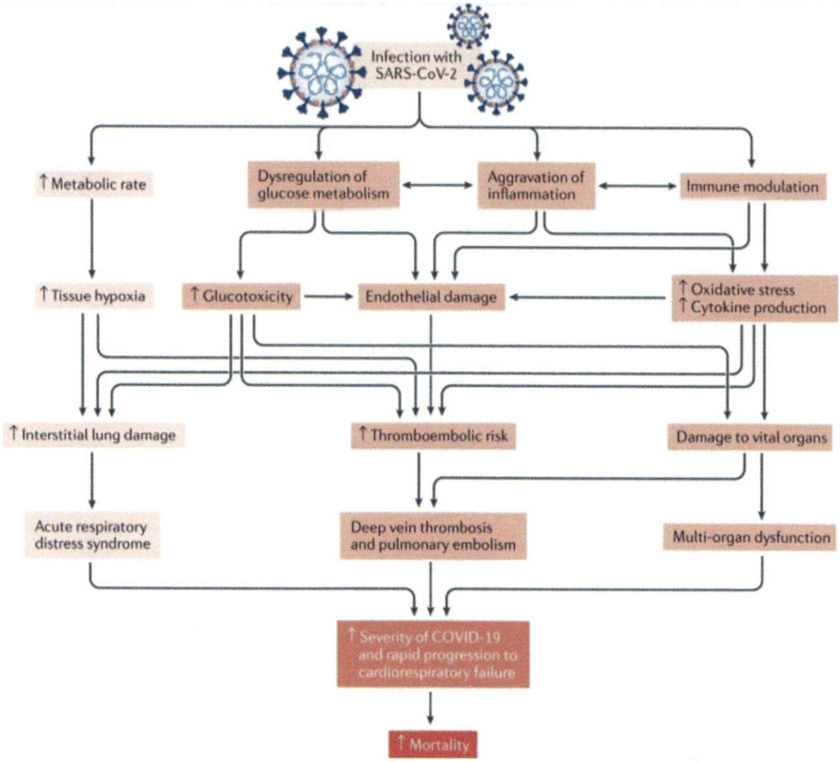

Fig. 16.2 Potential accentuated clinical processes after SARS-CoV-2 infection in people with diabetes mellitus. Darker red indicates processes that are accentuated in patients with type 2 diabetes mellitus (T2DM). Text from the figure Source Severe acute respiratory syndrome coronavirus 2 (SARS-CoV-2) infection increases metabolic rate, resulting in tissue hypoxia, which induces interstitial lung damage and acute respiratory distress syndrome (9,250). Patients with diabetes mellitus and coronavirus disease 2019 (COVID-19) exhibit dysregulation of glucose homeostasis, aggravation of inflammation and impairment in the function of the immune system (9,43,242,243). These conditions increase oxidative stress (243,247,248), cytokine production and endothelial dysfunction (243,254,255), leading to increased risk of thromboembolism and damage to vital organs. All these factors contribute to increased severity of COVID-19 and rapid progression to cardiorespiratory failure in patients with diabetes mellitus. *Source* Figure 3. Lim, S., Bae, J.H., Kwon, H.S. and Nauck, M.A., 2021. CoViD19 and diabetes mellitus: from pathophysiology to clinical management. Nature Reviews Endocrinology, 17(1), pp. 11–30. https://www.nature.com/articles/s41574-020-00435-4. By Springer Nature Group

US, the most common comorbidities were hypertension (56.6%) 3026, obesity (41.7%) 1737, and diabetes (33.8%) 1808 [24]. In a retrospective analysis of 1099 patients with CoViD19, from 552 hospitals in China, about 173 patients had severe disease. An increased association of diabetics was seen among the severe patients, as compared to the overall cohort, 16.2% (28/173) versus 7.4% (81/1099). Furthermore, a higher association of hypertensive patients was observed among the severe subjects at 23.7% (41/173), as compared to the 15% (165/1099) in the overall cohort [25]. The compounding of the risk factors strongly impacts the prognosis among CoViD19 subjects. According to a meta-analysis report of 281,461 individuals with CoViD19, from 11 countries/regions, the older age, male gender, diabetes, and hypertension were associated with higher mortality in CoViD19 patients (coefficient = 0.05 per year, 5.1, 8.2, 6.99, respectively; $P = 0.006$-0.0002) [26]. Raised body mass index (BMI) and obesity aggravate the risk of critical disease and death in diabetic CoViD19 patients. The characteristics and CoViD19–related outcomes (i.e. intubation for mechanical ventilation, death, and discharge by day 7) were analyzed according to the BMI status, in a retrospective study of 1,965 patients admitted with CoViD19, and T2D. The association of composite primary outcome rose progressively with increasing BMI, with odds ratios of (OR 1.65 [1.05–2.59]), class I (OR 1.93 [1.19–3.14]) and class II/III obesity (OR 1.98 [1.11–3.52]), for overweight, class I, and class II/III obesity, respectively, although the association was not confirmed in patients > 75 years of age [27]. The associations of 17 cardiometabolic traits with CoViD19 susceptibility and severity, was evaluated using 2-sample Mendelian randomization (MR) analyses. The authors suggested that obesity-related cardiometabolic diseases (type 2 diabetes, chronic kidney disease, stroke, and coronary heart disease), may be mediators of the relationship between body mass index and higher risk of hospitalization for COVID19 [28].

Diabetes mellitus appears to increase the risk of cardiac injury in CoViD19 patients. Studies show a higher occurrence of cardiac injury among diabetics with CoViD19, during hospitalization. It may be reflected by a more frequent association of markers of myocardial injury and heart failure among the diabetic CoViD19 patients, as compared to the non-diabetics. In a retrospective analysis of a cohort of 193 patients hospitalized with severe CoViD19, 148 were diabetics, and 45 were non-diabetics. The NT-proBNP (pg/mL) values were much higher in the diabetic patients 970 (323 to 2535), versus the non-diabetics 46 (31 to 267) < 0.001, (Normal < 285). Similarly, the Cardiac troponin I, (pg/mL) was also much higher, 43.1 (11.0 to 239.4) among the diabetics, as compared to the non-diabetics 1.9 (1.9 to 5.0) < 0.001, (Normal $\leq$ 15.60). In the overall cohort, the survival rate among the diabetic CoViD19 patients was much lower, n = 9/85 (10.6%), versus non-diabetics (n = 39/108 (36.1%)) $p < 0.001$, hazard ratio (HR) of 3.17 (95% confidence interval (CI) 1.93 to 5.20). After adjustment for age, hypertension, cardiovascular disease, and cerebrovascular disease a high HR 1.53 (95% CI 1.02 to 2.30); $p = 0.041$ was still significant [29].

A retrospective study of 7106 hospitalized CoViD19 patients, investigated the associations and prognostic power of circulating markers of cardiac injury CK-MB (creatinine phosphokinase-MB) or hs-cTnI levels (high sensitivity Troponin I) levels and others with the poor outcomes of CoViD19, and found that compared with the patient group without measurement of biomarkers (2814), the group with measured biomarker values (3219), had a higher percentage of diabetics, (413 (12.8%) versus non-diabetics 256 (9.1%) $p < 0.001$). The study showed a significant association of the biomarkers hs-cTnI, CK-MB, N-terminal pro-B-type natriuretic peptide or brain natriuretic peptide ((NT-pro)BNP), creatinine kinase (CK), and myoglobin (MYO) with the mortality risk [30].

Occurrence and outcomes of thrombo-embolic events in CoViD19 were assessed in a multicenter, observational cohort study of 1114 CoViD19 patients (from outpatient clinics, intensive care units, and non-intensive care hospital settings). The primary composite outcome was adjudicated major arterial or venous thromboembolism. Diabetes was commonly observed in all three groups of CoViD19 patients, intensive care 66/170 (38.8%), non-intensive care 68/229 (29.7%), outpatient clinics 67/715 (9.4%), and overall cohort 201/1114 (18.0%), who were found to have a high frequency of major arterial or venous thromboembolism, major adverse cardiovascular events, and symptomatic venous thromboembolism, especially in the intensive care settings [31].

Stressful conditions and infections often accompany hyperglycemia. The occurrence of hyperglycemia was observed in CoViD19 studies in both diabetic and non-diabetic subjects and was found to have poor outcomes, with worsening of prognosis in both groups [32]. A retrospective observational study evaluated glycemic and clinical outcomes, in 1122 hospitalized patients with COVID19, with and without diabetes and/or acutely uncontrolled hyperglycemia. The study concluded that diabetes and/or uncontrolled hyperglycemia occurred frequently. The COVID19 patients with diabetes and/or uncontrolled hyperglycemia had a longer LOS (length of stay) (5.7 vs 4.3 days, $P < 0.001$), and markedly higher mortality than patients without diabetes or uncontrolled hyperglycemia, 28.8% (n 184) versus 6.2% (n 386) ($P < 0.001$). Patients with uncontrolled hyperglycemia 40 of 96 (41.7%) had a particularly high mortality rate versus diabetic patients 13 of 88 (14.8%) ($P < 0.001$) [17].

The impact of glucose control may influence the outcomes of diabetic CoViD19 patients. Analysis of a large dataset of health analytics platform consisting of 17,278,392 adults and 10,926 CoViD19-related deaths, showed a %HbA1c > 7.5 (Hba1c $\geq$ 58 mmol mol^{-1}) within the previous 15 months, was associated with an increased rate of mortality [33]. Moreover, a tight glucose control in CoViD19 diabetic patients appears to have beneficial impact on the outcomes. Data from a retrospective, multi-centered study of 7,337 cases of COVID19, among which 952 had pre-existing T2D, indicate that improved glycemic control is associated with better outcomes, with markedly lower mortality in patients with CoViD19 and pre-existing T2D [34].

Moreover, elevated fasting plasma glucose levels have been observed in the older age adults testing positive for SARS CoV2. A retrospective study of outpatients aged 65 years old and above, analyzed data from a total of 135 older age subjects with T2D with baseline and follow-up fasting plasma glucose, and 50 older age subjects with T2D with baseline and follow-up HbA1c. The baseline and follow-up fasting plasma glucose were 7.08±1.80 and 7.48±2.14 mmol/L, respectively (P=0.008). The baseline and follow-up HbA1c were 7.2±1.7% and 7.4 ±1.8%, respectively (P=0.158). The study concluded that older age subjects with T2D had higher fasting plasma glucose levels during CoViD19 outbreak [35].

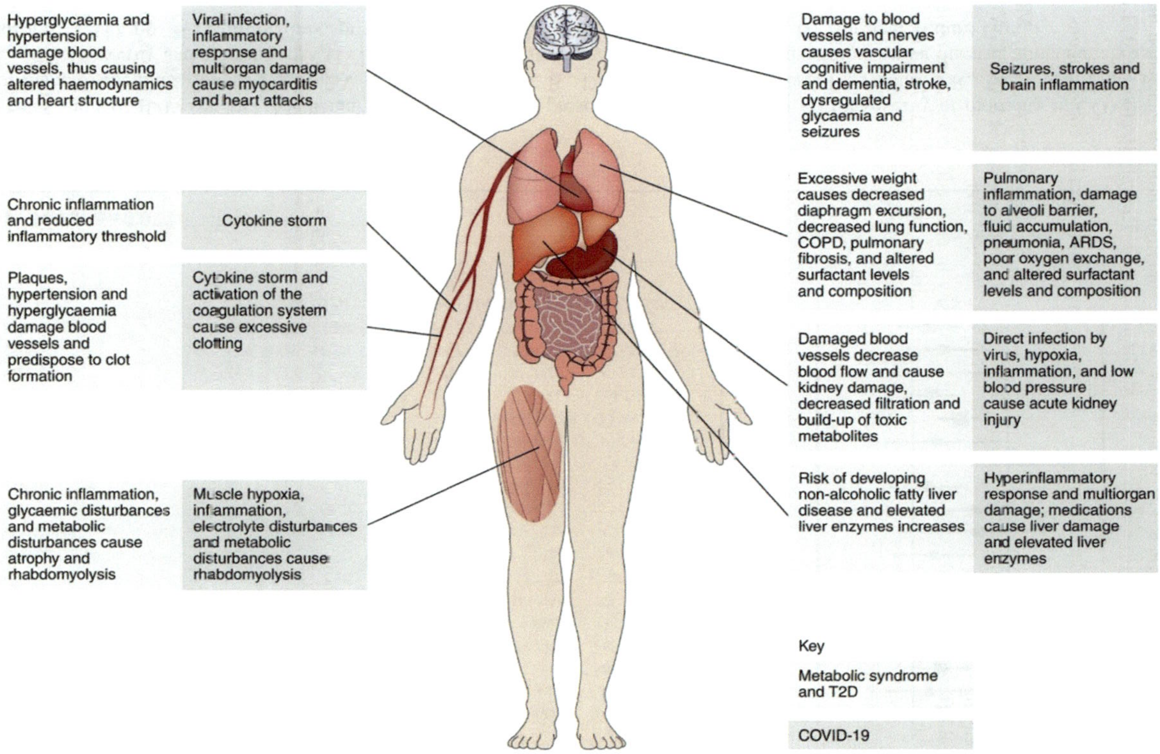

Fig. 16.3 The parallels among metabolic syndrome, T2D and COVID-19. *Source* Figure 2. Ayres, J.S., 2020. A metabolic handbook for the COVID-19 pandemic. Nature metabolism, 2(7), pp. 572–585 https://www.nature.com/articles/s42255-020-0237-2. By Springer Nature Group

Study name	Odds ratio	Lower limit	Upper limit	p-Value	DM	N-DM	Total	Relative weight
	Statistics for each study				Severe / Total			
Li J et al.	2,12	1,37	3,29	0,00	76 / 127	97 / 235	173 / 362	12,39
Giamarellos-Bourboulis et al.	1,50	0,37	6,06	0,57	6 / 10	22 / 44	28 / 54	3,02
Colombi D et al.	1,93	0,94	3,93	0,07	22 / 37	86 / 199	108 / 236	7,95
Li X et al.	1,92	1,19	3,10	0,01	52 / 83	217 / 465	269 / 548	11,61
Lei S et al.	5,67	0,94	34,03	0,06	6 / 8	9 / 26	15 / 34	1,96
Guo T et al.	4,56	1,98	10,51	0,00	16 / 28	36 / 159	52 / 187	6,55
Huang C et al.	0,25	0,03	2,28	0,22	1 / 8	12 / 33	13 / 41	1,33
Zhang JJ et al.	1,70	0,61	4,70	0,31	9 / 17	49 / 123	58 / 140	4,98
Liu W et al.	4,74	0,69	32,35	0,11	2 / 5	9 / 73	11 / 78	1,73
Wang D et al.	4,57	1,46	14,28	0,01	8 / 14	28 / 124	36 / 138	4,20
Zhang G et al.	1,47	0,57	3,81	0,43	7 / 22	48 / 199	55 / 221	5,47
Wang Z et al.	40,50	4,30	381,74	0,00	6 / 7	8 / 62	14 / 69	1,30
Zheng KI et al.	1,80	0,33	9,76	0,50	2 / 7	28 / 154	30 / 161	2,17
Guan WJ et al.	3,18	1,95	5,19	0,00	28 / 81	145 / 1018	173 / 1099	11,43
Feng Y et al.	1,59	0,85	2,98	0,15	17 / 49	107 / 427	124 / 476	9,15
Wan S et al.	8,90	2,27	34,99	0,00	9 / 12	31 / 123	40 / 135	3,12
Deng Q et al.	2,11	0,70	6,35	0,18	14 / 19	53 / 93	67 / 112	4,43
Mao L et al.	1,52	0,70	3,30	0,29	15 / 30	73 / 184	88 / 214	7,21
	2,35	1,80	3,06	0,00	296 / 564	1058 / 3741	1354 / 4305	

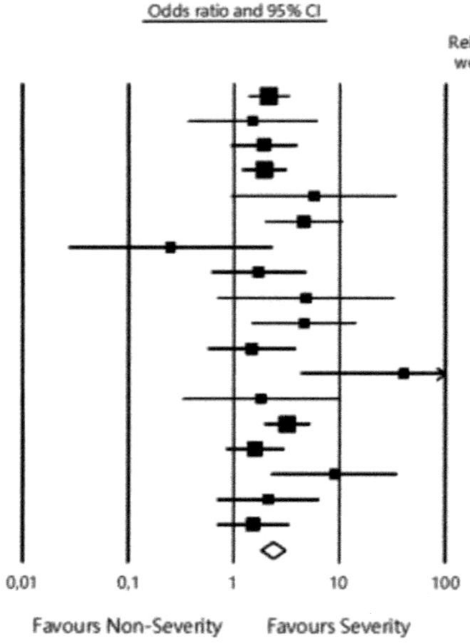

I^2: 34.78; p=0.073

Random Effects

Fig. 16.4 Diabetes and CoViD19 severity. Meta-analysis with forest plot presenting the OR and 95% CI for severity or mortality of COVID-19 according to the presence of diabetes mellitus. *Source* Figure 2A. de Almeida-Pititto, B., Dualib, P.M., Zajdenverg, L., Dantas, J.R., De Souza, F.D., Rodacki, M. and Bertoluci, M.C., 2020. Severity and mortality of COVID 19 in patients with diabetes, hypertension and cardiovascular disease: a meta-analysis. Diabetology & metabolic syndrome, 12(1), pp. 1–12. https://link.springer.com/article/10.1186/s13098-020-00586-4. By Springer Natur Group

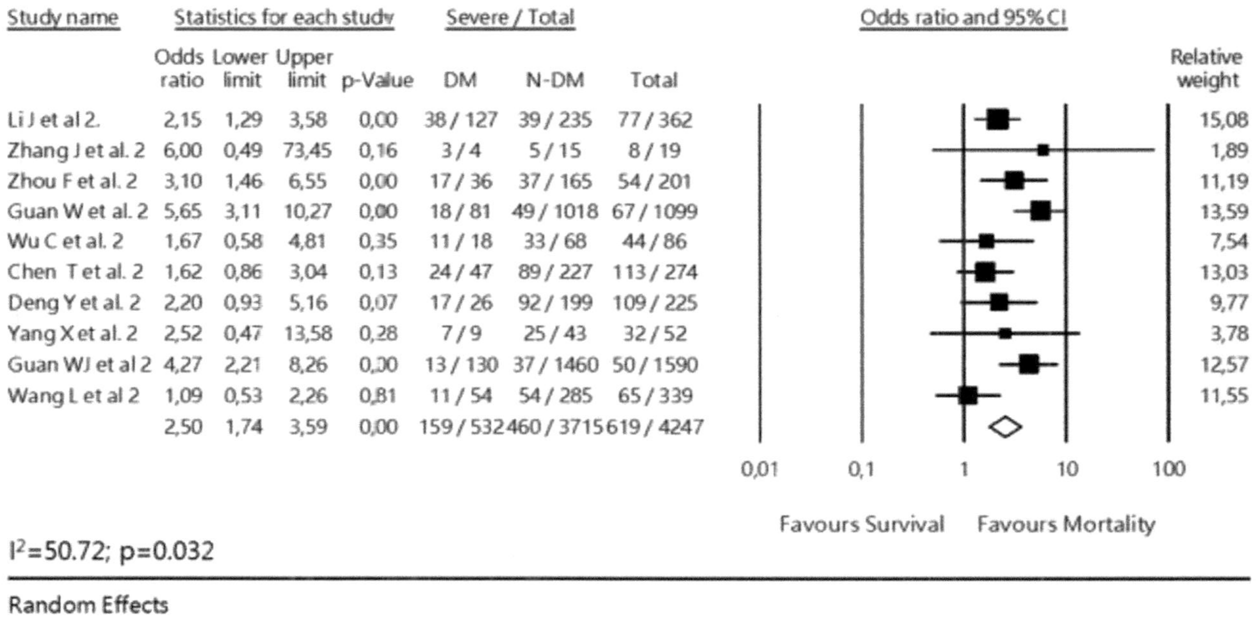

Fig. 16.5 Diabetes and CoViD19 mortalty. Meta-analysis with forest plot presenting the OR and 95% CI for severity or mortality of COVID-19 according to the presence of diabetes mellitus. *Source* Figure 2B. de Almeida-Pititto, B., Dualib, P.M., Zajdenverg, L., Dantas, J.R., De Souza, F.D., Rodacki, M. and Bertoluci, M.C., 2020. Severity and mortality of COVID 19 in patients with diabetes, hypertension and cardiovascular disease: a meta-analysis. Diabetology & metabolic syndrome, 12(1), pp. 1–12. https://link.springer.com/article/10.1186/s13098-020-00586-4

Although data are scarce, the occurrence of new-onset diabetes has been described in association with CoViD19. Studies suggest that new-onset hyperglycemia without diabetes and new-onset diabetes in CoViD19, may be associated with a poorer outcome, compared with normoglycemic individuals, and people with pre-existing diabetes [36]. Further studies are needed to establish the occurrence of new-onset diabetes in CoViD19 and a direct correlation between hyperglycemia and clinical outcomes in CoViD19 patients.

Diabetic ketoacidosis (DKA) is a known and serious complication of diabetes mellitus. Studies report the occasional occurrence of DKA among diabetics with CoViD19 in both type 1 and type 2 diabetics, and further indicate an association with poor outcomes. Report of an analysis based on studies reporting CoViD19 patients with DKA and combined DKA/ hyperglycemic hyperosmolar syndrome (HHS), observed DKA in CoViD19 portends a poor prognosis with mortality being higher in patients with combined DKA/HHS than isolated DKA [37]. Ethnic inequities have been described in the occurrence of DKA among CoViD19 subjects, along with the presence of additional risks among ethnic groups [37, 38].

CoViD19 has resulted in a significant burden on the health care systems worldwide and the association of diabetes with CoViD19 may contribute towards the burden. Several analyses suggest that diabetic patients with CoViD19 have longer hospital stay [39] and may have a higher estimated cost per hospital admission reflecting significant economic implications [40].

16.2 Pathogenesis

Hyperglycemia is an acute phase response to a critical illness [41], may be caused by several endogenous mechanisms including the stress, glucagon/cortisol/catecholamines, increased hepatic glucose production, reduced gastrointestinal (GI) absorption, impaired glucose clearance, or exogenous factors such as administration of drugs e.g., corticosteroids, intravenous (IV) nutrition or due to the infection or a combination of these factors. Hyperglycemia enhances ACE2 expression, and may facilitate SARS CoV2 replication [42]. Uncontrolled hyperglycemia may increase the risk of complications such as fluid and electrolyte disturbances, impaired adaptive immune response, and increased infection. Hyperglycemia induces gene expression of matrix metalloproteinases, which may promote further the spread of inflammation [43].

Pathogenetic chain of events following SARS CoV2 involving damage to the airway tracts, and pleiotropic invasion of the viral disease provoking intense immuno-modulatory, hyper-inflammatory, prothrombotic, vasoplegic, dysmetabolic as well as key cellular stress mechanisms and mechanisms related to the dysfunction of various homeostatic regulators, are described extensively in previous chapters in this book. Figures 16.1 and 16.2 highlight important mechanisms that are accentuated during the diabetes-CoViD19 interplay.

Dysglycemic states, immune dysfnction and CoViD19 display important interlnks. Impairment of the immune system secondary to hyperglycemia and CoViD19 during the acute phase may result in worsening of the infection. CoViD19 is a dysregulated immune-inflammatory condition that is likely to create a dysmetabolic state, which may further worsen immune inflammation in its turn. Multiple CoViD19 associated mechanisms may further aggravate the underlying risks in the diabetic subjects. Severe CoViD19, with the hyperimmune inflammatory response, accompanies an altered metabolic state, and poor glycemic control. Factors including elevated cytokines, acute inflammatory reactions, direct SARS CoV2-ACE2 binding, and indirect reactions potentiate the harmful impact of the adverse metabolic reactions.

Metabolism and immune responses have a bidirectional relationship [58] that may lead to a vicious cycle under the co-existence of diabetes and CoViD19. The dynamics of interaction between innate immune and metabolic systems may help to define this relationship. Both innate and adaptive immune mechanisms are impacted by diabetes leading to impaired host defense mechanisms [59] increasing the susceptibility to infections. An impaired immune state in the diabetic subjects further alters the balance in the immune response triggered by CoViD19.

Multiple virological and diabetic interconnections may be found that may elucidate the associated risks of CoViD19 and diabetes. Studies suggest that critical patients with type 2 diabetes mellitus, may have prolonged SARS CoV2 viral shedding [47], although contrary findings have been published [48]. Mechanisms related to weak innate immune mechanisms for instance among diabetics or other immuno-compromised states, exaggerated cytokine release in severe CoViD19, imbalance in protective and harmful RAS axes and ACE2 dysregulation, and several other mechanisms may impact viral shedding. Interestingly, studies have not shown unfavorable differences in the antibody response to SARS CoV2, between the diabetic and non-diabetic subjects [49–51]. Several mechanisms are related to the immune impairments in the diabetics that increase susceptibility to infections. Physicochemical changes such as rheological, alterations in the Na^+/K^+-ATPase activity, and others such as aggressive glycosylation including an accumulation of advanced glycation end products (AGE) associated with immunoglobulin dysfunction [44–46] may contribute towards the increased susceptibility. system secondary to hyperglycemia. SARS CoV2 [47, 48] SARS CoV2 [49–51]. Furthermore, the immune impairment, alterations in the lung structure, mechanisms related to ACE2 expression, may also contribute towards a higher predisposition of the diabetics towards pulmonary infections including CoViD19 [52–55]. Important pathognomonic features of diabetic patients include chronic inflammation, increased coagulation activity, impaired immune response, and glycemic instability. These mechanisms may increase the susceptibility of the diabetics towards severe immune manifestations of CoViD19. The molecular reactions related to energy metabolism, cellular energy deprivation, autophagy, oxidative stress, tissue hypoxia, also observed in patients with complicated CoViD19 with hyperactive and dysregulated inflammatory reactions, may trigger these pathogenetic mechanisms and form an important interlink between CoViD19 related complications and DM.

Diabetic subjects with CoViD19 have elevated markers of inflammation and coagulation. In a retrospective study of 174 patients admitted with CoViD19, diabetic patients had significantly higher ($P < 0.01$) serum inflammatory biomarkers IL-6, C-reaction protein (CRP), ferritin and coagulation index, D dimers, compared with non-diabetics [16]. Other studies also show an increase in high-sensitivity CRP (hsCRP), procalcitonin, IL-2 receptor, IL-6, IL-8, and TNF-α among the diabetic subjects with severe CoViD19 [29]. Severe CoViD19 is associated with the hyperimmune inflammatory response with exaggerated and persistent production of pro-inflammatory cytokines [19], including interleukins ((IL-2, IL-7), interferon-γ (IFN-γ), TNF-alpha (TNF-α), chemokines CCL2, and others, with IL-6 particularly predicting mortality [56]. Lymphopenia associated with worse CoViD19 regarded as a marker of risk, is distinctly observed among diabetics. Short term hyperglycemia and CoViD19 may induce lymphopenia [60], which may further aggravate the hyperimmune-inflammatory reactions of SARS CoV2 [61]. Data suggest that inflammation and lymphopenia resolve more slowly in T2DM patients with CoViD19 [62]. Exact mechanisms that promote the bidirectional connection of diabetes and CoViD19 need to be further explored.

Diabetes mellitus is an important cause of renal impairment. Patients with diabetes mellitus with CoViD19 appear to have elevated markers of renal injury. According to an observational cohort analysis of 316, older COVID19 patients hospitalized for COVID19 and 876 patients with non-COVID19 diagnoses, patients who developed AKI, were more frequently diabetic (55% vs 42%), had lower baseline eGFR (57 ± 26 vs 67 ± 21 mL/min), increased initial median CRP value (78 vs 42 mg/L) and were more often on treatment with antibiotics at hospitalization(60% vs 46%) compared to the COVID19 patients who did not develop AKI [57]. Besides worsening of a pre-existing renal disease, other causes such as thrombo-inflammatory damage, microvascular disease, systemic hemodynamic instability and several other factors associated with sepsis and hyper immune-inflammatory burden may accentuate renal deterioration in the diabetic subjects with CoViD19.

Diabetes is a pro-inflammatory condition, and involves a series of pathways and cellular mechanisms such as activation of Toll-like receptors (TLRs), Endoplasmic Reticulum Stress (ER stress), and inflammasome activation, leading to inflammation [63]. Metabolic changes strongly impact inflammation and homeostasis. Metabolism is linked with alterations in the immune cell metabolic configuration, and dynamics of the programming of functional properties (pro or anti-inflammatory) of immune cells [64]. Several mechanisms related to insulin resistance and insulin receptor dysfunction contribute to chronic inflammation in metabolic disorders [65, 66]. Elevation of inflammatory cells and cytokines may be seen in association with metabolic dysfunction that also accompanies insulin resistance. Macrophages play an important role in inflammation and insulin resistance in the adipose tissue [67, 68]. Overproduction of pro-inflammatory cytokines by innate immune cells affects metabolism and further induces cellular stress mechanisms [69]. Elevated levels of TNF-α in obesity reflect inflammation, particularly in association with insulin resistance and diabetes [70]. Immune-inflammatory and genetic mechanisms, linked with insulin resistance observed in the diabetics, are further aggravated by increased adiposity, known as active immune metabolic structure, may not only reflect an important connection between the increased risk of complications in diabetic subjects and CoViD19, but also are likely to play an important role in the association of obesity with diabetes mellitus observed in CoViD19 subjects.

The RAS mechanisms play a significant role in the development of insulin resistance in diabetics, in particular AngII [71], are also dysregulated in severe CoViD19. Angiotensin II increases capillary blood flow to increase insulin-mediated glucose disposal via AT_2 receptor, and AT_1 receptor activation leads to a reduced NO bioavailability, impaired insulin signaling, vasoconstriction, and insulin resistance [72].

Diabetes mellitus adversely impacts the cardiovascular system compromising vascular, myocardial, and electrical conduction systems. Pathogenetic mechanisms interconnecting diabetes mellitus and cardiovascular diseases found in the diabetics may exaggerate underlying susceptibility for CoViD19 related cardiovascular complications including arrhythmias, acute coronary events, heart failure, and others involving myocardial injury. The molecular transformations, cellular stress, extracellular matrix transformations, and several other factors related to the excessive generation of advanced glycated end products (AGE) in the diabetics, adversely impact the vascular and myocardial structures, immune cells, cytokines, and vaso-regulatory mechanisms [73]. Several other mechanisms associated with elevated glycemic levels have been linked to cardiac complications, including arrhythmias [44]. Almost two-thirds of heart failure (HF) patients have abnormal glucose homeostasis [74]. Glucose uptake and lipid metabolism are also impaired in the epicardial adipose tissue (EAT) of heart failure patients. The glucose uptake upon insulin stimulation, and lipolysis upon isoproterenol stimulation, are decreased in the EAT compared with subcutaneous adipose tissue (SAT) in HF patients [75]. Chronic glycemia damages the cardiovascular structures, and the underlying immune metabolic mechanisms enhance the cardiovascular vulnerability, which may explain the increase in markers of cardiac injury observed in diabetics in CoViD19.

Elevated body mass index (BMI) at an early age not only increases the risk of cardiovascular disease, type 2 diabetes mellitus [76, 77] and hypertension [77] but also development of adulthood obesity [78, 79]. Elevated adiposity in diabetic subjects and associated risk factors increase CoViD19 risks (Fig. 16.3). According to the report of a multicentre observational study in 1317 subjects with diabetes hospitalized for CoViD19, an increase in BMI was associated with increase in the criticality of the CoViD19 diabetic subjects, and the risk of death [80].

Data suggest that a higher expression of ACE2 in diabetes mellitus may be linked with higher susceptibility towards CoViD19, and increased complications [86]. Liver and pancreatic ACE2 locations may act as a target by the SARS CoV2 [81, 82]. Data suggest that the ACE2 expression may be observed both in the exocrine and islet cells, in acinar cells, and within subsets of islet cells in the pancreas, [81]. However, variations in the expression of ACE2 + cells in the pancreas exist across distinct pancreatic cell types. According to another analysis, localization of the ACE2 + cells may not be consistent in the pancreatic endocrine portion in the subjects, but the endothelial cells and pericytes of capillaries and interlobular ducts of the pancreas [83]. Report of a pooled analysis suggests that human pancreas may be a target of SARS CoV2 infection and β cell infection that could contribute to the metabolic dysregulation observed in patients with COVID19 [84]. Other factors may also play a role in the metabolic dysregulation associated with CoViD19 in diabetic subjects. Evidence shows the pathogenetic links of Furin (a type 1 transmembrane protein that promotes cell entry of coronaviruses) with diabetes and high mortality [85]. Like ACE2, DPP4 are coronavirus receptors [86], and control inflammation, and cardiometabolic physiology. ACE2 CoViD19, [87]. Furthermore, the potential role of ACE2 in insulin resistance and impaired secretion may be linked with diabetes [88], although no conclusive evidence establishes the significance of ACE2 for glucose control independent of the angiotensin pathway [89].

Development of diabetic ketoacidosis in CoViD19 patients [90] may implicate several mechanisms related to metabolic decompensation including viral-pancreatic beta-cell interactions and insulin deficiency, exaggerated counter-regulatory responses promoting ketone production, use of sodium-glucose cotransporter-2 inhibitors (SGLT2) inhibitors [91], and other factors. The viral pancreatic interactions suggesting possible beta pancreatic cell damage in CoViD19 patients that may result in diabetes in the non-diabetic patients, need to be further explored.

16.3 Treatment Implications

A precautious use of the drugs is warranted in diabetic patients with CoViD19. Drugs used in CoViD19 treatment, such as corticosteroids may induce hyperglycemia and impact the glycemic control in diabetics [92]. Other drugs, such as chloroquine, may cause hypoglycemia. Therefore, a frequent adjustment of the glucose-lowering medications, especially in combination with drugs used to treat CoViD19, may be needed. Aggressive treatment strategies might be needed for better and early control of the inflammatory and glycemic intensity in CoViD19 patients with diabetes. Although elevated glucose levels are observed in CoViD19 patients, the therapeutic threshold for insulin treatment in critical patients is not well understood [93], and needs to be defined. Insulin infusion has been suggested as an effective method for achieving glycemic targets and improving outcomes in patients with COVID19 [94].

The safety and efficacy of the antidiabetic treatment in CoViD19 diabetic subjects have been explored in various settings. Risks and benefits of antidiabetic drugs such as metformin, inhibitors of dipeptidyl peptidase 4 (DPP4i), SGLT2i, insulin have been identified in several studies. The observational, retrospective nature, small number of patients, heterogeneity, and methodological flaws, are among the important factors that make it difficult to draw concrete conclusions in studies investigating antidiabetic treatments in diabetic CoViD19 subjects, therefore, a cautious interpretation of these studies is warranted. National and local guidelines must be used to determine the best treatment options.

Certain antidiabetic drugs may offer better protection due to the additional benefits including anti-inflammatory actions. Metformin is known to reduce the TNF-α and other inflammatory adipokines in diabetics and obese subjects [95]. Antidiabetic agents such as DPP4i may have a potential anti-inflammatory role [96] through downregulation of cytokine storm and may benefit patients with CoViD19 [97], however conflicting reports about beneficial effects of DPP4i in CoViD19 patients have been published [98]. Similarly, anti-inflammatory actions have been described for glucagon-like peptide-1 (GLP1) receptor agonists [99] and insulin [100]. Although, studies show improvement in the outcomes in CoViD19 subjects with insulin treatment and even lowering of IL-6 and D-dimer levels [94], other studies have warned about the harmful effects of insulin in patients with diabetes and CoViD19 [101].

Use of metformin has been identified with risks in the severe diabetic CoViD19 subjects due to acute metabolic decompensation [102] however, metformin decreased mortality in COVID19 patients with diabetes [103] and improved the clinical outcomes of patients with mild to moderate SARSCoV2, especially in diabetic women [104]. A retrospective analysis further shows beneficial therapeutic value with reduced mortality with treatment with metformin in women with obesity or type 2 diabetes with CoViD19, however, no difference was seen among men [105].

Analyses show safety of DPP4i in CoViD19 subjects [106]. A population-based observational study of 8337 patients, has shown significant improvement in clinical outcomes associated with DPP4i use in COVID19 [107], however, weakness in the study design and methodology may pose significant limitations. The conflicting reports describing DPP4i, inconclusive results, and insufficient evidence may not allow recommendation of the use of DPP4i against COVID19. [98].

Similarly, use of SGLT2 inhibitors was identified with risk of ketoacidosis [108] and may limit its use in unstable CoViD19 patients. Studies provide reassurance about the safety of the SGLT2 inhibitors and DPP-4 inhibitors in type 2 diabetes with COVID19 [109], however, may be subject to limitations in the quality. Role of other antidiabetic drugs (SGLT2 i) in CoViD19 is under exploration in ongoing clinical trials [110, 111].

16.4 Summary

The frequent occurrence of diabetes mellitus with CoViD19, especially with severe disease, and impact on mortality appear significant. The trends can be observed worldwide across geographical boundaries and reflect a mixing epidemic of non-communicable diseases and the CoViD19 epidemic. Diabetes contributes towards potentiation of the viral disease and prolonged hospital stay. Sporadic occurrences of the DKA in diabetic patients have been reported in association with the viral disease. Regardless of CoViD19, diabetic patients are known to have worse outcomes when facing illnesses. Older patients and diabetics have higher mortality rates in cardiovascular diseases, cancer, or severe infections. Association of diabetes with potent risk factors, such as advanced age, hypertension, and obesity, further aggravate the risk of complications in CoViD19.

Hyperglycemia associated with CoViD19 may be transient or develop into new diabetes cases of new-onset diabetes have been reported in association with CoViD19. The exact association of new-onset diabetes with CoViD19 is poorly known, however, may reflect a diabetogenic potential of CoViD19. This has led to the exploration of new-onset diabetes in CoViD19 subjects in global initiatives, yet to be completed [112]. In an aggregate, diabetes mellitus appears to be frequently associated with CoViD19, and more frequently with the complicated disease. Although this association reflects a positive correlation with the severity and prognosis of CoViD19, definite conclusions must be drawn using robust study designs and methodology.

Reports describing the biochemical impact of diabetes in CoViD19, indicate a more intense inflammatory picture in the diabetics, as compared to the non-diabetic subjects with CoViD19. Similarly, elevated markers of cardiovascular risk in the diabetics with CoViD19 also reflect a higher risk of cardiovascular complications. The duration of pre-existing diabetes, previous glycemic control, associated complications, concomitant cardiometabolic risk factors reflect the actual gravity of diabetes and dictate the risks. These mechanisms are likely to be the major facilitators of CoViD19 related risks in diabetics. Association of immune impairment, micro and macrovascular disease, kidney damage, and cardiac involvement determine the vulnerability of the diabetic patients towards CoViD19 severity. On the other hand, the intensity of CoViD19, the severity of the immune-inflammatory reactions, direct viral actions, sepsis, are among several mechanisms that may aggravate diabetes-associated risks. The overall picture suggests that both diabetes and CoViD19 impact each other via potent pathogenetic links. Pathogenetic mechanisms, biochemical profile, and CoViD19 epidemiological data favor the role of diabetes mellitus in the development of complications, and the adverse impact of CoViD19 on diabetics. Inflammation may induce hyperglycemia and vice versa. Immunometabolism and met-inflammation play a key role in this association. The underlying burden of met-inflammation in the diabetics, local and systemic dysregulation of metabolism and RAS mechanisms, increased ACE2 activity, endothelial dysfunction, insulin resistance, prothrombotic mechanisms form an important pathogenetic substrate. Development of new-onset diabetes and hyperglycemia may reflect several underlying complex mechanisms, although implications of beta-pancreatic cell damage or exhaustion of poor reserve and ACE2 are plausible mechanisms. Furthermore, the inherent vulnerability of the diabetic patients for CoViD19 severity and complications appears realistic but does not define susceptibility towards the infection. The precise architectural composition of the concept of susceptibility of diabetics towards SARS CoV2 infection needs to be further determined. Moreover, the inherent weaknesses in the studies exploring viral shedding in the diabetic CoViD19 patients [47, 48], and lack of power, need to be addressed with further exploration of this phenomenon, using robust study designs and methodology.

Diabetics with CoViD19 require close monitoring and care in acute settings, and early therapeutic interventions to minimize the risks. Data indicate improvement in glycemic control results in better outcomes in diabetic patients with CoViD19 [34]. Prevention of CoViD19 in the diabetics and prompt treatment as well as maintaining a tight glucose control hold the principal stage when minimizing the risk of CoViD19 in the diabetics. Adherence to a healthy lifestyle, dietary measures, and exercise, remain the best principles in combatting CoViD19 in diabetics. Adaptations in diabetes care models are necessary to provide better care to the diabetic patients at risk of CoViD19 in the community. The use of telemedicine and remote guidance must be promoted during the times of the CoViD19 pandemic. Updated expert guidelines and protocols are needed to guide preventive measures to reduce the incidence of CoViD19 in patients with diabetes mellitus [113].

Summary Box

- CoViD19 studies confirm a higher association of diabetes across the geographical boundaries that associates with a variety of risk factors along the way and variations in the burden of CoViD19 and associated risks, adding to the woes of the health cares systems.
- Diabetes potentiates the risk of severity of the CoViD19, causes longer hospital stay, a delayed viral clearance, and may display an increased susceptibility. However, the notion of susceptibility of the diabetics for SARS CoV2 infection requires further exploration.
- Diabetic patients may have increased susceptibility for complications and adverse outcomes with CoViD19 that may reflect the vulnerability of diabetics.
- Several background risk factors accompanying diabetics elevate the risks of diabetes with CoViD19; older age and obesity are prominent.
- Pre-existing cardiovascular and metabolic conditions are associated with poor prognosis in CoViD19.
- Markers of cardiac injury are higher among diabetic CoViD19 patients.
- CoViD19 and diabetes hold a bidirectional relationship adversely impacting each other.
- Immunologic and metabolic pathways are important pathogenetic mechanisms linking diabetes and CoViD19.
- Hyperglycemia in both diabetic and non-diabetic CoViD19 subjects is associated with a worse prognosis.
- Hyperglycemia and inflammation promote each other.
- SARS CoV2 pancreatic interactions via ACE2 present a real risk, however, need further evaluation.

- Early and aggressive glucose management may save complications; the impact of lowering hyperglycemia in CoViD19 needs further exploration.
- The association of cardiometabolic risk factors with CoViD19 raises the significance of optimizing metabolic control.
- Current data provide a positive indication of the safety of antidiabetic drugs such as DPP4i and SGLT2i in CoViD19 patients.
- Diabetes mellitus and CoViD19 partnership carry significant health economic implications, and these may have a higher impact on the low-middle income economies.
- Further studies, with robust methodology and designs, are required to determine the efficacy and safety of the antidiabetic drugs and combinations in the CoViD19 diabetic subjects.

References

1. International Diabetes Federation. IDF Diabetes Atlas, 9th edn. https://diabetesatlas.org/en/.
2. Diabetes Facts and Figures. https://www.idf.org/aboutdiabetes/what-is-diabetes/facts-figures.html Accessed 12 Dec 2020.
3. Wang D, Hu B, Hu C, Zhu F, Liu X, Zhang J, Wang B, Xiang H, Cheng Z, Xiong Y, Zhao Y. Clinical characteristics of 138 hospitalized patients with 2019 novel coronavirus–infected pneumonia in Wuhan China. Jama. 2020;323(11):1061–69.
4. Grasselli G, Zangrillo A, Zanella A, Antonelli M, Cabrini L, Castelli A, Cereda D, Coluccello A, Foti G, Fumagalli R, Iotti G. Baseline characteristics and outcomes of 1591 patients infected with SARS-CoV-2 admitted to ICUs of the Lombardy Region Italy. JAMA. 2020;323(16):1574–81.
5. Bello-Chavolla OY, Bahena-López JP, Antonio-Villa NE, Vargas-Vázquez A, González-Díaz A, Márquez-Salinas A, Fermín-Martínez CA, Naveja JJ, Aguilar-Salinas CA. Predicting mortality due to SARS-CoV-2: A mechanistic score relating obesity and diabetes to COVID19 outcomes in Mexico. J Clin Endocrinol Metab. 2020;105(8):2752–61.
6. Docherty AB, Harrison EM, Green CA, Hardwick HE, Pius R, Norman L, Holden KA, Read JM, Dondelinger F, Carson G, Merson L. Features of 20 133 UK patients in hospital with CoViD19 using the ISARIC WHO clinical characterisation protocol: prospective observational cohort study. BMJ. 2020;369.
7. Yan Y, Yang Y, Wang F, Ren H, Zhang S, Shi X, Yu X, Dong K. Clinical characteristics and outcomes of patients with severe CoViD19 with diabetes. BMJ Open Diabetes Res Care .2020;8(1):e001343.
8. Richardson S, Hirsch JS, Narasimhan M, Crawford JM, McGinn T, Davidson KW, Barnaby DP, Becker LB, Chelico JD, Cohen SL, Cookingham J. Presenting characteristics, comorbidities, and outcomes among 5700 patients hospitalized with COVID19 in the New York City area. Jama. 2020;323(20):2052–2059.
9. Yang J, Zheng Y, Gou X et al. Prevalence of comorbidities and its effects in coronavirus disease 2019 patients: a systematic review and meta-analysis [published online ahead of print, 2020 Mar 12]. Int J Infect Dis. 2020;94:91–95. https://doi.org/10.1016/j.ijid.2020.03.017.
10. Burki T. COVID19 in Latin America. Lancet Infect Dis. 2020;20(5):547–548.

11. Drucker DJ. Diabetes, obesity, metabolism and SARS-CoV-2 infection: The end of the beginning. Cell Metab. 2021.
12. Kyazze AP, Bongomin F, Ninsiima S, Nattabi G, Nabakka W, Kukunda R, Odanga H, Ssekamatte P, Baluku JB, Kibirige D, Andia-Biraro I. Optimizing diabetes mellitus care to improve COVID19 outcomes in resource-limited settings in Africa. Ther Adv Infect Dis. 2021;8:20499361211009380.
13. Guan WJ, Ni ZY, Hu Y, Liang WH, Ou CQ, He JX, Liu L, Shan H, Lei CL, Hui DS, Du B. Clinical characteristics of coronavirus disease 2019 in China. N Engl J Med. 2020;382 (18):1708–2172.
14. Li B, Yang J, Zhao F, Zhi L, Wang X, Liu L, Bi Z, Zhao Y. Prevalence and impact of cardiovascular metabolic diseases on COVID19 in China. Clin Res Cardiol. 2020;109 (5):531–538. https://doi.org/10.1007/s00392-020-01626-9. Epub 2020 Mar 11. Review. PubMed PMID: 32161990; PubMed Central PMCID: PMC7087935).
15. Yan Y, Yang Y, Wang F, et al. Clinical characteristics and outcomes of patients with severe CoViD19 with diabetes. BMJ Open Diab Res Care. 2020;8:e001343. https://doi.org/10.1136/bmjdrc-2020-001343.
16. Guo W, Li M, Dong Y, et al. Diabetes is a risk factor for the progression and prognosis of COVID-19. Diabetes Metab Res Rev. 2020;e3319. https://doi.org/10.1002/dmrr.3319..
17. Bode B, Garrett V, Messler J, McFarland R, Crowe J, Booth R, Klonoff DC. Glycemic characteristics and clinical outcomes of COVID19 patients hospitalized in the United States. J Diab Sci Technol. 2020;14(4):813–21.
18. Centers for Disease Control and Prevention National Diabetes Statistics Report. Atlanta, GA: Centers for Disease Control and Prevention, US Department of Health and Human Services; 2020.
19. Huang C, Wang Y, Li X, Ren L, Zhao J, Hu Y, Zhang L, Fan G, Xu J, Gu X, Cheng Z. Clinical features of patients infected with 2019 novel coronavirus in Wuhan China. The lancet. 2020;395(10223):497–506.
20. Altonen BL, Arreglado TM, Leroux O, Murray-Ramcharan M, Engdahl R. Characteristics, comorbidities and survival analysis of young adults hospitalized with COVID19 in New York City. PloS one 2020;15(12):e024334.
21. Dennis JM, Mateen BA, Sonabend R, Thomas NJ, Patel KA, Hattersley AT, Denaxas S, McGovern AP, Vollmer SJ. Type 2 diabetes and COVID19–Related mortality in the critical care setting: a national cohort study in England, March–July 2020. Diabetes Care. 2021;44 (1):50–57.
22. McGurnaghan SJ, Weir A, Bishop J, Kennedy S, Blackbourn LA, McAllister DA, Hutchinson S, Caparrotta TM, Mellor J, Jeyam A, O'Reilly JE. Risks of and risk factors for COVID19 disease in people with diabetes: a cohort study of the total population of Scotland. Lancet Diab Endocrinol. 2021;9(2):82–93.
23. Holman N, Knighton P, Kar P, O'Keefe J, Curley M, Weaver A, Barron E, Bakhai C, Khunti K, Wareham NJ, Sattar N. Risk factors for COVID19 related mortality in people with type 1 and type 2 diabetes in England: a population-based cohort study. Lancet Diab Endocrinol. 2020;8(10):823–33.
24. Richardson S, Hirsch JS, Narasimhan M, et al. Presenting Characteristics, Comorbidities, and Outcomes Among 5700 Patients Hospitalized With COVID19 in the New York City Area. JAMA. 2020. https://doi.org/10.1001/jama.2020.6775.
25. Guan WJ, Ni ZY, Hu Y, Liang WH, Ou CQ, He JX, Liu L, Shan H, Lei CL, Hui DS, Du B. Clinical characteristics of coronavirus disease 2019 in China. N. Engl. J Med. 2020;382 (18):1708–20.
26. Li J, Huang DQ, Zou B, Yang H, Hui WZ, Rui F, Yee NTS, Liu C, Nerurkar SN, Kai JCY, Teng MLP. Epidemiology of COVID-19: a systematic review and meta-analysis of clinical characteristics, risk factors, and outcomes. J Med Virol. 2021;93(3):1449–58.
27. Smati S, Tramunt B, Wargny M, Caussy C, Gaborit B, Vatier C, Vergès B, Ancelle D, Amadou C, Bachir LA, Bourron O. Relationship between obesity and severe COVID-19

outcomes in patients with type 2 diabetes: results from the CORONADO study. Diab Obes Metab. 2021;23(2):391–403.
28. Leong A, Cole JB, Brenner LN, Meigs JB, Florez JC, Mercader JM. Cardiometabolic risk factors for COVID19 susceptibility and severity: a Mendelian randomization analysis. PLoS Med. 2021;18(3):e1003553.
29. Yan Y, Yang Y, Wang F, Ren H, Zhang S, Shi X, Yu X, Dong K. Clinical characteristics and outcomes of patients with severe CoViD19 with diabetes. BMJ Open Diab Res Care. 2021;8(1):e001343.
30. Qin JJ, Cheng X, Zhou F, Lei F, Akolkar G, Cai J, Zhang XJ, Blet A, Xie J, Zhang P, Liu YM. Redefining cardiac biomarkers in predicting mortality of inpatients with COVID19. Hypertension. 2020;76(4):1104–12.
31. Piazza G, Campia U, Hurwitz S, Snyder JE, Rizzo SM, Pfeferman MB, Morrison RB, Leiva O, Fanikos J, Nauffal V, Almarzooq Z. Registry of arterial and venous thromboembolic complications in patients with COVID19. J Am Coll Cardiol. 2020;76(18):2060–72.
32. Lee MH, Wong C, Ng CH, Yuen DCW, Lim AYL, Khoo CM. Effects of hyperglycaemia on complications of COVID19: a meta-analysis of observational studies. Diab Obes Metab. 2020.
33. Williamson EJ, Walker AJ, Bhaskaran K, Bacon S, Bates C, Morton CE, Curtis HJ, Mehrkar A, Evans D, Inglesby P, Cockburn J. Factors associated with COVID19-related death using OpenSAFELY. Nature. 2020;584(7821):430–6.
34. Zhu L, She ZG, Cheng X, Qin JJ, Zhang XJ, Cai J, Lei F, Wang H, Xie J, Wang W, Li H. Association of blood glucose control and outcomes in patients with COVID19 and pre-existing type 2 diabetes. Cell Metab. 2020;31(6):1068–77.
35. Xue T, Li Q, Zhang Q, Lin W, Weng J, Li L, Chen G. Blood glucose levels in elderly subjects with type 2 diabetes during COVID19 outbreak: a retrospective study in a single center. 2020.
36. Singh AK, Singh R. Hyperglycemia without diabetes and new-onset diabetes are both associated with poorer outcomes in COVID19. Diab Res Clin Prac. 2020;167:108382.
37. Pal R, Banerjee M, Yadav U, Bhattacharjee S. Clinical profile and outcomes in COVID19 patients with diabetic ketoacidosis: a systematic review of literature. Diab Metab Syndr Clin Res Rev. 2020;14(6):1563–9.
38. Ebekozien O, Agarwal S, Noor N, Neil AAO, Wong JC, Seeherunvong T, Sanchez J, DeSalvo D, Lyons SK, Majidi S, Wood JR. Full Inequities in Diabetic Ketoacidosis among Patients with Type 1 diabetes and COVID19: Data from 52 US Clinical Centers. J Clin Endocrinol Metab. 2021.
39. Kaminska H, Szarpak L, Kosior D, Wieczorek W, Szarpak A, Al-Jeabory M, Gawel W, Gasecka A, Jaguszewski MJ, Jarosz-Chobot P. Impact of diabetes mellitus on in-hospital mortality in adult patients with COVID19: a systematic review and meta-analysis. Acta diabetologica. 2021:1–10.
40. Bain SC, Czernichow S, Bøgelund M, Madsen ME, Yssing C, McMillan AC, Hvid C, Hettiarachchige N, Haagen Panton U. Costs of COVID19 pandemic associated with diabetes in Europe: a health care cost model. Curr Med Res Opin. 2020:1–1.
41. Marik PE, Bellomo R. Stress hyperglycemia: an essential survival response! Critical Care 2013;17(2):1–7.
42. Codo AC, Davanzo GG, de Brito Monteiro L, de Souza GF, Muraro SP, Virgilio-da-Silva JV, Prodonoff JS, Carregari VC, de Biagi Junior CAO, Crunfli F, Restrepo JLJ. Elevated glucose levels favor SARS-CoV-2 infection and monocyte response through a HIF-1α/glycolysis-dependent axis. Cell Metab. 2020;32(3):437–46.
43. Aljada A, Ghanim H, Mohanty P, Syed T, Bandyopadhyay A, Dandona P. Glucose intake induces an increase in activator protein 1 and early growth response 1 binding activities, in the expression of tissue factor and matrix metalloproteinase in mononuclear cells, and in plasma tissue factor and matrix metalloproteinase concentrations. Am J Clin Nutr. 2004;80(1):51–7.

44. Erickson JR, Pereira L, Wang L, Han G, Ferguson A, Dao K, Copeland RJ, Despa F, Hart GW, Ripplinger CM, Bers DM. Diabetic hyperglycaemia activates CaMKII and arrhythmias by O-linked glycosylation. Nature. 2013;502(7471):372–6.
45. Arnold JN, Wormald MR, Sim RB, Rudd PM, Dwek RA. The impact of glycosylation on the biological function and structure of human immunoglobulins. Annu Rev Immunol. 2007;25:21–50.
46. Wang TT. IgG Fc glycosylation in human immunity. Fc Mediated Act Antibodies. 2019: 63–75.
47. Buetti N, Trimboli P, Mazzuchelli T, Priore EL, Balmelli C, Trkola A, Conti M, Martinetti G, Elzi L, Ceschi A, Consonni V. Diabetes mellitus is a risk factor for prolonged SARS-CoV-2 viral shedding in lower respiratory tract samples of critically ill patients. Endocrine. 2020;70(3):454–60.
48. Cano E, Campioli CC, O'Horo JC. Nasopharyngeal SARS-CoV-2 viral RNA shedding in patients with diabetes mellitus. Endocrine. 2021;71(1):26–7.
49. Boonyaratanakornkit J, Morishima C, Selke S, Zamora D, McGuffin S, Shapiro AE, Campbell VL, McClurkan CL, Jing L, Gross R, Liang J. Clinical, laboratory, and temporal predictors of neutralizing antibodies against SARS-CoV-2 among COVID19 convalescent plasma donor candidates. J Clin Invest. 2021;131(3).
50. Zhao J, Yuan Q, Wang H, Liu W, Liao X, Su Y, Wang X, Yuan J, Li T, Li J, Qian S. Antibody responses to SARS-CoV-2 in patients with novel coronavirus disease 2019. Clin Infect Dis. 2020;71(16):2027–34.
51. Lampasona V, Secchi M, Scavini M, Bazzigaluppi E, Brigatti C, Marzinotto I, Davalli A, Caretto A, Laurenzi A, Martinenghi S, Molinari C. Antibody response to multiple antigens of SARS-CoV-2 in patients with diabetes: an observational cohort study. Diabetologia. 2020;63(12):2548–58.
52. Chávez-Reyes J, Escárcega-González CE, Chavira-Suárez E, León-Buitimea A, Vázquez-León P, Morones-Ramírez JR, Villalón CM, Quintanar-Stephano A, Marichal-Cancino BA. Susceptibility for some infectious diseases in patients with diabetes: the key role of glycemia. Front. Public Health. 2021;9.
53. Hulme KD, Yan L, Marshall RJ, Bloxham CJ, Upton KR, Hasnain SZ, Bielefeldt-Ohmann H, Loh Z, Ronacher K, Chew KY, Gallo LA. High glucose levels increase influenza-associated damage to the pulmonary epithelial-endothelial barrier. Elife. 2020;9: e56907.
54. Weynand B, Jonckheere A, Frans A, Rahier J. Diabetes mellitus induces a thickening of the pulmonary basal lamina. Respiration. 1999;66(1):14–9.
55. Sandler M. Is the lung a'target organ'in diabetes mellitus? Arch Intern Med. 1990;150 (7):1385–8.
56. Ruan Q, Yang K, Wang W, Jiang L, Song J. Clinical predictors of mortality due to COVID19 based on an analysis of data of 150 patients from Wuhan China. Intensive Care Med. 2020;46(5):846–8.
57. Xu H, Garcia-Ptacek S, Annetorp M, Bruchfeld A, Cederholm T, Johnson P, Kivipelto M, Metzner C, Religa D, Eriksdotter M. Acute kidney injury and mortality risk in older adults with COVID19. J Nephrol. 2021;34(2):295–304.
58. Raval FM. Nikolajczyk BS. The bidirectional relationship between metabolism and immune responses. Discoveries. 2013;1(1).
59. Berbudi A, Rahmadika N, Tjahjadi AI, Ruslami R. Type 2 diabetes and its impact on the immune system. Curr Diab Rev. 2020;16(5):442.
60. von Känel R, Mills PJ, Dimsdale JE. Short-term hyperglycemia induces lymphopenia and lymphocyte subset redistribution. Life Sci. 2001;69(3):255–62.
61. Fathi N, Rezaei N. Lymphopenia in COVID-19: Therapeutic opportunities. Cell Biol Int. 2020;44 9:1792–97.
62. Cheng Y, Yue L, Wang Z, Zhang J, Xiang G. Hyperglycemia associated with lymphopenia and disease severity of COVID19 in type 2 diabetes mellitus. J Diab Compl. 2021;35 2:107809.

63. Hameed I, Masoodi SR, Mir SA, Nabi M, Ghazanfar K, Ganai BA. Type 2 diabetes mellitus: from a metabolic disorder to an inflammatory condition. World Journal of Diabetes. 2015;6 (4):598.
64. Norata GD, Caligiuri G, Chavakis T, Matarese G, Netea MG, Nicoletti A, O'Neill LA, Marelli-Berg FM. The cellular and molecular basis of translational immunometabolism. Immunity. 2015;43(3):421–34.
65. Shimobayashi M, Albert V, Woelnerhanssen B, Frei IC, Weissenberger D, Meyer-Gerspach AC, Clement N, Moes S, Colombi M, Meier JA, Swierczynska MM. Insulin resistance causes inflammation in adipose tissue. J Clin Investig. 2018;128(4):1538–50.
66. Monteiro R, Azevedo I. Chronic inflammation in obesity and the metabolic syndrome. Mediat Inflamm. 2010.
67. Weisberg SP, McCann D, Desai M, Rosenbaum M, Leibel RL, Ferrante AW. Obesity is associated with macrophage accumulation in adipose tissue. J Clin Investig. 2003;112 (12):1796–808.
68. Odegaard JI, Ricardo-Gonzalez RR, Goforth MH, Morel CR, Subramanian V, Mukundan L, Eagle AR, Vats D, Brombacher F, Ferrante AW, Chawla A. Macrophage-specific PPARγ controls alternative activation and improves insulin resistance. Nature. 2007;447 (7148):1116–20.
69. Hahn WS, Kuzmicic J, Burrill JS, Donoghue MA, Foncea R, Jensen MD, Lavandero S, Arriaga EA, Bernlohr DA. Proinflammatory cytokines differentially regulate adipocyte mitochondrial metabolism, oxidative stress, and dynamics. Am J Physiol Endocrinol Metab. 2014;306(9):E1033–45.
70. Han JM, Patterson SJ, Speck M, Ehses JA, Levings MK. Insulin inhibits IL-10–mediated regulatory T cell function: implications for obesity. J Immunol. 2014;192(2):623–9.
71. Underwood PC, Adler GK. The renin angiotensin aldosterone system and insulin resistance in humans. Curr Hypertens Rep. 2013;15(1):59–70.
72. Muniyappa R, Yavuz S. Metabolic actions of angiotensin II and insulin: a microvascular endothelial balancing act. Mol Cell Endocrinol. 2013;378(1–2):59–69.
73. Goldin A, Beckman JA, Schmidt AM, Creager MA. Advanced glycation end products: sparking the development of diabetic vascular injury. Circulation. 2006;114(6):597–605.
74. Stratmann B, Tschoepe D. Sweet heart–contributions of metabolism in the development of heart failure in diabetes mellitus. Exp Clin Endocrinol Diab. 2008;116 01:S40-S45.
75. Burgeiro A, Fuhrmann A, Cherian S, Espinoza D, Jarak I, Carvalho RA, Loureiro M, Patrício M, Antunes M, Carvalho E. Glucose uptake and lipid metabolism are impaired in epicardial adipose tissue from heart failure patients with or without diabetes. Am J Physiol Endocrinol Metab. 2016;310(7):E550–64.
76. Kelly AS, Barlow SE, Rao G, Inge TH, Hayman LL, Steinberger J, Urbina EM, Ewing LJ, Daniels SR. Severe obesity in children and adolescents: identification, associated health risks, and treatment approaches: a scientific statement from the American Heart Association. Circulation. 2013;128(15):1689–712.
77. Field AE, Cook NR, Gillman MW. Weight status in childhood as a predictor of becoming overweight or hypertensive in early adulthood. Obes Res. 2005;13(1):163–9.
78. Krassas GE, Tzotzas T. Do obese children become obese adults: childhood predictors of adult disease. Pediatr Endocrinol Rev (PER). 2004;1:455–9.
79. Ball GD, Mushquash AR, Keaschuk RA, Ambler KA, Newton AS. Using Intervention Mapping to develop the Parents as Agents of Change (PAC©) intervention for managing pediatric obesity. BMC Res Notes. 2017;10(1):1–11.
80. Cariou B, Hadjadj S, Wargny M, Pichelin M, Al-Salameh A, Allix I, Amadou C, Arnault G, Baudoux F, Bauduceau B, Borot S. Phenotypic characteristics and prognosis of inpatients with COVID19 and diabetes: the CORONADO study. Diabetologia. 2020;63(8):1500–15.
81. Liu F, Long X, Zhang B, Zhang W, Chen X, Zhang Z. ACE2 expression in pancreas may cause pancreatic damage after SARS-CoV-2 infection. Clin Gastroenterol Hepatol. 2020;18 (9):2128.

82. Liu F, Long X, Zou W, Fang M, Wu W, Li W, Zhang B, Zhang W, Chen X, Zhang Z. Highly ACE2 expression in pancreas may cause pancreas damage after SARS-CoV-2 infection (Preprint) medRxiv: 2020. 02.2028.20029181.https://doi.org/10.1101/2020.02.28. 20029181.
83. Hikmet F, Méar L, Edvinsson Å, Micke P, Uhlén M, Lindskog C. The protein expression profile of ACE2 in human tissues. Mol Syst Biol. 2020;16 7:e9610.
84. Müller JA, Groß R, Conzelmann C, Krüger J, Merle U, Steinhart J, Weil T, Koepke L, Bozzo CP, Read C, Fois G. SARS-CoV-2 infects and replicates in cells of the human endocrine and exocrine pancreas. Nat Metab. 2021;3(2):149–65.
85. Fernandez C, Rysa J, Almgren P, Nilsson J, Engstrom G, Orho-Melander M, Ruskoaho H, Melander O. Plasma levels of the proprotein convertase furin and incidence of diabetes and mortality. J Intern Med. 2018;284:377–87.
86. Raj VS, Mou H, Smits SL, Dekkers DH, Müller MA, Dijkman R, Muth D, Demmers JA, Zaki A, Fouchier RA, Thiel V. Dipeptidyl peptidase 4 is a functional receptor for the emerging human coronavirus-EMC. Nature. 2013;495(7440):251–4.
87. Rao S, Lau A, So HC. Exploring diseases/traits and blood proteins causally related to expression of ACE2, the putative receptor of 2019-nCov: A Mendelian randomization analysis (Preprint) medRxiv: 2020.2003.2004.20031237, 2020. doi:https://doi.org/10.1101/ 2020.03.04.20031237.
88. Bindom SM, Lazartigues E. The sweeter side of ACE2: physiological evidence for a role in diabetes. Mol Cell Endocrinol. 2009;302:193–202. https://doi.org/10.1016/j.mce.2008.09. 020.
89. Drucker DJ. Coronavirus infections and type 2 diabetes—shared pathways with therapeutic implications. Endocr Rev. 2020;41(3):457–70.
90. Jie Chee Y, Jia Huey Ng S., Yeoh E. Diabetic ketoacidosis precipitated by CoViD19 in a patient with newly diagnosed diabetes mellitus. Diabetes Res Clin Pract. 2020:108166.
91. Batista DV, de Almeida Vieira CAF, Costa TA, Lima EG. COVID-19-associated euglycemic diabetic ketoacidosis in a patient with type 2 diabetes on SGLT2 inhibitor: a case report. Diabetology International. 2021;12(3):313–316.
92. Cai J, Li H, Zhang C, Chen Z, Liu H, Lei F, Qin JJ, Liu YM, Zhou F, Song X, Zhou J. The neutrophil-to-lymphocyte ratio determines clinical efficacy of corticosteroid therapy in patients with COVID19. Cell Metab. 2021;33(2):258–69.
93. Butler SO, Btaiche IF, Alaniz C. Relationship between hyperglycemia and infection in critically ill patients. Pharmacother J Human Pharmacol Drug Therapy. 2005;25 7:963–976.
94. Sardu C, D'Onofrio N, Balestrieri ML, Barbieri M, Rizzo MR, Messina V, Maggi P, Coppola N, Paolisso G, Marfella R. Outcomes in patients with hyperglycemia affected by COVID19. can we do more on glycemic control? Diabetes Care. 2020;43(7):1408 15.
95. Cameron AR, Morrison VL, Levin D, Mohan M, Forteath C, Beall C, McNeilly AD, Balfour DJ, Savinko T, Wong AK, Viollet B. Anti-inflammatory effects of metformin irrespective of diabetes status. Circ Res. 2016;119(5):652–65.
96. Mulvihill EE, Drucker DJ. Pharmacology, physiology, and mechanisms of action of dipeptidyl peptidase-4 inhibitors. Endocr Rev. 2014;35(6):992–1019.
97. Iacobellis G. COVID19 and diabetes: can DPP4 inhibition play a role?. Diab Res Clin Prac. 2020:162.
98. Bonora BM, Avogaro A, Fadini GP. Disentangling conflicting evidence on DPP-4 inhibitors and outcomes of COVID19: narrative review and meta-analysis. J Endocrinol Invest. 2021:1–8.
99. Drucker DJ. Mechanisms of action and therapeutic application of glucagon-like peptide-1. Cell Metab. 2018;27(4):740–56.
100. Hansen TK, Thiel S, Wouters PJ, Christiansen JS, Van den Berghe G. Intensive insulin therapy exerts antiinflammatory effects in critically ill patients and counteracts the adverse effect of low mannose-binding lectin levels. J Clin Endocrinol Metab. 2003;88(3):1082–8.
101. Yu B, Li C, Sun Y, Wang DW. Insulin treatment is associated with increased mortality in patients with COVID19 and type 2 diabetes. Cell Metab. 2021;33(1):65–77.

102. Hartmann-Boyce J, Morris E, Goyder C, Kinton J, Perring J, Nunan D. Managing diabetes during the COVID19 pandemic. 2020.
103. Luo P, Qiu L, Liu Y, Liu XL, Zheng JL, Xue HY, Liu WH, Liu D, Li J. Metformin treatment was associated with decreased mortality in COVID19 patients with diabetes in a retrospective analysis. Am J Trop Med Hyg. 2020;103(1):69–72.
104. Zangiabadian M, Nejadghaderi SA, Zahmatkesh MM, Hajikhani B, Mirsaeidi M, Nasiri MJ. The efficacy and potential mechanisms of metformin in the treatment of COVID19 in the diabetics: a systematic review. Front Endocrinol. 2021;12:263.
105. Bramante CT, Ingraham NE, Murray TA, Marmor S, Hovertsen S, Gronski J, McNeil C, Feng R, Guzman G, Abdelwahab N, King S. Metformin and risk of mortality in patients hospitalised with COVID19: a retrospective cohort analysis. Lancet Healthy Longevity. 2021;2(1):e34–41.
106. Roussel R, Darmon P, Pichelin M, Goronflot T, Abouleka Y, Ait Bachir L, Allix I, Ancelle D, Barraud S, Bordier L, Carlier A. Use of dipeptidyl peptidase-4 inhibitors and prognosis of COVID-19 in hospitalized patients with type 2 diabetes: A propensity score analysis from the CORONADO study. Diabetes Obes Metab. 2021;23(5):1162–72.
107. Rhee SY, Lee J, Nam H, Kyoung DS, Kim DJ. Effects of a DPP-4 inhibitor and RAS blockade on clinical outcomes of patients with diabetes and COVID19. 2020.
108. Hamblin PS, Wong R, Ekinci EI, Fourlanos S, Shah S, Jones AR, Hare MJ, Calder GL, Epa DS, George EM, Giri R. SGLT2 inhibitors increase the risk of diabetic ketoacidosis developing in the community and during hospital admission. J Clin Endocrinol Metab. 2019;104(8):3077–87.
109. Sainsbury C, Wang J, Gokhale K, Acosta-Mena D, Dhalla S, Byne N, Chandan JS, Anand A, Cooper J, Okoth K, Subramanian A. Sodium-glucose co-transporter-2 inhibitors and susceptibility to COVID-19: A population-based retrospective cohort study. Diabetes Obes Metab. 2021;23(1):263–9.
110. Dapagliflozin in Respiratory Failure in Patients With COVID-19 (DARE-19). Available on: www.clinicalTrials.gov. ClinicalTrials.gov Identifier: NCT04350593. Last updated on: 14 September 2021. Last accessed on 02 January 2022.
111. https://www.cochranelibrary.com/central/doi/10.1002/central/CN-02091756/full%3FhighlightAbstract%3D19%257Ccovid%257Cdiabet%257Cin%257Cdiabetics.
112. Rubino F, Amiel SA, Zimmet P, Alberti G, Bornstein S, Eckel RH, Mingrone G, Boehm B, Cooper ME, Chai Z, Del Prato S. New-onset diabetes in CoViD19. N Engl J Med. 2020;383(8):789–90.
113. https://www.idf.org/aboutdiabetes/what-is-diabetes/CoViD19-and-diabetes/1-CoViD19-and-diabetes.html.

Chapter 17
Obesity and COVID19

Key Questions

- What are the epidemiological links between obesity and CoViD19?
- What is the occurrence of obesity in CoViD19 and how does it vary among populations?
- What is the impact of elevated body mass index and obesity on outcomes in CoViD19?
- What are the implications of obesity and accompanying risk factors in CoViD19 subjects?
- Which pathogenetic mechanisms associated with obesity may impact the course of CoViD19?
- What are limitations in research quality in obesity studies in CoViD19 and what are their implications?

17.1 Introduction

Obesity is a complex multifactorial high-risk chronic condition with significant health economic implications. Global incidence of obesity is high with alarming trends [1, 2]. Obesity is considered to have reached pandemic levels, adversely impacting various regions across the globe. According to estimates, more than 13% of people may have been affected by obesity worldwide. In 2016, more than 1.9 billion adults aged 18 years and older were overweight. Of these, over 650 million adults were obese [3]. By 2025, global obesity prevalence is estimated to reach 18% in men, and surpass 21% in women; severe obesity is likely to surpass 6% in men and 9% in women [2]. Data indicate that over 40% of the population in Europe and the Americas may be obese [4]. According to a more recent analysis, overweight

U. Mallick, *Cardiovascular Complications of COVID-19*,
https://doi.org/10.1007/978-3-030-90065-6_17

and obesity may have affected more than half of the population in Europe [5]. The true prevalence of obesity, however, may be underestimated [6].

According to an estimate, high body mass index (BMI) accounted for 4.0 million deaths globally [7]. Variations in the classification of overweight and obesity with cutoff values of the BMI differing may impact risk estimation [8]. In adults, the classification systems [9] and obesity guidelines [10, 11] define healthy body weight as a BMI between 18.5 and 24.9 kg/m^2, overweight between 25.0 and 29.9 kg/m^2, and obesity $\geq$30 kg/m^2. Obesity is defined as having a body mass index (BMI) equal to or higher than 30 kg/m^2 for all populations worldwide, except for China, where according to the World Health Organization obesity is defined as having a BMI equal to or higher than 27.5 kg/m [12, 13].

The varying prevalence of obesity in different parts of the globe may influence CoViD19 differently. The impact of obesity on CoViD19 morbidity and mortality has been observed across various regions of the globe [14], especially in regions with high obesity burden including the Northern America, Latin America [15] and Europe. According to an analysis of characteristics that may influence CoViD19 outcomes, the African countries appear to have a consistently lower percentage of individuals (18–29%) with BMI > 25, as compared to the Western countries (34–68%), except for South Africa (52%) [16], and have lower CoViD19 impact [17].

Obesity and cardiometabolic risk factors are frequently observed among the CoViD19 subjects in the US. Report based on an analysis of a population-based surveillance program across 14 states representing approximately 10% of the US population, shows that obesity was the second most common underlying condition in the general population, closely the following hypertension, and first among younger individuals aged 18–49, among 1482 hospitalized patients with COVID19, [18]. A similar trend was observed in a case series of 5700 CoViD 19 patients admitted in hospital, in which most common comorbidities were hypertension (56.6%) 3026, obesity (41.7%) 1737, and diabetes (33.8%) 1808 [19].

Obesity is associated with a high burden of comorbidities (Fig. 17.2) and adversely impacts the outcomes of CoViD19 patients (Fig. 17.5). An association of obesity with poor outcomes among patients with cardiovascular or pulmonary diseases or infections, in particular, is well recognized. CoViD19 may precipitate exacerbation of the underlying comorbidities or an induce an exaggerated or disproportional organ dysfunction in obese subjects, for instance the need for invasive mechanical ventilation (Fig. 17.7). An interlink of obesity with death or hospitalization has been reported in previous viral pandemics [20]. Current data also appear to indicate an association of obesity with an increased risk of complications in CoViD19 patients [21], increased risk of ARDS (Fig. 17.4) and higher rate of ICU admissions (Fig. 17.6). According to a prospective observational study of 5279 CoViD19 hospitalized patients, obesity increased the risk for hospitalization and the development of a critical illness in CoViD19 patients. The study also showed a significant association of age, male sex, heart failure, and chronic kidney disease [22]. According to a report based on meta-analysis of 22 studies investigating obesity and CoViD19 outcomes and representing n = 30,141 patients from 7 countries, obesity is associated with an increased likelihood of presenting with more severe CoViD19 symptoms (OR 3.03, 95% CI 1.45–6.28, P = 0.003; 4 studies, n = 974), developing acute respiratory distress syndrome (ARDS; OR 2.89, 95% CI 1.14–7.34, P = 0.025; 2 studies, n = 96), requiring hospitalization (OR 1.68, 95% CI 1.14–1.59, P < 0.001; 4 studies, n = 6611), being admitted to an intensive care unit (ICU; OR 1.35, 95% CI 1.15–1.65, P = 0.001; 9 studies, n = 5298), and undergoing invasive mechanical ventilation (IMV; OR 1.76, 95% CI 1.29–2.40, P < 0.001; 7 studies, n = 1558) compared to non-obese patients. However, obese patients had similar likelihoods of death from CoViD19 as non-obese patients (OR 0.96, 95% CI 0.74–1.25, P = 0.750; 9 studies, n = 20,597) [23, 24]. Furthermore, data also show that patients with pre-existing metabolic fatty liver disease may have 6 times higher risk of developing severe CoViD19 in the presence of coexisting obesity [25]. Other analyses confirm the association of obesity with elevated risks in CoViD19 [26], including the risk of death [27–29] (Fig. 17.8). According to a report based on analyzed data from patients hospitalized with CoViD19 at 88 US hospitals enrolled in the American Heart Association's CoViD19 Cardiovascular Disease Registry, the obese subjects hospitalized with CoViD19 may have a higher risk of critical CoViD19 and in-hospital death and mechanical ventilation, in particular, if young (age ≤ 50 years), and more often have venous thromboembolism and dialysis. Obesity, and, in particular, class III obesity, was overrepresented in the registry in comparison with the US population, with the largest differences among adults ≤ 50 years. Among 7606 patients, in-hospital death or mechanical ventilation occurred in 2109 (27.7%), in-hospital death in 1302 (17.1%), and mechanical ventilation in 1602 (21.1%). After multivariable adjustment, classes I to III obesity were associated with higher risks of in-hospital death or mechanical ventilation (odds ratio, 1.28 [95% CI, 1.09–1.51], 1.57 [1.29–1.91], 1.80 [1.47–2.20], respectively), and class III obesity was associated with a higher risk of in-hospital death (hazard ratio, 1.26 [95% CI, 1.00–1.58]). Overweight and class I to III obese individuals were at higher risk for mechanical ventilation (odds ratio, 1.28 [95% CI, 1.09–1.51], 1.54 [1.29–1.84], 1.88 [1.52–2.32], and 2.08 [1.68–2.58], respectively). Significant BMI by age interactions were seen for all primary end points (P-interaction < 0.05 for each), such that the association of BMI with death or mechanical ventilation was strongest in adults ≤ 50 years, intermediate in adults 51 to 70 years, and weakest in adults >70 years. Severe obesity (BMI ≥ 40 kg/m^2) was associated with an increased risk of in-hospital death only in those ≤ 50 years (hazard ratio, 1.36 [1.01–1.84]) [24]. Moreover, an incremental association of the BMI was observed in related to death in CoViD19 patients; BMI of 30–35, 35–40, and over 40 kg/m^2 was associated with a 1.23-, 1.81- and 2.66-fold increased risk of death respectively [27]. In addition, dysmetabolism is known to favor the development of pulmonary complications [30, 31], and may elevate CoViD19 related risks. According to a prospective observational cohort study of CoViD19 patients, 46% (119/255) of patients had obesity among the critically ill subjects with acute hypoxemic respiratory failure [32]. Data suggest that raised BMI (>35 kg/m^2) increases the odds for requiring invasive ventilation seven times when compared with patients with lower BMI (<25 kg/m^2) [33, 34]. Similar associations may be observed in the relationship between obesity, cardiovascular, metabolic, or prothrombotic conditions and CoViD19. Raised BMI is a potent risk factor for cardiovascular diseases [35]. Concomitant presence of other risk factors such as diabetes mellitus, hypertension or others may aggravate risks among obese subjects with CoViD19. An elevated burden of cardiometabolic risk factors as observed in studies showing an increased association of hypertension (56.6%) 30,265,700, obesity (41.7%) 1737/5700, and diabetes (33.8%) 1808/5700 in CoViD19 hospitalized subjects [19], may increase the probability of CoViD19 related complications. In a restrospective analysis report of 1965 patients with type 2 diabetes mellitus (T2D) and CoViD19, clinical characteristics and CoViD19–related outcomes (i.e. intubation for mechanical ventilation [IMV], death and discharge by day 7 [D7]) were analysed according to BMI status. Increased BMI was found to heighten the criticality of the CoViD19 and the risk of death in diabetic subjects [36], which was consistent with the incremental value of the BMI: for overweight (odds ratio (OR) 1.65 [1.05–2.59]), class I obesity (OR 1.93 [1.19–3.14]) and class II/III obesity (OR 1.98 [1.11–3.52]), although the association was not confirmed in patients >75 years of age. The study concluded that overweight and obesity are associated with poor early prognosis in patients with T2D hospitalized for CoViD19 [37]. Analysis of the autopsy reports of 23 patients with CoViD19 from 5 centers in the US, showed a high burden of thrombotic disease with major involvement of the lungs and heart. All 3 patients with evidence of chronic cardiac enlargement had elevated BMI (BMIs of 33.8, 51.65, and 35.2 kg/m^2) [38].

The association of CoViD19 with older age individuals is well recognized, however studies show variability in association of age with CoViD19 in obese subjects. Studies have shown an association of obesity in younger subjects and CoViD19, with a significant risk associated with obesity in the younger subjects. Indications exist that overweight and obese patients with SARSCoV2 pneumonia, maybe younger than patients with normal weight [39]. Studies further indicate that obese patients, in particular, if young (age $\leq$ 50 years), are more likely to be hospitalized with CoViD19, and are at higher risk of in-hospital death or mechanical ventilation [24]. A large retrospective analysis of 6916 SARS CoV2 positive patients reporting risks associated with death, revealed a significant association of younger age and male gender. The study further indicated a leading role of severe obesity over the correlated risk factors [28].

The although several epidemiological studies provide a decent description of the association of subjects with elevated BMI and obesity with CoViD19, several inconsistencies may cloud the data quality, especially poor definitions of obesity and associated conditions. The inherent weaknesses of the study designs such as observation, or retrospective nature, may generate weaknesses that may compromise the validity of the results. CoViD19 pandemic may have limited the possibility of conducting well powered and well-conducted prospective studies with robust outcomes. CoViD19 is a heterogeneous condition with significant analytical and design challenges, and requires a complex approach during the research. The serious risk of confounding in CoViD19 may significantly compromise the results. A careful approach is needed in the interpretation of the data, especially related to the outcomes, or studies describing the causal relationship of obesity with CoViD19 and complications.

17.2 Pathogenetic Links – Obesity and CoViD19

A complex of risk factors known for their disease and mortality burden tag obesity and may complicate CoViD19 (Figs. 17.1 and 17.3). Conditions such as diabetes, kidney, and respiratory disease, are frequently found in association with obesity and have increased mortality risk [40]. The cardiovascular risk in obese patients or patients with elevated BMI is high, especially in association with hyperlipidemia, and elevated blood pressure [41]. The associations of 17 cardiometabolic traits with CoViD19 susceptibility and severity were evaluated using 2-sample Mendelian randomization (MR) analyses. The authors suggested that obesity-related cardiometabolic diseases (type 2 diabetes, chronic kidney disease, stroke, and coronary heart disease), may be mediators of the relationship between body mass index and higher risk of hospitalization for COVID19 [42]. The lower lung volumes and respiratory muscle strength, with impaired gas exchange, reflect altered pulmonary mechanics and ventilation although mark the obesity [43], several controversies related to the impact of obesity on mortality exist also described as "Obesity paradox" [44]. The role of lung pathology in obese patients in critical CoViD19, appears important [45]. The pathogenetic role of these risk factors in the development of severity of CoViD19 involves intricate immune-inflammatory, thrombogenic, metabolic, and toxic mechanisms that perturb homeostasis, causing tissue and organ dysfunction. The biological, clinical, and functional limitations in obese patients with elevated levels of metabolic and toxic stress, and immune impairment may amplify the adverse impact of CoViD19.

Obesity is a pro-inflammatory condition with significant immune compromise. Higher circulating interleukin 6 and C-reactive protein levels characterize the basal proinflammatory status of obesity. Biochemical changes associated with obesity include tissue hypoxia, high inflammatory burden, the elevation of markers of insulin resistance, hyperglycemia, elevated immune markers, etc. A cascade of

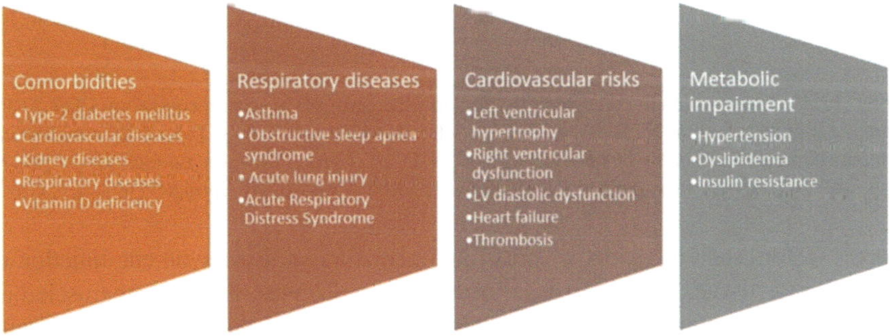

Fig. 17.1 Obesity and other comorbidities. *Source* Figure 1. Aghili, S.M.M., Ebrahimpur, M., Arjmand, B., Shadman, Z., Sani, M.P., Qorbani, M., Larijani, B. and Payab, M., 2021. Obesity in COVID-19 era, implications for mechanisms, comorbidities, and prognosis: a review and meta-analysis. International Journal of Obesity, 45(5), pp. 998–1016. https://www.nature.com/articles/s41366-021-00776-8. By Springer Nature Group

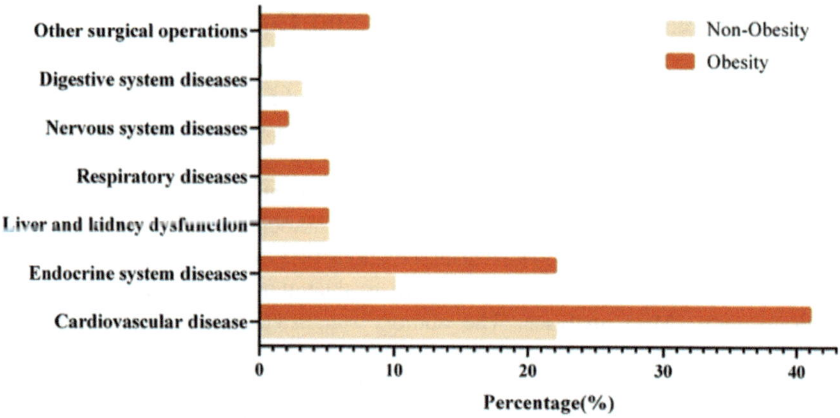

Fig. 17.2 Higher comorbidities in obese versus non-obese. Comparison of basic diseases between obesity and non-obesity patients. *Source* Figure 1. Kang, Z., Luo, S., Gui, Y., Zhou, H., Zhang, Z., Tian, C., Zhou, Q., Wang, Q., Hu, Y., Fan, H. and Hu, D., 2020. Obesity is a potential risk factor contributing to clinical manifestations of COVID-19. International Journal of Obesity, 44(12), pp. 2479–2485. https://www.nature.com/articles/s41366-020-00677-2. By Springer Nature Group

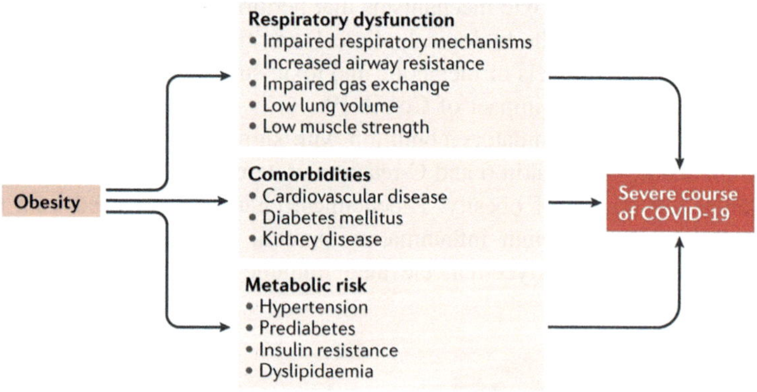

Fig. 17.3 Obesity-related comorbidities and mechanisms of a severe course of COVID-19. *Source* Figure 1. Stefan, N., Birkenfeld, A.L., Schulze, M.B. and Ludwig, D.S., 2020. Obesity and impaired metabolic health in patients with COVID-19. Nature Reviews Endocrinology, 16(7), pp. 341–342. https://www.nature.com/articles/s41574-020-0364-6. By Springer Publishers Group

stress factors such as oxidative stress and mediators shift the synthetic function of the adipose tissue, leading to insulin resistance, diabetes, and pro atherosclerotic cardiovascular complications. The high inflammatory burden associated with decreased circulation, poor oxygenation, augment the inflammatory stress in obesity. These mechanisms contribute to mitochondrial dysfunction, and increased oxidative stress, with an increase in free radicals and reactive oxygen species (ROS), ultimately resulting in exaggerated inflammatory stress [46].

Viral infections may reside in the adipose tissue [47, 48], and be prolonged in obese patients [49]. The adipose tissue has also been proposed to act as a reservoir for the SARS CoV2 [50], especially due to the ACE2 related tropism [51]. According to a report, obese CoViD19 subjects require longer hospitalization, more intensive and longer oxygen treatment, and they may have longer SARSCOV2 shedding [52]. The associations of 17 cardiometabolic traits with CoViD19 susceptibility and severity were evaluated using 2-sample Mendelian randomization (MR) analyses. The authors concluded that genetic evidence supports the higher BMI as a causal risk factor for CoViD19 susceptibility and severity [42].

Various studies confirm higher levels of inflammatory markers in obese CoViD19 subjects, including circulating ferritin, C-reactive protein (CRP), and tumor necrosis factor-α (TNF-α) on admission, and their impact on the severity of the viral disease [52, 53]. The CoViD19 associated hyperimmune reactions marked by significantly increased IL-6 levels are known to be directly proportional to the viral load and disease severity [54, 55]. Increased levels of pro-inflammatory cytokines are observed in obese patients, with a correlation between the increased IL-6 activity and the degree of obesity [56, 57].

Obesity is associated with impaired innate and adaptive immune responses. In obesity, adipose tissue accompanies proinflammatory mechanisms, with elevated cytokines and particularly adipokines, dysregulated tissue leukocyte expression, and inflammatory macrophage (and innate lymphoid) subsets replace tissue regulatory (M2) phenotypic cells. The inflammatory cytokines such as TNF-α, IL-1, IL-6, are main cytokines derived from the adipose tissue [58].

Dysfunctional immune responses in obese individuals may accentuate the SARSCoV2 pathogenicity. Macrophages regulate initiation and resolution of inflammation and tissue maintenance, and T cells, determine key antiviral defense. Raised BMI is corelated with number of macrophages, with macrophages representing as much as 25% of adipocyte cell numbers [59]. The "T cells" play an active role in obesity-related adipose tissue inflammation [60].

Impaired immune responses in patients with obesity may augment CoViD19 related immune irregularities. Data suggest that CoViD19 studies investigating immune responses did not detect meaningful differences in binding or neutralizing antibodies, T cell activity, or other functional humoral measures by BMI [61], although significant alterations in chronic inflammation, particularly driven by persistent innate immune response have been observed in obesity and CoViD19 settings [62]. Viral sensing delays may be an important cause [63]. SARS CoV2 immune response assessment accompanies challenges in assay standardization. The differences in antigen recognition, sensitivity, and specificity among the assays may impact the accuracy of the tests.

A dysregulated immune response in CoViD19 patients is marked by macrophage activation and T cell depletion [64, 65]. Leptin resistance [66], and mechanisms related to the adipose tissue macrophage, and lymphocyte dysfunction [67–69] may have pathogenetic implications in CoViD19. Leptin, an adipose tissue secretory cytokine and a key regulator of nutritional state and metabolism, is a modulator of immune system activation and innate-adaptive immune response that exerts positive effects on maturation, development, and function of B cells [70, 71]. Increased leptin resistance in obese patients [66] with elevated leptin levels may increase risks associated with the viral disease via alterations of the lymphocytes, and inhibition of CD8+ T cell response, and impaired memory T cell response. Reduced leptin response may be associated with adverse outcome in viral disease in obese patients [72]. Obese subjects are known to have inversed leptin/adiponectin ratio [73]. Adiponectin is a promotor of insulin sensitivity and anti-inflammatory activities with a protective impact on the vasculature, and heart. The adiponectin levels may be negatively impacted due to the hyper-immune inflammatory reactions associated with the severe COVID19. Exaggerated release of pro-inflammatory cytokines in COVID19 such as IL-6, TNF-alpha that also inhibits adiponectin [74], may contribute towards risk in CoViD19 patients with obesity.

Variations in the visceral and subcutaneous body fats have been linked with differences in cardiovascular risk [75]. White adipose tissue (WAT) produces numerous proinflammatory and pro-atherogenic cytokines and chemokines, Reports suggest that epicardial adipose tissue (EAT), a source of adipokines (including pro-inflammatory mediators) and harbor of ACE2, already recognized in association with elevated BMI and obesity, may play an important role in the cardiac complications in CoViD19 [76, 77]. Furthermore, the amount of EAT correlates with insulin resistance, metabolic syndrome [78], and cardiovascular diseases [75]. Viral-induced dysregulation of metabolic and vasoactive mechanisms may facilitate this process. Dysregulated RAS in CoViD19 may augment already depleted and dysfunctional counter-regulatory angiotensin-converting enzyme 2 Mas receptor axis in obese patients, and therefore may worsen the epicardial adipose tissue inflammation [77].

Obesity and vascular risk are interconnected. An increase in inflammation in perivascular adipose tissue may elevate coronary vascular risk [79, 80]. Reports suggest a possible link between the elevated B lymphocytes and macrophages in the perivascular adipose tissue may reflect increased vascular plaque instability [81]. An increased vascular risk in obese patients may contribute to an elevated risk of cardiovascular complications observed in association with obesity and CoViD19 including acute coronary syndromes.

Obesity accompanies an increased hypercoagulability and hypofibrinolytic activity and has an elevated venous and arterial thrombotic disease burden. CoViD19 patients, despite anticoagulation, may develop life-threatening prothrombotic complications [82]. Several mechanisms such as elevated expression of the prothrombotic molecules plasminogen activator inhibitor-1 [83], tissue factor (TF) [84], increased platelet activation [85], and others such as FVII [86], thrombin and antithrombin complexes (TAT) [87] contribute towards the obesity-associated prothrombotic inclinations, although the elevation in anti-thrombotic factors, such as tissue-type plasminogen activator (tPA) and protein C, have been described in obese subjects, which may be reactive [86]. CoViD19 is highly thrombogenic with significant therapeutic implications [88]. Prolonged activated partial thromboplastin time (APTT), delayed prothrombin time (PT), higher D-dimer and fibrin degradation products (FDP) levels, increased thrombin-antithrombin (TAT) complex, and decreased antithrombin (AT) are observed in CoViD19 patients [89], with CRP and D Dimers, among the obese subjects, associated with worse clinical outcomes [53]. Studies have also shown elevated fibrinogen, factor VIII (FVIII), von Willebrand factor levels, positive lupus anticoagulant, and antiphospholipid antibodies in critical CoViD19 patients [82], and elevated indicators of hypofibrinolytic activity such as plasminogen activator inhibitor-1 (PAI-1) levels and thrombin activatable fibrinolysis inhibitor (TAFI) and tissue plasminogen activator (tPA) [90]. The hemostatic dysfunction in CoViD19 appears to be a result of direct SARS CoV2 related mechanisms including SARS COV2-platelet interaction leading to platelet activation, or viral-induced inflammation led fibrinogen elevations via IL-6, endothelial activation, subsequently leading to tissue factor and contact activation pathways of the coagulation cascade further potentiating a hyper-coagulable state [91]. Mechanisms related to direct SARS COV2-endothelial injury have also been described [23]. Endothelial dysfunction in obese subjects, thrombo-inflammatory pathways, and immune dysregulation, are among salient mechanisms that determine the interplay and dynamics of coagulability augment the risk of thrombotic complication in obese patients who develop CoViD19. The balance between coagulation and fibrinolysis is altered in critical CoViD19 subjects [90]. Elevated levels of plasminogen activator inhibitor that is shed by the endothelial cells, may be linked with obesity and thrombotic cerebrovascular diseases [83]. The role of obesity in the alteration in the hemostatic balance in CoViD19 patients needs to be further explored.

Higher risk in the younger obese patients as compared to the older subjects with CoViD19 although requires further determination may reflect differential dynamics of the underlying risk factors associated with age. The all-cause relative risk of death associated with increasing BMI decreases with age [92]. A multitude of risk factors accompany older age that increases the risk of CoViD19, however, the decline in the adiposity with age, an increased cardiovascular vulnerability, immune-aging aspects, physical and psychological fitness, and several other biological and socio-economic factors, or even factors related to bias in the provision of healthcare may drive the risks.

17.3 Summary

Adipose tissue is a complex multifunctional structure, with an intense immune metabolic profile, and pleiotropic activities, and plays a vital role in endocrine, and immune functions. The structure is enriched not only with adipocytes but also immune cells that contribute to these functions, as well as several other vascular and regulatory processes. Excessive adiposity leads to a pathologic state. Obesity is a risk factor for multiple cardiovascular diseases, chronic pulmonary disorders, prothrombotic diseases, malignancies, and cerebrovascular diseases. Raised BMI and obesity appear to be closely associated with CoViD19, with increased severity of the disease as well as greater risk of complications. The burden of comorbidities associated with obesity including cardiovascular, metabolic, respiratory, and immune dysfunctions, are key high-risk elements that may compromise individual fitness thereby increased predisposition towards CoViD19 severity and the related risks. Geographical variations in the distribution of obesity across the globe may variably impact the CoViD19 outcomes across the populations and must be further explored.

Analysis of pathogenetic mechanisms involved in the development of obesity-related complications, reveals multiple mechanisms and pathways that may explain the strong CoViD19 -obesity interlink. Adipose inflammation significantly contributes towards cardiometabolic diseases, and metabolic risk factors not only promote cardiovascular diseases but also increase the burden of the morbidity related to cardiovascular diseases and increase mortality. Viral diseases are known for higher affinity for individuals with elevated BMI and may be prolonged in obese patients. Enhanced symptomatology (fever, myalgia, chills, and other compatible symptoms) in obese CoViD19 patients has been reported [61]. Whether obesity determines an increased risk of developing CoViD19 is not known. However, the risk of critical disease and worse outcomes in CoViD19 patients with obesity, appear to be important. It is not known whether the adipose tissue acts as a reservoir for SARS CoV2. SARS CoV2's direct interactions with the adipose tissue need to be further explored.

Among several important pathogenetic mechanisms that facilitate poor outcomes of CoViD19 in obese subjects, immune impairments that also weaken the antiviral defense mechanisms play an important role. Dysfunctional innate and adaptive immune responses in obesity, favor the critical viral disease. In obese subjects, the underlying immune-inflammatory dysfunction is like to further augment the imbalance in the cytokine response observed in CoViD19 resulting in hyper

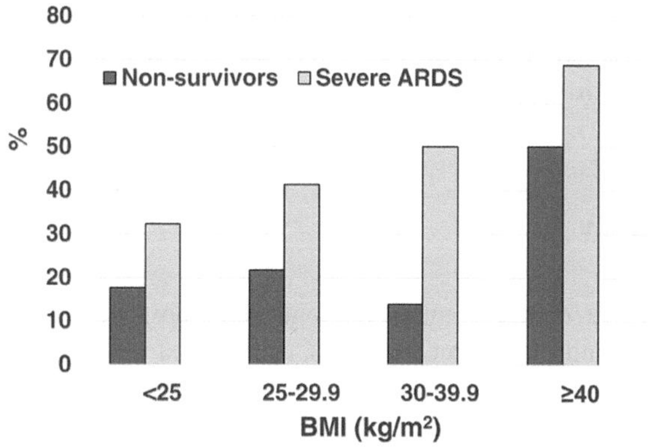

Fig. 17.4 Mortality rate (%) and prevalence of severe ARDS (%) according to BMI (kg/m^2) categories. *Source* Figure 1 Dana, R., Bannay, A., Bourst, P., Ziegler, C., Losser, M.R., Gibot, S., Levy, B., Audibert, G. and Ziegler, O., 2021. Obesity and mortality in critically ill COVID-19 patients with respiratory failure. International Journal of Obesity, pp. 1–10. https://www.nature.com/articles/s41366-021-00872-9. By Springer Nature Group

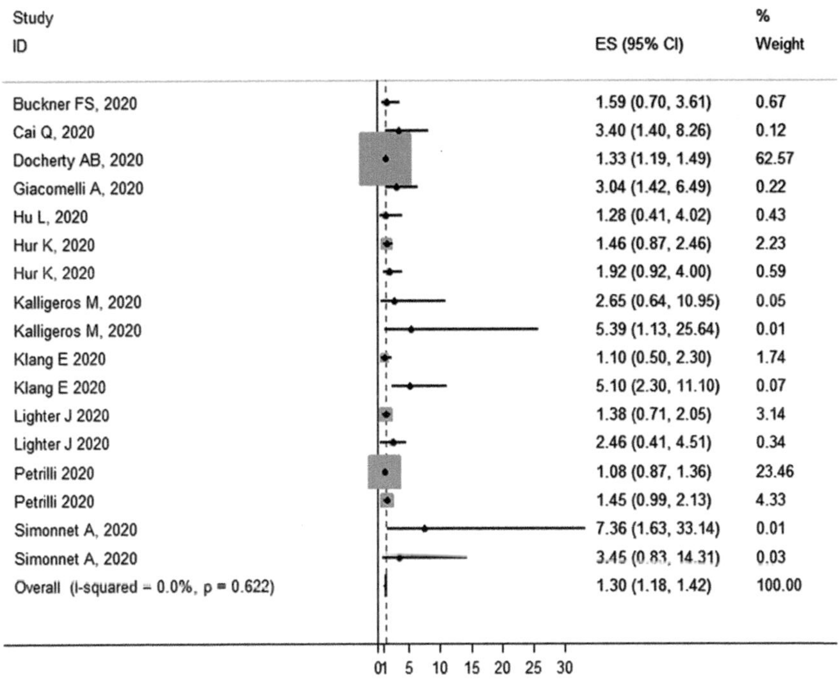

Fig. 17.5 A Forest-plot showing the association between obesity and poor outcome (95% CI 95% confidence interval). In a meta-analysis of 17 CoViD19 studies and obesity, obesity (BMI $\geq$ 30) was associated with poor outcome (OR: 1.297 [1.178–1.416], $p < 0.001$; I2: 0.0%, heterogeneity = 13.69). *Source* Figure 3a. Aghili, S.M.M., Ebrahimpur, M., Arjmand, B., Shadman, Z., Sani, M.P., Qorbani, M., Larijani, B. and Payab, M., 2021. Obesity in COVID-19 era, implications for mechanisms, comorbidities, and prognosis: a review and meta-analysis. International Journal of Obesity, 45(5), pp. 998–1016. https://www.nature.com/articles/s41366-021-00776-8. By Springer Nature Group

immune-inflammation. These mechanisms have a further deleterious impact on the vasculature, the coagulation system, and hemostasis. Inflammatory immune reactions. Increased visceral fat is associated with a higher risk of cardiovascular complications. Interlinks between cardiac and vascular risk and the perivascular and epicardial adipose tissues have been described. The epicardial adipose tissue and cardiac interactions involving immune, RAS, and other mechanisms explain the development of cardiac illnesses in obese patients. Dysregulation of these mechanisms in association with CoViD19 may explain the risks associated with obesity in CoViD19. There is growing evidence that inflammation is a key pathogenetic player in cardiovascular diseases and metabolic disorders including obesity and diabetes, a mechanism that is a frontrunner in severe and complicated CoViD19. Further research is needed to define the exact mechanisms responsible for interlinking obesity and CoViD19.

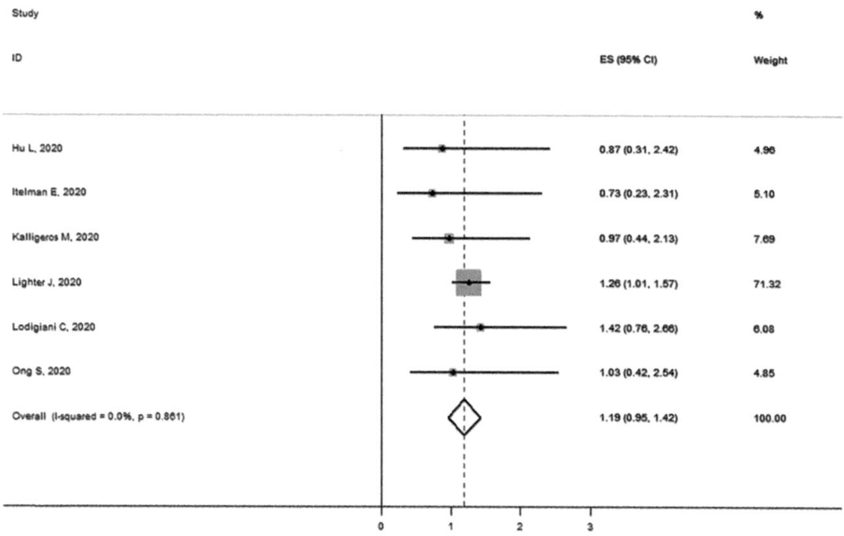

Fig. 17.6 Forest-plot showing lack of association between obesity and intensive care unit (ICU) admissions in CoViD19 (95% CI 95% confidence interval). In a meta-analysis of 17 CoViD19 studies and obesity, obesity (BMI $\geq$ 30) was not associated with ICU admission, and obesity did not significantly increase the ICU admission (OR: 1.189 [0.955–1.424], I2: 0.0%, heterogeneity = 1.92). *Source* Figure 3b. Aghili, S.M.M., Ebrahimpur, M., Arjmand, B., Shadman, Z., Sani, M.P., Qorbani, M., Larijani, B. and Payab, M., 2021. Obesity in COVID-19 era, implications for mechanisms, comorbidities, and prognosis: a review and meta-analysis. International Journal of Obesity, 45(5), pp. 998–1016. https://www.nature.com/articles/s41366-021-00776-8. By Springer Nature Group

Obese patients with CoVi19 may face increased challenges in the management, treatment response, prognosis, and outcomes. Implications of the metabolic, dietary, and lifestyle, genetic, iatrogenic, and psychosocial intricacies, further add to the complexities in understanding the risks associated with obesity, and its management. The compromised pulmonary mechanics with reduced lung vital capacity and functional capacity in obese patients may further aggravate CoViD19 lung injury. Reduced lung capacity aggravates an already diminished efficiency of ventilation in obese patients with complicated CoViD19 needing invasive support. The challenges related to the clinical, pathogenetic, psychosocial, and pharmacological factors in the management of obesity, in association with CoViD19, must be better understood. An aggressive approach is warranted when treating the obese patients with CoViD19, in special patients with a higher degree of obesity.

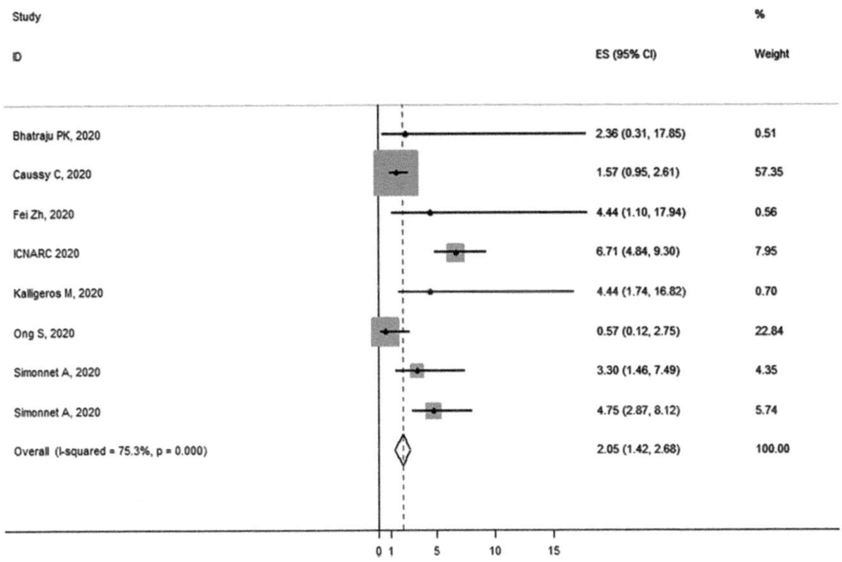

Fig. 17.7 Forest-plot showing the association between obesity and invasive mechanical ventilation (IMV) in CoViD19 (95% CI 95% confidence interval). In a meta-analysis of 17 CoViD19 studies and obesity, obesity (BMI $\geq$ 30) was associated with invasive mechanical ventilation (OR: 2.049 [1.420–2.678], I2: 75.3%, heterogeneity = 28.34). *Source* Figure 3c. S.M. M., Ebrahimpur, M., Arjmand, B., Shadman, Z., Sani, M.P., Qorbani, M., Larijani, B. and Payab, M., 2021. Obesity in COVID-19 era, implications for mechanisms, comorbidities, and prognosis: a review and meta-analysis. International Journal of Obesity, 45(5), pp. 998–1016. https://www.nature.com/articles/s41366-021-00776-8. By Springer Nature Group

In essence, obesity and CoViD19 have a close association. However, a better understanding of the epidemiological, clinical, pathogenetic, and management aspects of obesity is needed in relation to CoViD19. Although substantial data suggest obesity is a risk factor for the severity of CoViD19 and complications and contributes to mortality, data must be interpreted cautiously. The magnitude of the impact of obesity on CoViD19 needs to be further evaluated. The studies exploring obesity in association with CoViD19 have several limitations. The use of different diagnostic criteria for obesity, heterogeneity in the population considered obese, besides other limitations and confounding elements are notable. Studies using robust research methodology and designs must be conducted to explore the intricacies of the association of obesity with CoViD19 and the causal relationships. The pathophysiological mechanisms that define the interaction of heterogenous multi-systemic processes involved in obesity and CoViD19 must be better

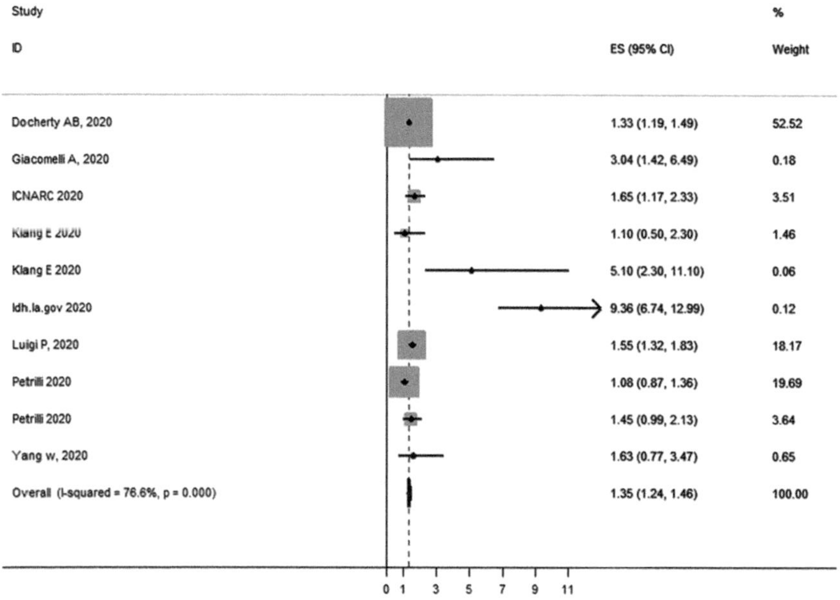

Fig. 17.8 Forest-plot showing the association between obesity and mortality in CoViD19 (95% CI 95% confidence interval). In a meta-analysis of 17 CoViD19 studies and obesity, obesity (BMI $\geq$ 30) was associated with mortality and obesity increased mortality (OR: 1.35 [1.241–1.459], I2: 76.6%, heterogeneity = 38.44). *Source* Figure 3d. Aghili, S.M.M., Ebrahimpur, M., Arjmand, B., Shadman, Z., Sani, M.P., Qorbani, M., Larijani, B. and Payab, M., 2021. Obesity in COVID-19 era, implications for mechanisms, comorbidities, and prognosis: a review and meta-analysis. International Journal of Obesity, 45(5), pp. 998–1016. https://www.nature.com/articles/s41366-021-00776-8. By Springer Nature Group

understood at the molecular levels. Complexities related to the highly prevalent special sub-population-group of patients with raised BMI and obesity at risk or with CoViD19 warrant aggressive and robust exploration, implementation of advanced preventive measures, and improved management and treatment strategies. Such efforts will facilitate the development of risk assessment strategies, and the development of better guidance for the clinicians treating vulnerable groups and help to make informed decisions.

Summary Box

- Obesity is a highly prevalent condition with significant geographical variations across the globe, and reflects a high disease burden with CoViD19.
- Obesity is associated with critical CoViD19 disease and a high risk of complications.
- Obese patients may have more severe symptoms, prolonged hospital delays, and prolong viral shedding in CoViD19.
- The intensity of the inflammatory markers is higher among obese CoViD19 subjects.
- Innate immune and inflammatory response appears to be predominantly elevated among obese subjects with CoViD19.
- Mechanisms involved in hypercoagulability and prothrombotic state in CoViD19 appear to have commonalities in obesity-related prothrombotic activities.
- Obesity often accompanies chronic cardiometabolic risk factors, which enhance potential risks with CoViD19.
- Compromised cardiorespiratory fitness in obese subjects may considerably elevate CoViD19 risks.
- Obese patients are more likely to need critical and invasive care and often face complex management challenges.
- Improved preventive and therapeutic interventions must be designed in patients with raised BMI and obesity at risk or with CoViD19.
- Studies investigating obesity in CoViD19 may be subject to confounding due to existing variations in the definition of obesity, heterogeneity associated with obesity, design, and methodological limitations, therefore, a cautious approach is needed in the interpretation of data.

References

1. Abarca-Gómez L, Abdeen ZA, Hamid ZA, Abu-Rmeileh NM, Acosta-Cazares B, Acuin C, Adams RJ, Aekplakorn W, Afsana K, Aguilar-Salinas CA, Agyemang C. Worldwide trends in body-mass index, underweight, overweight, and obesity from 1975 to 2016: a pooled analysis of 2416 population-based measurement studies in 1289 million children, adolescents, and adults. The Lancet. 2017;390(10113):2627–42.
2. NCD Risk Factor Collaboration. Trends in adult body-mass index in 200 countries from 1975 to 2014: a pooled analysis of 1698 population-based measurement studies with 19· 2 million participants. The Lancet, 2016;387(10026):1377–1396.
3. https://www.who.int/news-room/fact-sheets/detail/obesity-and-overweight.
4. Torres-Gil FM, Suh EH, Angel J. Working across borders: the social and policy implications of aging in the Americas. 2013.

5. Marques A, Peralta M, Naia A, Loureiro N, de Matos MG. Prevalence of adult overweight and obesity in 20 European countries, 2014. The European Journal of Public Health. 2018;28 (2):295–300.
6. Reilly JJ, El-Hamdouchi A, Diouf A, Monyeki A, Somda SA. Determining the worldwide prevalence of obesity. The Lancet. 2018;391(10132):1773–4.
7. Health Effects of Overweight and Obesity in 195 Countries over 25 Years. The GBD 2015 Obesity Collaborators. N Engl J Med. 2017;377:13–27. https://doi.org/10.1056/NEJMoa1614362.
8. Purnell JQ. Definitions, classification, and epidemiology of obesity. [Updated 2018 Apr 12]. In: Feingold KR, Anawalt B, Boyce A, et al., editors. Endotext [Internet]. South Dartmouth (MA): MDText.com Inc.; 2000. https://www.ncbi.nlm.nih.gov/books/NBK279167/.
9. Obesity: preventing and managing the global epidemic. Report of a WHO consultation. World Health Organ Tech Rep Ser. 2000;894:i–xii, 1–253. PMID: 11234459.
10. Jensen MD, Ryan DH, Apovian CM, Ard JD, Comuzzie AG, Donato KA, Hu FB, Hubbard VS, Jakicic JM, Kushner RF. 2013 AHA/ACC/TOS guideline for the management of overweight and obesity in adults. Circulation. 2014;129(25):S102–38.
11. Clinical guidelines on the identification, evaluation, and treatment of overweight and obesity in adults: executive summary. Expert panel on the identification, evaluation, and treatment of overweight in adults. Am J Clin Nutr. 1998;68(4):899–917. https://doi.org/10.1093/ajcn/68.4.899. PMID: 9771869.
12. de Siqueira JVV, Almeida LG, Zica BO, Brum IB, Barceló A, de Siqueira Galil AG. Impact of obesity on hospitalizations and mortality, due to COVID-19: a systematic review. Obes Res Clin Pract. 2020.
13. Anonymous. Estimating mortality from COVID-19: scientific brief World Health Organization; 2020. https://www.who.int/publications/i/item/WHO-2019-nCoV-Sci-Brief-Mortality-2020.1.
14. Hamed SM, Elkhatib WF, Khairalla AS, Noreddin AM. Global dynamics of SARS-CoV-2 clades and their relation to COVID-19 epidemiology. Sci Rep. 2021;11(1):1–8.
15. Halpern B, Louzada MLDC, Aschner P, Gerchman F, Brajkovich I, Faria-Neto JR, Polanco FE, Montero J, Juliá SMM, Lotufo PA, Franco OH. Obesity and COVID-19 in Latin America: a tragedy of two pandemics—official document of the Latin American Federation of obesity Societies. Obes Rev. 2021;22(3):e13165.
16. Blanton RE, Mock NB, Hiruy HN, Schieffelin JS, Doumbia S, Happi C, Samuels RJ, Oberhelman RA. African resources and the promise of resilience against COVID-19. Am J Trop Med Hyg. 2020;103(2):539.
17. Anjorin AA, Abioye AI, Asowata OE, Soipe A, Kazeem MI, Adesanya IO, Raji MA, Adesanya M, Oke FA, Lawal FJ, Kasali BA. Comorbidities and the COVID-19 pandemic dynamics in Africa. Tropical Med Int Health. 2021;26(1):2–13.
18. Garg S, Kim L, Whitaker M, O'Halloran A, Cummings C, Holstein R, Prill M, Chai SJ, Kirley PD, Alden NB, Kawasaki B. Hospitalization rates and characteristics of patients hospitalized with laboratory-confirmed coronavirus disease 2019—COVID-NET, 14 States, March 1–30, 2020. Morb Mortal Wkly Rep. 2020;69(15):458.
19. Richardson S, Hirsch JS, Narasimhan M, et al. Presenting Characteristics, Comorbidities, and Outcomes Among 5700 Patients Hospitalized With COVID-19 in the New York City Area. JAMA. Published online April 22, 2020. https://doi.org/10.1001/jama.2020.6775.
20. Louie JK, Acosta M, Winter K, Jean C, Gavali S, Schechter R, Vugia D, Harriman K, Matyas B, Glaser CA, Samuel MC. Factors associated with death or hospitalization due to pandemic 2009 influenza A (H1N1) infection in California. JAMA. 2009;302(17):1896–902.
21. Michalakis K, Ilias I. SARS-CoV-2 infection and obesity: common inflammatory and metabolic aspects. Diabetes Metab Syndr. 2020;14(4):469–71. https://doi.org/10.1016/j.dsx.2020.04.033. [Epub ahead of print] PubMed PMID: 32387864; PubMed Central PMCID: PMC7189186.
22. Petrilli CM, Jones SA, Yang J, Rajagopalan H, O'Donnell L, Chernyak Y, Tobin KA, Cerfolio RJ, Francois F, Horwitz LI. Factors associated with hospital admission and critical

illness among 5279 people with coronavirus disease 2019 in New York City: prospective cohort study. BMJ. 2020;369.
23. Hendren NS, de Lemos JA, Ayers C, Das SR, Rao A, Carter S, Rosenblatt A, Walchok J, Omar W, Khera R, Hegde AA. Association of body mass index and age with morbidity and mortality in patients hospitalized with COVID-19: results from the American Heart Association COVID-19 Cardiovascular Disease Registry. Circulation. 2021;143(2):135–44.
24. Zhang X, Lewis AM, Moley JR, Brestoff JR. A systematic review and meta-analysis of obesity and COVID-19 outcomes. Scientific reports. 2021;11(1):1–11.
25. Guan WJ, Ni ZY, Hu Y, Liang WH, Ou CQ, He JX, Liu L, Shan H, Lei CL, Hui DSC. Clinical characteristics of coronavirus disease 2019 in China. N Engl J Med. 2020 [Google Scholar] [Ref list].
26. Yang J, Hu J, Zhu C. Obesity aggravates COVID-19: a systematic review and meta-analysis. J Med Virol. 2021;93(1):257–61.
27. Williamson EJ, Walker AJ, Bhaskaran K, Bacon S, Bates C, Morton CE, Curtis HJ, Mehrkar A, Evans D, Inglesby P, Cockburn J. OpenSAFELY: factors associated with COVID-19 death in 17 million patients. Nature. 2020.
28. Tartof SY, Qian L, Hong V, Wei R, Nadjafi RF, Fischer H, Li Z, Shaw SF, Caparosa SL, Nau CL, Saxena T. Obesity and mortality among patients diagnosed with COVID-19: results from an integrated health care organization. Ann Intern Med. 2020;173(10):773–81.
29. Docherty AB, Harrison EM, Green CA, Hardwick HE, Pius R, Norman L, Holden KA, Read JM, Dondelinger F, Carson G, Merson L. Features of 20 133 UK patients in hospital with covid-19 using the ISARIC WHO Clinical Characterisation Protocol: prospective observational cohort study. BMJ. 2020;369.
30. Michalakis K, Panagiotou G, Ilias I, Pazaitou-Panayiotou K. Obesity and COVID-19: A jigsaw puzzle with still missing pieces. Clin Obes. 2021;11(1):p.e12420.
31. Puig-Domingo M, Marazuela M, Giustina A. COVID-19 and endocrine diseases. A statement from the European Society of Endocrinology. Endocrine. 2020;68(1):2–5.
32. Cummings MJ, Baldwin MR, Abrams D, Jacobson SD, Meyer BJ, Balough EM, Aaron JG, Claassen J, Rabbani LE, Hastie J, Hochman BR. Epidemiology, clinical course, and outcomes of critically ill adults with COVID-19 in New York City: a prospective cohort study. The Lancet. 2020;395(10239):1763–70.
33. Zhou F, Yu T, Du R, Fan G, Liu Y, Liu Z, Xiang J, Wang Y, Song B, Gu X. Clinical course and risk factors for mortality of adult inpatients with COVID-19 in Wuhan, China: a retrospective cohort study. The Lancet. 2020;395(10229):1054–1062. [Google Scholar] [Ref list].
34. Tang N, Bai H, Chen X, Gong J, Li D, Sun Z: Anticoagulant treatment is associated with decreased mortality in severe coronavirus disease 2019 patients with coagulopathy. Journal of Thrombosis and Haemostasis, n/a(n/a). [Ref list].
35. Eckel RH, Grundy SM, Zimmet PZ. The metabolic syndrome. The Lancet. 2005;365 (9468):1415–28.
36. Cariou B, Hadjadj S, Wargny M, Pichelin M, Al-Salameh A, Allix I, Amadou C, Arnault G, Baudoux F, Bauduceau B, Borot S. Phenotypic characteristics and prognosis of inpatients with COVID-19 and diabetes: the CORONADO study. Diabetologia. 2020;63(8):1500–15.
37. Smati S, Tramunt B, Wargny M, Caussy C, Gaborit B, Vatier C, Vergès B, Ancelle D, Amadou C, Bachir LA, Bourron O. Relationship between obesity and severe COVID-19 outcomes in patients with type 2 diabetes: Results from the CORONADO study. Diabetes Obes Metab. 2021;23(2):391–403.
38. Buja LM, Wolf DA, Zhao B, et al. The emerging spectrum of cardiopulmonary pathology of the coronavirus disease 2019 (COVID-19): Report of 3 autopsies from Houston, Texas, and review of autopsy findings from other United States cities [published online ahead of print, 2020 May 7]. Cardiovasc Pathol. 2020;48:107233. https://doi.org/10.1016/j.carpath.2020.107233.
39. Busetto L, Bettini S, Fabris R, Serra R, Dal Pra C, Maffei P, Rossato M, Fioretto P, Vettor R. Obesity and COVID-19: an Italian snapshot. Obesity. 2020;28(9):1600–5.

40. Prospective Studies Collaboration. Body-mass index and cause-specific mortality in 900 000 adults: collaborative analyses of 57 prospective studies. The Lancet. 2009;373(9669):1083–96.
41. Frühbeck G, Toplak H, Woodward E, Yumuk V, Maislos M, Oppert JM. Obesity: the gateway to ill health-an EASO position statement on a rising public health, clinical and scientific challenge in Europe. Obes Facts. 2013;6(2):117–20.
42. Leong A, Cole JB, Brenner LN, Meigs JB, Florez JC, Mercader JM. Cardiometabolic risk factors for COVID-19 susceptibility and severity: a Mendelian randomization analysis. PLoS Med. 2021;18(3):e1003553.
43. Dixon AE, Peters U. The effect of obesity on lung function. Expert Rev Respir Med. 2018;12 (9):755–67.
44. Nie W, Zhang Y, Jee SH, Jung KJ, Li B, Xiu Q. Obesity survival paradox in pneumonia: a meta-analysis. BMC Med. 2014;12(1):1–9.
45. Simonnet A, Chetboun M, Poissy J, Raverdy V, Noulette J, Duhamel A, Labreuche J, Mathieu D, Pattou F, Jourdain M, LICORN and the Lille COVID-19 and Obesity Study Group. High prevalence of obesity in severe acute respiratory syndrome coronavirus-2 (SARS-CoV-2) requiring invasive mechanical ventilation. Obesity. 2020;28(7):1195–1199.
46. Ellulu MS, Patimah I, Khaza'ai H, Rahmat A, Abed Y. Obesity and inflammation: the linking mechanism and the complications. Arch Med Sci. 2017;13:851–63. [PMC free article] [PubMed] [Google Scholar] [Ref list].
47. Ponterio E, Cangemi R, Mariani S, Casella G, De Cesare A, Trovato FM, Garozzo A, Gnessi L. Adenovirus 36 DNA in human adipose tissue. Int J Obes. 2015;39(12):1761–4.
48. Zwezdaryk KJ, Ferris MB, Strong AL, Morris CA, Bunnell BA, Dhurandhar NV, Gimble JM, Sullivan DE. Human cytomegalovirus infection of human adipose-derived stromal/stem cells restricts differentiation along the adipogenic lineage. Adipocyte. 2016;5(1):53–6.
49. Maier HE, Lopez R, Sanchez N, Ng S, Gresh L, Ojeda S, Burger-Calderon R, Kuan G, Harris E, Balmaseda A, Gordon A. Obesity increases the duration of influenza a virus shedding in adults. J Infect Dis. 2018;218(9):1378–82.
50. Ryan PM, Caplice NM. Is adipose tissue a reservoir for viral spread, immune activation, and cytokine amplification in coronavirus disease 2019? Obesity. 2020;28(7):1191–4.
51. Hoffmann M, Kleine-Weber H, Schroeder S, Krüger N, Herrler T, Erichsen S, Schiergens TS, Herrler G, Wu NH, Nitsche A, Müller MA. SARS-CoV-2 cell entry depends on ACE2 and TMPRSS2 and is blocked by a clinically proven protease inhibitor. Cell. 2020;181(2):271–280.
52. Moriconi D, Masi S, Rebelos E, Virdis A, Manca ML, De Marco S, Taddei S, Nannipieri M. Obesity prolongs the hospital stay in patients affected by COVID-19, and may impact on SARS-COV-2 shedding. Obes Res Clin Pract. 2020;14(3):205–9.
53. McNeill JN, Lau ES, Paniagua SM, Liu EE, Wang JK, Bassett IV, Selvaggi CA, Lubitz SA, Foulkes AS, Ho JE. The role of obesity in inflammatory markers in COVID-19 patients. Obes Res Clin Pract. 2021;15(1):96–9.
54. Chen X, Zhao B, Qu Y, Chen Y, Xiong J, Feng Y, Men D, Huang Q, Liu Y, Yang B, Ding J. Detectable serum SARS-CoV-2 viral load (RNAaemia) is closely correlated with drastically elevated interleukin 6 (IL-6) level in critically ill COVID-19 patients. Clin Infect Dis. 2020.
55. Zhu J, Pang J, Ji P, Zhong Z, Li H, Li B, Zhang J. Elevated interleukin-6 is associated with severity of COVID-19: a meta-analysis. J Med Virol. 2021;93(1):35–7.
56. Hotamisligil GS. Inflammation and metabolic disorders. Nature. 2006;444(7121):860–71.
57. Straub RH, Hense HW, Andus T, Schölmerich J, Riegger GA, Schunkert H. Hormone replacement therapy and interrelation between serum interleukin-6 and body mass index in postmenopausal women: a population-based study. J Clin Endocrinol Metab. 2000;85 (3):1340–4.
58. Kern L, Mittenbühler MJ, Vesting AJ, Ostermann AL, Wunderlich CM, Wunderlich FT. Obesity-induced TNFα and IL-6 signaling: the missing link between obesity and inflammation—driven liver and colorectal cancers. Cancers. 2019;11(1):24.

59. Cancello R, Henegar C, Viguerie N, Taleb S, Poitou C, Rouault C, Coupaye M, Pelloux V, Hugol D, Bouillot JL, Bouloumié A. Reduction of macrophage infiltration and chemoattractant gene expression changes in white adipose tissue of morbidly obese subjects after surgery-induced weight loss. Diabetes. 2005;54(8):2277–86.
60. Chatzigeorgiou A, Karalis KP, Bornstein SR, Chavakis T. Lymphocytes in obesity-related adipose tissue inflammation. Diabetologia. 2012;55(10):2583–92.
61. Nilles EJ, Siddiqui SM, Fischinger S, Bartsch YC, de Saint Aubin M, Zhou G, Gluck M, Berger S, Rhee J, Petersen E, Mormann B. Epidemiological and immunological features of obesity and SARS-CoV-2. medRxiv. 2020.
62. Méry G, Epaulard O, Borel AL, Toussaint B, Le Gouellec A. COVID-19: Underlying Adipokine Storm and Angiotensin 1–7 Umbrella. Front Immunol. 2020;11:1714.
63. McGonagle D, Ramanan AV, Bridgewood C. Immune cartography of macrophage activation syndrome in the COVID-19 era. Nat Rev Rheumatol. 2021:1–13.
64. Qin C, Zhou L, Hu Z, Zhang S, Yang S, Tao Y, Xie C, Ma K, Shang K, Wang W, Tian DS. Dysregulation of immune response in patients with coronavirus 2019 (COVID-19) in Wuhan China. Clin Infect Dis. 2020;71(15):762–8.
65. Izquierdo AG, Crujeiras AB, Casanueva FF, Carreira MC. Leptin, obesity, and leptin resistance: where are we 25 years later? Nutrients. 2019;11(11):2704.
66. Lee BC, Lee J. Cellular and molecular players in adipose tissue inflammation in the development of obesity-induced insulin resistance. Biochimica et Biophysica Acta (BBA)-Mol Basis Dis. 2014;1842(3):446–62.
67. Boutens L, Stienstra R. Adipose tissue macrophages: going off track during obesity. Diabetologia. 2016;59(5).879–94.
68. Misumi I, Starmer J, Uchimura T, Beck MA, Magnuson T, Whitmire JK. Obesity expands a distinct population of T cells in adipose tissue and increases vulnerability to infection. Cell Rep. 2019;27(2):514–24.
69. Francisco V, Pino J, Campos-Cabaleiro V, Ruiz-Fernández C, Mera A, Gonzalez-Gay MA, Gómez R, Gualillo O. Obesity, fat mass and immune system: role for leptin. Front Physiol. 2018;9:640.
70. Procaccini C, Jirillo E, Matarese G. Leptin as an immunomodulator. Mol Aspects Med. 2012;33(1):35–45.
71. Zhang AJ, To KK, Li C, Lau CC, Poon VK, Chan CC. Leptin mediates the pathogenesis of severe 2009 pandemic influenza A (H1N1) infection associated with cytokine dysregulation in mice with diet-induced obesity. J Infect Dis. 2013;207:1270–80. [PubMed] [Google Scholar] [Ref list].
72. Frühbeck G, Catalán V, Rodríguez A, Gómez-Ambrosi J. Adiponectin-leptin ratio: a promising index to estimate adipose tissue dysfunction Relation with obesity associated cardiometabolic risk. Adipocyte. 2018;7(1):57–62.
73. Fang H, Judd RL. Adiponectin regulation and function. Compr Physiol. 2011;8(3):1031–63.
74. Wronska A, Kmiec Z. Structural and biochemical characteristics of various white adipose tissue depots. Acta Physiol. 2012;205(2):194–208.
75. Zhao L. Obesity accompanying COVID-19: the role of epicardial fat. Obesity. 2020;28 (8):1367–1367.
76. Patel VB, Mori J, McLean BA, Basu R, Das SK, Ramprasath T, Parajuli N, Penninger JM, Grant MB, Lopaschuk GD, Oudit GY. ACE2 deficiency worsens epicardial adipose tissue inflammation and cardiac dysfunction in response to diet-induced obesity. Diabetes. 2016;65 (1):85–95.
77. Mazur A, Ostański M, Telega G, Malecka-Tendera E. Is epicardial fat tissue a marker of metabolic syndrome in obese children? Atherosclerosis. 2010;211(2):596–600.
78. Henrichot E, Juge-Aubry CE, Pernin A, Pache JC, Velebit V, Dayer JM, Meda P, Chizzolini C, Meier CA. Production of chemokines by perivascular adipose tissue: a role in the pathogenesis of atherosclerosis? Arterioscler Thromb Vasc Biol. 2005;25(12):2594–9.

79. Srikakulapu P, Upadhye A, Rosenfeld SM, Marshall MA, McSkimming C, Hickman AW, Mauldin IS, Ailawadi G, Lopes MBS, Taylor AM, McNamara CA. Perivascular adipose tissue harbors atheroprotective IgM-producing B cells. Front Physiol. 2017;8:719.
80. Farias-Itao DS, Pasqualucci CA, Nishizawa A, da Silva LFF, Campos FM, Bittencourt MS, da Silva KCS, Leite REP, Grinberg LT, Ferretti-Rebustini REDL, Jacob-Filho W. B lymphocytes and macrophages in the perivascular adipose tissue are associated with coronary atherosclerosis: an autopsy study. J Am Hear Assoc. 2019;8(24):e013793.
81. Helms J, Tacquard C, Severac F, Leonard-Lorant I, Ohana M, Delabranche X, Merdji H, Clere-Jehl R, Schenck M, Gandet FF, Fafi-Kremer S. High risk of thrombosis in patients with severe SARS-CoV-2 infection: a multicenter prospective cohort study. Intensive Care Med. 2020;46(6):1089–98.
82. Chen R, Yan J, Liu P, Wang Z, Wang C. Plasminogen activator inhibitor links obesity and thrombotic cerebrovascular diseases: the roles of PAI-1 and obesity on stroke. Metab Brain Dis. 2017;32(3):667–73.
83. Ayer JG, Song C, Steinbeck K, Celermajer DS, Freedman SB. Increased tissue factor activity in monocytes from obese young adults. Clin Exp Pharmacol Physiol. 2010;37(11):1049–54.
84. Santilli F, Vazzana N, Liani R, Guagnano MT, Davì G. Platelet activation in obesity and metabolic syndrome. Obes Rev. 2012;13(1):27–42.
85. De Pergola G, Pannacciulli N. Coagulation and fibrinolysis abnormalities in obesity. J Endocrinol Invest. 2002;25(10):899–904.
86. Şıklar Z, Öçal G, Berberoğlu M, Hacıhamdioğlu B, Erdeve ŞS, Eğin Y, Akar N. Evaluation of hypercoagulability in obese children with thrombin generation test and microparticle release: effect of metabolic parameters. Clin Appl Thromb Hemost. 2011;17(6):585–9.
87. Bikdeli B, Madhavan MV, Jimenez D, Chuich T, Dreyfus I, Driggin E, Nigoghossian CD, Ageno W, Madjid M, Guo Y, Tang LV. COVID-19 and thrombotic or thromboembolic disease: implications for prevention, antithrombotic therapy, and follow-up: JACC state-of-the-art review. J Am Coll Cardiol. 2020;75(23):2950–73.
88. Tang N, Li D, Wang X, Sun Z. Abnormal coagulation parameters are associated with poor prognosis in patients with novel coronavirus pneumonia. J Thromb Haemost. 2020;18 (4):844–7.
89. Nougier C, Benoit R, Simon M, Desmurs-Clavel H, Marcotte G, Argaud L, David JS, Bonnet A, Negrier C, Dargaud Y. Hypofibrinolytic state and high thrombin generation may play a major role in SARS-COV2 associated thrombosis. J Thromb Haemost. 2020;18 (9):2215–9.
90. Page EM, Ariëns RA. Mechanisms of thrombosis and cardiovascular complications in COVID-19. Thromb Res. 2021.
91. Varga Z, Flammer AJ, Steiger P, Haberecker M, Andermatt R, Zinkernagel A, Mehra MR, Scholkmann F, Schüpbach R, Ruschitzka F, Moch H. Electron microscopy of SARS-CoV-2: a challenging task–authors' reply. The Lancet. 2020;395(10238):e100.
92. Villareal DT, Apovian CM, Kushner RF, Klein S. Obesity in older adults: technical review and position statement of the American Society for Nutrition and NAASO, The Obesity Society. Am J Clin Nutr. 2005;82(5):923–34.

Chapter 18
The Older Age Adults and COVID19

Key Questions

- What are the epidemiological links between older age and CoViD19?
- Is there an association between critical CoViD19 and older age?
- Are older age adults at a higher risk of CoViD19 related cardiovascular complications?–How does older age impact the outcomes of CoViD19? What are the trends in fatality, worldwide, among the older age individuals?
- Do serum biomarkers have a role in determining CoViD19 related risks in the older age group?
- Which pathophysiological factors associated with age may contribute towards the severity of C0ViD19?
- During the CoViD19 pandemic, which age-associated challenges may be faced by the care providers, and the care receivers?

18.1 Epidemiology

Advanced age and male gender are considered as important risk factors for cardiovascular diseases amongst several other classical cardiovascular and metabolic factors commonly observed in association with CoViD19. Among these factors, older age appears to adversely impact the outcomes of CoViD19. Higher prevalence of CoViD19 complications has been reported in the older age group, with a more severe course, and higher rates of complications of COVID19 including mortality [1] (Fig. 18.1). The critical CoViD19 often requires advanced treatments, often poorly tolerated by older age adults. Data indicate that older age adults are less likely to survive on the invasive treatments [2]. Furthermore, the older

U. Mallick, *Cardiovascular Complications of COVID-19*,
https://doi.org/10.1007/978-3-030-90065-6_18

COViD19 patients may have a more atypical presentation that may include functional decline, acute mental change, and hypotension [3–5], and higher readmission rates [2]. The impact of the viral disease may be prolonged in older age adults. According to an analysis of data from 4,182 incident cases of COVID19 in which individuals self-reported their symptoms prospectively in the COVID Symptom Study app, older age and female sex were associated with long CoViD19 (4 weeks or 8 weeks threshold for defining the duration of long CoViD19) [6]. Furthermore, the susceptibility of older people to SARS CoV2 infection may be high and the gender disparity may be an important association. Analyses indicate that older people may be at higher risk of being infected with SARS CoV2 [1, 7], and the virus is more likely to infect older men with comorbidities [8]. The epidemiological dynamics of the association of older age adults and CoViD19, and the impact on outcomes, are further discussed in this chapter, along with salient pathogenetic features and possible associated mechanisms.

18.1.1 Oder Age and CoViD19 Criticality

According to a Centers for Disease Control and Prevention of the US (CDC) report, individuals older than age 65 made up 31% of COVID19 infections, 45% of hospitalizations, 53% of intensive care unit (ICU) admissions, and 80% of deaths caused by the infection [9]. According to a UK based prospective observational study involving 20,133 hospital in-patients with CoViD19, the median age of patients admitted to hospital with CoViD19, or with a diagnosis of CoViD19 made in the hospital, was 73 years (interquartile range 58–82, range 0–104) [1].

Several studies indicate the association of older age with critical disease and this is also observed among CoViD19 subjects. In a case series describing characteristics and early outcomes of 5700 hospitalized CoViD19 patients in New York, median age was 63 years [interquartile range {IQR}, 52–75; range, 0–107 years], 39.7% were females, and severe patients admitted in ICU (373 (14.2%) were older (median age, 68 years [IQR, 56–78]; 33.5% female) than the overall cohort [2]. According to a report of retrospective case series of 138 CoViD19 patients (median age 56 years (IQR, 42–68; range, 22–92 years), 75 (54.3%) males), the patients requiring ICU care (n = 36) were significantly older (median age, 66 years [IQR, 57–78] vs who did not receive ICU care (n = 102), 51 years [IQR, 37–62] $P < 0.001$, and were more likely to have underlying comorbidities [10]. A meta-analysis report of 212 studies involving 281461 individuals with CoViD19 from 11 countries/regions, revealed that individuals with severe disease were significantly older (60.4 years, 95% CI: 57.8–63.1) compared to those without the severe disease (44.6 years, 95% CI: 42.8–46.3), $P < 0.0001$ [11]. Other reports describe a lack of age correlation with the ICU admission among CoViD19 subjects. In an analysis of retrospective case series of 1591 CoViD19 patients admitted in the ICU, 363 patients (23% [95% CI, 21–25%]) were aged 71 years and older. Older patients (n = 786; age $\geq$ 64 years) had higher mortality than younger patients (n = 795; age $\leq$ 63 years) (36 vs. 15%; difference, 21% [95% CI, 17–26%]; $P < 0.001$). However, the analysis indicated a lack of difference in the median age, between the patients, admitted to the ICU (63 (IQR, 56–70)years old), and the median age of all the positive cases with COVID19 in the Italian subjects, further suggesting that older age may not be a risk factor for admission to the ICU [12].

The older age adults more often have a high burden of comorbidities, as compared to the younger subjects. Cardiovascular conditions are highly prevalent among older adults, as well as several other important comorbidities, such as diabetes, chronic kidney disease (CKD), and chronic obstructive pulmonary disease (COPD) also found in association with CoViD19 with an increase in age (Fig. 18.2). The effects of age and comorbidities have been described in several studies reporting CoViD19 [8, 10, 13]. Patients with CoViD19 in the older age groups with chronic disease burden appear to have an increased risk of complications. In an analysis report of a large-scale study of 72 314 cases with CoViD19 in China, morbidity, and mortality significantly increased with age. Mortality was higher in patients with pre-existing cardiovascular disease, diabetes, chronic respiratory disease, hypertension, and cancer, mostly older subjects [14]. According to a report analyzing characteristics of 168 patients who died of COVID19, median (IQR) age was 70 (64–78) years, 161 patients (95.8%) were older than 50 years, and 126 (75.0%) were men. Most patients (125 patients [74.4%]) had 1 or more comorbidities. Hypertension was the most common comorbidity (84 patients [50.0%]), followed by diabetes (42 patients [25.0%]), and ischemic heart disease (31 patients [18.5%]) [15]. These data suggest that the cardiovascular and pulmonary conditions hold a central position among the burden of comorbidities in the older age subjects with critical CoViD19.

Several multi-systemic complications may be observed among the CoViD19 patients. Data indicate that the rates of cardiovascular and other systemic critical complications such as ARDS, multi-organ failure, and death appear to be much higher in patients admitted with CoViD19 in the older age group [16]. In a retrospective study of 201 CoViD19 patients, admitted with pneumonia, older age was associated with a greater risk of development of acute respiratory distress syndrome (ARDS) and death, likely owing to less rigorous immune response (ARDS hazard ratio [HR], 3.26; 95% CI 2.08–5.11; and progression from ARDS to death HR, 6.17; 95% CI, 3.26–11.67) [17]. According to an analysis of 20 studies including 4965 older COVID19 patients ($\geq$ 60 years old), about 25.7% of patients developed renal injury or impairment as a complication of CoViD19 [18]. In an analysis of prospective cohort study of 4643 CoViD19 critically ill patients (median [IQR] age 63 [54–71] years) admitted in intensive care unit (ICU), conducted in 138 hospitals in France, Belgium, and Switzerland, early independent predictors of 90-day mortality were older age, immunosuppression, severe obesity, diabetes, higher renal and cardiovascular SOFA score components, among others. Mortality was higher in older, diabetic, obese, and severe ARDS patients [19].

18.1.2 CoViD19 Fatality in Older Age Adults

Association of older age with higher mortality in CoViD19 patients has been observed among various regions of the globe. According to the analysis of an observational database of 8910 patients with CoViD19 from 169 hospitals in Asia, Europe, and North America, the older age was associated with an increased risk of in-hospital death (age greater than 65 years (mortality of 10.0%, vs. 4.9% among those ≤ 65 years of age; odds ratio, 1.93; 95% confidence interval [CI], 1.60–2.41),) [20]. Analysis of UK data examining factors associated with COVID19-related death in primary care records of 17,278,392 adults and 10,926 COVID19-related deaths, indicated that increasing age was strongly associated with risk, with people aged 80 or over having a more than 20-fold-increased risk compared to 50–59-year-olds (fully adjusted HR 20.60; 95% confidence interval (CI) 18.70–22.68 [21].

In an analysis report of a large-scale study of 72 314 cases with CoViD19 in China, the percentage of older adults ≥ 80 years was 3% (1408 cases). Morbidity and mortality significantly increased with age. The CFR was <1% for patients <50 years of age, rose to 1.3% for 50-year-old patients, to 3.6% for 60-year-old patients, further rose to 8.0% (312 of 3918) among patients 70–79, and 14.8% (208 of 1408) in patients over 80 years [14]. Higher fatalities were also observed among older age Italian subjects. In an Italian cohort analysis of 12462 patients with CoViD19, about 827 deaths were reported. Fatalities were higher in the older age groups, 42·2% in 80–89 years, 32·4% in 70–79 years, 8·4% in 60–69 years, and 2·8% in 50–59 years. Significant gender disparity was observed with a male to female ratio of 80% to 20%, and older median age for women (83·4 years for women vs. 79·9 years for men) [22].

Similar trends in CoViD19 fatalities among older age subjects were observed in the US population. The preliminary reports in the US showed that among 4226 patients with CoViD19, the highest fatality was observed in persons aged 85 years and older (10–27%), followed by persons aged 65–84 years (3–11%), persons aged 55–64 years (1–3%), and persons aged 20–54 years (<1%), with no fatalities among persons 19 years and younger [23]. The long-term mortality risk may be higher with increasing age among CoViD19 patients. According to a retrospective case series study of 5700 CoViD19 hospitalized subjects in New York, the estimated 10-year survival estimated by "Charlson Comorbidity Index", was lower with increasing age decade, after the age of 50 years [2]. Data further indicate that among the older age adults from the ethnic groups, CoViD19 fatalities may occur in relatively younger individuals. A difference of 9–10 years in the median age has been observed in the US, among the Hispanic and non-white deceased (71 and 72 years, respectively) and the white counterparts (81 years) [24].

The relationship between age and CoViD19 mortality is consistent among population groups with a direct age-dependent risk correlation. The median age differences, however, may be observed in the ethnic groups or the populations. The age dependence of the risk associated with CoViD19 may differ across the populations and may be reflected by the differences in the infection fatality rate estimates across different geographical locations. Although multiple factors may drive the differences, age structure differences may be responsible for lower mortality rates in Asia and Africa, continents with a relatively larger proportion of the younger population [25].

18.1.3 Older Age and Cardiovascular Disease in CoViD19

Cardiovascular diseases commonly occur in the the older age adults and are an important cause of mortality in this group. Age is recognized as a powerful predictor of adverse events after Acute Coronary Syndrome [26–28]. Among patients with ACS, the odds for in-hospital mortality increase by 70% for each 10-year increase in age (odds ratio [OR] 1.70, 95% confidence interval, 1.52–1.82) after accounting for other factors [26]. The risk of cardiovascular events and death also increases with older age with viral infections [29]. CoViD19 appears to have increased cardiac risk, and older age is a significant association. According to an observational cohort study of 12,958 patients with CoViD19 in England, the patients in COVID19 and acute coronary syndromes (ACS) group were generally older, age 72.8 years versus 67.0 years non-ACS group. The black, Asian and minority ethnicity, more comorbid and had unfavorable presenting clinical characteristics such as elevated cardiac troponin, pulmonary edema, cardiogenic shock, and poor left ventricular systolic function, compared with the non-COVID19 ACS group. They were less likely to receive an invasive coronary angiography (67.7 vs. 81.0%), percutaneous coronary intervention (PCI) (30.2 vs. 53.9%) and dual antiplatelet medication (76.3 vs. 88.0%). After adjusting for all the baseline differences, patients with COVID19 ACS had higher in-hospital (adjusted odds ratio, aOR): 3.27; 95% confidence interval (CI): 2.41–4.42) and 30-day mortality (aOR: 6.53; 95% CI: 5.1–8.36) compared to patients with the non-COVID19 ACS [30].

The prevalence of hypertension increases with age. Elevated blood pressure affects approximately 70% of older adults [31] and often presents a challenge in the management of hypertension. Patients with advanced age usually have an increased prevalence of hypertension and have worse outcomes [32]. CoViD19 especially severe or fatal is frequently associated with hypertension [33], and frequently among the older age subjects [34]. However, data regarding the outcomes of hypertension in relation to the outcomes in CoViD19 subjects, especially to the age, may have controversies warranting further exploration. According to an analysis of an Italian report on CoViD19 related deaths, hypertension affected 73.8% of patients, the average age of patients was 78.5 years (median 80 years, range 31–103 years) (COVID19 [35]). Age and multimorbidity have been considered as the main confounding factors in several reports describing hypertension in connection with CoViD19 severity [17, 36, 37]. Although reports reaffirm that in the COVID19 outbreak, mortality is predicted by age and the presence of comorbidities, however, also suggest lack of significant interference of hypertension in the mortality [7]. The association of hypertension with CoViD19 outcomes has met several controversies that need to be addressed with further studies. Analyses, also show significant contribution of the cardiovascular and metabolic conditions, and hypertension, towards fatal CoViD19 outcomes, however, have indicated a higher impact on mortality in the younger subjects. Data from a large meta-analysis of 51 studies with a total of 48 317 patients with confirmed COVID19 infection suggest a higher prevalence of diabetes, hypertension, and CVD in the Korean population among the older subjects, however the relative risk of fatal outcome in young patients with hypertension, diabetes, and CVD was higher than in the older patients. The study shows a significant association of these conditions with fatal outcomes in patients with COVID19 across all age groups [38]. The reversal in risk affiliation may be related to higher prevalence of other risk factors including thrombotic diseases, metabolic risk factors, or impacted by confounding factors, use of mean age, or inclusion of a broader range of comorbidities.

Reports indicate the association of older age with diabetes in patients with CoViD19. According to an analysis, CoViD19 patients with diabetes and uncontrolled hyperglycemia, were older than their counterparts (median age of 65 vs. 61 years, $P = 0.005$) [39].). Reports further suggest that diabetes is a contributory factor towards mortality in older age subjects with CoViD19 [40]. According to another report from the US, among patients above age 65 years considered at higher risk of fatality, about 26.8% of patients appeared to be diabetics [41]. According to a report among 46 fatal cases of SARSCoV2, 84% of patients were older than age 60, diabetes was a likely association with increased mortality [42]. The interrelation between diabetes and CoViD19 outcomes in older age subjects requires further exploration.

18.2 CoViD19 Biomarkers in Older Adults

Older patients have the worse hematological and biochemical impact of CoViD19. Lymphocyte (LYM) count was progressively lower with increasing age in a retrospective case series study investigating 5700 CoViD19 hospitalized patients [2, 43] and an indicator of poor outcome [44]. According to a retrospective analysis of 244 patients with CoViD19, older age and lower LYM count on admission were independently associated with an increased risk for death. The association of age and LYM count was significant (odds ratio [OR] = 1.122; 95% confidence interval [CI] = 1.007–1.249; $P = 0.037$; and OR = 0.009; 95% CI = 0.001–0.138; $P = 0.001$, respectively). The area under the ROC curve in the logistic regression model was 0.913, and that for age and LYM count were 0.653 and 0.823, respectively, indicating that LYM count and age were the most important risk factors for death [45]. An association of high neutrophil count and troponin with mortality in CoViD19 patients aged 60 years and older was observed in a retrospective analysis of 204 elderly COVID19 patients ($\geq$ 60 years old, mean age 68 (60–95) years) [13]. The study also showed an increased incidence of hypoalbuminemia among the fatal cases. Other studies show an independent association of elevated serum levels of

D-Dimers and lactate dehydrogenase (LDH) with one-month mortality among older inpatients with CoViD19 [46]. According to an analysis of 20 studies of 4965 older CoViD19 patients (≥ 60 years old), lymphopenia and raised inflammation marked by elevated C-reactive protein (CRP) and erythrocyte sedimentation rate (ESR) were predominant among the study subjects. Limited number of studies reported elevated LDH, D Dimer, and IL6 serum levels [18].

Older age subjects with CoViD19 have elevated cardiac markers that are also associated with increased severity and poor outcomes. High troponin I more than 13.75 ng/L combined with either advanced age more than 60 years, or elevated aspartate aminotransferase (AST) level of more than 27.72 U/L was the best model to predict poor outcome in a meta-analysis 17794 patients, investigating the association of CoViD19 severity and mortality rate with the history of cardiovascular diseases and/or other comorbidities and cardiac injury laboratory markers. Pooled estimates revealed significantly higher age in critical/expired cases (SMD = 1.0, 95% CI = 0.72-1.31, $P < 0.001$) than the noncritical group [47]. In another analysis, Troponin and Beta Natriuretic Peptide/N-terminal Pro (BNP/NT Pro BNP) were found to be important biomarkers of in-hospital mortality in association with CoViD19 in older age adults, regardless of risk factors or cardiovascular disease background [48].

Analyses suggest a lack of correlation between biochemical markers of severity of CoViD19, and age or sex. According to a meta-analysis report of 64 studies of CoViD19 patients investigating 27 laboratory markers, the association of the markers of inflammation (Absolute Neutrophil Count (ANC), IL-6, ferritin, CRP, albumin), poor adaptive immune response (Absolute Lymphocyte Count (ALC)), intravascular coagulation (D-dimer), and tissue damage (LDH, hsTropI), was observed with a severe and fatal disease regardless of age or sex [49].

18.3 Risk Mechanisms in Older Age and CoViD19

Both, the viral and individual factors play an important role in the association of older age and CoViD19. The SARS CoV2 infection-related factors, such as viral severity, degree of invasion, or individual burden of comorbidities, the immune biological vulnerability of the older age adults, are likely to determine the higher association of the critical disease observed in CoViD19 patients. The clustering of the cardiometabolic risk factors compromised cardiac-vascular, and multi-organ fitness impacts the ability of the older age individuals to bear the burden of CoViD19. Elderly patients with CVD and CoViD19 face critical complications related to myocardial injury, arrhythmias, heart failure, or cardiogenic shock due to cardiac decompensation compounded with poor defense mechanisms, poor vascular and cardiac compliance aggravated by hyperinflammatory stress or direct viral damage a mechanism currently under exploration. The older age-related cardiometabolic conditions, vascular aging, the vulnerability of the cardiac structures, constitute the overlapping pathogenetic immune-inflammatory links between the age and CoViD19 risks. The increase in cardiometabolic demand due to the viral disease, age-associated deficits in control of hemodynamic mechanisms, together with immune-inflammatory and other biochemical and hematological reactions, may determine cardiovascular complications, especially in the presence of metabolic, cardiovascular risk factors.

18.3.1 Immune Dysfunction and Inflammation

Data show that aging negatively influences the immune response [50, 51], with variabilities between the individuals, and there appears to be an increasing heterogeneity among the individuals with aging [52]. A retrospective analysis of 201 CoViD19 patients with pneumonia, attributed the risk of ARDS and death among older age adults to the lack of rigorous immune response [17]. Accumulation of age-related inflammation also impacts the outcomes in advanced age and may be measured. According to a study up-regulation of inflammation was independently associated with worsened mobility functioning and frailty risk and that may be measured to evaluate the risk of functional loss [53]. Among 15 inflammatory biomarkers interleukin-6 (IL-6), and tumour necrosis factor-alpha (TNF-alpha) best-captured the risk of mortality due to chronic inflammation in the older adults (inflammation index score hazards ratio 1.33; 95% CI: 1.17–1.52), and predicated 10-year all-cause mortality [54].

The exaggerated or impaired immune-inflammatory processes observed with age may serve as important pathogenetic links with CoViD19 known with hyperimmune cytokine reactions. An ineffective pathogen recognition and macrophage activation, and a reduction in natural killer (NK) cell cytotoxicity, or decline in immune adaptive function associated with thymic atrophy and accumulation of anergic memory lymphocytes reflect impaired innate and adaptive mechanisms in the older individuals associated with immune-aging/immune-senescence. The intrinsic functional reduction in immune competence is associated with low-grade chronic inflammation, termed “inflamm-aging,” characterized by high levels of circulating cytokines and latent viral infections [55]. Similarly, impaired inflammatory functions as part of "inflamm-aging' may perpetuate immune dysfunction and facilitate the COVID19 susceptibility and severity, with chronic activation of innate immunity, accumulation of inflammation with growing age, and systemic low-grade inflammation associated with “inflamm-aging” [56–61]. In the older individuals, type I and III interferon responses are compromised, and inflammatory cytokines secretion by activated dendritic cells, is uncontrolled [62]. In the older subjects with severe CoViD19 infection, reduced viral clearance may be the result of the impaired type I interferon (IFN) responses, specifically reduced IFN-β and IFN-α mechanisms that may alter the immune balance and augment the cytokine storm. The behavior of immune markers in older subjects with CoViD19 may help identify risk and must be further explored. These mechanisms may have therapeutic value in the older age population with CoVi1D19 [63].

The compounding of impaired immune and inflammatory factors in the advanced age contributes towards susceptibility of the elderly patients towards complications in CoViD19 (Fig. 18.3). Viral factors may impact the epigenetic process that drives innate and adaptive defense mechanisms in the older via epigenome dysregulation (genomic instability through loss of heterochromatin and increased DNA damage, telomere attrition, and epigenetic alterations) [64]. The DNA methylation age of immune cells and other blood cell types can be measured before, during, and after infection could help elucidate both how the aged epigenome impacts disease severity and how the virus alters the aged epigenome [65]. The age-dependent defects in T-cell and B-cell function and the excess production of type 2 cytokines could lead to a deficiency in control of viral replication and more prolonged proinflammatory responses, potentially leading to poor outcome [66]. Aging may alter the LN (lymph node) stromal cell response to challenges, such as viral infections; age-related changes may be an underlying contributor to the impaired immune responses in older age adults [67]. In older subjects with CoViD19, a slow recovery may be associated with reduced muscle mass and fatigue, as a result of elevated cytokines, previously described, and interaction of cytokines such as IL-6 on the recovery process [68, 69].

The increased expression and activity of the NRLP3 inflammasomes is associated with aging, diabetes, and age-associated chronic conditions such as pulmonary fibrosis [70, 71]. The NLRP3 promotes inflammation via cleavage and activation of key inflammatory molecules including active caspase-1 (Casp1p20), IL-1β, and IL-18. Studies show that inflammasomes participate in the pathophysiology of CoViD19, and severity [72]. The NLR family pyrin domain containing 3 (NLRP3) in association with severe CoViD19 has implications in the hyperimmune reactions, appears to be a contributing factor towards the severity and complications [73]. The exact associations of these mechanisms need to be further examined.

18.3.2 ACE2 Mechanisms

ACE2 expression is downregulated in the older age individuals [74, 75]. SARS CoV2 infection downregulates the ACE2 [76] and may tilt the balance of the protective and harmful axes of the RAS, thereby enhancing the hyperactivity of the ACE/Ang II pathway that induces several proinflammatory, prothrombotic, pro-apoptotic, reactions as well as endothelial dysfunction, vascular damage and other adverse reactions [77–79]; as opposed to the protective ACE2/angiotensin-(1–7)/Mas receptor axis related mechanisms [79]. Downregulation of ACE2 with viral infection may predispose to relatively unopposed angiotensin II effects, such as hypertension, enhanced inflammation, and thrombosis [80].

An increase in ACE2 expression is associated with cardiovascular diseases, hypertension, heart failure, and other cardiovascular conditions [81, 82], and may be reactive. In established heart failure, there is an increase in circulating ACE2, while the cellular expression is downregulated [83]. ACE2 expression in the cardiac cells seems to be lower with older age, an important association of CoViD19 disease severity [75]. The lower expression of ACE2 reflects lower cardiac protection, thereby an increased cardiovascular risk. Furthermore, an age-associated increase in renin angiotensin system (RAS) signaling throughout the body perpetuate major proinflammatory changes, also a salient pathophysiologic feature of hypertension and diabetes, which are highly prevalent at older ages [84, 85]. The interaction of age and dysregulation in RAS mechanisms may contribute to the aggravation of the SARS CoV2 induced RAS imbalance, thereby increasing the risk of complications in the older age adults.

18.3.3 Miscellaneous Age Related Mechanisms

The aging processes involve enhanced oxidative and nitrative stress mechanisms and alterations in the conserved molecular pathways. Senescence is a state of gradual functional decline and stable growth arrest, with multiple pro-inflammatory and pro-disease processes. Involvement of senescence has been demonstrated in viral infections [86, 87] with hyperimmune inflammatory reactions [88] and the process of pyroptosis observed with SARS CoV2 [89] that may aggravate the process in older indviduals with CoViD19. Senescence impacts immune balance, hemostasis [90], vascular [91] and cardiac structures [92, 93] and contributes to multiple comorbidities associated with age. Measuring the burst of cellular senescence was proposed to be a contributor to COVID19 pathogenesis, and a predictor of COVID19 severity [94].

Changes in the vasculature with old age are reflected by micro and macrovascular dysfunction associated with arterial stiffness as a result of several processes such as calcification, glycosylation, pro-inflammatory processes, and endothelial dysfunction, or other processes related to anemia and thrombo-embolism [95, 96], may aggravate cardiovascular risk in the older subjects with CoViD19. Age-related changes in cardiovascular structures, such as central arterial stiffness, increase in left ventricular mass, and other cardiac and vascular measurements at elevated levels but not meeting criteria of classical cardiovascular conditions [97], may contribute to the development of complications in conditions such as CoViD19. Interconnections between senescence and pulmonary fibrosis [98, 99], may elevate respiratory vulnerability in the older subjects to CoViD19.

Similarly, several mechanisms related to glycosylation, age-related accumulation of glycated end products, demethylation patterns help understanding age-related risks related to the impact of unhealthy lifestyles that may increase susceptibility towards CoViD19 infection or complications. Advanced glycation end-products (AGEs) may modify the extracellular matrix (ECM); modify the action of hormones, cytokines, and free radicals via engagement of cell surface receptors; and impact the function of intracellular proteins [100]. The accumulation of AGEs in vascular, immune cells, intra- and extracellular environmental stress, endothelial dysfunction, and acceleration of the process under hyperglycemic conditions, lead to micro and macrovascular dysfunction and complications, is found with advancing age and associated metabolic conditions [101]. Role of the biomarkers of the biological age may predict CoViD19 severity [102]. Other mechanisms such as hypoalbuminemia, vitamin D deficiency, and other nutritional disorders [103, 104] may promote CoViD19 severity in older adults, and are under exploration.

18.4 Summary

The prevalence of older age adults varies across countries and continents, with geographical variations in the prevalence of CoViD19, however, the adverse association of old age and CoViD19 appears to be consistent across the world. Evidence suggests a more critical CoViD19 disease among older subjects. Differences in the mean age of subjects among different population groups may be observed among the studies however, most studies indicate a higher mean age among the critical subjects with CoViD19. The age dependence of the risk associated with CoViD19 may differ across the populations and may be reflected by the differences in the infection fatality rate estimates across different geographical locations.

CoViD19 may have more intense or atypical manifestations in the older age subjects, who appear to have a longer hospital stay and poor outcomes, and a poor recovery with possible long-term implications of the disease. Analyses suggest increased risk for developing protein-energy undernutrition, sarcopenia, and cachexia in CoViD19 patients [105]. The long-term data are not available, however, short-term mortality risk appears to be high in the older subjects, and the impact of age on mortality seems to be incremental. Risk models although may have several weaknesses appear to indicate long-term risk implications among older age adults. A combination of biochemical and clinical markers may determine the increased susceptibility to long-term implications of CoViD19 in older adults. A large analysis of 107 studies describing 145 prediction models based on living systematic review, reported several biases among the predicting models in CoViD19 studies, however, identified age, body temperature, lymphocyte count, and lung imaging features, as common factors among predictors of outcome that may be considered important [106]. Intricacies related to the estimation of the true impact of CoViD19 on mortality across the populations may have led to over or under estimation of the mortality risk, need to be further explored.

The elevated risk in the older subjects may be attributed to a higher burden of chronic comorbidities associated with age including cardiovascular, metabolic, renal, pulmonary, or dysfunctional hematological, and immunological systems. There is a higher prevalence of chronic comorbidities such as hypertension, coronary heart disease, heart failure, diabetes mellitus, or cancer in the older age subjects. The CoViD19 further adversely impacts vulnerable old adults, especially with a burden of comorbidities. The role of comorbidities in the determination of poor outcomes with CoViD19 in the older age subjects is complex and poorly understood. Several limitations exist in research data due to the presence of heterogeneity, design, methodology, and analytical biases that may confound the conclusions. Multiple biological and non-biological factors may play an equally important role in determining and aggravating the risks. Senescence, cellular stress processes, immune system deficiencies with immune-aging, processes related to inflamm-aging, and other molecular mechanisms that compromise cellular and tissue fitness are notable. A hypo-immune response with relative lymphopenia, impaired T-cell function, impaired interferon antiviral responses, reduced viral clearance, with elements of proinflammatory activity, may create an immune imbalance promoting increased susceptibility towards the disease and disease severity. Besides, genetic, or poor dietary habits, low psychophysical fitness, higher physical fragility, and others related to socioeconomic status, affordability, or lack of rapid access to a healthcare facility, appear extremely important factors that may impact the outcome of CoViD19 in older age adults. An improved understanding of inflamm-aging and immune senescence and related processes may help to unravel the interrelation between age and SARSCoV2 infection with practical implications in understanding the risks [65, 107].

Risk assessment models and algorithms in the older age subjects may help in identifying patients at higher risk of complications in CoViD19. Use of the risk frailty score has been advocated in the older age patients with CoViD19 [108]. The inflammation index score [54], hospital frailty risk score and other forms of frailty assessment methods may not only predict adverse risks, increased risk of hospitalization, nursing home admission, mortality and prolonged length of stay [109, 110]. These cost-effective methods may be excellent tools for the assessment of older age subjects with CoViD19 that need to be further explored.

The complexity of factors associated with poor outcomes in older age adults is further obscured by difficulties faced in providing optimum management. This may be due to the gaps in the evidence-based practice in this population group and poor clinical decision-making by the clinicians and carers involved in the management of the older age patients. The dilemma, of longevity versus quality-of-life facing interventions with aggressive treatment plans, best allocation of resources under extreme circumstances, patient preferences, and other factors constitute the clinical decision-making processes [111, 112]. Moreover, older age subjects may also face the dilemma of confusion, related to the inter-individual variability in the interpretation of the biological fragility in relation to the chronological age. Another important factor related to the poor outcome in older age adults may be related to their risk of facing age discrimination in the decision-making process related to the delivery of treatments or interventions. Such discriminations may lead to underestimating the benefits of a clinical intervention or failure in the delivery of the best care practices in this population group [111]. These scenarios are particularly reflected when making decisions for invasive interventions in older age adults, with the perception of lack of benefit vis a vis risk, as opposed to the younger patients.

Although there is increasing recognition of the use of advanced and evidence-based management strategies in the older patients in the Western world, when facing a serious threat of contagion like CoViD19 it appears to have failed to materialize [113–115]. Serious gaps have been seen in the provision of optimum healthcare services to the patients from the older age group, during the CoViD19 pandemic. This has been partially attributed to the lack of sufficient facilities, resources, medical infrastructure, or ability to cope with a high number of serious CoViD19 cases in the health care centers [116]. Nursing homes have also shown the presence of asymptomatic or pre-symptomatic cases of CoViD19, indicating the need for higher surveillance of the older age residents susceptible to the disease [117]. However, higher mortality in nursing homes indicates a strong need for improving standards of care and management practices [118]. According to a report describing data from 22 countries (as of October 21st, 2020), COVID19 contributed to about 46–47% of deaths among nursing home residents [119].

In recent years, a growing wealth of evidence has emerged advocating the use of more aggressive strategies in the management of patients in the older age group, strongly negating the common practices, and paving way for the use of a bigger variety of and more effective treatments in this population group. This has increased longevity and quality of life, especially in countries with advanced health care systems. However, subjects in the older age group remain vastly undertreated or poorly managed despite advancement in geriatrics, development of evidence-based treatment strategies, and expert guidelines for effective management of health conditions in the older age patients [120–122]. There is a strong need for disseminating the use of evidence-based practices for the management of older patients. The complexities of the clinical decision-making process under extreme

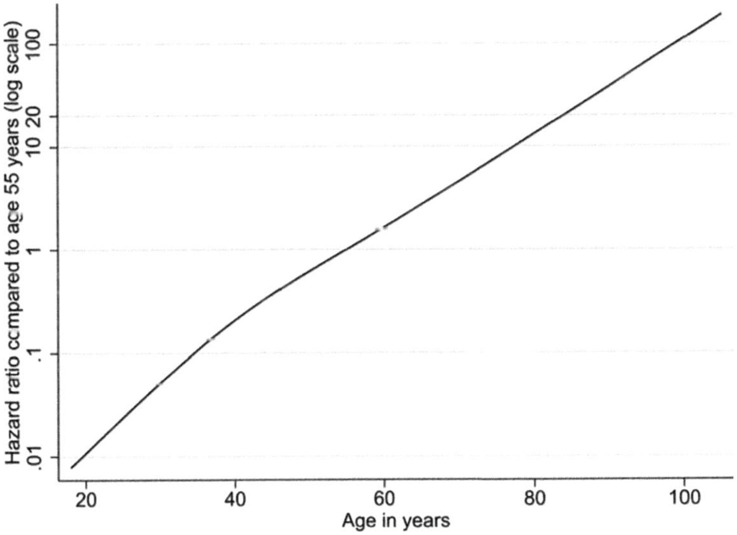

Fig. 18.1 Estimated log-transformed hazard ratio by age in years. *Source* Extended data figure 1. Williamson, E.J., Walker, A.J., Bhaskaran, K., Bacon, S., Bates, C., Morton, C.E., Curtis, H.J., Mehrkar, A., Evans, D., Inglesby, P. and Cockburn, J., 2020. Factors associated with COVID-19-related death using OpenSAFELY. Nature, 584(7821), pp. 430–436. https://www.nature.com/articles/s41586-020-2521-4. By Springer Nature Group

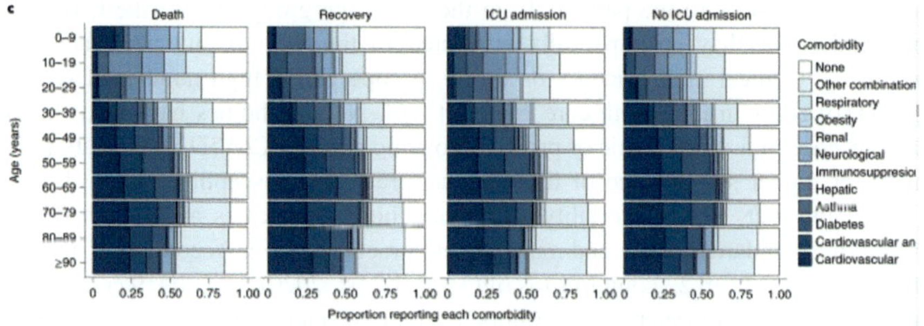

Fig. 18.2 Age–sex structure and clinical features of confirmed COVID-19 cases reported in the SIVEP-Gripe system. Comorbidities among confirmed COVID-19 cases according to age and outcome (n = 15,720 confirmed COVID-19 cases with complete comorbidity and outcome (death or recovery) information; n = 19,409 confirmed COVID-19 cases with complete information on comorbidities and ICU admission). Horizontal axes show the proportion of patients in each age/outcome stratified for each of the comorbidities recorded. *Source* Figure 6 c. de Souza, W.M., Buss, L.F., da Silva Candido, D., Carrera, J.P., Li, S., Zarebski, A.E., Pereira, R.H.M., Prete, C.A., de Souza-Santos, A.A., Parag, K.V. and Belotti, M.C.T., 2020. Epidemiological and clinical characteristics of the COVID-19 epidemic in Brazil. Nature human behaviour, 4(8), pp. 856-865. https://www.nature.com/articles/s41562-020-0928-4.By Springer Nature Group

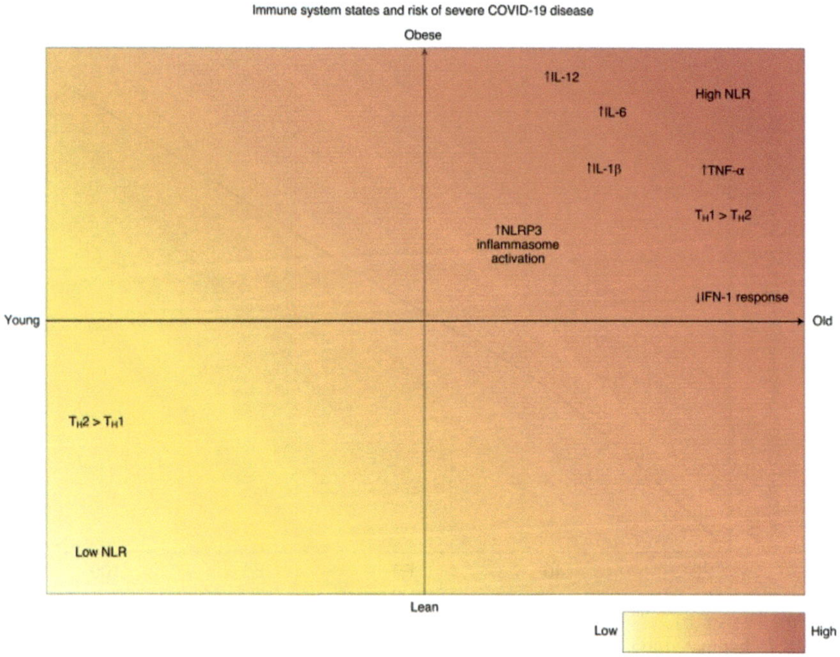

Fig. 18.3 Immune-system parameters associated with obesity, aging and severe COVID-19. The gradient illustrates the risk of developing severe COVID-19 in relation to known immune system changes with age (x axis) and obesity (y axis). *Source:*Figure 2. Brodin, P., 2021. Immune determinants of COVID-19 disease presentation and severity. Nature Medicine, 27(1), pp. 28-33. https://www.nature.com/articles/s41591-020-01202-8. By Springer Nature Group

circumstances must be recognized and addressed [123]. Further guidances are needed to be developed in the face of the pandemic of CoViD19, and the ever-growing threat of pandemics to help healthcare providers to take better decisions under the extreme environments [124]. These practices should be extended to other regions of the world to mitigate risks in such extreme situations.

Summary Box

- Older age preys upon CoViD19 that hunts older age adults with the disparate burden of co-morbidities.
- CoViD19 pandemic has particularly impacted older adults worldwide.
- CoViD19 patients with older age may experience worse infection, atypical symptoms, or may have poor treatment response.
- Critical CoViD19 is frequently associated with older age.
- In CoViD19, older age increases the risk of critical disease.
- Chronic disease burden is higher with older age and may contribute to the risk.
- Cardiovascular disease association as chronic comorbidities or as complications during CoViD19 are higher in older adults.
- Lymphopenia and raised inflammation are predominant lab markers in older age CoViD19 adults.
- Case fatality rates may differ among different populations, and age may be an important determinant.
- Markers of cardiac injury appear to be particularly elevated in older age adults although may be elevated without apparent cardiac history.
- Besides impaired immune function, the clustering of cardiometabolic risk factors compromised cardiovascular and multi-organ fitness impacts the ability of older age individuals to bear the burden of CoViD19.
- The older age CoViD19 interlink is a matrix of immune-inflammatory, chronic functional and structural decline, cellular stress mechanisms, senescence, genetic, dietary, physical, psychological, environmental, and viral factors that exploit each other.
- Cellular and extracellular stress mechanisms, chronic age-associated processes that impact the biological clock, cardiac and vascular aging, must be better understood in relation to viral diseases.
- Improved risk assessment models may improve outcomes in the older age subjects who often have elevated risk and require a higher level of care.
- Older age patients, in special, appear to have serious disadvantages when facing the challenges of CoViD19.

- Besides the clinical and medical factors, psychological, social care, and economic implications are also linked with the outcome of older age subjects with CoViD19.
- Psychosocial, nutritional support, fitness improvement programs, raised awareness among social and healthcare networks are important in minimizing risks in older adults and are effective measures for the prevention of infection.
- Overlapping pathogenetic immune-inflammatory links between age and cardiometabolic conditions, cardiac and vascular aging, that increase vulnerability of the cardiac structures, may particularly impact CoViD19 related cardiovascular risk in the older age.
- Above all, special acts of kindness, care, and affection in the community or hospital settings may do wonders for older adults.

References

1. Docherty AB, Harrison EM, Green CA, Hardwick HE, Pius R, Norman L, Holden KA, Read JM, Dondelinger F, Carson G, Merson L. Features of 20 133 UK patients in hospital with CoViD19 using the ISARIC WHO Clinical Characterisation Protocol: prospective observational cohort study. BMJ. 2020;369.
2. Richardson S, Hirsch JS, Narasimhan M, Crawford JM, McGinn T, Davidson KW, Barnaby DP, Becker LB, Chelico JD, Cohen SL, Cookingham J. Presenting characteristics, comorbidities, and outcomes among 5700 patients hospitalized with COVID19 in the New York City area. JAMA. 2020;323(20):2052–9.
3. Limpawattana P, Phungoen P, Mitsungnern T, Laosuangkoon W, Tansangworn N. Atypical presentations of older adults at the emergency department and associated factors. Arch Gerontol Geriatr. 2016;62:97–102.
4. Gómez-Belda AB, Fernández-Garcés M, Mateo-Sanchis E, Madrazo M, Carmona M, Piles-Roger L, Artero A. COVID-19 in older adults: what are the differences with younger patients? Geriatr Gerontol Int. 2021;21(1), 60–5.
5. Poco PCE, Aliberti MJR, Dias MB, Takahashi SDF, Leonel FC, Altona M, Venys AL, Shin-Ike IA, Garcia BA, Sumita LH, Lima LMDO. Divergent: age, frailty, and atypical presentations of COVID19 in hospitalized patients. The J Geronto: Ser A. 2021;76(3),e46–51.
6. Sudre CH, Murray B, Varsavsky T, Graham MS, Penfold RS, Bowyer RC, Pujol JC, Klaser K, Antonelli M, Canas LS, Molteni E. Attributes and predictors of long COVID. Nat Med. 2021;27(4):626–31.
7. Iaccarino G, Grassi G, Borghi C, Ferri C, Salvetti M, Volpe M. Age and multimorbidity predict death among COVID19 patients: results of the SARS-RAS study of the Italian society of hypertension. Hypertension. 2020;76(2):366–72.
8. Chen N, Zhou M, Dong X, Qu J, Gong F, Han Y, Qiu Y, Wang J, Liu Y, Wei Y, Yu T. Epidemiological and clinical characteristics of 99 cases of 2019 novel coronavirus pneumonia in Wuhan, China: a descriptive study. The Lancet. 2020;395(10223):507–13.
9. COVID19 CDC, Team R, COVID19 CDC, Team R, COVID19 CDC, Team R, Bialek S, Boundy E, Bowen V, Chow N, Cohn A, Dowling N, Ellington S, Gierke, R. Severe

outcomes among patients with coronavirus disease 2019 (COVID19)—United States, February 12–March 16, 2020. Morb Mortal Wkly Rep. 2020;69(12), 343–6.
10. Wang D, Hu B, Hu C, Zhu F, Liu X, Zhang J, Wang B, Xiang H, Cheng Z, Xiong Y, Zhao Y. Clinical characteristics of 138 hospitalized patients with 2019 novel coronavirus–infected pneumonia in Wuhan, China. JAMA. 2020;323(11):1061–9.
11. Li J, Huang DQ, Zou B, Yang H, Hui WZ, Rui F, Yee NTS, Liu C, Nerurkar SN, Kai JCY, Teng MLP. Epidemiology of COVID-19: a systematic review and meta-analysis of clinical characteristics, risk factors, and outcomes. J Med Virol. 2021;93(3):1449–58.
12. Grasselli G, Zangrillo A, Zanella A, Antonelli M, Cabrini L, Castelli A, Cereda D, Coluccello A, Foti G, Fumagalli R, Iotti G. Baseline characteristics and outcomes of 1591 patients infected with SARS-CoV-2 admitted to ICUs of the Lombardy Region, Italy. JAMA. 2020;323(16):1574–81.
13. Li P, Chen L, Liu Z, Pan J, Zhou D, Wang H, Gong H, Fu Z, Song Q, Min Q, Ruan S. Clinical features and short-term outcomes of elderly patients with COVID19. Int J Infect Dis. 2020;97:245–50.
14. Wu Z, McGoogan JM. Characteristics of and important lessons from the coronavirus disease 2019 (COVID19) outbreak in China: summary of a report of 72 314 cases from the Chinese center for disease control and prevention. JAMA Published Online First: 24 February 2020. https://doi.org/10.1001/jama.2020.2648.
15. Xie J, Tong Z, Guan X, Du B, Qiu H. Clinical characteristics of patients who died of coronavirus disease 2019 in China. JAMA Netw Open. 2020;3(4):e205619–e205619.
16. Yang X, Yu Y, Xu J, Shu H, Liu H, Wu Y, Zhang L, Yu Z, Fang M, Yu T, Wang Y. Clinical course and outcomes of critically ill patients with SARS-CoV-2 pneumonia in Wuhan, China: a single-centered, retrospective, observational study. The Lancet Respir Med. 2020;8 (5):475–81.
17. Wu C, Chen X, Cai Y, Zhou X, Xu S, Huang H, Zhang L, Zhou X, Du C, Zhang Y, Song J. Risk factors associated with acute respiratory distress syndrome and death in patients with coronavirus disease 2019 pneumonia in Wuhan, China. JAMA Intern Med. 2020;180 (7):934–94.
18. Neumann-Podczaska A, Al-Saad SR, Karbowski LM, Chojnicki M, Tobis S, Wieczorowska-Tobis K. COVID19-clinical picture in the elderly population: a qualitative systematic review. Aging Dis. 2020;11(4), 988.
19. Lambermont B. Clinical characteristics and day-90 outcomes of 4244 ctritically ill adults with COVID19: a prospective cohort study. Intensive Care Med. 2021.
20. Mehra MR, Desai SS, Kuy S, Henry TD, Patel AN. Cardiovascular disease, drug therapy, and mortality in CoViD19. New Engl J Med. 2020;382(25), e102.
21. Bhaskaran K, Bacon S, Evans SJ, Bates CJ, Rentsch CT, MacKenna B, Tomlinson L, Walker AJ, Schultze A, Morton CE, Grint D. Factors associated with deaths due to COVID19 versus other causes: population-based cohort analysis of UK primary care data and linked national death registrations within the OpenSAFELY platform. The Lancet Reg Health-Europe. 2021;6, 100109.
22. Remuzzi A, Remuzzi G. COVID19 and Italy: what next? The Lancet 2020;0. https://doi.org/10.1016/S0140-6736(20)30627-9.
23. US Centers for Disease Control and Prevention COVID19 Response Team. Severe Outcomes Among Patients with Coronavirus Disease 2019 (COVID19): United States, February 12-March 16, 2020. MMWR Morb Mortal Wkly Rep. Published online March 18, 2020. https://doi.org/10.15585/mmwr.mm6912e2.
24. Wortham JM. Characteristics of persons who died with COVID19—United States. 2020. MMWR. Morb Mortal Wkly Rep. 2020;6.
25. Ioannidis JP. Infection fatality rate of COVID19 inferred from seroprevalence data. Bull World Health Organ. 2021;99(1):19.
26. Granger CB, Goldberg RJ, Dabbous O, Pieper KS, Eagle KA, Cannon CP, Van De Werf F, Avezum A, Goodman SG, Flather MD, Fox KA; Global Registry of Acute Coronary Events

Investigators. Predictors of hospital mortality in the Global Registry of Acute Coronary Events. Arch Intern Med. 2003;163:2345–53.
27. Eagle KA, Lim MJ, Dabbous OH, Pieper KS, Goldberg RJ, Van de Werf F, Goodman SG, Granger CB, Steg PG, Gore JM, Budaj A, Avezum A, Flather MD, Fox KA; GRACE Investigators. A validated prediction model for all forms of acute coronary syndrome: estimating the risk of 6-month postdischarge death in an international registry. JAMA. 2004;291:2727–33.
28. Boersma E, Pieper KS, Steyerberg EW, Wilcox RG, Chang WC, Lee KL, Akkerhuis KM, Harrington RA, Deckers JW, Armstrong PW, Lincoff AM, Califf RM, Topol EJ, Simoons ML. Predictors of outcome in patients with acute coronary syndromes without persistent ST-segment elevation: results from an international trial of 9461 patients. Circulation. 2000;101:2557–67.
29. Nguyen JL, Yang W, Ito K, Matte TD, Shaman J, Kinney PL. Seasonal influenza infections and cardiovascular disease mortality. JAMA Cardiol. 2016;1(3):274–81.
30. Rashid M, Wu J, Timmis A, Curzen N, Clarke S, Zaman A, Nolan J, Shoaib A, Mohamed MO, de Belder MA, Deanfield J. Outcomes of COVID-19-positive acute coronary syndrome patients: a multisource electronic healthcare records study from England. J Internal Med. 2021.
31. Mozaffarian D, Benjamin EJ, Go AS, Arnett DK, Blaha MJ, Cushman M, De Ferranti S, Després JP, Fullerton HJ, Howard VJ, Huffman MD. Heart disease and stroke statistics—2015 update: a report from the American Heart Association. Circulation 2015;131(4), e29–322.
32. Vokonas PS, Kannel WB, Cupples LA. Epidemiology and risk of hypertension in the elderly: the Framingham Study. J Hypertens. Suppl: Official J Int Soc Hypertens. 1988;6(1), S3–9.
33. Kario K, Morisawa Y, Sukonthasarn A, Turana Y, Chia YC, Park S, Wang TD, Chen CH, Tay JC, Li Y, Wang JG. COVID-19 and hypertension—evidence and practical management: Guidance from the HOPE Asia Network. The J Clin Hypertens. 2020;22(7):1109–19.
34. Lippi G, Wong J, Henry BM. Hypertension and its severity or mortality in Coronavirus Disease 2019 (COVID19): a pooled analysis. Polish Arch Intern Med. 2020.
35. Surveillance Group, 2020. Characteristics of COVID19 patients dying in Italy: report based on available data on March 20th, 2020. Rome, Italy: Instituto Superiore Di Sanita. 2020. www.epicentro.iss.it/coronavirus/bollettino/Report-COVID-2019_20_marzo_eng.pdf. Accessed, 20.
36. Clerkin KJ, Fried JA, Raikhelkar J, Sayer G, Griffin JM, Masoumi A, Jain SS, Burkhoff D, Kumaraiah D, Rabbani L, Schwartz A. COVID19 and cardiovascular disease. Circulation. 2020;141(20):1648–55.
37. Guo T, Fan Y, Chen M, Wu X, Zhang L, He T, Wang H, Wan J, Wang X, Lu Z. Cardiovascular implications of fatal outcomes of patients with coronavirus disease 2019 (COVID19). JAMA Cardiol. 2020;5(7):811–8.
38. Bae S, Kim SR, Kim MN, Shim WJ, Park SM. Impact of cardiovascular disease and risk factors on fatal outcomes in patients with COVID19 according to age: a systematic review and meta-analysis. Heart. 2021;107(5):373–80.
39. Bode B, Garrett V, Messler J, McFarland R, Crowe J, Booth R, Klonoff DC. Glycemic characteristics and clinical outcomes of COVID19 patients hospitalized in the United States. J Diab Sci Technol. 2020;14(4):813–21.
40. Guo W, Li M, Dong Y, et al. Diabetes is a risk factor for the progression and prognosis of COVID-19. Diabetes Metab Res Rev. 2020;e3319. https://doi.org/10.1002/dmrr.3319.
41. Centers for Disease Control and Prevention National Diabetes Statistics Report, 2020. Atlanta, GA: Centers for Disease Control and Prevention, US Department of Health and Human Services, 2020.
42. Huang C, Wang Y, Li X, Ren L, Zhao J, Hu Y, Zhang L, Fan G, Xu J, Gu X, Cheng Z. Clinical features of patients infected with 2019 novel coronavirus in Wuhan, China. The Lancet. 2020;395(10223):497–506.

43. Richardson S, Hirsch JS, Narasimhan M. Clarification of mortality rate and data in abstract, results, and table 2. JAMA. 2020;10.
44. Wang L, He W, Yu X, Hu D, Bao M, Liu H, Zhou J, Jiang H. Coronavirus disease 2019 in elderly patients: characteristics and prognostic factors based on 4-week follow-up. J Infect. 2020;80(6):639–45.
45. Sun H, Ning R, Tao Y, Yu C, Deng X, Zhao C, Meng S, Tang F, Xu D. Risk factors for mortality in 244 older adults with COVID-19 in Wuhan, China: a retrospective study. J Am Geriatr Soc. 2020;68(6):E19–23.
46. Bousquet G, Falgarone G, Deutsch D, Derolez S, Lopez-Sublet M, Goudot FX, Amari K, Uzunhan Y, Bouchaud O, Pamoukdjian F. ADL-dependency, D-Dimers, LDH and absence of anticoagulation are independently associated with one-month mortality in older inpatients with CoViD19. Aging (Albany NY). 2020;12(12), 11306.
47. Toraih EA, Elshazli RM, Hussein MH, Elgaml A, Amin M, El-Mowafy M, El-Mesery M, Ellythy A, Duchesne J, Killackey MT, Ferdinand KC. Association of cardiac biomarkers and comorbidities with increased mortality, severity, and cardiac injury in COVID-19 patients: a meta-regression and decision tree analysis. J Med Virol. 2020;92(11), 2473–88.
48. Matsumoto S, Kuroda S, Sano T, Kitai T, Yonetsu T, Kohsaka S, Torii S, Kishi T, Komuro I, Hirata KI, Node K. Clinical and biomarker profiles and prognosis of elderly patients with coronavirus disease 2019 (COVID19) with cardiovascular diseases and/or risk factors. Circ J. 2021;85(6):921–8.
49. Khinda J, Janjua NZ, Cheng S, van den Heuvel ER, Bhatti P, Darvishian M. Association between markers of immune response at hospital admission and COVID-19 disease severity and mortality: a meta-analysis and meta-regression. J Med Virol. 2021;93(2):1078–98.
50. Govaert TM, Thijs CTMCN, Masurel N, Sprenger MJW, Dinant GJ, Knottnerus JA. The efficacy of influenza vaccination in elderly individuals: a randomized double-blind placebo-controlled trial. JAMA. 1994;272(21):1661–5.
51. Liu WM, van der Zeijst BA, Boog CJ, Soethout EC. Aging and impaired immunity to influenza viruses: implications for vaccine development. Human Vaccines. 2011;7 (sup1):94–8.
52. Shen-Orr SS, Furman D. Variability in the immune system: of vaccine responses and immune states. Curr Opin Immunol. 2013;25(4):542–7.
53. Bandeen-Roche K, Walston JD, Huang Y, Semba RD, Ferrucci L. Measuring systemic inflammatory regulation in older adults: evidence and utility. Rejuvenation Res. 2009;12(6), 403–10.
54. Varadhan R, Yao W, Matteini A, Beamer BA, Xue QL, Yang H, Manwani B, Reiner A, Jenny N, Parekh N, Fallin MD. Simple biologically informed inflammatory index of two serum cytokines predicts 10 year all-cause mortality in older adults. J Gerontol Ser A: Biomed Sci Med Sci. 2014;69(2):165–73.
55. Frasca D, Blomberg BB. Inflammaging decreases adaptive and innate immune responses in mice and humans. Biogerontology. 2016;17(1):7–19.
56. Fulop T, et al. Immunosenescence and inflamm-aging as two sides of the same coin: friends or foes? Front Immunol. 2018;8:1960.
57. Goronzy JJ, Weyand CM. Successful and maladaptive T cell aging. Immunity. 2017;46 (3):364–78.
58. Nikolich-Žugich J. T cell aging: naive but not young. J Exp Med. 2005;201(6):837–40.
59. Furman D, et al. Chronic inflammation in the etiology of disease across the life span. Nat Med. 2019;25(12):1822–32.
60. Cesari M, et al. Inflammatory markers and physical performance in older persons: the InCHIANTI study. J Gerontol Ser A Biol Med Sci. 2004;59(3):M242–8.
61. Franceschi C, Bonafè M, Valensin S, Olivieri F, De Luca M, Ottaviani E, De Benedictis G. Inflamm-aging: an evolutionary perspective on immunosenescence. Ann N Y Acad Sci. 2000;908(1):244–54.
62. Agrawal A, Agrawal S, Gupta S. Role of dendritic cells in inflammation and loss of tolerance in the elderly. Front Immunol. 2017;8:896.

63. Nidadavolu LS, Walston JD. Underlying vulnerabilities to the cytokine storm and adverse COVID19 outcomes in the aging immune system. The J Gerontol: Ser A. 2021;76(3):e13–8.
64. Keenan CR, Allan RS. Epigenomic drivers of immune dysfunction in aging. Aging Cell. 2019;18(1), e12878.
65. Mueller AL, McNamara MS, Sinclair DA. Why does COVID19 disproportionately affect older people? Aging (Albany NY). 2020;12(10):9959.
66. Opal SM, Girard TD, Ely EW. The immunopathogenesis of sepsis in elderly patients. Clin Infect Dis. 2005;41(Supplement_7), S504–12.
67. Masters AR, Hall A, Bartley JM, Keilich SR, Lorenzo EC, Jellison ER, Puddington L, Haynes L. Assessment of lymph node stromal cells as an underlying factor in age-related immune impairment. The J Gerontol: Ser A. 2019;74(11):1734–43.
68. Thoma A, Lightfoot AP. NF-kB and inflammatory cytokine signalling: role in skeletal muscle atrophy. Muscle Atrophy, 2018;267–79.
69. Belizário JE, Fontes-Oliveira CC, Borges JP, Kashiabara JA, Vannier E. Skeletal muscle wasting and renewal: a pivotal role of myokine IL-6. Springerplus. 2016;5(1), 1–15.
70. Stout-Delgado HW, Cho SJ, Chu SG, Mitzel DN, Villalba J, El-Chemaly S, Ryter SW, Choi AM, Rosas IO. Age-dependent susceptibility to pulmonary fibrosis is associated with NLRP3 inflammasome activation. Am J Respir Cell Mol Biol. 2016;55(2), 252–63.
71. Youm YH, Grant RW, McCabe LR, Albarado DC, Nguyen KY, Ravussin A, Pistell P, Newman S, Carter R, Laque A, Münzberg H. Canonical Nlrp3 inflammasome links systemic low-grade inflammation to functional decline in aging. Cell Metab. 2013;18(4):519–32.
72. Rodrigues TS, de Sá KS, Ishimoto AY, Becerra A, Oliveira S, Almeida L, Gonçalves AV, Perucello DB, Andrade WA, Castro R, Veras FP. Inflammasomes are activated in response to SARS-CoV-2 infection and are associated with COVID19 severity in patients. J Exp Med. 2020;218(3), e20201707.
73. Freeman TL, Swartz TH. Targeting the NLRP3 inflammasome in severe COVID19. Front Immunol. 2020;11, 1518.
74. Xudong X, Junzhu C, Xingxiang W, Furong Z, Yanrong L. Age-and gender-related difference of ACE2 expression in rat lung. Life Sci. 2006;78(19):2166–71.
75. Liu H, Gai S, Wang X, Zeng J, Sun C, Zhao Y, Zheng Z. Single-cell analysis of SARS-CoV-2 receptor ACE2 and spike protein priming expression of proteases in the human heart. Cardiovasc Res. 2020;116(10):1733–41.
76. Verdecchia P, Cavallini C, Spanevello A, Angeli F. The pivotal link between ACE2 deficiency and SARS-CoV-2 infection. Eur J Intern Med. 2020.
77. Brown NJ, Vaughan DE. Prothrombotic effects of angiotensin. Adv Intern Med. 2000;45:419–29.
78. Yildirim A, Russell J, Yan LSS, Senchenkova EY, Granger DN. Leukocyte-dependent responses of the microvasculature to chronic angiotensin II exposure. Hypertension. 2012;60 (6):1503–9.
79. Prestes TRR, Rocha NP, Miranda AS, Teixeira AL, Simoes-E-Silva AC. The anti-inflammatory potential of ACE2/angiotensin-(1-7)/Mas receptor axis: evidence from basic and clinical research. Curr Drug Targets. 2017;18(11), 1301–13.
80. Wang K, Gheblawi M, Oudit GY. Angiotensin converting enzyme 2: a double-edged sword [published online March 26, 2020]. Circulation. https://doi.org/10.1161/CIRCULATIONAHA.120.047049.
81. Gallagher PE, Ferrario CM, Tallant EA. Regulation of ACE2 in cardiac myocytes and fibroblasts. Am J Physiol-Heart Circulatory Physiol. 2008;295(6):H2373–9.
82. Mendoza-Torres E, Oyarzún A, Mondaca-Ruff D, Azocar A, Castro PF, Jalil JE, Chiong M, Lavandero S, Ocaranza MP. ACE2 and vasoactive peptides: novel players in cardiovascular/renal remodeling and hypertension. Ther Adv Cardiovasc Dis. 2015;9(4), 217–37.
83. Liu PP, Blet A, Smyth D, Li H. The science underlying COVID19: implications for the cardiovascular system. Circulation. 2020;142(1):68–78.
84. Lakatta EG. The reality of getting old. Nat Rev Cardiol. 2018;15(9):499–500.

85. Min LJ, Mogi M, Iwai M, Horiuchi M. Signaling mechanisms of angiotensin II in regulating vascular senescence. Ageing Res Rev. 2009;8(2):113–21.
86. Tang D, Kang R, Berghe TV, Vandenabeele P, Kroemer G. The molecular machinery of regulated cell death. Cell Res. 2019;29(5):347–64.
87. Keilich SR, Bartley JM, Haynes L. Diminished immune responses with aging predispose older adults to common and uncommon influenza complications. Cell Immunol. 2019;345:10399.
88. Acosta JC, Banito A, Wuestefeld T, Georgilis A, Janich P, Morton JP, Athineos D, Kang TW, Lasitschka F, Andrulis M, Pascual G. A complex secretory program orchestrated by the inflammasome controls paracrine senescence. Nat Cell Biol. 2013;15(8):978–90.
89. Yang M. Cell pyroptosis, a potential pathogenic mechanism of 2019-nCoV infection. 2020. Available at SSRN 3527420.
90. Bochenek ML, Schütz E, Schäfer K. Endothelial cell senescence and thrombosis: ageing clots. Thromb Res. 2016;147:36–45.
91. Ungvari Z, Tarantini S, Kiss T, Wren JD, Giles CB, Griffin CT, Murfee WL, Pacher P, Csiszar A. Endothelial dysfunction and angiogenesis impairment in the ageing vasculature. Nat Rev Cardiol. 2018;15(9):555–65.
92. Gude NA, Broughton KM, Firouzi F, Sussman MA. Cardiac ageing: extrinsic and intrinsic factors in cellular renewal and senescence. Nat Rev Cardiol. 2018;15(9):523–42.
93. Sheydina A, Riordon DR, Boheler KR. Molecular mechanisms of cardiomyocyte aging. Clin Sci. 2011;121(8):315–29.
94. Nehme J, Borghesan M, Mackedenski S, Bird TG, Demaria M. Cellular senescence as a potential mediator of COVID-19 severity in the elderly. Aging Cell. 2020;19(10), e13237.
95. Kovacic JC, Moreno P, Nabel EG, Hachinski V, Fuster V. Cellular senescence, vascular disease, and aging: part 2 of a 2-part review: clinical vascular disease in the elderly. Circulation. 2011;123(17):1900–10.
96. Wang M, Jiang L, Monticone RE, Lakatta EG. Proinflammation: the key to arterial aging. Trends Endocrinol Metab. 2014;25(2):72–9.
97. Lakatta EG, Levy D. Arterial and cardiac aging: major shareholders in cardiovascular disease enterprises: Part II: the aging heart in health: links to heart disease. Circulation. 2003;107(2):346–54.
98. Wiley CD, Brumwell AN, Davis SS, Jackson JR, Valdovinos A, Calhoun C, Alimirah F, Castellanos CA, Ruan R, Wei Y, Chapman HA. Secretion of leukotrienes by senescent lung fibroblasts promotes pulmonary fibrosis. JCI Insight. 2019;4(24).
99. Yanagi S, Tsubouchi H, Miura A, Matsuo A, Matsumoto N, Nakazato M. The impacts of cellular senescence in elderly pneumonia and in age-related lung diseases that increase the risk of respiratory infections. Int J Mol Sci. 2017;18(3):503.
100. Brownlee MDM. Advanced protein glycosylation in diabetes and aging. Annu Rev Med. 1995;46(1), 223–34.
101. Goldin A, Beckman JA, Schmidt AM, Creager MA. Advanced glycation end products: sparking the development of diabetic vascular injury. Circulation. 2006;114(6):597–605.
102. Lauc G, Sinclair D. Biomarkers of biological age as predictors of COVID19 disease severity. Aging (Albany NY). 2020;12(8):6490.
103. Acharya R, Poudel D, Bowers R, Patel A, Schultz E, Bourgeois M, Paswan R, Stockholm S, Batten M, Kafle S, Lonial K. Low serum albumin predicts severe outcomes in COVID19 infection: a single-center retrospective case-control study. J Clin Med Res. 2021;13(5):258–67.
104. Vasheghani M, Jannati N, Baghaei P, Rezaei M, Marjani M. The association of 25 (OH) Vitamin D levels and severity and outcome of COVID19: A Cross-sectional Study. 2021.
105. Bauer JM, Morley JE. COVID19 in older persons: the role of nutrition. Curr Opin Clin Nutr Metab Care. 2021;24(1):1.

106. Wynants L, Van Calster B, Collins GS, Riley RD, Heinze G, Schuit E, Bonten MM, Dahly DL, Damen JA, Debray TP, de Jong VM. Prediction models for diagnosis and prognosis of CoViD19: systematic review and critical appraisal. BMJ. 2020;369.
107. Bonafè M, Prattichizzo F, Giuliani A, Storci G, Sabbatinelli J, Olivieri F. Inflamm-aging: why older men are the most susceptible to SARS-CoV-2 complicated outcomes. Cytokine Growth Factor Rev. 2020;53, 33–7.
108. Gilis M, Chagrot N, Koeberle S, Tannou T, Brunel AS, Chirouze C, Bouiller K. Older adults with SARS-CoV-2 infection: utility of the clinical frailty scale to predict mortality. J Med Virol. 2021;93(4):2453–3246.
109. Jørgensen R, Brabrand M. Screening of the frail patient in the emergency department: a systematic review. Eur J Intern Med. 2017;45:71–3.
110. Gilbert T, Neuburger J, Kraindler J, Keeble E, Smith P, Ariti C, Arora S, Street A, Parker S, Roberts HC, Bardsley M. Development and validation of a hospital frailty risk score focusing on older people in acute care settings using electronic hospital records: an observational study. The Lancet. 2018;391(10132):1775–82.
111. Ivey DC, Wieling E, Harris SM. Save the young—the elderly have lived their lives: ageism in marriage and family therapy. Fam Process. 2000;39(2):163–75.
112. Ben-Harush A, Shiovitz-Ezra S, Doron I, Alon S, Leibovitz A, Golander H, Ayalon L. Ageism among physicians, nurses, and social workers: Findings from a qualitative study. European Journal of Ageing. 2017. https://doi.org/10.1007/s10433-016-0389-9.
113. Iosa M, Paolucci S, Morone G. CoViD19: a dynamic analysis of fatality risk in Italy. Front Med. 2020;7:185.
114. Brooke J, Jackson D. Older people and COVID-19: isolation, risk and ageism. 2020.
115. Cox C. Older adults and CoViD19: social justice, disparities, and social work practice. J Gerontological Soc Work. 2020;63(6–7), 611–24.
116. Rosenbaum L. Facing CoViD19 in Italy—Ethics, Logistics, and Therapeutics on the Epidemic's Front Line. N Engl J Med. 2020. https://doi.org/10.1056/NEJMp2005492. [Epub ahead of print] PubMed PMID: 32187459.
117. Kimball A, Hatfield KM, Arons M, James A, Taylor J, Spicer K, et al., Asymptomatic and Presymptomatic SARS-CoV-2 Infections in Residents of a Long-Term Care Skilled Nursing Facility.
118. Boodman E, Branswell H. First CoViD19 outbreak in a US nursing home raises concerns. 2020. https://www.statnews.com/2020/02/29/new-CoViD19-death-raisesconcerns-about-virus-spread-in-nursing-homes/GoogleScholar.
119. Comas-Herrera A, Zalakaín J, Litwin C, Hsu AT, Lane N, Fernández JL. Mortality associated with COVID19 outbreaks in care homes: early international evidence. Article in LTCcovid. org, international long-term care policy network, CPEC-LSE. 2020;26.
120. Ng R, de Boer R, Green MD. Undertreatment of elderly patients with non-small-cell lung cancer. Clin Lung Cancer. 2005;7(3):168–74. Review. PubMed PMID: 16354310.
121. Robb C, Chen H, Haley WE. Ageism in mental health and health care: a critical review. J Clin Geropsychol. 2002;8(1):1–12. https://doi.org/10.1023/A:1013013322947.
122. Courtney M, Tong S, Walsh A. Acute-care nurses' attitudes towards older patients: a literature review. Int J Nurs Pract. 2000; 6(2):62–9.
123. Vandrevala T, Hampson SE, Daly T, Arber S, Thomas H. Dilemmas in decision-making about resuscitation–a focus group study of older people. Soc Sci Med. 2006; 62(7):1579–93.
124. Lloyd-Sherlock P, Ebrahim S, Geffen L, et al. Bearing the brunt of CoViD19: older people in low and middle income countries. BMJ 2020;368. https://doi.org/10.1136/bmj.m1052.

Chapter 19
Gender Disparity in CoViD19

Key Questions

- What is the burden of gender bias in CoViD19?
- How is gender bias related to CoViD19 in different parts of the globe?
- Does gender disparity impact cardiovascular outcomes in CoViD19?
- Which gender-related mechanisms may determine the cardiovascular associations in CoViD19?
- What are the challenges in understanding the gender bias in CoViD19?
- What are the pathogenetic links that may promote gender disparity in CoViD19?

19.1 Epidemiology

The sex and gender differences are reflected in multiple biological and non-biological aspects of human health and other aspects of life. Whether related to a disease, predisposition towards a disease, disease outcomes, or in relationship with response to pharmaceutical or non-pharmaceutical interventions, or even diagnostics or interactions with healthcare systems. Analysis of the CoViD19 studies reveals a gender dichotomy, with a higher prevalence of the disease among the male subjects, although deviations have emerged. Several analyses describe gaps and limitations in the initial data from the CoViD19 pandemic and indicate a lack of disaggregated age and sex data in multiple studies that may blur the plausibility. However, the evolving data and overall indicators, consistently reflect a gender disparity in the CoViD19 occurrence, and the related mortality, especially in the older age groups, and across the geographical regions of the globe. Data indicate

U. Mallick, *Cardiovascular Complications of COVID-19*,
https://doi.org/10.1007/978-3-030-90065-6_19

a sex predisposition to COVID19, with men more susceptible to the disease and its complications [1–3]. According to a retrospective analysis report of 1099 patients with CoViD19, from 552 hospitals in 30 provinces in China, about 58% of the patients were men [4]. In a retrospective case series of 1591 consecutive CoViD19 patients, in the Lombardy region in Italy, the prevalence of males was much higher 83% (1304), and also had severe disease. In this study older patients (n = 786; age $\geq$ 64 years) had higher mortality than younger patients (n = 795; age $\leq$ 63 years) (36% vs 15%; difference, 21% [95% CI, 17%-26%]; P < 0.001) [2].

The association of gender with CoViD19 severity and mortality (Figs. 19.6 and 19.7) was revealed in several analyses. Analysis of retrospective observational study of 52 critically ill patients with CoViD19, revealed a high proportion of males 67% (35) [5]. A retrospective analysis of 487 severe CoViD19 patients, showed an independent association of male sex with severe disease at admission (OR 3.68 [95% CI 1.75–7.75], $P = 0.001$) [6]. Furthermore, the association of cardiometabolic factors, in severely ill male CoViD19 subjects, was linked with the severity of CoViD19 and death [7].

However, analyses further indicate, there may be an equal gender distribution, and a lack of significant association of severity of CoViD19 with male gender, although confirm the significance of higher mortality. In a large systematic review, data of 281,461 CoViD19 patients, from 212 studies from 11 countries, both sexes were equally distributed however, among patients with severe disease, 61% were males. Male gender was not significantly associated with severity of the illness, however, there was a significant association with mortality (coefficient 5.1, CI 2.4–7.9, p.0002) [8]. A meta-analysis of 3,111,714 reported global CoViD19 cases demonstrated that male sex is associated with the development of severe disease i.e. almost three times the odds of requiring intensive treatment unit (ITU) admission (OR = 2.84; 95% CI = 2.06, 3.92; $p = 1.86 \times 10^{-10}$) and death (OR = 1.39; 95% CI = 1.31,1.47; $p = 5.00 \times 10^{-30}$) (Figs. 19.4 and 19.5). The authors also observed that males and females are at equivalent risk of infection (Fig. 19.3) [9].

Further CoViD19 data show trends indicating a higher mortality in association with gender disparity. Analysis of the initial CoViD19 data from China revealed a death rate of 4.7% in males, and 2.8% in females [10], and larger global CoViD19 datasets, further confirmed presence of severe disease and higher mortality in males as compared to the females [11]. A report of 16 countries reporting 178,568 COVID19 deaths, from a total population of approximately 2.4 billion people over 6 weeks, recorded in May 2020, showed mortality rates from COVID19 were 77% higher in men than in women (IRR = 1.77, 95%CI = 1.74, 1.79) [12]. Another multinational analysis of CoViD19 data covering an estimated population of 194 349 591 men and 201 715 364 women (deaths: 77 652 men and 59 591 women) from the beginning of the pandemic until June 21, 2020, describes unequal male to female mortality sex ratio per 100,000 across different age groups: the overall ratio was 1·4 (crude ratio 1·3); the ratio in age 0–9 years age group was 0·81; in 40–49 years age group 1·9; in the 50–59 years age group 2·3; in the 60–69 years age group 2·6, and 1·65 in people older than 80 years [13]. Studies further describe the characteristics of the deceased CoViD19 patients in relation to the gender disparity.

In a retrospective report analyzing characteristics of 168 patients, who died of COVID19, 126 (75.0%) were men, and median (IQR) age was 70 (64–78) years, 161 patients (95.8%) were older than 50 years [14]. Later data, covering a longer period, confirm the gender gap in CoViD19. According to a report describing mortality data in the US for the year Jan-December 2020, the age-adjusted death rates remained higher among males (990.5) than among females (689.2). The death rates were lowest among persons aged 5–14 years (13.6), and highest among persons aged $\geq$ 85 years (15,007.4) [15].

Regional reports from various parts of the globe, confirm similar epidemiological patterns of association of gender disparity with CoViD19. According to a report of an Italian cohort of 12,462 patients with CoViD19, about 827 deaths were reported. Significant gender disparity was observed with male to female ratio of 80% to 20%, and the older median age for women (83·4 years for women vs 79·9 years for men). Fatalities were higher among the older age groups, 42·2% in 80–89 years, 32·4% in 70–79 years, 8·4% in 60–69 years, and 2·8% in 50–59 years [16]. A large UK based report from the primary care records of 17,278,392 adults describing 10,926 CoViD19-related deaths, revealed association of male gender with death (hazard ratio (HR) 1.59 (95% confidence interval 1.53–1.65)) [17]. According to a government-reported time series of CoViD19 cases and deaths in Peru, stratified by age group and gender, a higher mortality burden per 100,000 was recorded among men, 279.2 for men age 80 years, versus 108.8 for women of the same age; 207.6 for men age 70–79 years, versus 85.1 for women of the same age. The cumulative morbidity ratio among men was higher than women, across all age groups (proportion test, p-value < 0.001), except for the individuals aged 0–9 years (proportion test, p-value = 0.85) [18]. Similarly, in a retrospective case series of 5700 CoViD19 hospitalized patients in New York, about 60.3% were males, and 39.7% females. Mortality rates were higher for male compared with female patients at every 10-year age interval older than 20 years [3].

19.2 Discrepancies in the Epidemiological Data

Several discrepancies in the data may be observed in CoViD19 related to the distribution of gender and associated risk. The pattern of risk distribution according to gender may vary. According to a report describing gender disparity trends in CoViD19 cases in India, early evidence indicates a higher overall burden in males, but a higher relative risk of COVID19 mortality in females. Elderly males and females both display a high mortality risk. The study further showed a significantly higher case fatality rate in the females, age 40–49 years [19]. The study pointed to a higher relative risk of mortality in the females among CoViD19 subjects, as compared to the male subjects. The analysis was based on crowdsourcing data, with significant gaps in reporting age and sex-specific data, and observed similar gaps in the studies reporting CoViD19 in the Indian population.

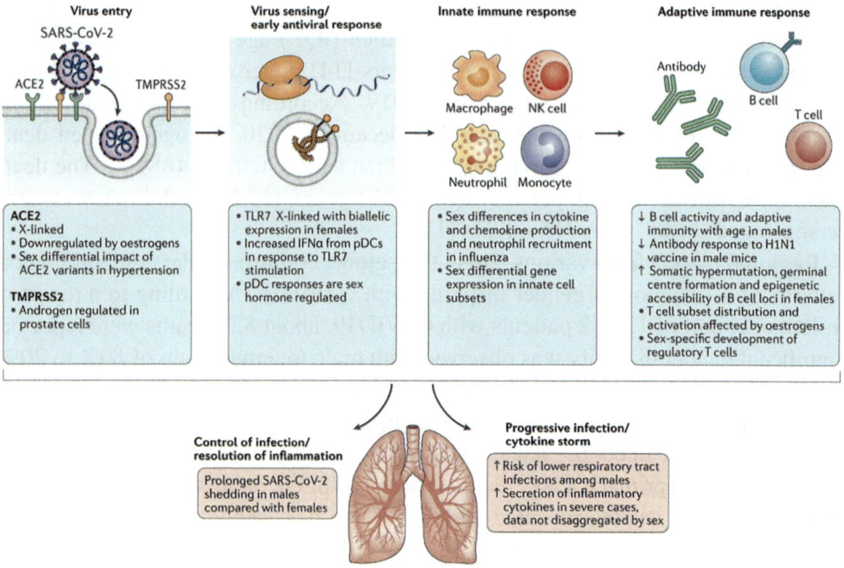

Fig. 19.1 Known sex differences that may impact immune responses to SARS-CoV-2 and COVID-19 progression. An illustrative summary of the sequence of events in severe acute respiratory syndrome coronavirus 2 (SARS-CoV-2) infection and the associated immune responses. Broadly speaking (from left to right), there are the initial steps of virus entry, innate recognition of the virus with activation of antiviral programs, the recruitment of innate immune cells and induction of an adaptive immune response. These major steps culminate either in successful control of infection and pathogen elimination or in a pathological inflammatory state. Sex differences that may be operative at multiple points along these pathways are indicated in the blue boxes. ACE2, angiotensin-converting enzyme 2; H1N1, H1N1 influenza virus; IFNα, interferon-α; NK, natural killer; pDC, plasmacytoid dendritic cell; TLR7, Toll-like receptor 7; TMPRSS2, transmembrane protease serine 2. *Source* Figure 2. Scully, E.P., Haverfield, J., Ursin, R.L., Tannenbaum, C. and Klein, S.L., 2020. Considering how biological sex impacts immune responses and COVID-19 outcomes. *Nature Reviews Immunology*, pp. 1–6. https://www.nature.com/articles/s41577-020-0348-8. By Springer Nature Group

The initial CoViD19 reports showed an equal gender distribution [20, 21] that was also observed in further analyses [21], however, lack of sex-disaggregated data analyzed from a gender perspective, and several gaps and limitations may exist in the initial CoViD19 studies. A data analysis report from 20 countries with the highest numbers of confirmed CoViD19 cases, revealed that few countries had reported sex aggregated data, and further concluded that sex and age data were inconclusive for the determination of health outcomes in patients with CoViD19 [21]. Inaccuracies in data have been linked with a lack of data reporting deaths. An analysis suggested inconsistency in data reporting, concluding, lack of fatality data related to deaths from COVID19 in non-hospitalized patients, may have resulted in the under-reporting of deaths in women. And further suggested a negative impact of invisibility of data by sex and gender, on women with CoViD19 more than men

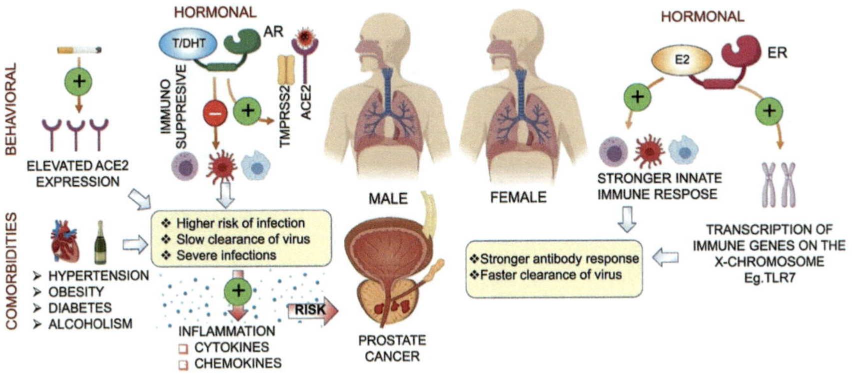

Fig. 19.2 Sex differences in COVID-19. Illustration highlights potential biological (hormone signaling, immunological) and behavioral differences between males and females that contribute to sex divergence in response to SARS-CoV-2. Estrogens have protective functions that contribute to stronger innate immune response in females resulting in faster clearance of virus loads. Androgens and AR regulate tissue level expression of TMPRSS2; serine protease involved in SARS-CoV-2 infection combined with immunosuppressive effects and comorbidities can contribute to the severity of disease in males. Inflammation, an outcome of COVID-19 associated with severe infection, is a potential risk factor for prostate cancer and can augment progression of active disease. *Source* Figure 4. Chakravarty, D., Nair, S.S., Hammouda, N., Ratnani, P., Gharib, Y., Wagaskar, V., Mohamed, N., Lundon, D., Dovey, Z., Kyprianou, N. and Tewari, A.K., 2020. Sex differences in SARS-CoV-2 infection rates and the potential link to prostate cancer. Communications biology, 3(1), pp. 1–12. https://www.nature.com/articles/s42003-020-1088-9?elqTrackId=eecce2f1a1ee4a3c9abf199c258e7795. By Springer Nature Group

[22]. Besides, several other factors such as differences in the demographics, health systems, CoViD19 detection and reporting systems, or social or cultural differences may play an important role in the discrepancies. There were significant variations in the number of countries in reporting disaggregated gender data related to cases, phenotypic variations, morbidities, or death. An analysis found a wide range of disparity in the format, sex, and or age disaggregation, and amount and accessibility of data made available to the public and scholars, with most countries lacking data on confirmed CoViD19 cases, and outcomes stratified by sex [23].

Post CoViD19 syndromes have been reported, although concrete definitions are lacking. A trend describing a higher proportion of female subjects may be observed in these syndromes. A surveillance report from an ambidirectional cohort study of 1733 patients with confirmed COVID19 who had been discharged, revealed significant sex differences, with women more likely to experience fatigue and anxiety/depression at 6 months follow-up [24]. Although currently under debate, "prolonged CoViD19 with the duration of symptoms stretching over a few weeks to months", has been reported to have a more frequent association with the female gender [25]. In a prospective observational cohort study of 4,182 SARS CoV2 positive patients using the COVID Symptom Study app, symptom duration was compared with that in age-, sex- and body mass index (BMI)-matched symptomatic

Source	Infected males	Total infections	Proportion	95%-CI	Weight
Australia, 21/05/2020 (7)	3598	7087	0.51	[0.50; 0.52]	1.1%
Belgium, 22/05/2020 (8)	20,683	56,511	0.37	[0.36; 0.37]	1.1%
China, 11/02/2020 (9)	22,981	44,672	0.51	[0.51; 0.52]	1.1%
Denmark, 19/05/2020 (12)	4672	11,044	0.42	[0.41; 0.43]	1.1%
France, 23/03/2020 (13)	2998	6378	0.47	[0.46; 0.48]	1.1%
Germany, 21/05/2020 (14)	84,841	176,752	0.48	[0.48; 0.48]	1.1%
Iran, 15/03/2020 (15)	8545	14,991	0.57	[0.56; 0.58]	1.1%
Italy, 14/05/2020 (16)	102,628	222,074	0.46	[0.46; 0.46]	1.1%
Netherlands, 26/05/2020 (17)	16,755	45,578	0.37	[0.36; 0.37]	1.1%
Norway, 25/05/2020 (18)	4151	8352	0.50	[0.49; 0.51]	1.1%
Portugal, 25/05/2020 (19)	12,975	30,788	0.42	[0.42; 0.43]	1.1%
South Korea, 26/05/2020 (20)	4664	11,225	0.42	[0.41; 0.42]	1.1%
Spain, 22/05/2020 (21)	106,970	248,953	0.43	[0.43; 0.43]	1.1%
Switzerland, [illegible]	13,989	30,601	0.46	[0.45; 0.46]	1.1%
Republic of Ireland, 31/05/2020 (23)	10,601	24,924	0.43	[0.42; 0.43]	1.1%
Chile, 07/05/2020 (24)	13,654	25,972	0.53	[0.52; 0.53]	1.1%
Sweden, 26/05/2020 (25)	14,140	34,440	0.41	[0.41; 0.42]	1.1%
Finland, 26/05/2020 (26)	3248	6628	0.49	[0.48; 0.50]	1.1%
Czech Republic, 26/05/2020 (27)	4336	8778	0.49	[0.48; 0.50]	1.1%
Romania, 24/05/2020 (28)	7559	18,283	0.41	[0.41; 0.42]	1.1%
Austria, 26/05/2020 (29)	8083	16,496	0.49	[0.48; 0.50]	1.1%
Saudi Arabia, 25/05/2020 (30)	54,600	74,795	0.73	[0.73; 0.73]	1.1%
Greece, 25/05/2020 (31)	1585	2882	0.55	[0.53; 0.57]	1.1%
Estonia, 11/05/2020 (32)	783	1741	0.45	[0.43; 0.47]	1.1%
Philippines, 26/05/2020 (33)	7930	14,595	0.54	[0.54; 0.55]	1.1%
New Zealand, 26/05/2020 (34)	667	1503	0.44	[0.42; 0.47]	1.1%
Slovenia, 25/03/2020 (35)	274	562	0.49	[0.45; 0.53]	1.0%
England, 20/05/2020 (36)	66,186	145,808	0.45	[0.45; 0.46]	1.1%
Scotland, 18/05/2020 (37)	5636	14,594	0.39	[0.38; 0.39]	1.1%
Pakistan, 23/05/2020 (38)	44,720	57,690	0.78	[0.77; 0.78]	1.1%
Colombia, 27/05/2020 (39)	13,540	24,104	0.56	[0.56; 0.57]	1.1%
Ecuador, 26/05/2020 (40)	15,964	28,700	0.56	[0.55; 0.56]	1.1%
Mexico, 27/05/2020 (41)	44,473	78,023	0.57	[0.57; 0.57]	1.1%
Thailand, 24/05/2020 (42)	1654	3040	0.54	[0.53; 0.56]	1.1%
Luxembourg, 27/05/2020 (43)	2041	4001	0.51	[0.49; 0.53]	1.1%
Indonesia, 27/05/2020 (44)	13,496	24,538	0.55	[0.54; 0.56]	1.1%
Dominican Republic, 26/05/2020 (45)	8576	15,723	0.55	[0.54; 0.55]	1.1%
Argentina, 27/05/2020 (46)	7091	13,920	0.51	[0.50; 0.52]	1.1%
Northern Ireland, 22/05/2020 (47)	1747	4565	0.38	[0.37; 0.40]	1.1%
Ghana, 01/06/2020 (48)	4842	8070	0.60	[0.59; 0.61]	1.1%
Somalia, 01/06/2020 (49)	1423	1976	0.72	[0.70; 0.74]	1.1%
Sierra Leone, 27/05/2020 (50)	410	829	0.49	[0.46; 0.53]	1.1%
Haiti, 30/05/2020 (51)	1270	2124	0.60	[0.58; 0.62]	1.1%
Jamaica, 31/05/2020 (52)	248	586	0.42	[0.38; 0.46]	1.0%
Nigeria, 30/05/2020 (53)	6631	9855	0.67	[0.66; 0.68]	1.1%
Bangladesh, 01/06/2020 (54)	35,169	49,534	0.71	[0.71; 0.71]	1.1%
New York State, 20/05/2020 (55)	181,437	354,370	0.51	[0.51; 0.51]	1.1%
Texas, 21/05/2020 (56)	7583	14,456	0.52	[0.52; 0.53]	1.1%
Illinois, 21/05/2020 (57)	48,821	102,686	0.48	[0.47; 0.48]	1.1%
Pennsylvania, 22/05/2020 (58)	29,153	66,258	0.44	[0.44; 0.44]	1.1%
Massachusetts, 18/05/2020 (59)	39,658	90,084	0.44	[0.44; 0.44]	1.1%
New Jersey, 20/05/2020 (60)	75,073	151,472	0.50	[0.49; 0.50]	1.1%
Michigan, 21/05/2020 (61)	25,150	53,510	0.47	[0.47; 0.47]	1.1%
California, 20/05/2020 (62)	43,450	86,197	0.50	[0.50; 0.51]	1.1%
Washington, 20/05/2020 (63)	8794	19,117	0.46	[0.45; 0.47]	1.1%
Louisiana, 21/05/2020 (64)	14,602	36,504	0.40	[0.39; 0.41]	1.1%
Maryland, 22/05/2020 (65)	21,283	44,424	0.48	[0.47; 0.48]	1.1%
Virginia, 22/05/2020 (66)	17,285	34,950	0.49	[0.49; 0.50]	1.1%
North Carolina, 22/05/2020 (67)	10,418	21,262	0.49	[0.48; 0.50]	1.1%
South Carolina, 22/05/2020 (68)	4067	9638	0.42	[0.41; 0.43]	1.1%
Alabama, 29/05/2020 (69)	6800	16,530	0.41	[0.40; 0.42]	1.1%
Mississippi, 27/05/2020 (70)	4915	12,147	0.40	[0.40; 0.41]	1.1%
Ohio, 29/05/2020 (71)	16,445	31,625	0.52	[0.51; 0.53]	1.1%
Arkansas, 29/05/2020 (72)	3906	6538	0.60	[0.59; 0.61]	1.1%
Indiana, 29/05/2020 (73)	15,230	33,068	0.46	[0.46; 0.47]	1.1%
Wisconsin, 29/05/2020 (74)	8657	16,974	0.51	[0.50; 0.52]	1.1%
Minnesota, 28/05/2020 (75)	11,051	22,947	0.48	[0.48; 0.49]	1.1%
Florida, 28/05/2020 (76)	25,611	51,918	0.49	[0.49; 0.50]	1.1%
Kentucky, 29/05/2020 (77)	4328	9185	0.47	[0.46; 0.48]	1.1%
Iowa, 29/05/2020 (78)	9583	18,791	0.51	[0.50; 0.52]	1.1%
Missouri, 29/05/2020 (79)	6826	12,673	0.54	[0.53; 0.55]	1.1%
Connecticut, 28/05/2020 (80)	18,662	41,559	0.45	[0.44; 0.45]	1.1%
Rhode Island, 29/05/2020 (81)	6439	14,635	0.44	[0.43; 0.45]	1.1%
New Hampshire, 18/05/2020 (82)	2006	3652	0.55	[0.53; 0.57]	1.1%
Vermont, 29/05/2020 (83)	458	975	0.47	[0.44; 0.50]	1.1%
Maine, 29/05/2020 (84)	1072	2226	0.48	[0.46; 0.50]	1.1%
Oklahoma, 29/05/2020 (85)	2986	6338	0.47	[0.46; 0.48]	1.1%
Alaska, 29/05/2020 (86)	220	430	0.51	[0.46; 0.56]	1.0%
Arizona, 29/05/2020 (87)	8679	18,465	0.47	[0.46; 0.48]	1.1%
Colorado, 29/05/2020 (88)	12,088	25,121	0.48	[0.47; 0.49]	1.1%
Delaware, 29/05/2020 (89)	4117	9236	0.45	[0.44; 0.46]	1.1%
West Virginia, 29/05/2020 (90)	911	1951	0.47	[0.44; 0.49]	1.1%
Oregon, 19/05/2020 (91)	1727	3660	0.47	[0.46; 0.49]	1.1%
North Dakota, 29/05/2020 (92)	1188	2520	0.47	[0.45; 0.49]	1.1%
New Mexico, 29/05/2020 (93)	3462	7364	0.47	[0.46; 0.48]	1.1%
Nevada, 29/05/2020 (94)	3887	8350	0.47	[0.45; 0.48]	1.1%
Montana, 15/05/2020 (95)	225	468	0.48	[0.43; 0.53]	1.0%
Kansas, 29/05/2020 (96)	5358	9719	0.55	[0.54; 0.56]	1.1%
Idaho, 29/05/2020 (97)	1249	2769	0.45	[0.43; 0.47]	1.1%
Wyoming, 29/05/2020 (98)	331	667	0.50	[0.46; 0.53]	1.1%
Random effects model		**3,111,714**	**0.50**	**[0.48; 0.51]**	**100.0%**

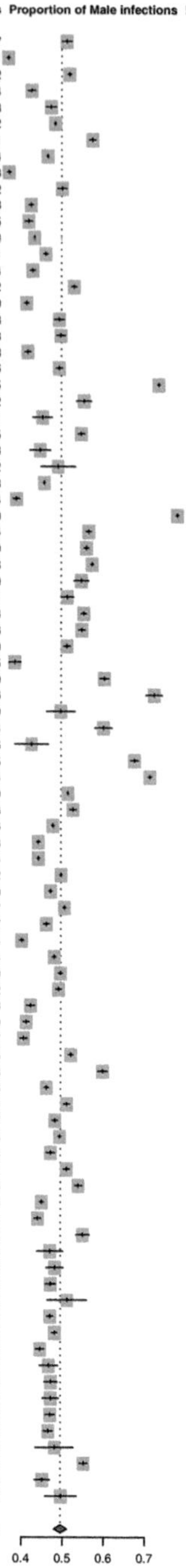

◂**Fig. 19.3** There is no observed sex difference in the proportion of people with COVID-19. There is no observed sex difference in the proportion of people with COVID-19. The table summarizes the number of confirmed male COVID-19 cases and the total number of COVID-19 cases in 90 reports. The forest plot illustrates the estimated proportion of male cases for each report (grey boxes), with 95% confidence intervals (CI; horizontal black lines). The estimated pooled proportion of male cases (dark grey diamond) was 0.5 (95% CI = 0.48,0.51). A two-sided test confirmed the estimated pooled proportion was not significantly different from 0.5 (p = 0.56), indicating no difference between the proportions of male and female infections. Meta-analysis used a random effects model, which accounted for variance across reports and used the indicated weights for each report. *Source* Figure 2. Peckham, H., de Gruijter, N.M., Raine, C., Radziszewska, A., Ciurtin, C., Wedderburn, L.R., Rosser, E.C., Webb, K. and Deakin, C.T., 2020. Male sex identified by global COVID-19 meta-analysis as a risk factor for death and ITU admission. Nature communications, 11(1), pp. 1–10. https://www.nature.com/articles/s41467-020-19741-6. By Springer Nature Group

controls who tested negative for COVID19. The duration of 4 weeks or 8 weeks long CoViD19 was more commonly reported among the females. Long COVID was characterized by symptoms of fatigue, headache, dyspnea, and anosmia and was more likely with increasing age and body mass index, and female sex. However, the study has several limitations related to design and the methodology [26]. Further data are needed to characterize the post CoViD19 syndromes or long CoViD19 and assess possible associations of gender disparity.

19.3 Factors Associated with Gender Dichotomy

The gender differences in CoViD19 may be associated with a variety of factors related to the hormonal environment, immune function, regulatory mechanisms, the aging process, or the structural and functional status of cardiovascular structures. The interactions and synergism of several mechanisms impact gender-based associations of CoViD19. Historically, women have a lesser risk of viral infections, better immune response (both innate and adaptive), more efficient, intense, and prolonged [27–29]. Data show that hormonal factors, lifestyle differences, associated co morbidities, and genetic factors play an important role in gender dichotomy [30, 31]. These factors are also involved in age-specific gender variations seen in cardiovascular diseases. Since CoViD19 is associated with cardiovascular complications, exploring these factors is of paramount importance.

Multiple factors contribute to the elevated health risks in advanced age, including a frequent association of comorbidities. In a multinational registry of 14,712 patients with CoViD19, of whom 6387 (43%) were men, exploring the relationship between male sex and CoViD19 mortality and age dependency, men had significantly higher mortality than did women, and this difference was not completely explained by the higher prevalence of comorbidities in men. In this study, the cumulative probability of survival remained significantly lower in the propensity score-matched men than in women after excluding patients younger than

Source	Males Deaths	Males Total	Females Deaths	Females Total	OR	95%-CI	Weight
Australia, 21/05/2020 (7)	56	3598	44	3489	1.24	[0.83; 1.84]	0.9%
Belgium, 22/05/2020 (8)	3318	20,683	3234	35,598	1.91	[1.82; 2.01]	1.7%
China, 11/02/2020 (9)	653	22,981	370	21,691	1.69	[1.48; 1.92]	1.6%
Denmark, 19/05/2020 (12)	314	4672	237	6372	1.87	[1.57; 2.22]	1.5%
France, 23/03/2020 (13)	94	2998	67	3380	1.60	[1.17; 2.20]	1.1%
Germany, 21/05/2020 (14)	4515	84,841	3627	91,911	1.37	[1.31; 1.43]	1.7%
Iran, 15/03/2020 (15)	503	8545	350	6446	1.09	[0.95; 1.25]	1.5%
Italy, 14/05/2020 (16)	17,877	102,628	11,815	119,267	1.92	[1.87; 1.97]	1.7%
Netherlands, 26/05/2020 (17)	3240	16,755	2616	28,733	2.39	[2.26; 2.53]	1.7%
Norway, 25/05/2020 (18)	128	4151	107	4201	1.22	[0.94; 1.58]	1.2%
Portugal, 25/05/2020 (19)	649	12,975	681	17,813	1.32	[1.19; 1.48]	1.6%
South Korea, 26/05/2020 (20)	142	4664	127	6561	1.59	[1.25; 2.03]	1.3%
Spain, 22/05/2020 (21)	11,608	10,6970	8928	141,983	1.81	[1.76; 1.87]	1.7%
Switzerland, 26/05/2020 (22)	948	13,989	697	16,612	1.66	[1.50; 1.84]	1.6%
Chile, 07/05/2020 (24)	175	13,654	119	12,318	1.33	[1.05; 1.68]	1.3%
Sweden, 26/05/2020 (25)	2274	14,140	1851	20,300	1.91	[1.79; 2.04]	1.7%
Finland, 26/05/2020 (26)	134	3248	151	3380	0.92	[0.73; 1.17]	1.3%
Czech Republic, 26/05/2020 (27)	185	4336	132	4442	1.46	[1.16; 1.83]	1.3%
Romania, 24/05/2020 (28)	699	7559	487	10,724	2.14	[1.90; 2.41]	1.6%
Austria, 26/05/2020 (29)	367	8083	276	8413	1.40	[1.20; 1.64]	1.5%
Greece, 25/05/2020 (31)	121	1585	51	1297	2.02	[1.44; 2.83]	1.1%
Estonia, 11/05/2020 (32)	30	783	31	958	1.19	[0.71; 1.99]	0.7%
Philippines, 26/05/2020 (33)	571	7930	315	6665	1.56	[1.36; 1.80]	1.5%
England, 20/05/2020 (36)	18,684	66,186	13,134	77,540	1.93	[1.88; 1.98]	1.7%
Scotland, 18/05/2020 (37)	1791	5636	1755	8950	1.91	[1.77; 2.06]	1.6%
Pakistan, 23/05/2020 (38)	811	44,720	256	12,970	0.92	[0.80; 1.06]	1.5%
Colombia, 27/05/2020 (39)	495	13,540	308	10,564	1.26	[1.09; 1.46]	1.5%
Ecuador, 26/05/2020 (40)	2139	15,964	1082	12,736	1.67	[1.54; 1.80]	1.6%
Mexico, 27/05/2020 (41)	5760	44,473	2837	33,550	1.61	[1.54; 1.69]	1.7%
Thailand, 24/05/2020 (42)	43	1654	13	1386	2.82	[1.51; 5.26]	0.6%
Luxembourg, 27/05/2020 (43)	62	2041	48	1960	1.25	[0.85; 1.83]	1.0%
Indonesia, 27/05/2020 (44)	942	13,496	554	11,042	1.42	[1.27; 1.58]	1.6%
Dominican Republic, 26/05/2020 (45)	332	8576	142	7147	1.99	[1.63; 2.42]	1.4%
Argentina, 27/05/2020 (46)	294	7091	202	6784	1.41	[1.17; 1.69]	1.4%
Northern Ireland, 22/05/2020 (47)	260	1747	243	2750	1.80	[1.50; 2.17]	1.4%
New York State, 20/05/2020 (55)	13,352	181,437	9615	171,161	1.33	[1.30; 1.37]	1.7%
Texas, 21/05/2020 (56)	268	7583	190	6593	1.23	[1.02; 1.49]	1.4%
Illinois, 21/05/2020 (57)	2560	48,821	2042	51,690	1.35	[1.27; 1.43]	1.7%
Pennsylvania, 22/05/2020 (58)	2406	29,153	2578	36,420	1.18	[1.11; 1.25]	1.7%
Massachusetts, 18/05/2020 (59)	2954	39,658	3189	49,077	1.16	[1.10; 1.22]	1.7%
Michigan, 21/05/2020 (61)	2718	25150	2411	28360	1.30	[1.23; 1.38]	1.7%
California, 20/05/2020 (62)	1926	43,450	1521	42,252	1.24	[1.16; 1.33]	1.7%
Washington, 20/05/2020 (63)	574	8794	470	9941	1.41	[1.24; 1.60]	1.6%
Louisiana, 21/05/2020 (64)	1363	14,602	1143	20,077	1.71	[1.57; 1.85]	1.6%
Maryland, 22/05/2020 (65)	1054	21,283	1038	23,141	1.11	[1.02; 1.21]	1.6%
Virginia, 22/05/2020 (66)	573	17,285	560	17,425	1.03	[0.92; 1.16]	1.6%
North Carolina, 22/05/2020 (67)	378	10,418	349	10,844	1.13	[0.98; 1.31]	1.5%
South Carolina, 22/05/2020 (68)	218	4067	201	5339	1.45	[1.19; 1.76]	1.4%
Alabama, 29/05/2020 (69)	319	6800	270	9600	1.70	[1.44; 2.01]	1.5%
Mississippi, 27/05/2020 (70)	341	4915	352	7232	1.46	[1.25; 1.70]	1.5%
Ohio, 29/05/2020 (71)	1092	16,445	1004	14,864	0.98	[0.90; 1.07]	1.6%
Indiana, 29/05/2020 (73)	954	15,230	904	17,040	1.19	[1.09; 1.31]	1.6%
Wisconsin, 29/05/2020 (74)	312	8657	238	8317	1.27	[1.07; 1.51]	1.5%
Minnesota, 28/05/2020 (75)	492	11,051	465	11,433	1.10	[0.97; 1.25]	1.6%
Florida, 28/05/2020 (76)	1372	25,611	1074	26,262	1.33	[1.22; 1.44]	1.6%
Kentucky, 29/05/2020 (77)	181	4328	228	4608	0.84	[0.69; 1.02]	1.4%
Iowa, 29/05/2020 (78)	270	9583	250	8832	1.00	[0.84; 1.18]	1.5%
Connecticut, 28/05/2020 (80)	1858	18,662	1962	22,702	1.17	[1.09; 1.25]	1.7%
Rhode Island, 29/05/2020 (81)	326	6439	367	8196	1.14	[0.98; 1.33]	1.5%
New Hampshire, 18/05/2020 (82)	92	2006	80	1617	0.92	[0.68; 1.26]	1.1%
Vermont, 29/05/2020 (83)	31	458	24	513	1.48	[0.85; 2.56]	0.7%
Oklahoma, 29/05/2020 (85)	171	2986	158	3338	1.22	[0.98; 1.53]	1.3%
Arizona, 29/05/2020 (87)	486	8679	398	9756	1.39	[1.22; 1.60]	1.5%
Colorado, 29/05/2020 (88)	789	12,088	628	12,759	1.35	[1.21; 1.50]	1.6%
Delaware, 29/05/2020 (89)	169	4117	187	5091	1.12	[0.91; 1.39]	1.4%
Oregon, 19/05/2020 (91)	80	1727	58	1929	1.57	[1.11; 2.21]	1.0%
Nevada, 29/05/2020 (94)	237	3887	171	4142	1.51	[1.23; 1.84]	1.4%
Montana, 15/05/2020 (95)	9	225	7	243	1.40	[0.51; 3.84]	0.3%
Kansas, 29/05/2020 (96)	107	5358	101	4180	0.82	[0.63; 1.08]	1.2%
Idaho, 29/05/2020 (97)	39	1249	43	1513	1.10	[0.71; 1.71]	0.8%
Random effects model		**1,319,094**		**1,416,420**	**1.39**	**[1.31; 1.47]**	**100.0%**

Mortality Odds Ratio

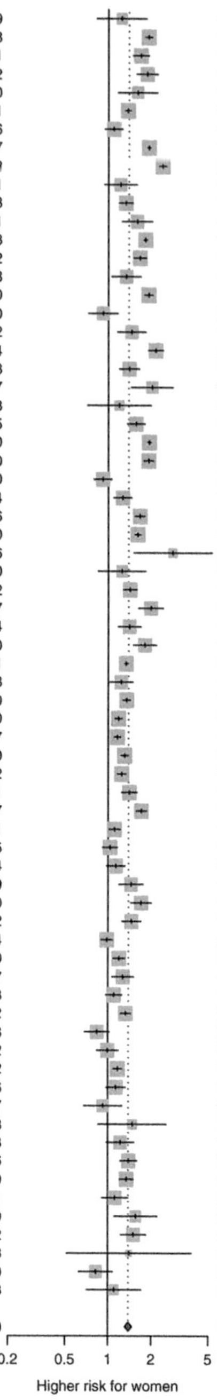

◄**Fig. 19.4** Male sex is associated with a significantly increased risk of mortality within COVID-19 patients. Male sex is associated with a significantly increased risk of mortality within COVID-19 patients. The table summarizes the number of deaths and total number of confirmed COVID-19 cases for each sex for n = 70 reports with complete data on infection and mortality in males and females. The forest plot illustrates the estimated odds ratio (OR) for the association of death with male sex for each report (grey boxes) with 95% confidence intervals (CI; horizontal black lines). The estimated pooled OR (dark grey diamond) was 1.39 (95% CI = 1.31, 1.47). A two-sided test confirmed the estimated pooled OR was significantly different from 1 (p = 5.00e-30). Meta-analysis used a random effects model with individual reports weighted using the indicated weights. *Source* Figure 4 Peckham, H., de Gruijter, N.M., Raine, C., Radziszewska, A., Ciurtin, C., Wedderburn, L.R., Rosser, E.C., Webb, K. and Deakin, C.T., 2020. Male sex identified by global COVID-19 meta-analysis as a risk factor for death and ITU admission. Nature communications, 11(1), pp. 1–10. https://www.nature.com/articles/s41467-020-19741-6. By Springer Nature Group

Source	Males ITU	Males Total	Females ITU	Females Total	OR	95%-CI	Weight
China, 24/02/2020 (10)	35	35	17	17			0.0%
China, 07/02/2020 (11)	22	75	14	63	1.45	[0.67; 3.15]	8.3%
Denmark, 19/05/2020 (12)	243	4672	91	6372	3.79	[2.97; 4.83]	14.7%
France, 23/03/2020 (13)	190	2998	95	3380	2.34	[1.82; 3.01]	14.6%
Spain, 22/05/2020 (21)	5358	106,970	2343	141,983	3.14	[2.99; 3.30]	16.0%
Chile, 07/05/2020 (24)	714	13,654	456	12,318	1.44	[1.27; 1.62]	15.7%
Sweden, 26/05/2020 (25)	1474	14,140	513	20,300	4.49	[4.05; 4.98]	15.8%
Scotland, 18/05/2020 (37)	361	5636	141	8950	4.28	[3.51; 5.21]	15.1%
Random effects model		**148,180**		**193,383**	**2.84**	**[2.06; 3.92]**	**100.0%**

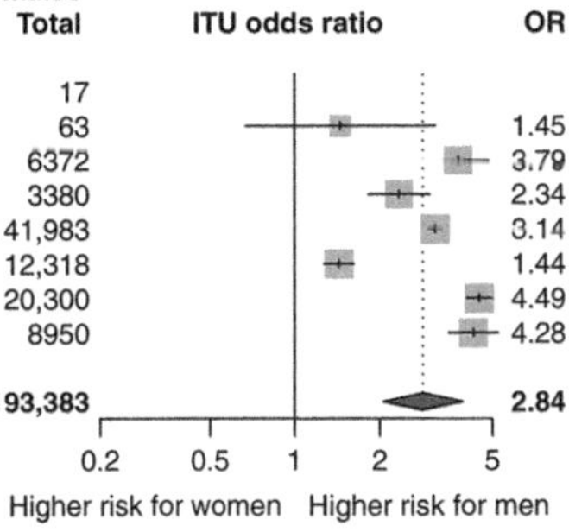

Fig. 19.5 Male sex is associated with a significantly increased risk of ITU admission within COVID-19 patients. The table summarizes the number of ITU admissions and total number of confirmed COVID-19 cases for each sex for n = 8 reports with complete data on SARS-CoV-2 infections and ITU admissions in males and females. The forest plot represents the estimated odds ratio (OR) for the association of ITU admission with male sex for each report (grey boxes), with 95% confidence intervals (CI; horizontal black lines). The estimated pooled OR (dark grey diamond) was 2.84 (95% CI = 2.06, 3.92). A two-sided test confirmed the estimated pooled OR was significantly different from 1 (p = 1.86e-10). Meta-analysis used a random effects model with individual reports weighted using the indicated weights. *Source* Figure 3. Peckham, H., de Gruijter, N.M., Raine, C., Radziszewska, A., Ciurtin, C., Wedderburn, L.R., Rosser, E.C., Webb, K. and Deakin, C.T., 2020. Male sex identified by global COVID 19 meta-analysis as a risk factor for death and ITU admission. Nature communications, 11(1), pp. 1–10. https://www.nature.com/articles/s41467-020-19741-6. By Springer Nature Group

50 years [32]. The factors related to the loss of hormonal protection past middle age, particularly in females, appear important and may contribute to an increased risk. The age-associated decreases in sex steroid hormones, namely, estrogen and testosterone, may mediate proinflammatory increases in older adults that could increase their risk of COVID19 adverse outcomes [33].

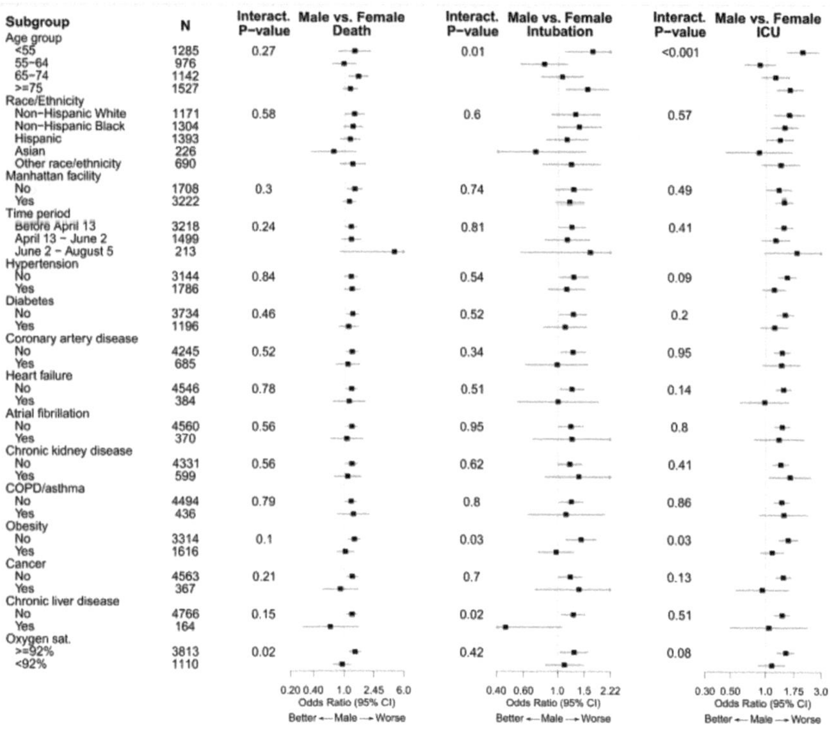

Fig. 19.6 Subgroup analysis for male sex as a predictor of mortality, intubation, or ICU care. In a sex-stratified analysis of a cohort of 4930 hospitalized COVID-19 patients highlighting clinical factors that may contribute to sex differences in the outcome of COVID-19, the forest plot depicts the odds ratio associated with male sex (versus female sex) within the subgroup specified in a multivariable logistic regression model, including an interaction term between the subgroup variable and sex and adjusting for the other variables listed. The interaction p value for sex and each subgroup variable is shown. *Source* Figure 1. Jun, T., Nirenberg, S., Weinberger, T., Sharma, N., Pujadas, E., Cordon-Cardo, C., Kovatch, P. and Huang, K.L., 2021. Analysis of sex-specific risk factors and clinical outcomes in COVID-19. Communications Medicine, 1(1), pp. 1–8. https://www.nature.com/articles/s43856-021-00006-2. By Springer Nature Group

19.4 Gender Disparity in Immune Response

Gender based differences in the immune system may impact CoViD19 (Fig. 19.1). Gender dichotomy related to factors related to immunity and the immune response is an extremely well documented sexually dimorphic biological process in humans [34, 35]. Sex-disparities have been often observed in response to communicable diseases [36, 37]. A significant number of genes that regulate our immune response and inflammation reside on the X chromosome. A high number of immune-related genes responsible for innate and adaptive immune responses to infection are on the X chromosome. Evidence suggests that the X-chromosome and

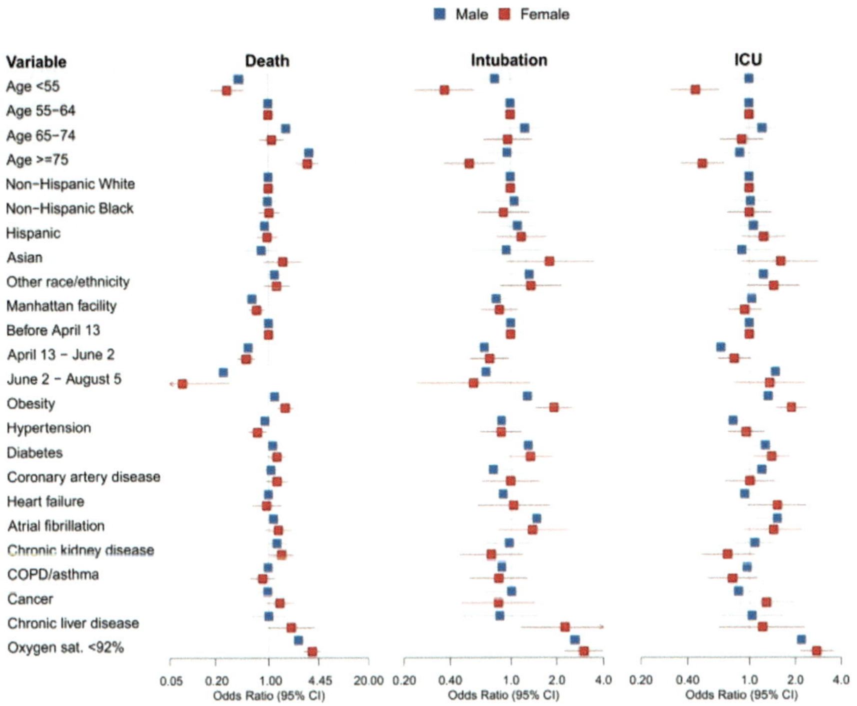

Fig. 19.7 Forest plots depicting sex-stratified multivariable logistic regression models predicting mortality (Male N = 2657; Female N = 2099), intubation (Male N = 2669; Female N = 2108), or ICU care (Male N = 2669; Female N = 2108). A sex-stratified analysis of a cohort of 4930 hospitalized COVID-19 patients highlighting clinical factors that may contribute to sex differences in the outcome of COVID-19. The odds ratio associated with each variable is depicted in blue for the male-specific models and in red for the female-specific models. *Source* Figure 2. Jun, T., Nirenberg, S., Weinberger, T., Sharma, N., Pujadas, E., Cordon-Cardo, C., Kovatch, P. and Huang, K.L., 2021. Analysis of sex-specific risk factors and clinical outcomes in COVID-19. Communications Medicine, 1(1), pp. 1–8. https://www.nature.com/articles/s43856-021-00006-2. By Springer Nature Group

X-linked genes mainly determine sex dimorphism in disease susceptibility and prognosis [38, 39]. Sex hormones such as testosterone and estrogen, play important roles in immune responses, and differences in sex hormones may be correlated with age-specific and age-dependent immune responses. The immune-related X-linked genes appear to be more activated in the female immune cells. Certain estrogen receptors (ERα and ERβ) are expressed in a variety of immune cells (lymphocyte T, B, natural killer cells, macrophages, dendritic cells (DCs), neutrophils). The E2 has anti-inflammatory effects, and elevated expression attenuates the production of chemokines and recruitment of leukocytes and monocytes into several tissues, including the lungs [40, 41]. The anti-inflammatory effects of high E2 are mediated by signaling through ERs, which inhibit activation of

NF-κB-mediated inflammatory responses [42]. Evidence shows that the effect of sex hormones on immune cell functions may be dose-dependent [43]. Testosterone has suppressive effects on immune function possibly increasing susceptibility to infectious diseases observed in men [44] or increase pro-inflammatory cytokine levels [45].

Data also suggest a stronger antibody response in women in the early phase in CoViD19 [46], a possible mechanism in gender disparity. Although controversies exist, women may have lower IL-6 levels than men [47], and IL-6 levels might increase with age [48, 49] or with association of metabolic conditions [50]. Higher IL-6 levels in older age females correlate with poor functioning [51]. The gender differences in IL-6 expression may aggravate male predisposition towards CoViD19 severity, however, these mechanisms need further exploration.

19.5 Gender Disparity in ACE2 Mechanisms

Viral cell entry in CoViD19 is mediated by ACE2 located at cell surface membrane (mACE2) in multiple tissues in different proportions and is also found in the circulatory form (sACE2). Gender disparity in the expression of ACE2 has been validated in multiple studies indicating predominance in the male subjects, although genetic mechanisms favor the elevated ACE2 expression in females due to the location of the ACE2 gene on the X chromosome [52]. The X chromosome also harbors genes related to immune mechanisms that determine gender dimorphism responsible for the enhanced immune response in females.

Data from various studies and analyses suggest higher ACE2 expression in male subjects [53–55], although reports have also suggested that ACE2 expression may be higher among women [56].

The expression of ACE2 is low in healthy individuals [54] and decreases with age [57, 58].

Various hypothetical models have been proposed linking higher ACE2 expression in females benefiting women against CoViD19 and its complications [59]. It has been argued that the location of the ACE2 gene on the X chromosome might lead to higher ACE2 levels in females, therefore offering better protection against more severe disease compared to men [52]. However, since ACE2 acts as a gateway for viral cell entry assisted by TMRPSS2 co protein and increased ACE2 expression promotes increased viral affinity, the argument that ACE2 expression is linked with a high risk of CoViD19 appears to be strong.

Recent research has indicated the genetic polymorphism of ACE2, revealing ACE2 variants with a higher affinity to bind with the virus. These variants appear to be more common in the male gender, and certain populations such as Asians. Studies suggest ACE2 expression may be higher in Asian males [60]. Furthermore, various hypotheses have emerged questioning the correlation between factors and mechanisms that influence homeostasis via regulatory and counter-regulatory arms of the renin angiotensin system (RAS). Such specific hemizygous viral-entry booster ACE2 variants and associated mechanisms might be linked with the higher impact of the viral disease in the male gender [61].

Smoking increases ACE2 expression [62]. Association of smoking, ACE2 expression and burden of CoViD19 in males, especially in the Asian population is subject to debate due to the controversies in data [63]. A higher proportion of male smokers seen in certain populations with a higher burden of severe CoViD19 and ACE2 expression variations, provide an argument for such debate [64]. Methodological limitations of the research related to the incidence and severity of CoViD19 in male subjects and ACE2 expression, restrict drawing plausible conclusions.

19.6 Gender Disparity in Cardiovascular Diseases

Gender impacts the occurrence, treatment response, and outcomes in cardiovascular diseases [65–67]. Among patients with CoViD19, an association of pre-existing cardiometabolic diseases and the occurrence of cardiovascular complications is notable among CoViD19 complications. These are frequently associated with the male gender, as compared to the female gender. Women in their midlife years have historically been at a lower risk for overall vascular events than similarly aged men. It is well known that women develop cardiovascular diseases 7 to 10 years later than men. Overall, atherosclerotic plaque burden and markers of inflammation appear to be greater in men than women, and are predictive of cardiovascular events, rendering men at a greater risk. Many factors may account for the gender differences observed in association with cardiovascular diseases. These include differences in the vascular risk, presence of factors determining resilience against cardiovascular diseases in females, and several others that account for the gender bias seen in cardiovascular complications in CoViD19 subjects.

On the other hand, certain cardiac conditions may have a higher prevalence in females with features of age dependency. More women have high blood pressure as compared to men, the prevalence being greater in women >65 years of age [68]. Although it is generally considered that females exhibit lower levels of cardiovascular diseases, as compared with males, the age adjusted prevalence of uncontrolled blood pressure is higher in females compared with males [69].

Females with heart conditions generally do better regardless of age. According to an analysis of the observation database of 8962 CoViD19 patients from 169 hospitals in Asia, Europe, and North America, the relationship of cardiovascular disease and drug therapy with in-hospital death among hospitalized patients with CoViD19 was assessed. For the female sex, the odds ratio for dying in the hospital was 0.79 (95% confidence interval [CI], 0.65 to 0.95), suggesting an association between survival and female sex, independent of older age [70].

19.6.1 Cardiovascular Pathogenetic Features and Gender

The gender-related pathogenicity of cardiovascular associations and complications, in COViD19 and associated mechanisms, are not fully understood. Multiple mechanisms appear to facilitate the cardiovascular risk in CoViD19, however, the association of certain regulatory, hormonal, and other factors may have specific gender-related implications. Analyses indicate an association of inflammatory, immune, thrombotic, and regulatory mechanisms that may be influenced by the hormonal factors related to the female gender [71–74].

The role of RAS-related mechanisms appears crucial in the gender-related implications in the pathogenesis of CoViD19. The dynamics of ACE2 expression seem to be linked with sex and age differences observed in the CoViD19 severity. These are linked with genetic predispositions, membranous ACE2 shedding, AngII/ADAM17 activity, and other factors. The expression and variations in the distribution of ACE2 among several tissues, such as the cardiac and testicular tissues, and age-related dynamics may be of particular interest [75, 76].

The analysis exploring the expression of ACE2 in adult heart tissue has shown a high expression of ACE2 in the pericytes that might act as the target cardiac cell of SARS CoV2 [77]. The male gender may exhibit a decreased cardiac ACE2 expression and age-related decline. According to a study, cells in the male adult heart showed a lower ACE2+ rate than in females (5.93% vs. 9.32%, $P < 0.01$), and ACE2 expression in the cardiac cells seems to be lower with older age, and TMPRSS2, is rarely expressed in the human adult heart [59]. Furthermore, the cardiac tissue appears to have a lower TMPRSS2 expression [78], that may diminish the chances of direct viral-cardiac interaction.

An increase in ACE2 expression is associated with several cardiovascular conditions and may have predictive value. Elevated levels of circulating ACE2 have also been associated with heart failure [79] and hypertension [80] and coronary artery disease [81]. According to a study higher levels of ACE2 were observed in the females with coronary heart disease (CHD), independently predicting the CHD in the female subjects, especially those with multivessel disease [82]. Higher circulatory ACE2 expression in heart failure has been validated in a recent study. A large multi-center prospective study in 11 European countries, investigated ACE2 concentrations in an index cohort of 1485 men and 537 women with heart failure. Results were validated in a cohort of 1123 men and 575 women. The male sex was strongest predictor of elevated serum ACE2 concentrations, in both cohorts (estimate = 0.26, $P < 0.001$; and 0.19, $P < 0.001$, respectively). The authors concluded, in both independent cohorts of patients with heart failure, plasma concentrations of ACE2 were higher in men than in women [83]. These findings confirm previous knowledge that circulating ACE2 levels in patients are sex-dependent, being 50% higher in men than in women in heart failure [84]. Heart failure patients are generally older and accompany multiple comorbidities. In a CoViD19 study, heart failure was more common among older subjects with comorbidities [85]. An analysis suggested that the heart may suffer less owing to the reduced expression of TMPRSS2 [78]. Loss of ACE2 expression with age and a decreased ACE2 cardiac expression may predispose male subjects towards a higher risk of cardiovascular complications. However, these associations need further exploration. The elevation in ACE2 expression in cardiovascular diseases, particularly higher in the male subjects, may reflect a robust protective response in male subjects, a compensatory mechanism [79], reflexive to the failing cardiovascular structural and functional parameters, and mark the higher risk in this gender group, or perhaps reflect a higher tissue expression that may expose to a higher CoViD19 risk, however that remains to be further determined.

Besides the RAS, gender dimorphism also appears to be associated with other hemodynamic regulatory systems such as the endothelin system implicated in cardiovascular diseases [86, 87]. Elevated endothelin-1 levels are associated with cardiac failure and may reflect cardiovascular risk in CoViD19 patients [88, 89]. Data show that serum endothelin 1 levels are higher in male subjects, compared to the females, and are higher in older females compared to the lower age group [90–93, 110].

Estrogens protect females and an increase in CoViD19 risk in female subjects with age, associated with the decline in estrogens, may contribute to the cardiac risk. The protective role of estrogen against heart disease has been revealed in several studies [94, 95]. Analyses suggest, the incidence of coronary artery disease (CAD) increases in women as the estrogen levels decline with age, and following menopause, suggesting a protective role for estrogen in the heart [96, 97]. The disintegrin ADAM 17 TACE that regulates ACE2 expression associated with cardiovascular diseases, is regulated by the estrogens. Evidence suggests that estrogens may offer a protective role against CVD in females through upregulation of ADAM17 and ADAM10 expression involved in ectodomain cleavages in atherosclerosis [98].

Multiple comorbidities are often associated with older age. Older age male CoViD19 patients often have positive cardiac history and higher risk [99]. Gender associated impact on multiple cardiovascular and metabolic conditions is extensively described [100]. The impact of gender dichotomies is associated with comorbidities, such as diabetes mellitus, obesity, and coronary heart disease, although variation in risk distribution may exist, in different populations or subgroups according to ethnicity, cardiovascular disease phenotype, or other factors. The gender interaction with comorbidities in CoViD19 and outcomes needs further exploration.

19.7 Summary

In summary, despite limitations, the overall data appear to indicate a gender disparity in the occurrence of CoViD19 and mortality. The gender bias in CoViD19 has an age-specific character, however, the male to female ratio may not be similar across subgroups. There appears to be a higher burden of CoViD19 among male subjects across several regions of the globe, although variations may not be huge. The gender-related variations have been observed during previous pandemics [101], and are known with cardiovascular diseases [100]. Controversies have been reported about gender related data in CoViD19 studies. Several factors appear to be responsible for the discrepancies observed in the gender-based data in CoViD19 studies. Among these, the lack of standardization in capturing data, gaps in data cleaning and processing, publication of age and gender-disaggregated data, use of data from controversial sources or evolving characteristics of the disease, or even limited testing, are notable. However, with the evolving pandemic, and improvements in study methodologies. study designs and reporting, and in other aspects of research conduct as well as with a better understanding of the CoViD19, encouraging trends are seen.

Despite controversies, gender disparity in CoViD19 has remained an important characteristic of the CoViD19 pandemic, with age-related dependency. The overall mortality risk appears to be higher among males. In CoViD19 risks are reported to be higher with the advancing age. Although females also manifest elevated risk in the advanced age, there appears to be a lack of uniformity in the age dependency. The male gender appears to remain at a higher risk, especially for the increased mortality, as compared to the females. In CoViD19, the mortality risk continues to increase with age in males as compared to females. Although, older men have a higher risk than women, the risk differences may narrow with age. The findings of gender disparity and gender-based health experiences have led to potential sex-based therapeutic measures in CoViD19, with hormonal therapy a potential protective intervention [73, 102]. The usefulness of these therapies needs to be further validated. The relationship between CoViD19 and gender disparity is not straightforward. The intricacies related to the age and sex-dependent variations in CoViD19 remain to be further explored. The discrepancies in data must be addressed using robust research designs and methodology. Further studies are needed to assess the age and sex-specific differences in the disease occurrence, phenotypic variations, and associated comorbidities including cardiovascular diseases in CoViD19, as well as the trends. The variations in gender-based associations with risk, and risk distribution, and magnitude of impact need to be better described in various world populations for a better global understanding of the gender disparity in CoViD19. Furthermore, post covid19 syndromes that seem to reflect the prolonged impact of the viral disease post recovery, although are described in the literature require further characterization, especially in relation to the gender. Gender disparity interactions in such post CoViD19 complications, need to be assessed.

A variety of pathophysiological factors and mechanisms highlighted in research although may explain the vulnerability of the male gender in CoViD19 and its complications. Similarly, multiple gender associated lifestyle and behavioral factors may play a part. Behavioral factors including others such as increase alcohol consumption [103] and smoking (with differences between high and low-middle-income countries [104, 105] are well recognized in a higher association among male subjects (Fig. 19.2). Several aspects of gender-based characteristics may impact exposure to the viral disease, vulnerability, ability to fight the pathogen, or others related to the treatment and care, must be recognized. These include hygiene practices [106], gender differences in behaviors related to a preventive approach [107] as well as occupational factors [108].

A robust immune system in males may not be as effective in the older age, and promotes increasing vulnerability towards the viral disease. among other mechanisms. The extent of immune-senescence appears to be bigger among the older age males, as compared to the older age females. According to an analysis, the age-related decline of various immunological parameters is less pronounced in females than in males [109]. Among gender linked factors, genetic factors such as X-linked inflammatory mechanisms and features of the immune system, the role of sex hormones, regulatory proteins including ACE2, and factors involved in the maintenance of regulatory and counter-regulatory balance necessary for homeostasis are important. The mechanisms involving coagulative, immunopathological, fibroproliferative processes may be interlinked with sex dimorphism seen in CoViD19 and the risk of developing cardiovascular complications. In CoViD19, variations in the gender-related factors may unevenly determine dysregulated hyperinflammatory, and prothrombotic responses. Synergistic actions of these mechanisms may potentiate variations in risk associated with a specific gender. It is important to investigate gender-based disease profiles highlighting the importance of these factors and determine age-specific and age-dependent immune characteristics, genetic variations, and factors related to RAS and other regulatory proteins involved in homeostasis.

The gender implications of the dual role of ACE2, as a principal machine for SARS CoV2 cell entry, and an important regulatory protective mechanism of RAS, need to be further analyzed. The ACE2 downregulation with infection, loss of protective mechanisms involved in viral lung injury repair, exposure to adverse AngII/AT1R axis, adversely impact the equipoise of RAS regulated homeostatic balance, are key mechanisms that determine the pathogenicity of SARS CoV2. Specific ACE2 variants, their distribution, and linking mechanisms [109], may carry unfavorable gender-related implications, and need to be further explored.

CoViD19 has a significant association with cardiovascular diseases. Gender disparity appears to project an important corelation with preexisting cardiovascular and metabolic conditions and the risk of developing cardiovascular complications observed in CoViD19. The exact position of gender and sex implications in cardiovascular complications in CoViD19 remains unexplored or underreported. The association of the male gender as a cardiovascular risk factor may further potentiate the cardiovascular risk associated with CoViD19. These associations, however, require further exploration. There is a lack of dis-aggregated age and sex data in CoViD19 studies in general, and in particular, investigating cardiovascular diseases. Studies stratifying age and sex data are needed to establish true associations and trends in sex and gender-related impact in CoViD19 patients.

The role of RAS mechanisms appears particularly important linking gender disparity and CoViD19, as well as the higher rates of cardiovascular complications. Definite mechanisms are not fully understood. Female X link genetic superiority over males may offer protection against CoViD19, the associations of the mechanisms and intricacies of the molecular processes involved need to be further determined. The dynamics and interactions of elevated serum ACE2 expression, a compensatory reaction in cardiovascular diseases, need to be further explored concerning the gender disparities, in cardiovascular complications of CoViD19.

A robust exploration of these mechanisms, cellular and molecular pathways, may help further tailoring the age and gender-specific treatments in CoViD19, prevent complications and improve the outcomes. The development of effective public health strategies, risk monitoring, assessment, and disease prevention models, may help to reduce the health inequity, associated with CoViD19 and in several other health conditions that display the gender disparity, especially disadvantaging the female gender.

Summary Box

- CoViD19 appears to accompany a gender disparity in general and also in relation to the cardiovascular complications. The association of age and male gender, as a risk in CoViD19 patients, is consistently reflected among the studies throughout the pandemic in 2019 to date, as of the middle of 2021.
- Gender disparity in CoViD19 appears to have an age-specific character, although the overall risk appears to remain higher among males.
- In CoViD19, the mortality is higher among males.
- Various global populations reflect gender disparity in association with CoViD19, although differences may be reported.
- Several factors including behavioral. life style, biological, genetic and others determine the gender based differences in risks among CoViD19 subjects.
- The expression and activity of angiotensin-converting enzyme 2 (ACE2), immune function, genetic, hormonal, behavioral, cultural, and social factors impact gender-related outcomes in CoViD19.
- Females exhibit better immunity compared to men, have hormonal protection, and may have advantages linked with genetic factors.
- Gender and sex implications in the cardiovascular complications in CoViD19 need better exploration, although male predominance is observed.
- There is a strong need for sex and gender-disaggregated data in CoViD19, even more for determining the gender-specific cardiovascular links.

References

1. Jin JM, Bai P, He W, Wu F, Liu XF, Han DM, Liu S, Yang JK. Gender differences in patients with COVID19: focus on severity and mortality. Front Public Health. 2020;8:152.
2. Grasselli G, Zangrillo A, Zanella A, et al. Baseline characteristics and outcomes of 1591 patients infected with SARS-CoV-2 admitted to ICUs of the Lombardy Region, Italy [published online ahead of print, 2020 Apr 6]. JAMA. 2020;323(16):1574–1581. https://doi.org/10.1001/jama.2020.5394.
3. Richardson S, Hirsch JS, Narasimhan M, Crawford JM, McGinn T, Davidson KW, Barnaby DP, Becker LB, Chelico JD, Cohen SL, Cookingham J. Presenting characteristics, comorbidities, and outcomes among 5700 patients hospitalized with COVID19 in the New York City area. JAMA. 2020;323(20):2052–9.
4. Guan W, Ni Z, Liang W, et al. Clinical characteristics of coronavirus disease 2019 in China. N Engl J Med. 2020 (published online Feb 28). https://doi.org/10.1056/NEJMoa2002032.
5. Yang X, Yu Y, Xu J, et al. Clinical course and outcomes of critically ill patients with SARS-CoV-2 pneumonia in Wuhan, China: a single-centered, retrospective, observational study. Lancet Respir Med. 2020; (published online Feb 24) https://doi.org/10.1016/S2213-2600(20)30079-5.
6. Shi Y, Yu X, Zhao H, Wang H, Zhao R, Sheng J. Host susceptibility to severe COVID19 and establishment of a host risk score: findings of 487 cases outside Wuhan. Crit Care. 2020;24(1):1–4.
7. Li X, Xu S, Yu M, Wang K, Tao Y, Zhou Y, Shi J, Zhou M, Wu B, Yang Z, Zhang C. Risk factors for severity and mortality in adult COVID19 inpatients in Wuhan. J Allergy Clin Immunol. 2020;146(1):110–8.
8. Li J, Huang DQ, Zou B, Yang H, Hui WZ, Rui F, Yee NTS, Liu C, Nerurkar SN, Kai JCY, Teng MLP. Epidemiology of COVID-19: A systematic review and meta-analysis of clinical characteristics, risk factors, and outcomes. J Med Virol. 2021;93(3):1449–58.
9. Peckham H, de Gruijter NM, Raine C, Radziszewska A, Ciurtin C, Wedderburn LR, Rosser EC, Webb K, Deakin CT. Male sex identified by global COVID-19 meta-analysis as a risk factor for death and ITU admission. Nature Communications, 2020;11(1):1–10.
10. https://www.worldometers.info/coronavirus/coronavirus-age-sex-demographics/.
11. http://globalhealth5050.org/covid19. Accessed 18 Apr 2020.
12. Yanez ND, Weiss NS, Romand JA, Treggiari MM. COVID19 mortality risk for older men and women. BMC Public Health. 2020;20(1):1–7.
13. Bhopal SS, Bhopal R. Sex differential in COVID19 mortality varies markedly by age. Lancet (London, England) 2020.
14. Xie J, Tong Z, Guan X, Du B, Qiu H. Clinical characteristics of patients who died of coronavirus disease 2019 in China. JAMA Netw Open. 2020;3 4:e205619–e205619.
15. Ahmad FB, Cisewski JA, Miniño A, Anderson RN. Provisional mortality data—united states, 2020. Morb Mortal Wkly Rep. 2021;70(14):519.
16. Remuzzi A, Remuzzi G. COVID19 and Italy: what next? The Lancet 2020.https://doi.org/10.1016/S0140-6736(20)30627-9.
17. Williamson EJ, Walker AJ, Bhaskaran K, Bacon S, Bates C, Morton CE, Curtis HJ, Mehrkar A, Evans D, Inglesby P, Cockburn J. Factors associated with COVID19-related death using OpenSAFELY. Nature 2020; 584 7821:430–436.
18. Munayco C, Chowell G, Tariq A, Undurraga EA, Mizumoto K. Risk of death by age and gender from CoViD19 in Peru, March-May, 2020. Aging (Albany NY). 2020;12(14):13869.
19. Joe W, Kumar A, Rajpal S, Mishra US, Subramanian SV. Equal risk, unequal burden? Gender differentials in COVID19 mortality in India. J Glob Health Sci. 2020;2 1.
20. Zhang JJ, Dong X, Cao Y, et al. Clinical characteristics of 140 patients infected with SARS-CoV-2 in Wuhan, China. Allergy. 2020; (published online Feb 19). https://doi.org/10.1111/all.14238.

21. BMJ Global Health Blogs. Sex, gender and COVID19: Disaggregated data and health disparities. BMJ Global Health. https://blogs.bmj.com/bmjgh/2020/03/24/sex-gender-and-CoViD19-disaggregated-data-and-health-disparities/. Published 2020. Accessed 24 Mar 2020.
22. Gebhard C, Regitz-Zagrosek V, Neuhauser HK, Morgan R, Klein SL. Impact of sex and gender on COVID19 outcomes in Europe. Biol Sex Differ. 2020;11 1:29. Published 2020 May 25. https://doi.org/10.1186/s13293-020-00304-9.
23. Kocher K, Delot-Vilain A, LoTempio J, Délot EC. Paucity and disparity of publicly available sex-disaggregated data for the COVID19 epidemic hamper evidence-based decision-making. Arch Sex Behav. 2021;50(2):407–26.
24. Huang C, Huang L, Wang Y, Li X, Ren L, Gu X, Kang L, Guo L, Liu M, Zhou X, Luo J. 6-month consequences of COVID19 in patients discharged from hospital: a cohort study. The Lancet. 2021.
25. Marx V. Scientists set out to connect the dots on long COVID. Nat Methods. 2021;18 5:449–453.
26. Sudre CH, Murray B, Varsavsky T, Graham MS, Penfold RS, Bowyer RC, Pujol JC, Klaser K, Antonelli M, Canas LS, Molteni E. Attributes and predictors of Long-COVID: analysis of COVID cases and their symptoms collected by the Covid Symptoms Study App. 2020.
27. Giefing-Kröll C, Berger P, Lepperdinger G, Grubeck-Loebenstein B. How sex and age affect immune responses, susceptibility to infections, and response to vaccination. Aging Cell. 2015;14(3):309–21.
28. Ruggieri A, Anticoli S, D'Ambrosio A, Giordani L, Viora M. The influence of sex and gender on immunity, infection and vaccination. Annali dell'Istituto superiore di sanita. 2016;52(2):198–204.
29. Ruggieri A, Gagliardi MC, Anticoli S. Sex-dependent outcome of hepatitis B and C viruses infections: synergy of sex hormones and immune responses? Front Immunol. 2018;9:2302.
30. Bartz D, et al. Clinical advances in sex-and gender-informed medicine to improve the health of all: a review. JAMA Int Med. 2020. 29.
31. Klein SL, Flanagan KL. Sex differences in immune responses. Nat Rev Immunol. 2016;16 (10):626.
32. Alkhouli M, Nanjundappa A, Annie F, Bates MC, Bhatt DL. Sex differences in case fatality rate of COVID19: Insights from a multinational registry. In: Mayo clinic proceedings, vol 95, No 8, pp. 1613–1620. Elsevier; 2020.
33. Al-Lami RA, Urban RJ, Volpi E, Algburi AM, Baillargeon J. Sex hormones and novel corona virus infectious disease (COVID19). In: Mayo clinic proceedings. Elsevier; 2020.
34. Klein SL, Flanagan KL. Sex differences in immune responses. Nat Rev Immunol. 2016. https://doi.org/10.1038/nri.2016.9025.
35. Ortona E, Pierdominici M, Rider V. Editorial: Sex Hormones and Gender Differences in Immune Responses. Front Immunol. 2019;10(1076):1–2. https://doi.org/10.3389/fimmu.2019.01076.
36. Gemmati D; Varani K, Bramanti B, Piva R, Bonaccorsi G, Trentini A, Manfrinato MC, Tisato V, Care A, Bellini T. "Bridging the Gap" everything that could have been avoided if we had applied gender medicine, pharmacogenetics and personalized medicine in the gender-omics and sex-omics era. Int J Mol Sci. 2019;21:296.
37. Syrett CM, Anguera MC. When the balance is broken: X-linked gene dosage from two X chromosomes and female-biased autoimmunity. J Leukoc Biol. 2019;106:919–32.
38. Casimir GJ, Lefevre N, Corazza F, Duchateau J. Sex and inflammation in respiratory diseases: a clinical viewpoint. Biol Sex Differ. 2013;4 16:148.
39. Meester I, Manilla-Munoz E, Leon-Cachon RBR, Paniagua-Frausto GA, Carrion-Alvarez D, Ruiz-Rodriguez CO, Rodriguez-Rangel X, Garcia-Martinez JM. Sexy chromosomes and the immune system: Reflections after a comparative study. Biol Sex Differ. 2020;11:3.

40. Giraud SN, Caron CM, Pham-Dinh D, Kitabgi P, Nicot AB. Estradiol inhibits ongoing autoimmune neuroinflammation and NFκB-dependent CCL2 expression in reactive astrocytes. Proc Natl Acad Sci. 2010;107(18):8416–21.
41. Chotirmall SH, Greene CM, Oglesby IK, Thomas W, O'Neill SJ, Harvey BJ, McElvaney NG. 17β-estradiol inhibits IL-8 in cystic fibrosis by up-regulating secretory leucoprotease inhibitor. Am J Respir Crit Care Med. 2010;182(1):62–72.
42. Biswas DK, Singh S, Shi Q, Pardee AB, Iglehart JD. 2005. Crossroads of estrogen receptor and NF-κB signaling. Science's STKE. 2005;288:pe27–pe27.
43. Klein SL, Marriott I, Fish EN. Sex-based differences in immune function and responses to vaccination. Trans R Soc Trop Med Hyg. 2015;109(1):9–15.
44. Bartz D, Chitnis T, Kaiser UB, Rich-Edwards JW, Rexrode KM, Pennell PB, Goldstein JM, O'Neal MA, LeBoff M, Behn M, Seely EW. Clinical advances in sex-and gender-informed medicine to improve the health of all: a review. JAMA Intern Med. 2020;180(4):574–83.
45. Bianchi VE. The anti-inflammatory effects of testosterone. J Endocr Soc. 2019;3(1):91–107.
46. Zeng F, Dai C, Cai P, Wang J, Xu L, Li J, Hu G, Wang Z, Zheng F, Wang L. A comparison study of SARS-CoV-2 IgG antibody between male and female COVID-19 patients: a possible reason underlying different outcome between sex. J Med Virol. 2020;92(10): 2050–4.
47. Conti P, Younes A. Coronavirus COV-19/SARS-CoV-2 affects women less than men: clinical response to viral infection. J Biol Regul Homeost Agents. 2020;34(2):339–43.
48. Wei J, Xu H, Davies JL, Hemmings GP. Increase of plasma IL-6 concentration with age in healthy subjects. Life Sci. 1992;51(25):1953–6.
49. Young DG, Skibinski G, Mason JI, James K. The influence of age and gender on serum dehydroepiandrosterone sulphate (DHEA-S), IL-6, IL-6 soluble receptor (IL-6 sR) and transforming growth factor beta 1 (TGF-β1) levels in normal healthy blood donors. Clin Exp Immunol. 1999;117(3):476.
50. Geerlings SE, Brouwer EC, Van Kessel KC, Gaastra W, Stolk RP, Hoepelman AI. Cytokine secretion is impaired in women with diabetes mellitus. Eur J Clin Invest. 2000;30(11):995–1001.
51. Ferrucci L, Penninx BW, Volpato S, Harris TB, Bandeen-Roche K, Balfour J, Leveille SG, Fried LP, Md JMG. Change in muscle strength explains accelerated decline of physical function in older women with high interleukin-6 serum levels. J Am Geriatr Soc. 2002;50 (12):1947–54.
52. Bhatia K, Zimmerman MA, Sullivan JC. Sex differences in angiotensin-converting enzyme modulation of Ang (1–7) levels in normotensive WKY rats. Am J Hypertens. 2013;26: 591–8.
53. Sama IE, Ravera A, Santema BT, van Goor H, Ter Maaten JM, Cleland JGF, Rienstra M, Friedrich AW, Samani NJ, Ng LL, Dickstein K, Lang CC, Filippatos G, Anker SD, Ponikowski P, Metra M, van Veldhuisen DJ, Voors AA. Circulating plasma concentrations of angiotensin-converting enzyme 2 in men and women with heart failure and effects of renin–angiotensin–aldosterone inhibitors. Eur Heart J. 2020;41 19:1810–1817. https://doi.org/10.1093/eurheartj/ehaa373.
54. Patel SK, Velkoska E, Burrell LM. Emerging markers in cardiovascular disease: where does angiotensin-converting enzyme 2 fit in? Clin Exp Pharmacol Physiol. 2013;40:551–9. https://doi.org/10.1111/1440-1681.12069.
55. Swärd P, Edsfeldt A, Reepalu A, Jehpsson L, Rosengren BE, Karlsson MK. Age and sex differences in soluble ACE2 may give insights for COVID19. Crit Care. 2020;24(1):221. Published 2020 May 14. https://doi.org/10.1186/s13054-020-02942-2.
56. Ciaglia E, Vecchione C, Puca AA. COVID19 infection and circulating ACE2 levels: protective role in women and children. Front Pediatr. 2020;8:206.
57. Xudong X, Junzhu C, Xingxiang W, Furong Z, Yanrong L. Age-and gender-related difference of ACE2 expression in rat lung. Life Sci. 2006;78(19):2166–71.

58. Liu H, Gai S, Wang X, Zeng J, Sun C, Zhao Y, Zheng Z. Single-cell analysis of SARS-CoV-2 receptor ACE2 and spike protein priming expression of proteases in the human heart. Cardiovasc Res. 2020;116(10), 1733–1741.
59. Gemmati D, Bramanti B, Serino ML, Secchiero P, Zauli G, Tisato V. COVID19 and Individual Genetic Susceptibility/Receptivity: Role of ACE1/ACE2 Genes, Immunity, Inflammation and Coagulation. Might the Double X-chromosome in Females Be Protective against SARS-CoV-2 Compared to the Single X-Chromosome in Males?. Int J Mol Sci. 2020;21(10):E3474. Published 2020 May 14. https://doi.org/10.3390/ijms21103474.
60. Wu C, Zheng S, Chen Y, Zheng M. Single-cell RNA expression profiling of ACE2, the putative receptor of Wuhan 2019-nCoV, in the nasal tissue. 2020.
61. Darbani B. The expression and polymorphism of entry machinery for COVID19 in human: Juxtaposing population groups, gender, and different tissues. Int J Environ Res Public Health. 2020;17:3433.
62. Smith JC, Sheltzer JM. Cigarette smoke triggers the expansion of a subpopulation of respiratory epithelial cells that express the SARS-CoV-2 receptor ACE2. bioRxiv. 2020;2020:013672.
63. Cai H. Sex difference and smoking predisposition in patients with COVID19 [published correction appears in Lancet Respir Med. 2020 Apr;8(4):e26]. Lancet Respir Med. 2020;8 (4):e20. https://doi.org/10.1016/S2213-2600(20)30117-X.
64. Guan W, Ni Z, Liang W, et al. Clinical characteristics of coronavirus disease 2019 in China. N Engl J Med. 2020; (published online Feb 28.) https://doi.org/10.1056/NEJMoa2002032.
65. Regitz-Zagrosek V. Therapeutic implications of the gender-specific aspects of cardiovascular disease. Nat Rev Drug Discovery. 2006;5(5):425–39.
66. Glaser R, Herrmann HC, Murphy SA, Flather MD, Mallick U. Women responded to an early invasive strategy as well as men in the acute coronary syndrome/Commentary. ACP J Club. 2003;139(1):3.
67. EUGenMed, Cardiovascular Clinical Study Group, Regitz-Zagrosek V, Oertelt-Prigione S, Prescott E, Franconi F, Gerdts E, Foryst-Ludwig A, Maas AH, Kautzky-Willer A, Knappe-Wegner D. Gender in cardiovascular diseases: impact on clinical manifestations, management, and outcomes Eur Heart J. 2016;37 1:24-33.
68. National Center for Health Statistics. Health, United States, 2009: with special feature on medical technology. https://www.cdc.gov/nchs/data/hus/hus09.pdf. Published 2010. Accessed on Jun 12 2021.
69. Ong KL, Tso AW, Lam KS, Cheung BM. Gender difference in blood pressure control and cardiovascular risk factors in Americans with diagnosed hypertension. Hypertension. 2008;51:1142–8.
70. Mehra MR, Desai SS, Kuy S, Henry TD, Patel AN. Cardiovascular disease, drug therapy, and mortality in CoViD19. N Engl J Med. 2020;382 25:e102.
71. Channappanavar R, Fett C, Mack M, Ten Eyck PP, Meyerholz DK, Perlman S. Sex-based differences in susceptibility to severe acute respiratory syndrome coronavirus infection. J Immunol. 2017;198(10):4046–53.
72. Brosnihan KB, Hodgin JB, Smithies O, Maeda N, Gallagher P. Tissue-specific regulation of ACE/ACE2 and AT1/AT2 receptor gene expression by oestrogen in apolipoprotein E/ oestrogen receptor-α knock-out mice. Exp Physiol. 2008;93(5):658–64.
73. Mauvais-Jarvis F, Klein SL, Levin ER. Estradiol, progesterone, immunomodulation, and COVID19 outcomes. Endocrinology. 2020;161 9:bqaa127.
74. Aune B, Øian P, Omsjø I, Østerud B. Hormone replacement therapy reduces the reactivity of monocytes and platelets in whole blood—a beneficial effect on atherogenesis and thrombus formation? Am J Obstet Gynecol. 1995;173(6):1816–20.
75. Donoghue M, Hsieh F, Baronas E, Godbout K, Gosselin M, Stagliano N, Donovan M, Woolf B, Robison K, Jeyaseelan R, Breitbart RE. A novel angiotensin-converting enzyme–related carboxypeptidase (ACE2) converts angiotensin I to angiotensin 1–9. Circ Res. 2000;87(5):e1–9.

76. Hamming I, Timens W, Bulthuis MLC, Lely AT, Navis GV, van Goor H. Tissue distribution of ACE2 protein, the functional receptor for SARS coronavirus. A first step in understanding SARS pathogenesis. J Pathol J Pathol Soc Great Britain Ireland. 2004;203 2:631–37.
77. Chen L, Li X, Chen M, Feng Y, Xiong C. The ACE2 expression in human heart indicates new potential mechanism of heart injury among patients infected with SARS-CoV-2. Cardiovasc Res. 2020;116 6:1097–1100. https://doi.org/10.1093/cvr/cvaa078.
78. Liu H, Gai S, Wang X, Zeng J, Sun C, Zhao Y, Zheng Z. Single-cell analysis of SARS-CoV-2 receptor ACE2 and spike protein priming expression of proteases in the human heart. Cardiovasc Res. 2020;116 10:1733–41.
79. Epelman S, Tang WW, Chen SY, Van Lente F, Francis GS, Sen S. Detection of soluble angiotensin-converting enzyme 2 in heart failure: insights into the endogenous counter-regulatory pathway of the renin-angiotensin-aldosterone system. J Am Coll Cardiol. 2008;52(9):750–4.
80. Uri K, Fagyas M, Siket IM, Kertesz A, Csanadi Z, Sandorfi G, Clemens M, Fedor R, Papp Z, Edes I, Toth A. New perspectives in the renin-angiotensin-aldosterone system (RAAS) IV: circulating ACE2 as a biomarker of systolic dysfunction in human hypertension and heart failure. PLoS One. 2014;9 4:e87845.
81. Ocaranza MP, Godoy I, Jalil JE, Varas M, Collantes P, Pinto M, Roman M, Ramirez C, Copaja M, Diaz-Araya G, Castro P, Lavandero S. Enalapril attenuates downregulation of Angiotensin-converting enzyme 2 in the late phase of ventricular dysfunction in myocardial infarcted rat. Hypertension. 2006;48 4:572–8.
82. Zhou X, Zhang P, Liang T, Chen Y, Liu D, Yu H. Relationship between circulating levels of angiotensin-converting enzyme 2-angiotensin-(1–7)-MAS axis and coronary heart disease. Heart Vessels. 2020;35(2):153–61.
83. Iziah E Sama, Alice Ravera, Bernadet T Santema, Harry van Goor, Jozine M ter Maaten, John G F Cleland, Michiel Rienstra, Alex W Friedrich, Nilesh J Samani, Leong L Ng, Kenneth Dickstein, Chim C Lang, Gerasimos Filippatos, Stefan D Anker, Piotr Ponikowski, Marco Metra, Dirk J van Veldhuisen, Adriaan A Voors, Circulating plasma concentrations of angiotensin-converting enzyme 2 in men and women with heart failure and effects of renin–angiotensin–aldosterone inhibitors, European Heart Journal, Volume 41, Issue 19, 14 May 2020, Pages 1810–1817, https://doi.org/10.1093/eurheartj/ehaa373.
84. Fagyas M, Úri K, Siket IM, Fülöp GÁ, Csató V, Daragó A, Boczán J, Bányai E, Szentkirályi IE, Maros TM, Szerafin T. New perspectives in the renin-angiotensin-aldosterone system (RAAS) II: albumi n suppresses angiotensin converting enzyme (ACE) activity in human. PLoS One. 2014; 9 4:e87844.
85. Yang X, Yu Y, Xu J, Shu H, Liu H, Wu Y, Zhang L, Yu Z, Fang M, Yu T, Wang Y. Clinical course and outcomes of critically ill patients with SARS-CoV-2 pneumonia in Wuhan, China: a single-centered, retrospective, observational study. Lancet Respir Med. 2020;8 (5):475–81.
86. Lawton JS. Sex and gender differences in coronary artery disease. Semin Thorac Cardiovasc Surg. 2011;23(2):126–30.
87. Gohar EY, Giachini FR, Pollock DM, Tostes RC. Role of the endothelin system in sexual dimorphism in cardiovascular and renal diseases. Life Sci. 2016 Aug 15;159:20–29. doi: https://doi.org/10.1016/j.lfs.2016.02.093. Epub 2016 Mar 3. Review. PubMed PMID: 26939577; PubMed Central PMCID: PMC4992599.
88. Badagliacca R, Sciomer S, Petrosillo N. Endothelin receptor antagonists for pulmonary arterial hypertension and COVID19: Friend or foe? J Heart Lung Transplant. 2020;39 (7):729–30.
89. Franco V, Bradley EA, Badagliacca R, Sabanayagam A, Rajpal S, Lastinger LT, Daniels CJ, Smith JS, Benza RL. Pulmonary vasodilators: beyond the bounds of pulmonary arterial hypertension therapy in COVID19. Pulm Circ. 2020;10(4):2045894020970369.
90. Barton M, Cosentino F, Brandes RP, Moreau P, Shaw S, Lüscher TF. Anatomic heterogeneity of vascular aging: role of nitric oxide and endothelin. Hypertension. 1997; 30 4:817–24.

91. Polderman KH, Stehouwer CD, van Kamp GJ, Dekker GA, Verheugt FW, Gooren LJ. Influence of sex hormones on plasma endothelin levels. Ann Intern Med. 1993; 118 6:429–32.
92. Miyauchi T, Yanagisawa M, Iida K, Ajisaka R, Suzuki N, Fujino M, Goto K, Masaki T, Sugishita Y. Age- and sex-related variation of plasma endothelin-1 concentration in normal and hypertensive subjects. Am Heart J. 1992; 123 4 Pt 1:1092–3.
93. Maeda S, Tanabe T, Miyauchi T, Otsuki T, Sugawara J, Iemitsu M, Kuno S, Ajisaka R, Yamaguchi I, Matsuda M. Aerobic exercise training reduces plasma endothelin-1 concentration in older women. J Appl Physiol 1985. 2003; 95 1:336–41.
94. Barrett-Connor E, Bush TL. Estrogen and coronary heart disease in women. JAMA. 1991;265(14):1861–7.
95. Mendelsohn ME, Karas RH. The protective effects of estrogen on the cardiovascular system. N Engl J Med. 1999;340(23):1801–11.
96. Tan YY, Gast GC, van der Schouw YT. Gender differences in risk factors for coronary heart disease. Maturitas. 2010;65(2):149–60.
97. Lee LV, Foody JM. Women and heart disease. Cardiol Clin. 2011; 29(1):35–45.
98. Zhou M, Dai W, Cui Y, Li Y. Estrogen downregulates gp130 expression in HUVECs by regulating ADAM10 and ADAM17 via the estrogen receptor. Biochem Biophys Res Commun. 2020;523:753–758.
99. Petrilli CM, Jones SA, Yang J, Rajagopalan H, O'Donnell L, Chernyak Y, Tobin KA, Cerfolio RJ, Francois F, Horwitz LI. Factors associated with hospital admission and critical illness among 5279 people with coronavirus disease 2019 in New York City: prospective cohort study. BMJ. 2020:369.
100. Mosca L, Barrett-Connor E, Kass Wenger N. Sex/gender differences in cardiovascular disease prevention: what a difference a decade makes. Circulation. 2011;124(19):2145–54.
101. Davies SE, Bennett B. A gendered human rights analysis of Ebola and Zika: locating gender in global health emergencies. Int Aff. 2016;92(5):1041–60.
102. Lipsa A, Prabhu JS. Gender disparity in COVID19: Role of sex steroid hormones. Asian Pacific J Trop Med. 2021;14 1:5.
103. Ely M, Hardy R, Longford NT, Wadsworth ME. Gender differences in the relationship between alcohol consumption and drink problems are largely accounted for by body water. Alcohol Alcohol. 1999;34(6):894–902.
104. Zeman MV, Hiraki L, Sellers EM. Gender differences in tobacco smoking: higher relative exposure to smoke than nicotine in women. J Women's Health Gender Based Med. 2002;11 2:147–53.
105. Han J, Chen X. A meta-analysis of cigarette smoking prevalence among adolescents in China: 1981–2010. Int J Environ Res Public Health. 2015;12(5):4617–30.
106. Johnson HD, Sholcosky D, Gabello K, Ragni R, Ogonosky N. Sex differences in public restroom handwashing behavior associated with visual behavior prompts. Percept Mot Skills. 2003; 97 3:805–10.
107. Bertakis KD, Azari R, Helms LJ, Callahan EJ, Robbins JA. Gender differences in the utilization of health care services. J Fam Pract. 2000;49(2):147–147.
108. Global Health 5050. COVID-19 Sex-disaggregated data tracker. 2020. The Sex, Gender and COVID19 Project | Global Health 50/50 (globalhealth5050.org). Accessed 12 June 2021.
109. Caruso C, Accardi G, Virruso C, Candore G. Sex, gender and immunosenescence: a key to understand the different lifespan between men and women? 2013.
110. Lekontseva O, Chakrabarti S, Davidge ST. Endothelin in the female vasculature: a role in aging? Am J Physiol Regul Integr Comp Physiol. Mar 2010;298(3):R509–16.

Chapter 20
An Overview of Quality of Research in COVID19

Key Questions

- What are the key measures of quality in clinical research?
- Which key quality limitations have been reported in the CoViD19 research?
- What are the main implications of the limitations in research quality, on CoViD19?
- Which research quality improvement measures. related to CoViD19 research, have been initiated?

20.1 Introduction

The global pandemic of CoViD19 presents a grave challenge to the care providers, patients, and health care system, and warrants robust high-quality evidence for the complex clinical decision-making process. Several thousand research publications have emerged in the scientific databases since the beginning of the CoViD19 pandemic publishing scientific, clinical, and epidemiological, laboratory, and other relevant data. CoViD19 literature published since January 2020 showed rapid growth. A publicly available database, set up by the World Health Organization (WHO) with a collection of articles about CoViD19, had included 3294 articles by March 30, 2020, and 25 607 by June 02, 2020 and 286,543 by June 17, 2021 [1].

Poor quality research presents a challenge to the scientific world. It is vital to identify and differentiate poor quality research from robust, well designed, well-conducted, and soundly analyzed research studies. Several internal and external factors impact the quality of a clinical research study, therefore the research must be carefully assessed for validity purposes. The internal validity is the extent

U. Mallick, *Cardiovascular Complications of COVID-19*,
https://doi.org/10.1007/978-3-030-90065-6_20

to which the observed results represent the truth in the population under study (are not due to methodological errors). Random errors and systematic errors impact the internal validity of epidemiological studies. A lack of accuracy in the estimation of the exposure-disease relationship reflects a random error. Bias is any systematic error that occurs in the design or the conduction of clinical research or the analysis or publication. Bias reflects a compromise in the internal validity of the study, for instance, due to the selection or information bias. Another factor that may compromise the internal validity of an epidemiological study is "confounding". Confounding biases occur when a measure of an intervention is distorted due to the association of intervention with other factor(s) that influence the outcome investigated. When a variable is associated with both the exposure and the disease under study, the effect of the exposure on the outcome blends with the effects of other risk and protective factors for the outcome that are present differentially by the exposure status. On the other hand, external validity of a study refers to how well the outcome of the study can be applied to other settings. For instance, the extent to which the results of a study are generalizable to patients in routine practice and include scientific and statistical generalization [2]. Several measures may be introduced to increase the internal and external validity of the studies. For instance, to enhance the internal validity of a study, measures such as a correct definition of exposure and disease, meticulous study planning, careful data collection and handling, adequate quality control, adequate implementation strategies-including adequate recruitment strategies, data analysis, and sample size, reducing attrition and others, may be used. Confounding must be identified and controlled to imrpove the internal validity of a study. The external validlty of a study can be enhanced by carefully considering the interactions of variables in the real world i.e. ensuring broad inclusion criteria to have a study population as close as possible to the real-life population, and carefully chosen exclusion criteria.

A variety of biases related to different study phases and components may influence the quality of a research study and its outcomes. Study design, methodology, analysis, and reporting are subject to flaws and biases. Flawed study design may result from poorly defined risk and outcome, non-validated methodology, lack of standardization, and non-blinded data collection. Methodological limitations may be related to inappropriate sample size calculations, lack of power, sparse or inconsistent reporting on the methodology used in the observational studies or randomized control trials. The notable examples of common biases that may occur in the studies include those related to an inappropriate randomization process due to unclear or lack of randomization, concealment, blinding process, and techniques, or confounding biases such as selection biases, information biases, etc., or related to data attrition such as poor or lack of follow up. The variations in death rates in different studies related to the complications of CoViD19 may point to biases, flaws, or inconsistencies in the epidemiological data, and maybe due to small sample sizes or even regional restrictions as observed in studies conducted in a single region (Wuhan). Similarly, such biases may be observed in studies reporting cardiac biomarkers in CoViD19. Although the diagnostic and prognostic significance of the cardiac biomarkers is extremely well-validated, indication bias associated with the serum cardiac biomarkers such as beta natriuretic peptide (BNP), Troponin may result in confounding due to the possibility of the elevation of these biomarkers due to a variety of reasons.

Randomized controlled trials (RCTs) are considered the highest level of evidence amongst other study designs. Observational study designs are descriptive and non-experimental with high variability in the quality and quantity of the evidence. Although observational study designs carry inherited flaws may produce extremely useful data to help to answer important scientific and clinical questions. Observational studies are useful in determining the long-term outcomes and associated factors, in describing rare adverse events or rare diseases, and in determining characteristics of diagnostic tests. Due to several difficulties and limitations associated with the pandemic, CoViD19 studies may not have had an adequate follow-up period. Reasonably large sample size and meticulous clinically relevant data may compensate for these biases to a certain extent and improve the reliability.

In observational studies, a cohort design may be used that allows observing of a population at risk for a specific disease or the population that has uniformly distributed risk factors or the disease. Therefore, such study design allows studying the incidence and history of a disease, and incidence rates, relative risks and confidence intervals (CI 95%) can be calculated. The design allows investigating the associations between multiple exposures and multiple outcomes in one cohort including the rare exposures and may offer the advantage of hypothesis generation. Cohort studies have usually broader inclusion criteria and fewer exclusion criteria, are more generalizable to clinical practice as compared to the RCTs that are known to lack generalizability.

According to the observation period, the observational studies can be, for example, cross-sectional (at a single time point) or longitudinal (with follow-up) for tracking the risk factors and outcomes. With regards to the timing of measurements, in observational studies, measurements can be made concurrently as the investigation proceeds with time, or non-concurrently when the measurements have already been recorded in past, and are simply extracted for instance from the medical records. Concurrent investigation allows for the implementation of measures to obtain better quality data allowing for standardization of definitions and methodology, whereas the non-concurrent measurements are confined for these measures. With regards to perspective related to the risk factors and outcomes, observational studies can be prospective and retrospective. Cohort studies retrospective (conducted backward in time) or prospective (conducted forward in time) are considered among the higher ranks of the study designs. Cohort themes may have variations, such as the before-after study and nested case–control study (within a cohort study).

Exposure to confounding and bias warrants a cautionary approach in the designing and analytical processes. The presence of confounding in the cohort studies hampers the ability of the study design to establish causal effects. Confounding may be caused by non-random allocation to the exposure, and the possibility of the presence of other variables that may differ between the subjects exposed and non-exposed, and have an association with the outcome measured. Such factors may or may not be identified or measured or inappropriately measured. Known confounders can be controlled with study design (case–control design or randomization) or during data analysis via regression (multivariate analyses can adjust potential confounders). Lack of adjustment of results for important co-variates can produce misleading results. Furthermore, in retrospective study designs, since data are collected retrospectively, can be less costly, however remain subject to specific bias such as limitations in data (variety, quality), selection bias, recall bias, and others. Prospective studies allow more accurate data collection with regards to the exposures, confounders, and endpoints and allow follow-up. These designs can be costly and time-consuming, however offer strength to the evidence. Several factors such as uncertainties associated with largely unexplored disease, complex heterogeneity of CoViD19, especially when associated with complications, warrant an even more careful approach in the study design, with judicious selection of the endpoints, adequate sample size, and an appropriate follow-up period. Furthermore, these factors may impact the analytical process and lead to conclusions that may be subject to significant biases.

20.2 Quality Issues in CoViD19 Research and Improvement Initiatives

The urgency of the pandemic may imply alterations in the protocols, cause deviations from standard quality assurance measures or interfere in the practical aspects of trials such as resulting in pausing the recruitment process, or the analytical process that may compromise the quality of research. CoViD19 research reflects a variety of research study designs, both conventional and non-conventional [3]. Studies reporting clinical characteristics and features of the disease appear to be mostly cohort studies, retrospective studies, or a few prospective studies and very few case series. According to an analysis aimed to reviewing and categorizing CoViD19-related medical research and to critically appraise peer-reviewed original articles. A total of 11,452 peer-reviewed or preprints references made available from 1 November 2019 to 1 May 2020 have been identified with our search strategy. After removing duplicates, studies not related to CoViD19, studies written in a language different than English or Chinese, and protocols, 10,516 references remained of which 7468 (71.0%) were peer-reviewed articles. Among these, 4190 (56.1%) articles were opinions that did not include any data or analytics (comprising viewpoints, editorials, perspectives, expert opinions). Instead, original studies accounted for 1109 articles (14.9%), case reports 697 (9.3%), research letters 786 (10.5%), reviews 638 (8.5%) and systematic reviews 48 (0.6%). The authors concluded that the majority of CoViD19 research is composed of publications without original data. Peer-reviewed original articles with data showed a high risk of bias and included a limited number of patients [4]. Basic characteristics of CoViD19-related, peer-reviewed original articles is provided in Table 20.2.

A systematic review evaluated the methodological quality of currently available CoViD19 studies compared to historical controls. A total of 14787 CoViD19 papers were identified as of May 14, 2020 and 4892 duplicate articles were removed. In total, 9895 titles and abstracts were screened, and 9101 articles were excluded due to the study being pre-clinical in nature, case report, case series <5 patients, in a language other than English, reviews (including systematic reviews), study protocols or methods, and other coronavirus variants with an overall inter-rater study inclusion agreement of 96.7% ($\kappa = 0.81$; 95% CI, 0.79–0.83). A total number of 794 full texts were reviewed for eligibility. Over 108 articles were excluded for ineligible study design or publication type (such as letter to the editors, editorials, case reports or case series <5 patients), wrong patient population, non-English language, duplicate articles, wrong outcomes, and publication in a non-peer-reviewed journal. The final analysis included 686 CoViD19 articles identified with an inter-rater agreement of 86.5% ($\kappa = 0.68$; 95% CI, 0.67–0.70) out of a total of 9895 titles and abstracts screened. According to the results, the comparative analysis of CoViD19 to historical articles reveals a shorter time to acceptance (13.0[IQR, 5.0–25.0] days vs. 110.0[IQR, 71.0–156.0] days in CoViD19 and control articles, respectively; $p < 0.0001$). The methodological quality scores are lower in CoViD19 articles across all study designs. The authors concluded that CoViD19 clinical studies have a shorter time to publication and have lower methodological quality scores than control studies in the same journal [5]. Methodological quality scores of different study types stratified by CoViD19 and historical control articles are provided in Table 20.1. Differences in methodological quality scores in CoViD19 compared to historical control articles are provided in Fig. 20.1.

In an exercise to critically appraise the evidence related to the effectiveness of chloroquine and hydroxychloroquine (with azithromycin) in CoViD19, about 6 studies, 3 randomized control trials, and 3 observational studies were analyzed. The authors concluded that CoViD19 research methodology is very poor in the area of chloroquine/hydroxychloroquine research and potential treatments. Limitations included, poor and sparse reporting and underreporting of important patient outcomes needed to discern decision-making priorities [6].

Poor reporting and methodology, as well as flaws related to the endpoints, have been reported in several trials investigating chloroquine and hydroxychloroquine in CoViD19 [7]. Another trial, an open-label randomized controlled trial investigating the efficacy of hydroxychloroquine in 150 mild to moderately ill CoViD19 patients showed significant flaws and inconsistencies. These biases were related to poor randomization and allocation concealment, under recruitment of the target population resulting in a significant reduction in sample size rendering the trial underpowered, at risk of greater random error, and inconsistent and selective outcome reporting for the difference between manuscript and the published trial protocol [8]. Similarly, a non-comparative, observational study showed a decline in the viral load in a cohort of 80 relatively mildly infected patients treated with a combination of hydroxychloroquine and azithromycin [9], was found to have a poor design with an

Table 20.1 Methodological quality scores of different study types stratified by COVID-19 and historical control articles

	COVID-19 articles (*n* = 686)	Matched articles (*n* = 1078)		P-value*
		COVID-19 (*n* = 539)	Control (*n* = 539)	
	N (%)	*N* (%)	*N* (%)	
Study design				
Case series	380 (55.4)	277 (51.4)	277 (51.4)	
Cohort	199 (29.0)	174 (32.3)	174 (32.3)	
case control	38 (5.5)	32 (5.9)	32 (5.9)	
Diagnostic	63 (9.2)	53 (9.8)	53 (9.8)	
Randomized controlled trial	6 (0.9)	3 (0.6)	3 (0.6)	
Geographic region				<0.0001
Asia/Oceania	469 (68.4)	377 (69.9)	167 (31.0)	
Europe	139 (20.3)	99 (18.4)	176 (32.7)	
Americas	78 (11.4)	63 (11.7)	196 (36.4)	
Types of article				0.91
Original research	614 (89.5)	486 (90.2)	484 (89.8)	
Letter	35 (5.1)	26 (4.8)	29 (5.4)	
Communication	37 (5.4)	27 (5.0)	26 (4.8)	
Retrospective study	590 (86.0)	459 (85.2)	386 (71.6)	<0.0001
Sex reported	620 (90.4)	484 (89.8)	483 (89.6)	0.92
Sample size calculated without case series	(*n* = 306)	(*n* = 262)	(*n* = 262)	
	7 (2.3)	4 (1.5)	30 (11.5)	<0.0001
Method of SARS-CoV-2 diagnosis				
PCR	548 (79.9)	437 (81.1)	–	–
ELISA	2 (0.3)	1 (0.2)	–	
Physical exam only	5 (0.7)	4 (0.7)	–	
Multiple	3 (0.4)	2 (0.4)	–	–
Unknown	128 (18.7)	95 (17.6)	–	–
Ethics approval				0.48
Received	566 (81.0)	433 (80.3)	451 (83.7)	
Not required/received	91 (13.3)	73 (13.5)	60 (11.1)	
Not mentioned	39 (5.7)	33 (6.1)	28 (4.1)	
Impact factor—median (IQR) (*n* = 652)	4.7 (2.9–7.6)	–	–	–
Time to acceptance—median (IQR) (*n* = 450)	13.0 (5.0–25.0)	13.0 (5.0–25.0)	11.0 (71.0–156.0)	<0.0001

COVID-19 articles were 1:1 matched with control articles from the same journal (identical impact factor) and study design. PCR: polymerase chain reaction; ELISA: enzyme-linked immunosorbent assay
*Statistical analysis was conducted to compare COVID-19 to historical control articles with their corresponding P-values
Source Table 1. Jung, R.G., Di Santo, P., Clifford, C., Prosperi-Porta, G., Skanes, S., Hung, A., Parlow, S., Visintini, S., Ramirez, F.D., Simard, T. and Hibbert, B., 2021. Methodological quality of COVID-19 clinical research. Nature communications, 12(1), pp. 1–10. https://www.nature.com/articles/s41467-021-21220-5. By Springer Nature Group

Table 20.2 Basic characteristics of COVID-19-related, peer-reviewed original articles

Type of original article studies involving patients	Number of studies (%)	Number of patients median (IQR)	Number of studies at risk of bias (%)			Patients consent			
			Low	Intermediate	High	Written informed consent *N* (%)	Oral consent *N* (%)	Open data *N* (%)	No consent *N* (%)
Case–control	68 (9.5)	108 (62–211)	11 (16.2)	25 (36.7)	32 (47.1)	22 (32.4)	2 (2.9)	2 (2.9)	42 (61.8)
Cohort	50 (7.0)	110 (54–327)	7 (14.0)	20 (40.0)	23 (46.0)	15 (30.0)	1 (2.0)	4 (8.0)	30 (60.0)
Cross-sectional	306 (42.9)	217 (80–730)	10 (3.3)	43 (14.0)	253 (82.7)	89 (29.1)	18 (5.9)	75 (24.5)	112 (40.5)
case series	129 (18.1)	18 (9–53)	9 (6.9)	26 (20.2)	94 (72.9)	24 (18.6)	15 (11.6)	3 (2.3)	87 (67.4)
Diagnostic	37 (5.2)	84 (49–215)	0 (0)	0 (0)	37 (100.0)	3 (8.1)	0 (0)	0 (0)	34 (91.9)
Prognostic	8 (1.1)	143 (66–217)	3 (37.5)	1 (12.5)	4 (50.0)	0 (0)	0 (0)	0 (0)	8 (100.0)
Simulation	185 (25.9)	1428 (14–40,695)	16 (8.6)	47 (25.4)	122 (66.0)	3 (1.6)	1 (0.5)	131 (70.8)	50 (27.0)
Non-randomized trial	8 (1.1)	35 (29–58)	1 (12.5)	1 (12.5)	6 (75.0)	4 (50.0)	0 (0)	0 (0)	4 (50.0)
Randomized controlled trial	4 (0.6)	56 (29–111)	0 (0)	2 (50.0)	2 (50.0)	2 (50.0)	0 (0)	0 (0)	2 (50.0)

This table displays the basic characteristics of the 713 clinical, peer-reviewed, COVID-19-related, original articles we critically appraised based on several risk of bias tools, according to the type of studies. Eighty-two studies were assessed using two tools, to better reflect their design. Shown are the number of studies, the median number of patients, the overall risk of bias after quality assessment, and how patient consent was addressed by authors.

Source Table 1. Raynaud, M., Zhang, H., Louis, K., Goutaudier, V., Wang, J., Dubourg, Q., Wei, Y., Demir, Z., Debiais, C., Aubert, O. and Bouatou, Y., 2021. COVID-19-related medical research: a meta-research and critical appraisal. BMC Medical Research Methodology, 21(1), pp. 1–11. https://link.springer.com/article/10.1186/s12874-020-01190-w. By Springer Nature Group

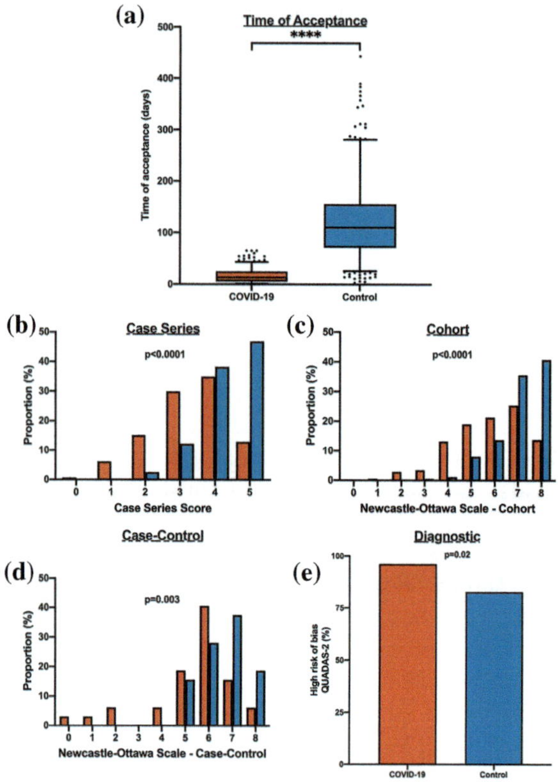

Fig. 20.1 Differences in methodological quality scores in COVID-19 compared to historical control articles. **a** Time to acceptance was reduced in COVID-19 articles compared to control articles (13.0 [IQR, 5.0–25.0] days versus 110.0 [IQR, 71.0–156.0] days, n = 347 for COVID-19 and n = 414 for controls; $p < 0.0001$). **b** When compared to historical control articles, COVID-19 articles were associated with lower case series score (n = 277 for COVID-19 and n = 277 for controls; $p < 0.0001$). **c** COVID-19 articles were associated with lower NOS cohort score compared to historical control articles (n = 174 for COVID-19 and n = 174 for controls; $p < 0.0001$). **d** COVID-19 articles were associated with lower NOS case–control score compared to historical control articles (n = 32 for COVID-19 and n = 32 for controls; $p = 0.003$). **e** COVID-19 articles were associated with higher diagnostic risk of bias (QUADAS-2) compared to historical control articles (n = 53 for COVID-19 and n = 53 for controls; $p = 0.02$). For panel A, boxplot captures 5, 25, 50, 75 and 95% from the first to last whisker. Orange represents COVID-19 articles and blue represents control articles. Two-sided Mann–Whitney U-test was conducted to evaluate differences in time to acceptance between COVID-19 and control articles. Differences in study quality scores were evaluated by two-sided Kruskal–Wallis test. Differences in diagnostic risk of bias were quantified by Chi-squares test. $p < 0.05$ was considered statistically significant. *Source* Fig. 4. Jung, R.G., Di Santo, P., Clifford, C., Prosperi-Porta, G., Skanes, S., Hung, A., Parlow, S., Visintini, S., Ramirez, F.D., Simard, T. and Hibbert, B., 2021. Methodological quality of COVID-19 clinical research. Nature Communications, 12(1), pp. 1–10. https://www.nature.com/articles/s41467-021-21220-5. By Springer Nature Group

irrelevant choice of endpoints, a variety of confounding issues, and biases including selection bias, data attrition, poor reporting, and several other flaws [10, 11].

A rapid systematic review and critical appraisal of studies that developed or validated a multivariable CoViD19 related prediction model from PubMed and Embase through Ovid, Arxiv, medRxiv, and bioRxiv, up to 24 March 2020, was analyzed. About 2696 titles were screened, and 27 studies describing 31 prediction models were included. The review showed that proposed models were poorly reported, had a high risk of bias, with optimistic reported performance [12]. The analysis pointed to several biases such as the bias for the participants' domain (participants enrolled in the studies not representative of the models' targeted populations), the bias for the predictor's domain (predictors not available at the models' intended time of use, not clearly defined, or influenced by the outcome measurement), or bias induced by the outcome measurement (use of subjective or proxy outcomes (e.g., non-covid-19 severe respiratory infections)), and bias for the analysis domain (such as small sample sizes). Other analyses have detected data source variability as a potential contributor of bias in the distributed research networks [13] indicating quality issues in the scientific datasets, or have found uniformly poor quality in COVID-19 predictive models, discouraging their clinical use [14]. Others have raised concerns regarding citation bias and a predilection of reporting beneficial over harmful effects in the CoViD19 treatment research, potentially in the context of white hat bias [15], indicating possible distortion of evidence towards the promotion of what is widely perceived as fair ends, associated with certain treatments.

Flaws in the methodology and sub-optimal reporting of research findings may lead to biased estimates of the treatment effect, further leading to inappropriate treatment decisions that may be harmful to the patients. Analysis of two clinical trials, four retrospective cohort studies, and a systemic review selected from 69 articles through Pubmed, 55 through medrxiv, 13 through Trip, and 519 through Google Scholar, was performed. The review aimed to investigate the evidence for the use of lopinavir/ritonavir (LPVr) as a treatment for CoViD19. The limitations identified indicated lack of randomized trials, or lack of blinding in RCTs, underpowered studies with smaller sample size, and observational studied with lack of adjustment of results for important co-variates leading to misleading results. The authors concluded, there was no strong evidence for the efficacy of lopinavir/ritonavir in the treatment of CoViD19. Overall, the limited studies identified were subject to methodological flaws [16].

Several types of study limitations are self-reported by the researchers in publications may indicate types of bias these studies have been exposed to. A large observational retrospective case series of 1591 CoViD19 hospitalized patients reported enrollment of consecutive patients between February 20 and March 18, 2020, in any of the 72 participating hospitals [17]. Several biases including selection bias, interviewer bias, recall bias may be observed regarding the data collection (limited data, mood of data collection, missing data for some outcomes). Other methodological limitations include a lack of standardization, short follow-up, and mortality data, and the length of stay data that are subject to change.

Furthermore, the analysis had not been adjusted for multiple comparisons. Given the possibility of a type I error, the authors advised cautiously interpreting the data due to its exploratory and descriptive nature.

Gender-related data in CoViD19 appears to have drawn criticism. An analysis of data reviewed from 20 countries with the highest numbers of confirmed CoViD19 cases revealed, few countries reported sex aggregated data and concluded that sex and age data were inconclusive for the determination of health outcomes in patients with CoViD19 [18]. Another analysis of gender-based trends in CoViD19 revealed a paucity of usable raw data sets and a generalized lack of standardization of the captured data, making comparisons difficult and a wide range of sex ratios among confirmed cases, which changed over time [19]. Inconsistencies in data reporting have been suggested in an analysis, concluding the lack of fatality data related to CoViD19 deaths in non-hospitalized patients may have resulted in the under-reporting of deaths in women [20].

Expedition of the peer-review process may have led to omissions in key quality measures in published clinical research related to CoViD19. In an analysis of papers reporting clinical trials involving CoViD19 patients searched either randomized or non-randomized (indexed by 4th April 2020) terms, about 521 papers were identified and four studies were included. The authors concluded that the quality of sample size calculation in clinical trials on CoViD19 patients indexed in PubMed was not acceptable [21].

Several analyses and reports highlight the issues and challenges faced during the pandemic and provide a variety of practical recommendations to help improve research methodology, reduce bias, and improve the study quality [13, 22, 23]. Adaptation in research infrastructure and operations, improvement in study designs, data collection methods, analytical techniques, as well as the development of multi-national collaborations, the standardization of protocols, data sharing, and several other measures can help to improve research standards, research and data quality, and reliability in CoViD19. Lessons learned from the initial experiences during the pandemic can lead to the achieve the next higher level of data quality.

Protocols have become publications in their own right, allowing for peer review and feedback on trial assumptions at an early stage in the conduct of a trial [24]. To achieve standardization in protocols for CoViD19 research with only closed CoViD19 cases, two main initiatives have created protocols for the investigators, the 'International Severe Acute Respiratory and emerging Infection Consortium (ISARIC)' (isaric.tghn.org) and the 'Lean European Open Survey on SARS-CoV-2 Infected Patients (LEOSS)' (leoss.net).

As part of CoViD19 R&D Blueprint, the WHO has proposed a master protocol for researchers involved in the development and assessment of therapeutics against SARS-CoV-2 [25]. Master protocols are used to test different investigational agents against a shared control arm with a uniform set of clinical endpoints, enrollment criteria, predefined data collection, and statistical methods. Researchers aligning their methodology to WHO's master protocol will surely improve the quality of the COVID19 research [26, 27]. In order to provide a tailored global research response to facilitate cross-border collaborations and partnerships across professional disciplines worldwide, the World Health Organization (WHO) working with the Global Research Collaborative for Infectious Disease Preparedness (GLOPID-R) has also established a CoViD19 research roadmap (www.glopid-r.org).

The EMEA (European Medicines Agency), has issued guidance with points to consider on implications of CoViD19 on methodological aspects of ongoing clinical trials [28]. Adhering to the CONSORT (Consolidated Standards of Reporting Trials) checklist for optimal clinical trial reporting [29] and the STROBE (STrengthening the Reporting of OBservational studies in Epidemiology) statement that outlines the guidance for optimal reporting of observational studies [30] (Fig. 20.1).

20.3 Summary

In summary, several gaps and limitations may be observed in CoViD19 related research describing the disease characteristics, risks, treatments, and outcomes. Throughout the pandemic, various analyses have been conducted that have highlighted these limitations. These limitations comprise a range of study design-related, methodological, and analytical biases and flaws. The emergency, as a result of a largely unfamiliar pathogen, resulting in the global pandemic of CoViD19, caused unprecedented clinical chaos, and further prompted the researchers to investigate and explore the complex clinical, laboratory, epidemiological characteristics of CoViD19, in a relatively short period. Complex ethical challenges are associated with the CoViD19 pandemic impacting research, healthcare systems, and patients [31], and may not be easily met during the emergencies such as the CoViD19 pandemic.

A variety of design and methodological limitations, biases related to data collection or reporting that may adversely impact the quality of research, maybe observed in CoViD19 research. The retrospective nature of analyses, or unconventional designs, or multiple types of biases related to various stages of a study warrant a precautious approach in data interpretation. Furthermore, cautions must be applied when using unconventional study designs [32] including those investigating prevention and therapeutic options in CoViD19, for instance, vaccines [33]. The data relating to the efficacy and safety of drugs of potential treatment value may be subject to misinterpretations due to the flaws and biases in the research design or methodology. The lack of strong evidence for the efficacy of lopinavir/ritonavir in the treatment of CoViD19 was associated with flaws in methodology and sub-optimal reporting of the research findings, as observed in an analysis [16]. Such flaws may lead to biased estimates of the treatment effect, further leading to inappropriate treatment decisions that may be harmful to the patients. Furthermore, the lack of standardization of definitions, such as observed in the obesity trials or the studies investigating cardiac injury, or the lack of standardized antibody assays, or the non-availability of sex, and age disaggregated data, are a few examples indicating lack of uniformity in research in CoViD19 research in various stages of the research. The risks can be minimized using robust designs, methodological safeguards, using standardized definitions, laboratory assays, and appropriate analytical methods and statistical techniques. The trial designs must be harmonized and the use of master protocols must be implemented in CoViD19 research internationally. Adherence to the expert guidelines may help reduce the lack of standardization in the conduct of trials and improve the quality of reporting. The expert guidelines, models introduced by international expert initiatives, and other forms of concerted efforts may help improve the quality and conduct of clinical research.

The extraordinary circumstances as observed in the CoViD19 pandemic, demand a meticulous approach when analyzing data. The uncertainties related to the variety of risks of developing the novel disease, diversity of associated comorbidities, pathophysiological complexities require detailed analysis. It becomes even more important to question, explore, and critically appraise the data. The clinical, and diagnostic features and markers of disease severity are complex, therefore, recognition, associations, and implications of factors that impact these parameters, necessitate a detailed approach while examining the data. The complexities associated with prognostication and assessment of outcomes imply the use of robust designs and analytical methods must be evaluated and interpreted carefully. The robust peer-reviewing process is critical to maintaining the quality of research data to be published and must be ensured during the pandemic. The study retractions of the CoViD19 published research papers [34] may have resulted in financial losses [35] in an already tense environment burdened by the financial pressures due to the pandemic on the institutions. Efforts must be made to minimize such risks. Problematic substandard research may ultimately cause harm to the patients, scientific integrity, as well as productivity [36]. A robust peer-reviewing process, critical to maintaining the quality of research data to be published, must be ensured during the pandemic. The ethical challenges associated with the global pandemic must be met despite obstacles.

The rapid spread of the disease across the globe led to the development of research studies exploring CoViD19 to understand the disease, minimize the disease burden, and reduce the fatality in the endeavor to offer protection to the populations. Numerous multinational initiatives and sharing of datasets and research findings led to the generation of vast amounts of data and publications. Several factors including the geographical diversity of the healthcare systems, and a variety of approaches, resulted in the inundation of research data with variations in the quality and significant diversities in the conduct, analysis, and reporting. These factors further determined the need for the development of concerted efforts to minimize the consequent risks and adverse impact of the massive amount of data, and improve the research efforts, to better combat the new coronavirus disease. The development of global initiatives to streamline and standardize the research internationally, based on these efforts, are likely to be effective and lead the improvements. More efforts are needed to improve the research infrastructure, regulatory setup, and research expertise globally, in special in the low-middle-income countries, where the high burden of CoViD19 has resulted in disproportional health and economic woes.

Summary Box

- In the endeavor to combat the CoViD19 pandemic, as part of research activities, a wealth of evidence has been generated globally, which has tremendously contributed to a greater understanding of the novel coronavirus disease and minimizing the burden.
- Several gaps and limitations may exist in the CoViD19 research in the process of designing conducting, and analysis stages.
- In the quality of CoViD19 research, key limitations appear to be related to the study designs, lack of standardization of definitions, laboratory assays, incomplete follow-up, confounding, analytical biases, and data attrition, among others.
- Pandemic-related pressures may have influenced the quality of research publications in CoViD19.
- Pressures for a rapid publication of research, hastening of the peer review process, use of less robust designs are notable factors that may have compromised the data quality in some CoViD19 research.
- The complexities related to the heterogeneity of CoViD19 are likely to have significant implications on the research designs, methodology, and analytical process, which may be addressed using meticulous approaches in various stages of research such as designing, analysis etc.
- The readers should apply precautions in the interpretation of research reports, especially due to the uncertainties related to the pandemic of CoViD19, and must scrutinize the studies and recognize the potential biases related to different stages and levels of the studies.
- Bias in the studies assessing treatments in CoViD19 must be assessed cautiously to avoid the misinterpretations of data that may lead to an over or underestimation of the treatment benefits or harms.
- Global and national research quality assurance initiatives that may help to generate improved data are welcome.
- Lessons must be learned from the initial CoViD19 related research experiences to improve the standard of research and fill in the gaps for a better characterization, diagnostics, and prognostication of CoViD19.

References

1. CoViD19: global literature on coronavirus disease. World Health Organization. https://search.bvsalud.org/global-literature-on-novel-coronavirus-2019-ncov/?lang=en. Accessed 17 Jun 2021.
2. Rothman KJ: Epidemiology. An Introduction. New York, Oxford University Press. 2002; 20–21.
3. Sudre CH, Murray B, Varsavsky T, Graham MS, Penfold RS, Bowyer RC, Pujol JC, Klaser K, Antonelli M, Canas LS, Molteni E. Attributes and predictors of Long-COVID: analysis of COVID cases and their symptoms collected by the Covid Symptoms Study App. medRxiv. 2020.
4. Raynaud M, Zhang H, Louis K, Goutaudier V, Wang J, Dubourg Q, Wei Y, Demir Z, Debiais C, Aubert O, Bouatou Y. COVID-19-related medical research: a meta-research and critical appraisal. BMC Medical Research Methodology. 2021;21(1):1–11.
5. Jung RG, Di Santo P, Clifford C, Prosperi-Porta G, Skanes S, Hung A, Parlow S, Visintini S, Ramirez FD, Simard T, Hibbert B. Methodological quality of COVID-19 clinical research. Nature Communications. 2021;12(1):1–10.
6. Alexander PE, Debono VB, Mammen MJ, et al. COVID-19 coronavirus research has overall low methodological quality thus far: case in point for chloroquine/hydroxychloroquine [published online ahead of print, 2020 Apr 21]. J Clin Epidemiol. 2020; S0895-4356(20) 30371-1. https://doi.org/10.1016/j.jclinepi.2020.04.016.
7. Ferner Robin E, Aronson Jeffrey K. Chloroquine and hydroxychloroquine in covid-19. BMJ. 2020; 369:m1432.
8. Tang W, Cao Z, Han M, Wang Z, Chen J, Sun W, et al. Hydroxychloroquine in patients with mainly mild to moderate coronavirus disease 2019: open label, randomised controlled trial. BMJ. 2020; 369:m1849.
9. Gautret P, Lagier JC, Parola P, et al. Clinical and microbiological effect of a combination of hydroxychloroquine and azithromycin in 80 covid-19 patients with at least a six-day follow up: a pilot observational study. Travel Med Infect Dis. 2020; 34:101663. https://doi.org/10.1016/j.tmaid.2020.101663.
10. Eliesbik. Thoughts on the Gautret et al. paper about hydroxychloroquine and azithromycin treatment of COVID-19 infections. Science Integrity Digest. 2020. https://scienceintegritydigest.com/2020/03/24/thoughts-on-the-gautret-et. Accessed 17 May 2020.
11. https://pubpeer.com/publications/B4044A446F35DF81789F6F20F8E0EE. Last Accessed on 5 Jan 2022.
12. Wynants L, Van Calster B, Bonten Marc MJ, Collins GS, Debray Thomas PA, De Vos M, et al. Prediction models for diagnosis and prognosis of covid-19 infection: systematic review and critical appraisal. BMJ. 2020; 369:m1328.
13. Sáez C, Romero N, Conejero JA, García-Gómez JM. Potential limitations in COVID-19 machine learning due to data source variability: a case study in the nCov2019 dataset. J Am Med Inform Assoc. 2021;28(2):360–4.
14. Wynants L, Van Calster B, Collins GS, Riley RD, Heinze G, Schuit E, Bonten MM, Dahly DL, Damen JA, Debray TP, de Jong VM. Prediction models for diagnosis and prognosis of covid-19: systematic review and critical appraisal. BMJ. 2020; 369.
15. Bellos I. A metaresearch study revealed susceptibility of Covid-19 treatment research to white hat bias: first, do no harm. J Clin Epidemiol. 2021;136:55–63.
16. Dorward J, Gbinigie K. Lopinavir/ritonavir: a rapid review of effectiveness in COVID-19. 2020.
17. Grasselli G, Zangrillo A, Zanella A, et al. Baseline characteristics and outcomes of 1591 patients infected with SARS-CoV-2 admitted to ICUs of the Lombardy region, Italy [published online ahead of print, 2020 Apr 6]. JAMA. 2020; 323(16):1574–81. https://doi.org/10.1001/jama.2020.5394.

18. BMJ Global Health Blogs. Sex, gender and COVID-19: disaggregated data and health disparities. BMJ Global Health. 2020. https://blogs.bmj.com/bmjgh/2020/03/24/sex-gender-and-covid-19-disaggregated-data-and-health-disparities/. Accessed 24 Mar 2020.
19. Kocher KM, Délot-Vilain A, Spencer DA, LoTempio J, Délot EC. Paucity and disparity of publicly available sex-disaggregated data for the COVID-19 epidemic hamper evidence-based decision-making. medRxiv. 2020. 04.29.20083709. https://doi.org/10.1101/2020.04.29.20083709.
20. Gebhard C, Regitz-Zagrosek V, Neuhauser HK, Morgan R, Klein SL. Impact of sex and gender on COVID-19 outcomes in Europe. Biol Sex Differ. 2020; 11(1):29. https://doi.org/10.1186/s13293-020-00304-9.
21. Lee PH. The quality of the reported sample size calculation in clinical trials on COVID-19 patients indexed in PubMed [published online ahead of print, 2020 Apr 30]. Eur J Intern Med. 2020; S0953-6205(20)30178-3. https://doi.org/10.1016/j.ejim.2020.04.057.
22. Fleming TR, Labriola D, Wittes J. Conducting clinical research during the COVID-19 pandemic: protecting scientific integrity. JAMA. 2020;324(1):33–4.
23. Kunz CU, Jörgens S, Bretz F, Stallard N, Van Lancker K, Xi D, Zohar S, Gerlinger C, Friede T. Clinical trials impacted by the COVID-19 pandemic: adaptive designs to the rescue? Stat Biopharm Res. 2020;12(4):461–77.
24. Mallick U, et al. Protocol development. Pract Guid Des Anal Report. 2006:23.
25. https://www.who.int/blueprint/priority-diseases/key-action/COVID-19_Treatment_Trial_Design_Master_Protocol_synopsis_Final_18022020.pdf
26. Stegall MD, Smith B, Bentall A, Schinstock C. The need for novel trial designs, master protocols, and research consortia in transplantation. Clin Transplant. 2020; 34(1):e13759. https://doi.org/10.1111/ctr.13759.
27. WHO R&D blueprint novel coronavirus COVID-19 therapeutic trial synopsis. https://www.who.int/blueprint/priority-diseases/keyaction/COVID19_Treatment_Trial_Design_Master_Protocol_synopsis_Final_18022020.pdf. Accessed 02 April 2020.
28. Points to consider on implications of Coronavirus disease (COVID-19) on methodological aspects of ongoing clinical trials; 25 March 2020, EMA/158330/2020, Committee for Human Medicinal Products (CHMP). https://www.ema.europa.eu/en/documents/scientific-guideline/points-consider-implications-coronavirus-disease-covid-19-methodological-aspects-ongoing-clinical_en.pdf. Accessed 02 Jun 2020.
29. Schulz KF, Chalmers I, Hayes RJ, Altman DG. Empirical evidence of bias. Dimensions of methodological quality associated with estimates of treatment effects in controlled trials. JAMA.1995; 273(5):408–12.
30. von Elm E, Altman DG, Egger M, Pocock SJ, Gøtzsche PC, Vandenbroucke JP. STROBE initiative. The strengthening the reporting of observational studies in epidemiology (STROBE) statement: guidelines for reporting observational studies. Int J Surg. 2014; 12 (12):1495–9. https://doi.org/10.1016/j.ijsu.2014.07.013.
31. Meagher KM, Cummins NW, Bharucha AE, Badley AD, Chlan LL, Wright RS. COVID-19 ethics and research. In: Mayo clinic proceedings, vol. 95, no. 6. Amsterdam: Elsevier;2020. pp. 1119–23.
32. Bhandari N, Upadhyay RP, Chowdhury R, Taneja S. Challenges of adopting new trial designs in LMICs. Lancet Glob Health. 2021;9(5):e575–6.
33. Johnson R, Jackson C, Presanis A, Villar SS, De Angelis D. Quantifying efficiency gains of innovative designs of two-arm vaccine trials for COVID-19 using an epidemic simulation model. Statistics in Biopharmaceutical Research, (just-accepted). 2021;1–22.
34. Bramstedt KA. The carnage of substandard research during the COVID-19 pandemic: a call for quality. J Med Ethics. 2020;46(12):803–7.
35. Stern AM, Casadevall A, Steen RG, Fang FC. Financial costs and personal consequences of research misconduct resulting in retracted publications. Elife, 2014; 3:e02956.
36. Oswald AJ, Proto E, Sgroi D. Happiness and productivity. J Law Econ. 2015;33(4):789–822.

Index

U. Mallick, *Cardiovascular Complications of COVID-19*,
https://doi.org/10.1007/978-3-030-90065-6

D

E

F

G

H

GPSR Compliance

The European Union's (EU) General Product Safety Regulation (GPSR) is a set of rules that requires consumer products to be safe and our obligations to ensure this.

If you have any concerns about our products, you can contact us on ProductSafety@springernature.com

In case Publisher is established outside the EU, the EU authorized representative is:

Springer Nature Customer Service Center GmbH
Europaplatz 3
69115 Heidelberg, Germany

Batch number: 10726058

Printed by Printforce, the Netherlands